Forensic DNA Evidence Interpretation

Second Edition

Forensic DNA Evidence Interpretation

Second Edition

Edited by

John S. Buckleton
Institute of Environmental Science and Research
Auckland, New Zealand

Jo-Anne Bright
Institute of Environmental Science and Research
Auckland, New Zealand

Duncan Taylor
Forensic Science SA
Adelaide, South Australia

CRC Press
Taylor & Francis Group
Boca Raton London New York

CRC Press is an imprint of the
Taylor & Francis Group, an **informa** business

CRC Press
Taylor & Francis Group
6000 Broken Sound Parkway NW, Suite 300
Boca Raton, FL 33487-2742

First issued in paperback 2021

© 2016 by Taylor & Francis Group, LLC
CRC Press is an imprint of Taylor & Francis Group, an Informa business

No claim to original U.S. Government works

ISBN 13: 978-0-367-77810-1 (pbk)
ISBN 13: 978-1-4822-5889-9 (hbk)

**Visit the Taylor & Francis Web site at
http://www.taylorandfrancis.com**

**and the CRC Press Web site at
http://www.crcpress.com**

Contents

Contents

Preface

Forensic science is, to some extent, a derived science. It is happy to borrow technology and ideas from other sciences. There is, however, a 'forensic mindset' and ethos that is peculiar to our science. When DNA technology was launched, the interpretation was attempted by forensic scientists such as Ian Evett and John S. Buckleton. Eventually it became clear, or indeed we had it rammed into our heads, that there was a great amount of classical population genetic work that needed to be considered by forensic scientists. This situation was brought to the world's attention by David Balding, Peter Donnelly, Richard Nichols and Bruce Weir. Forensic science is very fortunate to have these fine minds working on their problems and we are personally deeply indebted to Bruce Weir, who has contributed so much to the field and several, otherwise unpublished sections to this book, in areas that we could not solve ourselves. We recognize very considerable assistance over many years from David Balding. We also acknowledge a very considerable intellectual debt to Ian Evett; large sections of this book are influenced by him.

Much of the work described in this book has been undertaken collaboratively. We have tried to reference areas that can be specifically acknowledged. However in working with people one picks up concepts and ideas almost by osmosis. In this regard we specifically acknowledge a debt to Chris Triggs, Simon Walsh, James M. Curran, Bonnie Law and Hannah Kelly. This work was supported in part by grant 2011-DN-BX-K541 from the US National Institute of Justice. Points of view in this document are those of the authors and do not necessarily represent the official position or policies of the U.S. Department of Justice.

This book is written from the perspective of less mathematically attuned caseworkers although we suspect that some sections may give the reader cause to doubt this. We have also made some effort to review pertinent areas that have arisen during court proceedings. We have attempted to tabulate formulae needed for forensic DNA casework given many different scenarios and applications. We have found many errors in the literature (including in our own work) and have sought to correct these. No one is error-free however and we would welcome any corrections to these tables.

The text is heavily referenced and in many cases these references are personal communications or restricted material. This fact may be frustrating for the reader who wants to obtain these texts and we have previously been criticized in reviews for doing this.

There are several reasons to reference a piece of work, whether it is published or not. One is to direct the reader to further reading. However another is to give credit to the author of an idea. Therefore in many cases we have tried to attribute an idea to the originator. Where we have failed to do this, we apologize and would welcome correction. We have also quoted the original texts extensively. Often the original authors stated the matter better than we possibly could, and it is often interesting to see how early some illuminating comments were made.

We have had sections of texts read to us in court many times. Any caseworker who has this happen should direct the prosecutor or defence counsel to this Preface. No author is perfect and writing a text does not make one an authority. In many cases the caseworker has studied the case in question to an extent that advice from some 'quoted authority' is completely irrelevant.

Preface

Above all our goal is to provide a link between the biological, forensic and interpretative (or statistical) domains of the DNA profiling field. It is a challenge for caseworkers to keep apace of the ever-changing technological and operational demands of their role, as well as accurately assess the strength of the evidence under these fluctuating circumstances. We hope this book can act as a guide, or template, through which many of the complex issues can be tackled.

John S. Buckleton
Institute of Environmental Science and Research

Jo-Anne Bright
Institute of Environmental Science and Research

Duncan Taylor
Forensic Science South Australia

Editors

John S. Buckleton has a PhD and DSc from the University of Auckland, New Zealand. He is a fellow of the Royal Society of New Zealand, a member of the Scientific Working Group on DNA Analysis Methods and is on the International Society for Forensic Genetics DNA Commission. His caseworking experience covers 32 years in the United Kingdom, United States, Australia and New Zealand. He has examined over 2000 cases and testified possibly over 200 times. This includes testimony in New Zealand, Australia and the United States. Dr Buckleton has co-authored over 170 significant publications in the forensic field (shoeprints, firearms, DNA, blood grouping, tool marks, fire debris analysis, glass and paint) and presented DNA and glass courses in the United Kingdom, United States, Australia, Asia and New Zealand from 1988 to the present to practising professional forensic scientists. He has supervised four PhD students in the field of forensic interpretation and been involved in international research and development programmes in the area of the forensic interpretation of glass and DNA, including expert systems.

Jo-Anne Bright is a science leader at the Institute of Environmental Science and Research Limited in Auckland, New Zealand. She has 16 years of experience in casework and quality management within the forensic biology laboratory. In 2015, she earned her PhD in forensic science from the University of Auckland, New Zealand. She has over 50 publications in the area of forensic DNA analysis and interpretation. Dr Bright is a co-developer of the DNA profile interpretation software STRmix and has undertaken many presentations and workshops on DNA profile interpretation in Australasia, the United States and Europe.

Duncan Taylor is the principal scientist of forensic statistics at Forensic Science South Australia, Adelaide, Australia. He earned his PhD in molecular biology and a diploma in biostatistics, and has worked in the forensic field for over a decade. Dr Taylor has produced numerous DNA reports and presented evidence in magisterial and district courts in Australian states, as well as in the High Court of Australia. He is a member of the Australasian Statistics Scientific Working Group and the Scientific Working Group on DNA Analysis Methods for Y-STRs and has published a number of works in both areas. Dr Taylor is one of the developers of STRmix, a DNA interpretation software being used in forensic labs in Australia and New Zealand. He is an associate professor in biology at Flinders University, Bedford Park, Australia, and supervises honours and PhD students.

Contributors

Mikkel Meyer Andersen
Department of Mathematical Sciences
Faculty of Engineering and Science
Aalborg University
Aalborg, Denmark

Jo-Anne Bright
Forensic Biology Group
Institute of Environmental Science
    and Research
Auckland, New Zealand

John S. Buckleton
Institute of Environmental Science
    and Research
Auckland, New Zealand

Michael Coble
Applied Genetics Group
National Institute of Standards and Technology
Gaithersburg, Maryland

James M. Curran
Department of Statistics
Faculty of Science
University of Auckland
Auckland, New Zealand

Peter Gill
Department of Forensic Biology
Norwegian Institute of Public Health
Nydalen, Norway
and
Department of Forensic Medicine
University of Oslo
Oslo, Norway

Tacha Hicks
School of Criminal Justice
Faculty of Law, Criminal Justice and Public
    Administration
Fondation pour la formation continue
    l'Université de Lausanne
University of Lausanne
Lausanne-Dorigny, Switzerland

Duncan Taylor
Forensic Science South Australia
Adelaide, South Australia, Australia

Simon J. Walsh
Specialist Operations
Australian Federal Police
Canberra, Australia

Biological Basis for DNA Evidence

Duncan Taylor, Jo-Anne Bright and John S. Buckleton[*]

Contents

This book deals in large part with the interpretation of DNA evidence, mixed or unmixed, after it has been collected, stored, transferred and finally analyzed in the laboratory. The supposition throughout is that the earlier stages in the chain that leads to evidence in court have been undertaken correctly. The inference at the final end of the chain is practically useless unless all these earlier aspects have been undertaken with due attention to continuity and integrity.[1]

---

[*] Based on an earlier version by Peter Gill and John Buckleton.

This chapter gives a brief background to the biotechnology relevant to the interpretation of short tandem repeat (STR) samples. For an extended discussion see the excellent work by Rudin and Inman[2,3] as well as Butler.[4]

Historical and Biological Background

Modern forensic DNA history begins with the first DNA case, which was processed by the then-34-year-old professor Sir Alec Jeffreys from Leicester University, UK. This case involved the murders of two 15-year-old girls, Lynda Mann and Dawn Ashworth.[5] The police were convinced that the perpetrator was a local man. Consequently, blood samples were requested from all males of a certain age group from three villages within the area of the two murders. These samples were analyzed using a combination of classical blood-typing techniques and multi-locus probe DNA profiling. The first mass screening of individuals using DNA technology led to the arrest and confession of Colin Pitchfork, a cake decorator with a history of flashing.[6]

This pioneering case demonstrated the potential of DNA profiling[7-10] and firmly pointed towards its future as the most important forensic investigative tool to be developed in the twentieth century.

DNA is the genetic code of most organisms. The DNA of humans and many other organisms has been used in forensic work. Human primers can also be used to amplify the DNA from some other primates.[11] Much of the work discussed here focuses on the analysis of modern human DNA. However many of the principles apply to all organisms and to ancient DNA.[12]

Most human DNA is present in the nucleus of the cell. It is packaged in the 46 chromosomes of most cells. This DNA is termed *nuclear DNA*. However a small portion of the DNA complement of each cell is housed in the mitochondria. This mitochondrial DNA is inherited by a different mechanism and is treated differently in the forensic context. A separate section in a subsequent chapter 10, non-autosomal forensic markers is devoted to this topic.

Most human cells are diploid, meaning that they have two copies of each chromosome. Exceptions include the sex cells (sperm or ova), which are haploid (having a single copy of each chromosome), and liver cells, which are polyploid. Diploid cells contain 46 chromosomes in 23 pairs (the count was given as 48 for over 40 years). The human chromosomes are numbered from 1 to 22 starting with the largest numbered 1 and the second largest numbered 2. The 23rd pair is the X and Y chromosomes, which dictate the sex of the individual. This pair may be referred to as *non-autosomal* or as *gonosomal*.

Each chromosome possesses a centromere. This structure is involved in organizing the DNA during cell division. It is always off-centre and hence produces the short arm and long arm of the chromosome.

A normal female has two X chromosomes, whereas a normal male has one X and one Y chromosome. One of the female X chromosomes is deactivated in each cell, forming a *Barr body* structure visible through the microscope. The X chromosome that is deactivated may differ for each cell.[13] In mammals possession of the Y chromosome determines the organism to be male. In fact possession of even a small section of the short arm of the Y chromosome will result in a male. Other orders of life, such as reptiles, determine sex using other mechanisms. One chromosome of each of the 23 pairs has been inherited from the mother and one from the father.

It was historically not possible, from the examination of a single individual, to tell which chromosome had come from which parent, with the exception that a Y chromosome must have come from a male individual's father and hence the X chromosome of a male must have come from his mother. However there are reports utilizing paternally imprinted allele typing that suggest that the ability to determine the parental origin of a chromosome may be possible for some loci.[13-16] In mammals some genes undergo parental imprinting and either the maternal or the paternal allele may be preferentially expressed in the offspring. The reason for this is currently unknown. Imprinting appears to be associated with differential methylation upstream from the allele. This difference gives the potential to determine the parental origin of some alleles in the vicinity of any imprinted gene. Seventy-six human genes have been identified as undergoing paternal imprinting, although more are under investigation.[17]

When most individuals are DNA profiled, they show either one or two alleles at each locus. If they show one we assume that they are homozygotic, meaning that they have received two copies of the same allele, one from each parent. If an individual shows two alleles, he or she is usually assumed to be heterozygotic. In such cases the individual has inherited different alleles from each parent. An exception is caused by null or silent alleles. Heterozygotic individuals bearing one silent allele may easily be mistaken for homozygotes. Silent alleles most probably occur when an allele is actually present but the system is unable to visualize it. Alternative methods may in fact be able to visualize the allele. Hence the term *silent allele* is preferable instead of the term *null*, although uptake of this preferred term is patchy.

There are a few genetic exceptions that may lead to people having more than two alleles. These include trisomy (three chromosomes), translocation of a gene (a copy of the gene has been inserted somewhere else on the genome), somatic mutation (the individual has different genotypes in different cells) and chimerism (coexistence of two genetically distinct cell populations).[18]

It is thought that all humans except identical twins differ in their nuclear DNA. Even identical twins may differ in minor ways. There is no formal proof of this concept of underlying uniqueness and it has little influence on forensic work as all technologies examine only a very few points or loci on the entire human genome. Recent studies however are using DNA methylation profiling to investigate epigenetic differences between monozygotic twins.[19] The areas of the human genome used for DNA STR profiling are largely intronic. This means that they are non-coding DNA segments between areas of DNA that code for proteins. They were initially presumed to be functionless; however evidence is accruing that non-coding DNA may indeed have a function.[20–22] A function for some non-coding DNA regions may include regulating development in eukaryotes. Interestingly large areas of non-coding DNA, many of which are not implicated in regulation, are strongly conserved between species. This may be strong evidence that they too are, indeed, functional.

Introns are peculiar to eukaryotes and are thought to have developed late in eukaryotic evolution. They have a propensity to contain polymorphic regions, which means that they have many differing forms. This is thought to be because there is little or no selective pressure on some of these loci and hence different forms may persist in populations, side by side.

In most of the ensuing chapters it is assumed that the genotype of people does not change throughout their lives and is the same in all their diploid cells. In general the genotype of an individual is set at the moment of gamete fusion. Minor changes may occur during a lifetime as a result of somatic mutation, and an adult individual is expected to show some level of mosaicism. It is possible that some genetic changes may be encouraged by practices during a lifetime. For example, allelic alteration has been reported in the cells of oral or colorectal cancer patients and betel quid chewers.[23–25] Such an alteration may affect genotyping when a reference DNA sample is taken from a different body tissue to the scene sample.

DNA Profiling Technology

DNA profiling has gone through three major stages of technological advancement and is on the brink of a fourth. Loosely speaking the first three were the multi-locus, single locus and STR stages. The emerging fourth stage is sequencing. The advent of large-scale, low-cost parallel sequencing means this fourth stage is becoming practical in a forensic laboratory. Protocols for extracting DNA and constructing single locus profiles are described by Budowle et al.[26] and Butler.[4] These stages have not been discussed further in this book.

Short Tandem Repeat Analysis

In the mid-1990s, the technology changed to encompass the use of polymerase chain reaction (PCR) of STR loci.[27] The PCR reaction has been likened to a molecular photocopier. It enables the exponential amplification of very small amounts of DNA. Previous methods typically required 500 ng for a successful test. With PCR, 1 ng or less could be analyzed. The STR loci selected had much smaller alleles, typically between 100 and 400 bp. Resolution of small fragments by polyacrylamide gel electrophoresis (PAGE) was much improved compared with previous methods that analyzed fragments of several kilobases. Consequently, the difference between STR alleles differing by one repeat was sufficient to allow unambiguous assignment of genotypes. This was perceived as a considerable advantage. Smaller alleles were also more suitable for the PCR reaction as it is more efficient with low molecular weight DNA fragments.

PCR involves a number of replication cycles. Each cycle has the potential to double the amount of DNA, although the actual amplification is slightly less than a doubling. In many cases standard casework using STRs is undertaken at 27–34 cycles. At perfect amplification this theoretically should amplify the starting template by a factor of 134 million to 17 billion (10^9). However, perfect amplification is not achieved.

It is possible to amplify the DNA of a single cell.[28] The analysis of trace DNA evidence was initially described by the term *low copy number* (LCN) in the United Kingdom. This has led to confusion[29-34] and a plausible better set of terms is to reserve LCN for a specific 34-cycle technology and use LTDNA ('low template DNA') for any low-level profile.[35,36]

The suggested guidelines for reporting LTDNA evidence are different to 'conventional' DNA profiling because of the increased uncertainty in the origin of the DNA and the increase in artefactual issues. These difficulties can be dealt with in a binary sense by introducing interpretation rules, or in a continuous sense by modelling the behaviour of LTDNA profiles. Both of these concepts are dealt with separately in subsequent chapters.

The introduction of PCR-based STR analysis was the major innovation that expanded the utility of DNA profiling (Figure 1.1). In summary:

- The development of PCR improved the sensitivity of the analysis.

- The time taken per analysis was reduced to less than 24 hours.

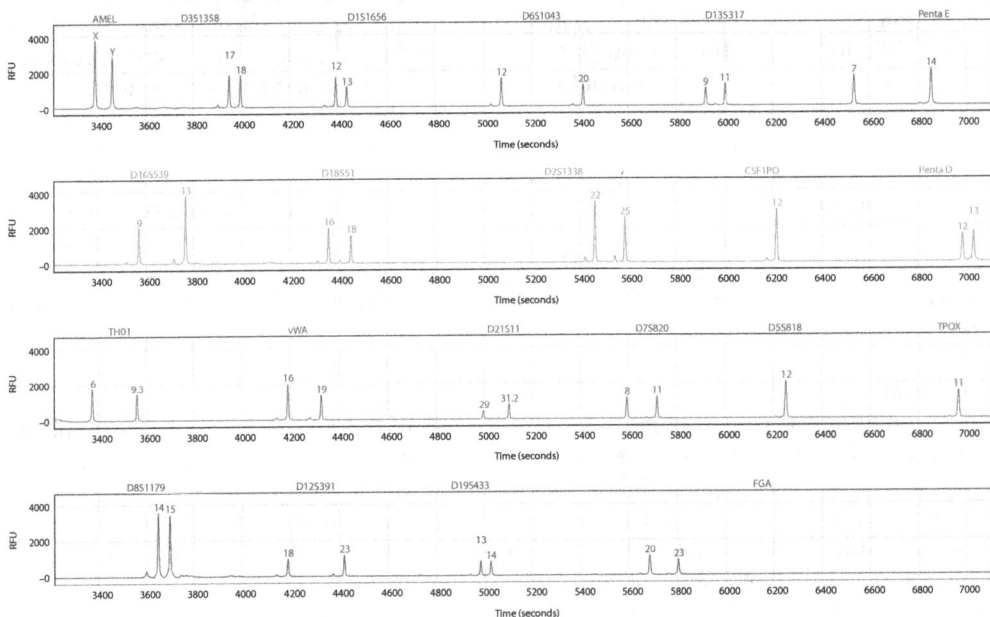

Figure 1.1   The PowerPlex® 21 short tandem repeat profile of a male individual analysed in OSIRIS (http://www.ncbi.nlm.nih.gov/projects/SNP/osiris/). The dye in the top pane is fluorescein (blue), the second JOE (green), third TMR-ET (yellow) and fourth pane CXR-ET (red).

4

- The cost-effectiveness of the method was greatly improved due to a reduction in the labour required.

- The shorter STR loci allowed the analysis of degraded DNA samples, which are frequently encountered by forensic scientists. Such analysis was possible because these short segments of DNA stood a higher chance of being intact after degradation.

- STR loci could be multiplexed together using several different STR primer pairs to amplify several loci in one reaction. Multiplexing was further facilitated by the development of dye-labelled primers that could be analyzed on automated DNA sequencers.

- The collection of data was automated, and the analysis and interpretation of data was amenable to automation. A discussion of common nomenclature is in Box 1.1.

BOX 1.1   NOMENCLATURE*

The trace produced by most modern DNA analyses is a plot of signal (measured in relative fluorescent units, rfu) versus time. This is termed an *electropherogram* (epg). Below is John Buckleton's epg. The timescale has been converted, using standards, to molecular weight.

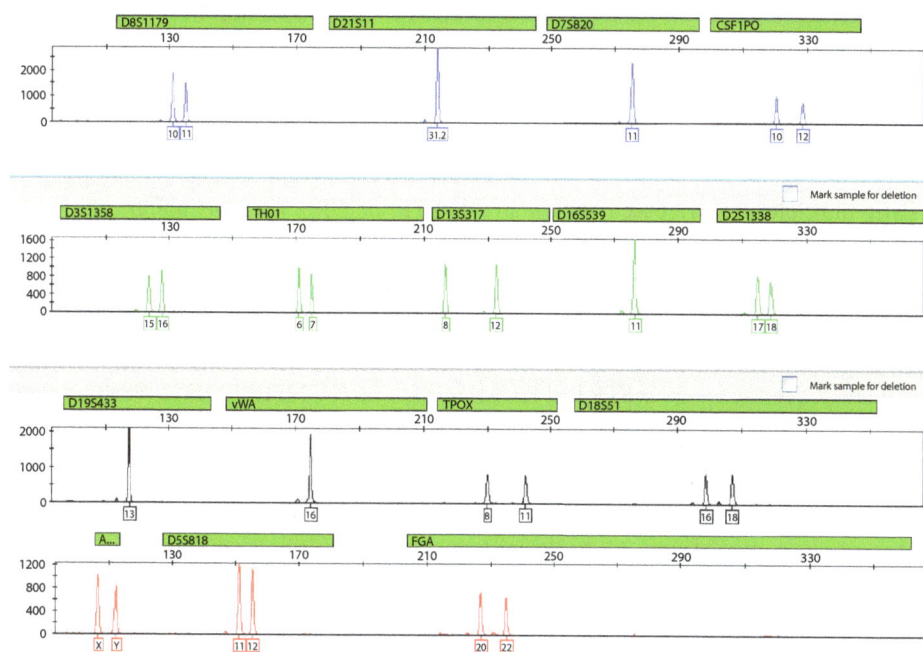

The genotype of an individual is represented as a string of numbers. Looking at the epg above we infer that John Buckleton's genotype for the Identifiler™ loci is 10,11; 31.2,31.2; 11,11; 10,12; 15,16; 6,7; 8,12; 11,11; 17,18; 13,13; 16,16; 8,11; 16,18; XY; 11,12; 20,22. The epg is not a genotype and the genotype is not an epg, although they are closely related. What then is a *profile*? The nearest definition we can deduce from common usage is that it is used as a synonym for either the *genotype* (e.g. John Buckleton's profile) or the *epg* (e.g. the crime scene profile). The use of this word to mean two things blurs the fact that the genotype is inferred from the epg.

---

* This section was enhanced by discussion with Dr Simone Gittelson.

It may be worth noting that even though the analysis takes less than 24 hours, routine turn-around times of five days for volume crime are not trivial to maintain. Forensic DNA analysis is dominated by note taking, form filling and paperwork.

Selection of Autosomal STR Loci for Forensic Multiplexing

STR loci consist of repeated segments of two to eight bases. These are termed *dimeric, trimeric* and so on. Dimeric loci are not used for forensic applications because excessive slippage during amplification (termed *stuttering*) results in a large number of spurious bands that are difficult to interpret. Trimeric, tetrameric and pentameric loci are less prone to this problem.

Several factors are considered when choosing candidate STR loci:

- A high level of variability within a locus is desired so that the locus has a low match probability.

- The length of alleles should be in the range 90–500 bp. Typically, the higher the molecular weight of the alleles, the lower the precision of their measurement. Smaller alleles are less affected by degradation and are therefore less likely to drop out.

- Loci could have been selected based on chromosomal location to ensure that closely linked loci are not chosen; however this possibility has not been carried into practice. See Table 1.1 for the chromosomal location of some common STR loci. As a quick guide to the nomenclature of the locus locations, those that begin with, say, D5 are on chromosome 5.

- Robustness and reproducibility of results are essential.

- In order to ease interpretation it is desirable that loci do not stutter excessively.

Early multiplexes were based on few simple STR loci. The four loci *quadruplex* was probably the first to be widely used for court reporting purposes.[37] The match probability was high by modern standards, in the order of 10^{-4}; hence initially the evidence was often supported by single locus probe evidence. In 1996 a six-locus STR system combined with the amelogenin sex test[38] was introduced.[39,40] This system, known as the *second-generation multiplex* (SGM), superseded single locus probe analysis in the United Kingdom and New Zealand. The SGM had more loci and included the complex STR loci HUMD21S11 and HUMFIBRA/FGA,[41] which are highly polymorphic. The expected match probability was decreased to approximately 1 in 5×10^7.

The introduction of SGM in 1995 narrowly preceded the launches of national DNA databases in the United Kingdom (1995) and New Zealand (1996).[42,43] More than five million samples are now stored in the UK database and over 10 million in the US database,[44] established in 1998. As databases become much larger, it is necessary to manage and minimize the possibility of matches to innocent people (adventitious matches). This goal may be achieved by increasing the discriminating power of the STR systems in use. Such additional discrimination may be utilized either in the database itself or in post-hit confirmation. Multiplexes with more loci and more discriminating power are becoming available. For a complete list of different commercially available multiplexes, their STR loci, chromosomal locations, repeat sequence and much more, the reader is referred to the STR database, STRBase, managed by the US National Institute of Standards and Technology.[45]

Some harmonization of STR loci used in forensic work has been achieved by collaboration at the international level (see Table 1.1). In April 2009, the European Network of Forensic Science Institutes (ENFSI) adopted an extended set of core loci to enable matching between countries.[46,47] The United States has plans to adopt additional core loci to facilitate matching with many of the new loci consistent with the European set.[48-50]

Linked STR Loci

The measure of distance between two loci is termed a *centiMorgan* (cM). This is defined as the distance between genes at which there is a 1% chance that a marker at one genetic locus will

Table 1.1 Core Set of Loci Used in Certain Jurisdictions

Locus	Chromosome	Chromosomal Location	Physical Position Mb May 2004 NCBI Build 35	CODIS	Proposed US Extended Set	ENFSI Original Standard Set	Extended European Standard Set	Interpol Standard Set	Australian Standard Set
D1S1656	1	1q42			*		*		*
TPOX	2	2p25.3 thyroid peroxidase 10th intron	1.472	*	*		*		*
D2S1338	2	2q35	218.705		*				*
D2S441	2	2p14			*		*		
D3S1358	3	3p21.31	45.557	*	*	*	*	*	*
FGA	4	4q31.3 α-fibrinogen 3rd intron	155.866	*	*	*	*	*	*
D5S818	5	5q23.2	123.139	*	*				*
CSF1PO	5	5q33.1c-fms proto-oncogene 6th intron	149.436	*	*				*
ACTBP2SE33	6	6q14 beta-actin-related pseudogene	89.043		*				
D7S820	7	AC004848-13 7q21.11	83.433	*	*				*
D8S1179	8	8q24.13	125.976	*	*	*	*	*	*

(Continued)

Table 1.1 (Continued) Core Set of Loci Used in Certain Jurisdictions

Locus	Chromosome	Chromosomal Location	Physical Position Mb May 2004 NCBI Build 35	CODIS	Proposed US Extended Set	ENFSI Original Standard Set	Extended European Standard Set	Interpol Standard Set	Australian Standard Set
D10S1248	10				*		*		
TH01	11	11p15.5 tyrosine hydroxylase 1st intron	2.149	*	*	*	*	*	*
vWA	12	12p13.31 von Willebrand Factor 40th intron	5.963	*	*	*	*	*	*
D12S391	12	12p12			*		*		*
D13S317	13	13q31.1	81.620	*	*				
Penta E	15	15q26.2	95.175		*				
D16S539	16	16q24.1	84.944	*	*			*	*
D18S51	18	18q21.33	59.100	*	*	*	*	*	*
D19S433	19	19q12	35.109		*				
D21S11	21	21q21.1	19.476	*	*	*	*	*	*
Penta D	21	21q22.3	43.880						
D22S1045	22	22q12.3					*		
DYS391	Y				*				

Source: Butler, J.M., *Journal of Forensic Sciences*, 51(2), 253–265, 2006.
ENFSI, European Network of Forensic Science Institutes; CODIS, Combined DNA Index System.

be separated from a marker at another locus due to a recombination event in a single generation (meiosis). One centiMorgan equates to a recombination fraction of 0.01. It is a commonly held belief that a distance of 50 cM is sufficient to assure independence. However the relationship between physical distance and recombination is not linear and a distance of 50 cM does not equate to a recombination fraction of 0.5.[51,52]

The simplest relationship between distance and recombination fraction is described by Haldane.[51] Consider two loci, A and B; denote the genetic distance between them as x and their recombination fraction as R

$$R = \frac{1}{2} \times \left(1 - e^{-2x}\right)$$ Haldane

Kosambi took into account the fact that the strands of the DNA molecule are to some extent rigid and hence that the occurrence of a crossover will inhibit the possibility of a second nearby recombination event. He gives the relationship between the recombination fraction, R, and the map distance by

$$R = \frac{1}{2} \times \frac{1 - e^{-4x}}{1 + e^{-4x}}$$ Kosambi

If the distance between two loci on the same chromosome is 'short', the loci are said to be linked and are not inherited independently. The two loci may be described as syntenic. The recombination fraction, R, is 0.5 for genes that assort independently; i.e. they are located on different chromosomes or separated by sufficient distance on the same chromosome. In practice the value of R can be measured directly by experiment or estimated from the physical distance separating the two loci.[51,52]

When discussing linkage it is necessary to consider the concept of phase. The gametic phase represents the original allelic combinations an individual inherits from their parents. *Phase* is a specific association of alleles at different loci on the same chromosome. The actual phase of the alleles is often unknown.

While the loci chosen for inclusion in forensic multiplexes are predominantly on different chromosomes, for some time these multiplexes have contained a few pairs of loci on the same chromosome (Table 1.2).[53] Therefore the subject of linked loci is important to the forensic arena.

Linkage of this level is unlikely to lead to linkage disequilibrium in the population unless there is a recent evolutionary event.[56] This is simply because sufficient generations have typically elapsed to allow the recombination, albeit reduced, to reassort the alleles.

An elegant empirical investigation and confirmation of this theoretical prediction comes from a study of syntenic STR loci on 12 chromosomes in 145 two-generation families. This includes all the loci listed in Table 1.2. The authors conclude, 'Linkage disequilibrium between pairs of 30 syntenic STR markers located on 12 autosomes was analyzed. No significant linkage disequilibrium was detected'.[57]

Linkage equilibrium would not be true if there was a recent evolutionary event. The most obvious candidate for such an event would be recent admixture of two populations such as Caucasian and African American or Caucasian and Maori.

The effect of linkage in pedigrees spanning a few generations is well known in genetics, but in forensic work it is a less common consideration. If we assume linkage equilibrium at the population level, then linkage has no effect at all in a pedigree unless the following two conditions are met:

1. At least one individual in the pedigree (the central individual) is involved in at least two meioses, either as a parent or as a child.

2. That individual is a double heterozygote at the loci in question.

Even these requirements are insufficient. There are examples where both these conditions are met and yet there is still no effect. One example would be when the single available ancestor

Table 1.2 Examples of Loci Located on the Same Chromosome, Their Distance Apart and Common Commercial STR Multiplexes

Locus Pairs	Chromosomal Location	Distance (cM)	Recombination Fraction (Kosambi Function)	Multiplex
vWA	12p13.31			NGM and NGM SElect™, Sinofiler, PowerPlex ESX, ESI 16 and 17 and PowerPlex 21, Qiagen ESSplex, GlobalFiler™, PowerPlex Fusion
D12S391	12p12	11.94	0.117	
D5S818	5q23.2			CODIS, Identifiler, Sinofiler, PowerPlex 16, 18D and 21, Qiagen IDplex, GlobalFiler, PowerPlex Fusion
CSF1PO	5q33.1	27.76	0.252	
D2S1338	2q35	Different arms, unlinked. Note that this corrects an error in Gill et al.[54] and Bright et al.[55]		Identifiler and PowerPlex 18D and 21, Qiagen IDplex, GlobalFiler, PowerPlex Fusion
TPOX	2p25			
D21S11	21q21.1			PowerPlex 16, 21 and Fusion
Penta D	21q33.1	44.73	0.357	
D2S1338	2q35			NGM and NGM SElect, PowerPlex ESX and ESI 17 and PowerPlex 18D and 21, GlobalFiler, PowerPlex Fusion
D2S441	2p14	Different arms, unlinked		
TPOX	2p25			GlobalFiler and PowerPlex Fusion
D2S441	2p14	88.81	0.472	

Source: Bright, J.A., et al., A Guide to forensic DNA interpretation and linkage. *Profiles in DNA*, 2014. Available from: http://www.promega.com/resources/profiles-in-dna/2014/a-guide-to-forensic-dna-interpretation-and-linkage/.
STR, short tandem repeat; CODIS, Combined DNA Index System.

of the central individual is the same heterozygote at one of the loci in question, thereby giving no phase information. O'Connor et al.[58] give a simulation study that shows that the potential effect may vary from very little to considerable.

The Forensic Science Regulator Guidelines[59] recommend consideration of these effects. 'Recommendation 8: The method for calculating match probabilities when relatives are considered as potential sources should be adjusted to account for linkage between syntenic loci. [The Regulator endorses this as a requirement.]'

Recently commentators have advocated alternate ways of dealing with syntenic loci.[58,60] These approaches include dropping a locus or treating the pair of loci as a diplotype. Neither approach is sustainable. This is discussed in Chapters 3 and 4.

STR Locus Nomenclature

Several different classes of STR loci have been defined. Urquhart et al.[61] classified different loci according to the complexity of their sequences. One of the most ubiquitous STR loci used is HUMTH01.[62,63] This consists of a simple repeating sequence $(AATG)_{5-11}$ with a common non-consensus allele $[AATG]_6ATG[AATG]_3$. Compound STR loci such as HUMVWFA31[64] consist of repeating sequences $(ATCT)_2(GTCT)_{3-4}(ATCT)_{9-13}$, whereas complex repeats such as HUMD21S11[65] are less uniform. Detailed information may, again, be obtained from STRBase.[45,66]

This nomenclature system has found widespread application. However, as technologies advance, deficiencies in the system are being found and we may see a revision in the future.[67]

These sequences are based on a tetrameric repeating sequence interspersed with invariant di- and trinucleotides. Complex hypervariable $(AAAG)_n$ repeats such as human beta-actin-related pseudogene (ACTBP2)[68,69] are much more difficult to accommodate to a nomenclature based upon the number of tetrameric repeat sequences. This difficulty results because variant mono-, di-, tri- and tetramers are scattered throughout the locus. These latter STRs have found limited use in a few European countries.

STR Allele Designation

The greatest advantage of fluorescence-automated sequencer technology is the ability to detect several different dye-labelled moieties. For example, current systems are able to detect five colours. The determination of DNA fragment sizes is dependent upon the use of two types of standard markers. In every sample that is electrophoresed, a series of dye-labelled DNA fragments of known size are included. This internal size standard may be composed of restricted bacteriophage-labelled DNA (for instance the Applied Biosystems GS 500 product) or, alternatively, artificial DNA concatemers (for instance the Applied Biosystems HD 400 product).

The second kind of standard marker is the *allelic ladder* (Figure 1.2). This marker comprises all the common alleles for each locus and is compared with each lane on an electrophoretic run.[70] Allelic ladders should span the entire range of the common alleles of a locus. However it is not necessary that every allele be represented in the ladder. Many rare alleles have been discovered and some of these are outside the range of the ladder. If possible there should be no gap larger than four bases between the rungs of the ladder for tetrameric and dimeric STR loci. If the STR repeat is greater than four bases, then the maximum gap should be the size of the repeat.

The allelic ranges of some loci may overlap. These loci are labelled with different dyes, therefore allowing each locus to be identified. Loci that are labelled with the same dye have to be separated sufficiently to minimize the possibility of overlap of the allele ranges.

Allele sizes are measured relative to the internal size standard, often by using the Elder and Southern local method.[71,72] The size of the unknown alleles in the questioned sample is then

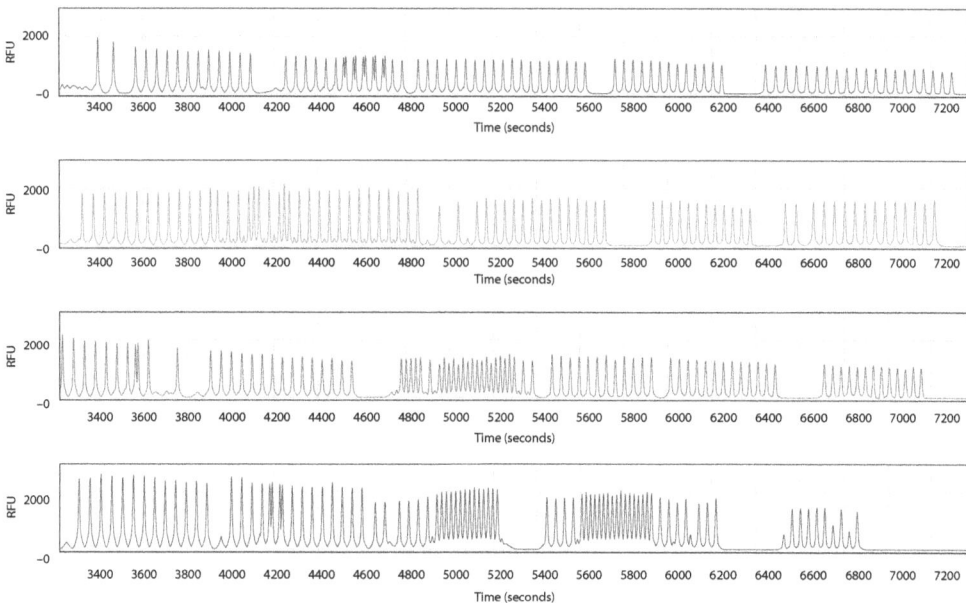

Figure 1.2   Allelic ladders from the PowerPlex® 21 system (Promega Corporation, Madison, Wisconsin).

11

compared with the size of the known alleles of the allelic ladder. The units are typically base pairs (bp) or bases.

Provided that a questioned allele is within ±0.5 bp of a corresponding ladder peak, allelic designation may be undertaken. In all electrophoretic systems it is usual for a small amount of aberrant migration to occur such that the migration rate may be either slower or faster than expected. This phenomenon is termed *band shift*. Band shift tends to be in the same direction for two alleles in the same lane. This shift can be measured to ensure consistency,[70] acting as an additional quality control check and also as a means to designate off-ladder or 'rare' alleles.[73]

STR Allelic Nomenclature

The International Society of Forensic Genetics (ISFG) DNA Commission[74–76] has recommended an STR allelic nomenclature based upon the number of repeat sequences present in an allele. If a partial repeat sequence is present, then the size of the partial repeat is given in bases after a decimal point* – for example, the common allele HUMTH01 9.3 consists of 9 repeats followed by a partial repeat of 3 bases. This method is suitable for typing simple STR loci.

Complex hypervariable repeats such as ACTBP2 (SE33) do not possess a simple repeating structure. The designation of complex STR repeats such as ACTBP2, D11S554 and APOAI1 follows from the size of specific alleles. The size is dependent upon the primers utilized and hence different primers will produce a differently named allele. The allelic size may also be dependent upon the internal structure of the allele. Hence designations are prefixed with the term 'type-'.

The designation scheme to be used for a given locus is dependent upon the characteristics of the locus itself. If possible, the designation should follow the recommendations of the ISFG DNA commission unless this approach is precluded by allelic structure at this locus.

Linking the allelic ladder and the nomenclature of STR loci provides the key to standardization. In principle the platform used (capillary electrophoresis or PAGE) is not particularly important. Direct comparisons can be made between different instruments, provided that allelic sizing is consistent. In addition comparisons can also be made between different multiplexes derived from different manufacturers using different primer sets. The allelic ladders act as control reference standards that enable laboratories using different hardware and multiplexes to compare results.

Y Chromosome STR

STR also exists on the Y chromosome and the same typing technology can be used. Y-STR marker nomenclature names the loci as *DYS* followed by a number, for example *DYS455*. Y-STR analysis differs from autosomal in that Y-STR

- Are often amplified for more PCR cycles
- Show more locus to locus imbalance
- Present largely one allele per locus
- Do not recombine[77]

Next-Generation Sequencing

With the recent advances in DNA sequencing methodology and bioinformatics (the storage, retrieval and analysis of biological data), next-generation sequencing (NGS) technologies are becoming more available. NGS technologies are already being applied to fields such as medical genetics and evolutionary biology and were instrumental in the sequencing of the human genome.

The application of NGS technologies to forensic DNA problems is still under investigation.[78–83] NGS may be useful for analyzing standard autosomal DNA markers (STRs and SNPs), haplotypes (mitochondrial DNA sequences and Y-chromosomal markers) and mRNA markers, which are increasingly being used for the identification of body fluids and cell types. Before

---

* This mark is termed a *decimal point* by biochemists but strictly speaking it is just a dot. There is no hint of the decimal system in what comes after the dot.

widespread use, NGS technologies will require the application of strict quality measures and development of analysis and interpretation guidelines as for any new forensic technology.[84]

Understanding STR Profiles

In this section we begin the process of interpreting electropherograms. It is necessary to understand the effects of some genetic anomalies and the outputs of the PCR and electrophoresis systems to understand both simple unmixed profiles and, more crucially, mixtures. Some anomalies and outputs are introduced briefly here.

Genetic Anomalies

Trisomy and Gene Duplication

The first trisomy 'discovered' was that associated with Down's syndrome at chromosome 21, reported by Lejeune in 1959.[85] Subsequently trisomies were discovered at chromosomes 13 and 18 but always associated with severe disorders. Trisomies appear more common in spontaneously aborted foetuses. Chromosomal duplication of ChrX appears to be more common and to have fewer effects possibly due to the deactivation of all X chromosomes bar one.

Both chromosome and gene duplication affect all cells in an individual. In practice it is impossible to tell the difference between these two phenomena without resorting to genetic analysis. If a deletion or insertion of a repeat unit accompanies duplication, then three bands of similar size are generated (see Figure 1.3).

If a gene is duplicated without additional mutation, then two bands are visible in a 2:1 ratio. In the example in Figure 1.4 an XXY individual has two copies of the X chromosome. Note that the other loci are balanced and this argues against the possibility that this sample is a mixture. In the multiplex described by Sparkes et al.[39,40] trisomy or gene duplication was observed in 1 in 2000 samples at each locus (see Table 1.3). Johnson et al.[86] reported three gene duplication events in a sample of 525 males. Crouse et al.[87] reported 18 three-banded patterns at TPOX and 1 at CSF1PO in over 10,000 samples. There is emerging evidence that the relatively common three-banded patterns at TPOX result from a gene duplication and that the extra copy may be on the X chromosome far from the TPOX locus itself (on chromosome 2).[88] The extra allele is almost always allele 10 and is thought to be on the q arm of the X chromosome.[89-94] This unusual situation has been used effectively in paternity.[93] STRBase[45,66] gives up-to-date counts of three-banded patterns at some loci. Unfortunately we cannot turn these into rates because we do not know how many samples were examined to find them. Valuable reports continue to appear.[95,96]

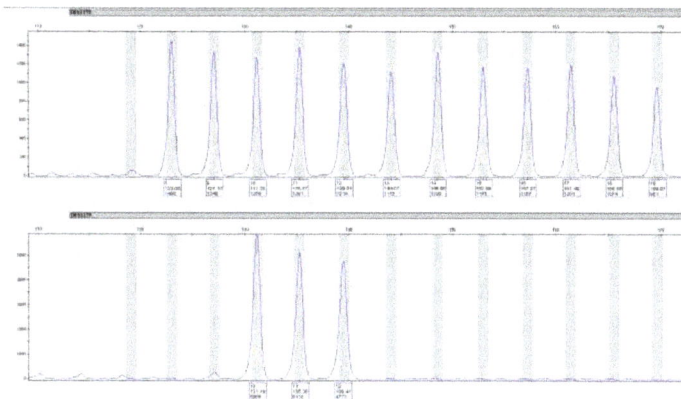

Figure 1.3   Example of a D8S1179 trisomy or translocation appears in the lower pane. Note that the peaks are equivalent in height. This is often referred to as the *Clayton Type 2 pattern*. The allelic ladder is in the upper pane.

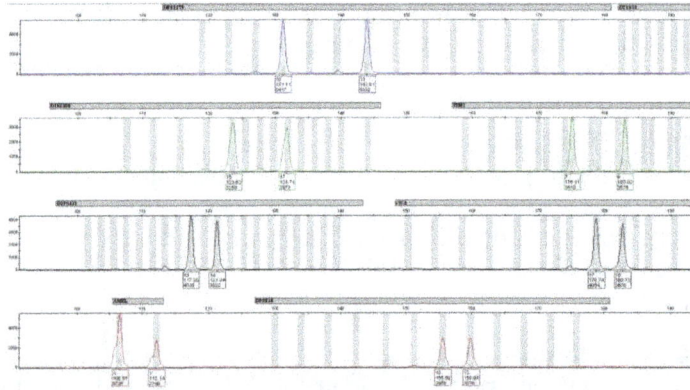

Figure 1.4 XXY individual (lower pane left) showing an X peak twice the size of the Y peak. The remaining loci of the Identifiler multiplex are balanced.

Table 1.3 The Occurrence of Trisomy or Gene Duplication at Some STR Loci in ~600,000 Profiles	
Locus	Count
Amelogenin	1191
D21S11	9
D18S51	7
D8S1179	24
FGA	12
vWA	8
THO1	1

Somatic Mutation

Somatic mutation occurs during embryological development or later in life. A mutation occurs in one line of cells and hence cells with two slightly different but closely related genotypes coexist. The earlier in the development of the organism that this occurs, the larger the number of cells likely to be descendants of the mutated cell. This leads to a three-banded profile (Figure 1.5) when samples of these cells are typed. Further examples can be seen in Mertens et al.[94] This phenomenon should not be confused with chimerism, which occurs when two separate cell lines coexist in one organism (often produced by the merger of two fertilized eggs).

The peak heights will be dependent upon the relative proportion of the two cell types in the sample and need not be equivalent. This is arguably the most difficult condition to elucidate since it is possible that not all tissues will demonstrate somatic mutation. It is possible that some somatic mutations will not be distinguishable from stutters. Hence these figures are probably underestimates since mutations are recorded only if they are unambiguous.

PCR Effects

The PCR amplification process is imperfect. In each amplification round most often a correct copy of the allele is made but occasionally a miscopy occurs. The most common miscopy is to produce an allele one repeat shorter, termed a *back stutter*, or simply a *stutter*. Even less frequently the miscopy may be an allele one repeat longer, termed a *forward stutter*.

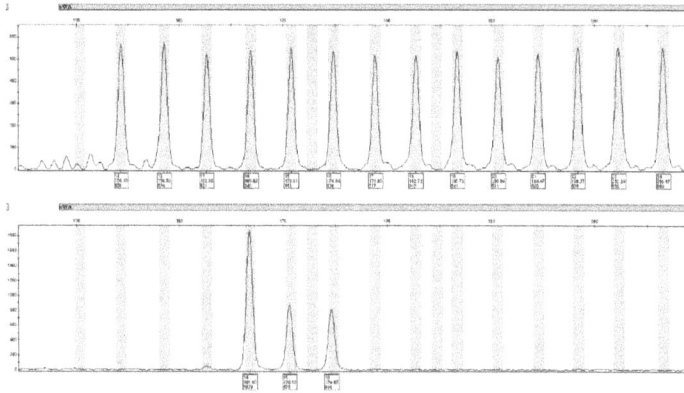

Figure 1.5 Somatic mutation at the vWA locus, lower pane. Note that three peaks of different heights are present. This is often referred to as the *Clayton Type 1 pattern*. The upper pane shows vWA allelic ladders.

The two peaks of a heterozygote are typically slightly different in height or area. This difference may be due to different amplification efficiencies, different stuttering rates or different sampling of template at the start of the process.[97] The difference in the height of the two peaks of a heterozygote is termed *heterozygote balance* (Hb) in the United Kingdom and Europe and *peak height ratio* (PHR) in the United States. This is an example of the unfortunate habit of things being renamed on each side of the Atlantic which unnecessarily widens the divide. Hb has precedence and maybe gives a better indication of what is being considered (the balance of two peaks of a heterozygote). PHR could, for example, apply to the ratio of any two peaks, say, an allelic peak and its stutter product. We will use Hb but acknowledge no special right for Europe to name things. We also acknowledge the aversion that mathematicians understandably have towards multi-letter symbols. For example, what is the difference between PHR and $P \times H \times R$?

Low template levels are known to lead to substantial changes to profile morphology, such as extreme peak imbalance or dropout, and the almost unavoidable appearance of contaminant alleles.[98,99] The effects can be largely predicted by computer simulations modelling the sampling and PCR process.[97] In 1999 standard methods for interpretation appeared inadequate for some LTDNA work and new methods and safeguards appeared desirable.[29,30,34,100–102]

Such changes to profile morphology are likely to be due to sampling effects in the template.[97] While sampling is thought to be the main driver of stochastic effects, an early PCR 'event' such as a stutter in the first cycle when there are very few templates might theoretically have a large effect on subsequent peak areas (although in practice stutters are not excessively common at such low levels of DNA).[97]

Heterozygote imbalance increases as the amount of DNA template is reduced.[103,104] The number and size of stutter peaks increase at all loci as the cycle number increases.

Analytical Threshold

A peak in the electropherogram (epg) may be allelic, a PCR by-product, artefactual such as pull-up, or electronic noise. Back stutter is almost unavoidable and we can assume that almost every allelic peak has an associated back stutter peak. Forward stutter and double back stutter are also produced by the PCR process, less frequently and in smaller amounts. Since back stutter, forward stutter and double back stutter are allelic products, they do not differ from a true allelic peak in any way and cannot be differentiated by visual examination. These are not the only artefactual PCR products. For example, there is a –2 bp stutter at SE33 which is a complex locus with largely tetranucleotide repeats.

To apply a rational decision process it is necessary to consider both the probability that the peak is allelic and the costs and benefits of wrong or correct decisions. The consideration of the costs and benefits is called *utility*, and we begin with that.

There are four possible outcomes and it is helpful to arrange them in a square:

	Peak is Allelic	Peak is Not Allelic
Peak is assigned as allelic	This is a correct decision and will improve the analysis.	This is an incorrect decision and the damage can be severe, ranging from the addition of a false contributor to false exclusion.
Peak is assigned as not allelic	This is an incorrect decision but the damage is moderate. Most probably we will lower the power of our analysis by a small amount.	This is a correct decision and will improve the analysis.

Let us proceed to considering the probability that an observed peak of height, O, is allelic. Call the event of it being truly allelic A and hence the event of it being not allelic as $\bar{A}$. By studying the non-allelic background between peaks that are allelic or −4 stutter, we can obtain a probability density for $p(O,\bar{A})$. This is the probability density that a peak is non-allelic and of this height. Bayes' theorem gives us

$$\Pr(A\,|\,O) = \frac{p(O,A)}{p(O,A) + p(O,\bar{A})} \tag{1.1}$$

This equation is not trivial to implement. Consider the term $p(O|A)\Pr(A)$, which is the one we need to complete the calculation. This is the probability that an allelic peak is present of exactly this height. Our opinion on this would be very strongly affected by the presence of other peaks in the profile of about this height. This would lead us to believe that there was a low-level contributor present and hence $p(O|A)\Pr(A)$ might be quite high. Conversely, if there were no other low-level peaks in the profile, we might think that $p(O|A)\Pr(A)$ is low.

Two interpretation strategies are available:

1. An approach based on analytical threshold (AT)

2. Systems that deal with potential noise at the interpretation stage and require no AT

Discussions of the position of the AT usually concentrate on the electronic noise and it is suggested that the AT should not be used to manage artefacts. For example, SWGDAM[105] states: '3.1.1.2. ... the analytical threshold should be established based on signal-to-noise considerations (i.e. distinguishing potential allelic peaks from background). The analytical threshold should not be established for purposes of avoiding artefact labelling as such may result in the potential loss of allelic data'.

Valid efforts have been made to model electronic noise and we give a feel of these types of efforts below. These approaches usually consider the probability of a peak of height O_A if it is electronic noise, $\Pr(O_A|\text{electronic noise})$. They suggest selecting an AT at some point when $\Pr(O_A|\text{electronic noise})$ is expected to be small. We embrace the validity of the sentiment about not using AT to manage artefacts, but in a brutal pragmatic sense it is necessary to consider the downstream effects of the position of the AT. This needs a lot more than a consideration of

Pr(O_A|electronic noise) and we might suggest that electronic noise is the least difficult of the factors needing consideration.

It is of primary importance to recognize that artefactual peaks such as forward stutter and double back stutter do not carry any label that they are artefactual. They look in every way allelic and the only clues are position and height. Statements such as 'remove all artefactual peaks' assume some insight not possessed by science.

Consider initially a threshold-based approach. Peaks above the AT are often examined manually for morphology. At this stage pull-up and electronic spikes will be removed. Any peak above the AT that passes manual inspection is passed to the interpretation phase. Lowering the AT will detect more allelic peaks but will also pass more back stutter, forward stutter and double back stutter peaks. The total utility of a lowering of the AT is therefore the sum of these effects and depends crucially on how significant are the consequences of passing such peaks. This, in turn, depends on how they are treated at the interpretation phase.

In previous binary systems the passing of peaks falsely assigned as potentially allelic had a very significant negative effect (negative utility) on the interpretation. Hence historically ATs were set high. The modern probabilistic systems, especially the continuous ones, have a greater tolerance to false peaks and hence the utility function is changed. More specifically there is now less risk associated with lower ATs.

The semi-continuous models in widespread use (LRmix,[106] Lab Retriever,[107] LikeLTD[108]) do not utilize peak heights directly in the software.* All of these systems currently function with a threshold-based strategy and currently peaks in stutter positions are either removed or dealt with as ambiguous (either partly allelic or totally stutter). Peaks that are above this threshold and passed to the software must be explained as allelic, ambiguous or drop-in. Peaks dealt with using the drop-in function would include true drop-ins, that is, allelic peaks that appear singly in the extract, and non-allelic peaks not treated as ambiguous. To emphasize that the software should be run by an expert,† we will refer to the software–expert pair (SEP). The effect of dropping the AT would be more true allelic peaks detected, which has a strongly positive utility. However there will also be more peaks needing manual removal, treatment as ambiguous or drop-in, or which may suggest the addition of a trace contributor. These have a negative utility. The net effect is unstudied. In Box 1.2 we give a case report with identifying details removed but containing the essence. This case hammers home the potential negative effects of small peaks.

The continuous software programmes in current use (STRmix™[109] and TrueAllele[110]) can treat noise peaks directly, modelling the probability of these peaks if they arise from a contributor as allelic or stutter or if they do not arise from a contributor (encompassing noise or drop-in). STRmix does not currently model forward stutter or double back stutter (or the –2 bp stutter for SE33).

**BOX 1.2   AN EXAMPLE OF THE NEGATIVE EFFECTS
OF REPORTING SMALL PEAKS IN A PROFILE**

A woman reports that she is raped by a single assailant. She lives alone and has no consensual partners.

The profile has a major and a minor that can be explained by the victim and the person of interest. Very small peaks lead the report to state that this is a mixture of at least three people. This destroys the victim's credibility and the person of interest is acquitted.

---

* However expert intervention allows for the manual extraction of a clear major and Lab Retriever utilizes peak height in forming the probability of dropout (D).
† Following Gill and Haned.[106]

If a drop-in function is used for semi-continuous SEP or STRmix, the AT value does not need to be set as conservatively as with traditional interpretation methods. The setting of an AT will affect both the probability of dropout and drop-in.

If forward stutter and double back stutter are not manually removed or treated as ambiguous, then the drop-in function will now be used to model true drop-ins and also other peaks that pass AT and manual inspection. It will therefore need to be higher than if it was simply modelling drop-in. When used in this way the drop-in rate cannot be set from negative controls but needs to be set from positive samples with known ground truth.

It is therefore advantageous for the semi-continuous SEP and STRmix to manually remove forward and double back stutter. We discuss forward stutter in a later section but at this stage cannot add to the discussion on double back stutter.

Electronic Noise

A study of GeneMapper ID-X baselines suggests small but significant effects of colour and machine on both the mean and the standard deviation of noise. There appears to be an effect of template on the standard deviation.

Table 1.4 gives the predicted values of the mean +10 sd and 0.99999 quantile of the gamma distribution for two different machines, for the different colours, at 10 and 500 pg template. The value of the mean +10 sd has been suggested as one way to inform the AT.[111] The data in Table 1.4 under the gamma distribution 0.99999 quantile have been developed by fitting a gamma distribution to the data using maximum likelihood estimation (MLE). The parameters of the gamma were allowed to vary with template.

Looking at the values in the mean +10 sd columns in Table 1.4 it would be possible to pick one AT for both machines and all colours and most templates. This value could be 30 rfu or even lower values could be considered. No actual data in our demonstration set actually exceed this value. The actual maximum observed was 14 rfu.

Table 1.4   Mean +10 sd and the Gamma Distribution 0.99999 Quantile for Two Different Machines, for the Different Colours, at 10 and 500 pg Template

Machine	Colour	10 pg		500 pg	
		Mean +10 sd	Gamma 0.99999 Quantile	Mean +10 sd	Gamma 0.99999 Quantile
1	Blue	19	17	24	17
	Green	24	19	29	26
	Orange	19	15	25	15
	Purple	22	16	27	20
	Red	19	20	25	22
	Yellow	18	19	23	19
2	Blue	16	15	21	15
	Green	21	20	26	19
	Orange	16	13	22	15
	Purple	19	15	24	16
	Red	16	15	22	19
	Yellow	14	14	20	15

Modelling baseline in this manner assumes normality of the noise, and this assumption has been suggested as approximately true.[112] In Figure 1.6 we give a plot of the observed data across all colours, template amounts and machines. This graph also includes the best fit normal distribution. The data show a very slight positive skew as evidenced by the small departures of the observed from the best fit normal distribution. The best fit gamma is also shown in Figure 1.6 and looks subjectively to be no better a fit than the normal, except that it has the advantage of being bounded by 0 and hence has no density at negative values. We are likely to be interested in the positive tail. On these data the gamma slightly overestimates the density at the positive tail, whereas the normal slightly underestimates it.

The Osiris* software uses a different baseline algorithm. Figure 1.7 gives the distribution of peak heights of noise peaks in five positive samples. In these five samples there were 25 regions above 10 rfu, with the largest being 21 rfu. At least some of these had acceptable morphology.

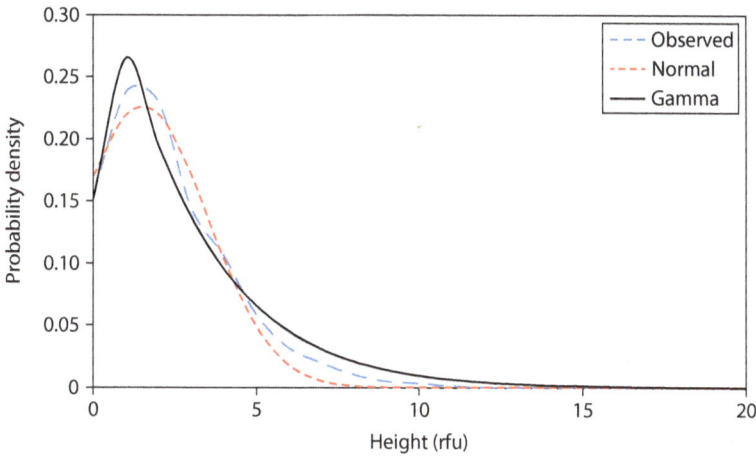

Figure 1.6   Observed heights of noise peaks on two 3130 machines using GeneMapper ID-X software with a normal and a gamma distribution overlaid.

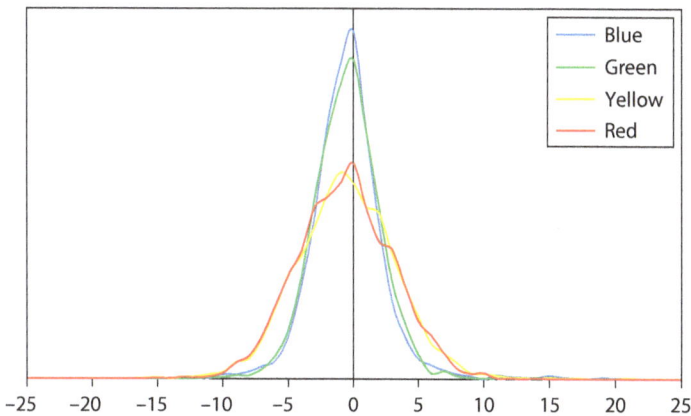

Figure 1.7   Observed heights of noise peaks using Osiris software on one 3130 machine in five positive Identifiler Plus samples. The colours are the Identifiler Plus dye colours. (Data kindly supplied by Dr Tim Kalafut, USACIL.)

---

* Available at http://www.ncbi.nlm.nih.gov/projects/SNP/osiris/

This example demonstrates the factors that we have identified that should be examined during validation. Specifically the baseline noise should be examined for every colour, each machine in use and over template ranges. The differences observed in this dataset were in many cases statistically significant but small. It would be reasonable when setting an AT to have one of the following:

1. One AT for all machines, colours and templates

2. Different values for each machine and colour, plausibly set near the top template

When setting an AT operator time can be considered. For very low ATs time is spent manually removing bad morphology peaks. As stated in the main text, electronic noise is only one part of a larger problem.

Heterozygote Balance

The factors affecting Hb are thought to be both random and systematic. We are aware of two definitions of *heterozygote balance* and both are known by the term Hb. These are as follows:

$$Hb_1 = \frac{O_{HMW}}{O_{LMW}}$$

where HMW and LMW refer to the higher and lower molecular weight allele, respectively, and O is peak height, and

$$Hb_2 = \frac{O_{smaller}}{O_{larger}} \text{ (also termed PHR)}$$

where *smaller* and *larger* refer to the height of the alleles. Hb_1 is the preferred definition as it preserves more of the initial information. Note that it is possible to obtain Hb_2 from Hb_1 but not vice versa. Unfortunately Hb_2 is in prevalent use and has led to erroneous conclusions in the past.[111]

At LTDNA levels one peak of a heterozygote may be so imbalanced that it either does not exceed the threshold set for the declaration of an allele or it is simply not detected at all. This allele is said to have dropped out. A situation where the person of interest has an allele not present in the resulting epg is termed a *non-concordance*[113] and is difficult to interpret at LTDNA levels using the binary model.[114] The more elegant solution lies with probabilistic methods.[115,116]

Previous work has identified several factors that are thought to affect heterozygote balance. The mean of Hb is thought to be affected by the difference in the number of repeat sequences, δ, between the alleles at a heterozygote locus. Alleles with a larger number of repeat sequences are thought to produce relatively smaller height peaks.[98]

The variability in Hb in Applied Biosystems' SGMPlus, Identifiler™,[117] MiniFiler™,[118] GlobalFiler™ and NGM SElect™,[119] as well as Profiler Plus and PowerPlex 21 multiplexes has been examined.

It was found that at lower peak heights variability was much greater. Figure 1.8 shows the shape of a typical plot of Hb versus average peak height, APH. The data fit a model where the variance of logHb is proportional to $\frac{k^2}{APH}$, where k is a constant (black dotted lines). Traditional Hb thresholds are plotted on Figure 1.8 as red dotted lines.

The DNA extraction and amplification processes have been modelled and the effect on Hb predicted[97,120–123] (see also the open source programme SimPCR 2). This modelling suggests that a major factor in Hb at LTDNA levels is the initial sampling of template.

An increase of one cycle in the PCR process increases peak heights by approximately a factor of 2 for the same capillary machine. Comparison of graphs such as Figures 1.9 and 1.10 across different multiplexes suggests that an increase in cycle number moves the curve to the right so that the variability observed is approximately the same if APH is scaled according to the cycles. If multiplex 2 has two more cycles than multiplex 1, then the effect seen at APH = 100

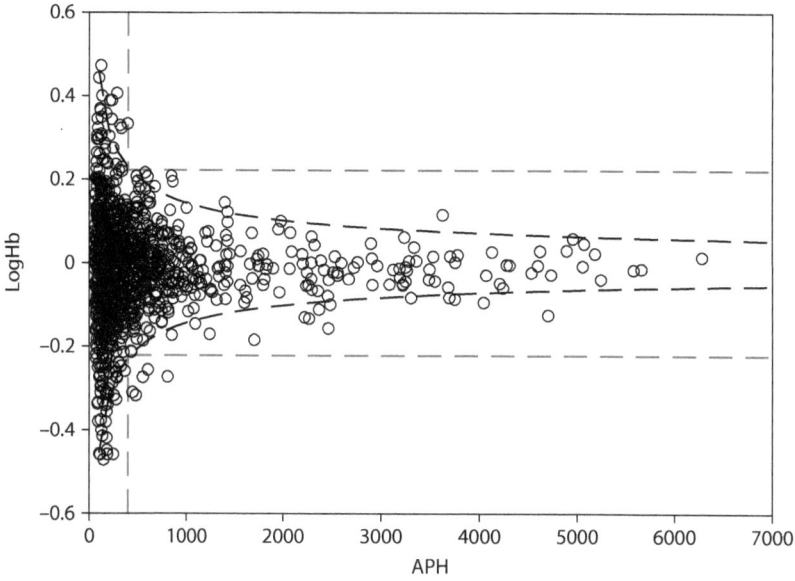

Figure 1.8   A plot of $\log_{10}$Hb versus average peak height for GlobalFiler™ data.

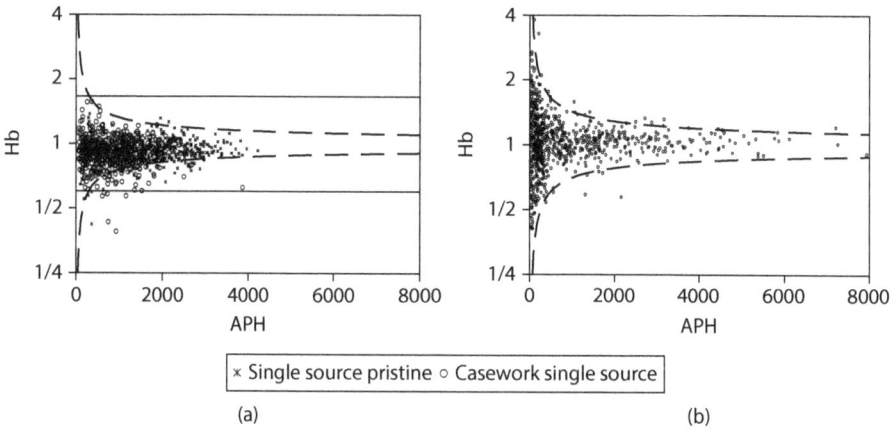

× Single source pristine ∘ Casework single source

(a)   (b)

Figure 1.9   (a) A plot of heterozygote balance (Hb) versus average peak height (APH) for Identifiler single source pristine DNA and casework samples at 28 cycles. A sample of 500 points from Bright et al.[124] is plotted. Also plotted are the traditional bounds of 1.66 and 0.60 and the lines $Hb = 10^{\pm\sqrt{14.6/APH}}$. (b) A plot of Hb versus APH for PowerPlex 21 data at 30 cycles. The dotted lines are $Hb = 10^{\pm\sqrt{23.6/APH}}$.

in multiplex 1 will be similar to the effect at APH = 400 rfu in multiplex 2. This effect is probably a manifestation of the hypothesis of Gill et al.[97] that sampling of initial template is a significant factor in variability in Hb.

We note the following:

1. The variance of a sum is the sum of the variances.

2. $\log Hb = \log O_{HMW} - \log O_{LMW}$.

3. The variance in the log of the HMW and LMW peaks should be similar.

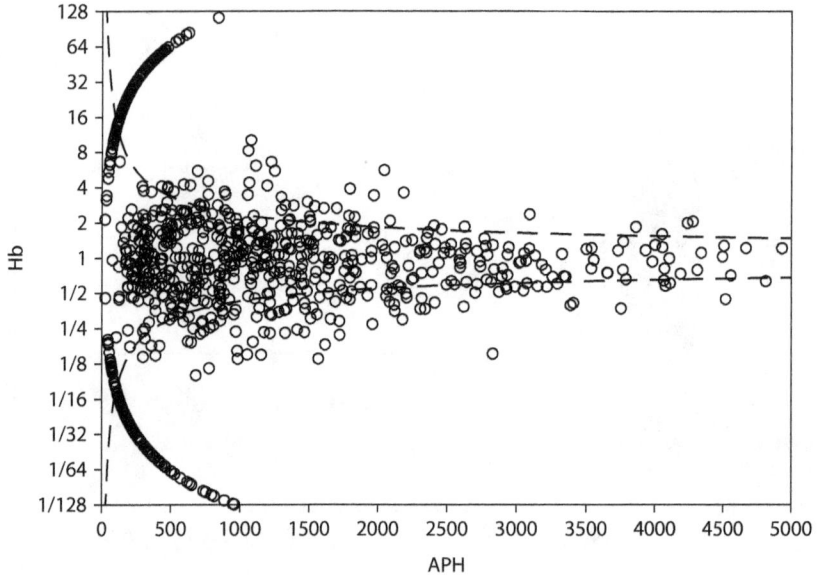

Figure 1.10 A plot of heterozygote balance (Hb) versus average peak height (APH) for the Petricevic et al.[104] data with normal injection conditions. The trilobite genal spines are the dropped alleles. The two dotted lines are Hb $= 10^{\pm\sqrt{138/APH}}$.

We may conclude that the variance in logHb should be twice the variance in the individual peaks. This may seem a rather theoretical conclusion but it does provide an avenue to estimating the variance in peak heights from readily available data.

There has been some justifiable criticism that the data behind an assessment of such variability is developed from samples constructed from pristine DNA.[30] The criticism is that this practice does not adequately mimic casework conditions. Bright et al.[124] compared pristine and casework samples and did not find a difference.

Allelic Dropout

Most laboratories define some threshold, T, below which a single peak is deemed to potentially have a dropped-out partner (i.e. a partner below the peak detection threshold, Z). This threshold is variously called the *stochastic threshold*, the *homozygote threshold* or the *mixture interpretation threshold* (MIT). An allele with a potentially dropped partner is usually marked with some identification; for example, aF stands for the a allele and a potentially dropped partner. Hence aF could be an aa homozygote or a heterozygote with the a allele and any other. *Allele dropout* is defined as the condition where an allele cannot be visualized. Findlay et al.[125,126] suggest that dropout is a separate phenomenon to heterozygote balance, not simply an extreme form of it. However the studies on Hb described above tend to suggest that this is not so. Note that in these graphs there is no discontinuity in the increase of variability as APH lessens. We must therefore expect that this variability eventually means that a peak may be sufficiently small not to be observed.

Degradation Slopes

It is empirically noted that high molecular weight loci usually have smaller peaks than lower molecular weight loci. This is typically referred to as a *degradation slope* or a *ski slope*. It is supposed that this is caused by smaller alleles being more resistant to degradation (refer to Box 1.3).

BOX 1.3   KELLY, BRIGHT AND BUCKLETON

Consider that the degradation of the DNA strand was random with respect to location. Consider a fragment of length l. If the probability of a break is p, at any of the locations $1 \ldots l$ the chance of the full fragment being amplified is $(1 - p)l$. Since $1 - p$ is less than 1, this equation describes an exponential decline in peak height.

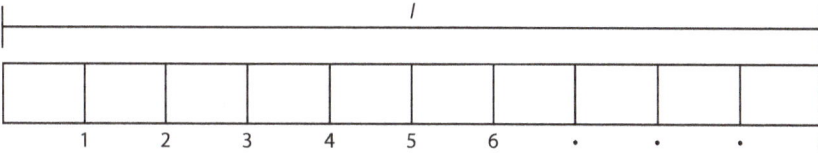

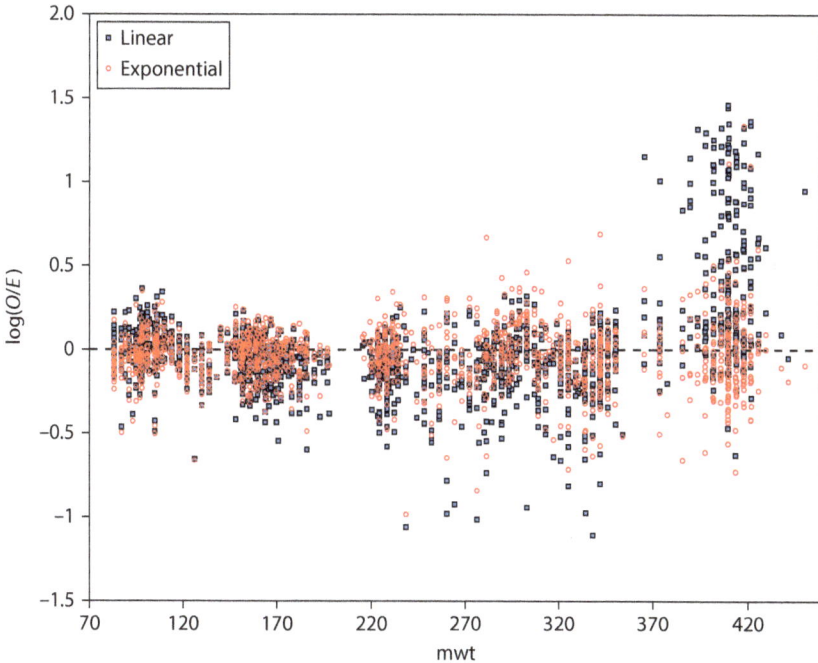

Figure 1.11   A plot of $\log\left(O_a / E_a'\right)$ versus m_a in base pairs using the exponential and linear fitting. (©Australian Academy of Forensic Sciences, reprinted by permission of Taylor & Francis, www.tandfonline. com. Bright, J.-A., et al. *Australian Journal of Forensic Sciences* 45(4): 445–449, 2013.)

Figure 1.11 gives a plot $\log\left(O_a / E_a'\right)$ for the PowerPlex 21 multiplex versus molecular weight (m_a) in base pairs.[127] E_a' is the expected value using either a linear or an exponential model. The more extreme positive departures from expectation occur at the high molecular weight end, approximately 350 bp and above, and extreme negative departures occur in the mid-zone. This is expected if we force a straight line on an exponential curve. The exponential fit reduces the number of these types of departure.

Back Stutter

Stuttering refers to the production of peaks at positions other than the parental allelic position. Stuttering is presumed to be due to miscopying or slippage during the PCR process. The proposed mechanism slipped strand mispairing involves the polymerase enzyme stalling and disassociating from the DNA during replication. After disassociation, a loop of one or more repeats may form in either the nascent or template strand, causing the addition or deletion of one or more repeats, respectively. The deletion to addition ratio has been calculated as between 14 $(CA)_n$ repeats in vitro.[128] Deletions are thought to be more common as they require fewer nucleotides to disassociate since it is the nascent strand that dissociates. This is therefore more 'energetically favourable'.[129]

The term *back stutter* is reserved for the loss and *forward stutter* for the addition of complete repeat units. Refer to Box 1.4 for a further discussion of these terms. For tetrameric loci the loss of one unit can be thought of as the $N - 4$ stutter and the loss of two units is the $N - 8$ stutter. The addition of one unit can be thought of as $N + 4$ stutter.

It is useful to define stutter ratio $SR = \dfrac{O_{a-1}}{O_a}$, where O_{a-1} is the height of the stutter peak and O_a the height of the parent allele. SR is routinely investigated by laboratories prior to implementing new multiplexes.[119,130–132] From these studies thresholds are determined below which peaks in stutter positions are removed. These thresholds may be locus specific or applied to all loci within a multiplex.

SR was empirically found to be approximately linearly proportional to the longest uninterrupted sequence (LUS).[133,134] This relationship is demonstrated in Figure 1.10 for the TH01 locus. As discussed previously in this chapter, TH01 is a simple repeat with the structure $[AATG]_{3-12}$ with a common non-consensus allele $[AATG]_6ATG[AATG]_3$ which is typed as a 9.3 allele. The LUS value for the 9.3 variant allele is 6. From Figure 1.12 it can be seen that LUS is a better predictor of SR than allele.

Stutter ratios for more complex STR loci, notably SE33, are poorly explained by a model based on LUS. SE33 has some alleles with two or three long sequences. This locus better fits a model where all repeat sequences are considered as contributing to stuttering after subtraction of a factor, x, of repeats. This has been termed the multi-sequence model.

$$SR = m \sum_i \max(l_i - x, 0)$$

BOX 1.4   WHY ARE BACKWARD AND FORWARD STUTTER SO NAMED?

We recently had a discussion with a referee about what directions are forward or backward when describing stutter: 'Numenclature [sic]: *Stutter* often is used to refer to $(n - 1)$ stutters (i.e. stutters that appears [sic] in *front* of the parental peak). Stutters in $n + 1$ appears [sic] *after* the parental peak and is therefore naturally referred to as *backstutters*'.

This gave us cause to evaluate the nomenclature. The forward stutter product $(N + 4)$ is larger than the allele and comes out after it during electrophoresis. Hence it is forward in time and also 'to the right' on a standard epg, which could easily be called 'reading forward'. The referee obviously thinks of forward as 'before' or 'to the left'. If we think about slipped strand mispairing, looping out of the nascent strand makes a longer product, the template strand a shorter one.

But why would either of these be termed *backward* or *forward*? We follow common usage and see no value and much confusion in renaming.

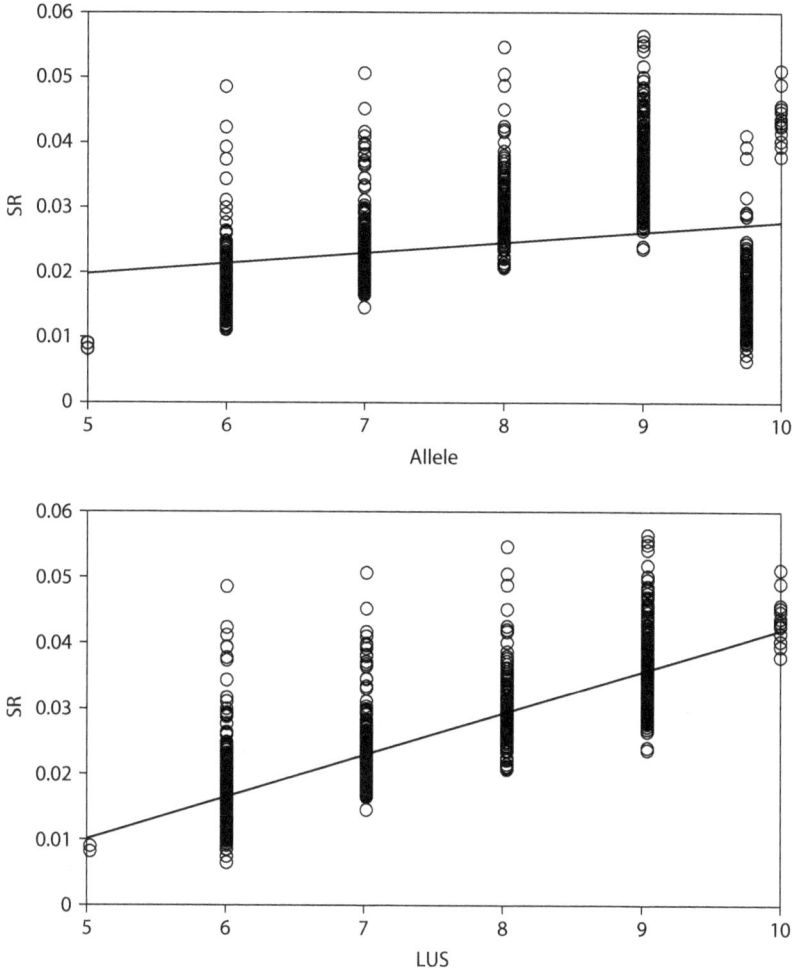

Figure 1.12   A plot of SR versus allele and LUS for the THO1 allele.

where m and x are constants and l_i is the length of sequence i. Figure 1.13 shows a plot of the observed SR – the predicted SR using the LUS and the multi-sequence model for the SE33 locus.

The term x in the multi-sequence model was interpreted as the number of repeats before stuttering begins and was termed the lag. In the above dataset $x = 5.83$ for SE33. This means that the short sequences contribute nothing to stuttering. Our experience with SE33 is limited but we have found acceptable but poorer fits than that described above in other SE33 datasets.

There is no difference between allele, LUS and a multi-sequence approach for the simple repeat loci.

For a locus such as THO1 there is one common allele, the 9.3, which has an interrupt. The sequence contains a stretch of 6 and one of 3. The multi-sequence model returns $x = 3.32$, which means that the three repeat sequences contribute nothing to the modelled SR. Hence, for THO1, there is no difference between the LUS and the multi-sequence models although both are superior to using allele. This is also true for FGA where no secondary sequence exceeds the value for x of 4.80. For vWA and D21S11 some secondary and tertiary sequences are of a moderate length. For these two loci the multi-sequence model showed a reduction in the average error in estimation of 17% and 5%, respectively, compared with the LUS model. This is consistent with

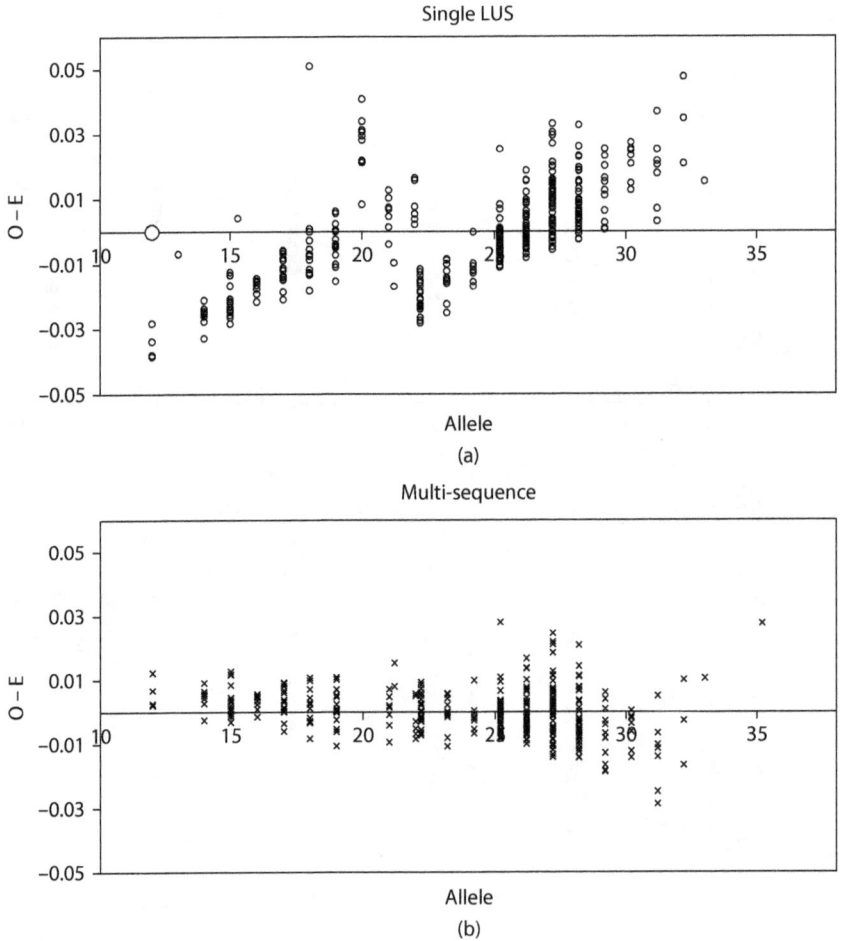

Figure 1.13 Observed stutter ratio (SR) – the predicted SR (O – E) versus allele for the SE33 locus using the LUS model (a) and multi-sequence model (b).

the small effect of secondary and tertiary sequences above the lags of $x = 3.46$ and 4.66. However again the first dataset we examined appeared to be the best one for this model. In other datasets we have found it necessary to modify the multi-sequence model to

$$SR = m \sum_i \max(l_i - x, 0) + c$$

where c is a constant.

Using this amendment the multi-sequence model can therefore completely replace the LUS model for all loci studied to date.

Theoretical modelling suggests that SR should be proportional to cycle number (compare Figures 1.11 and 1.12).

Variance about the predicted SR appears to be well explained by the parent allele height. Weusten and Herbergs[135] (hereafter the WH model) examined this theoretically and suggest that variation should be inversely proportional to the square root of the expected number of DNA strands entering the amplification. This suggests that the 95% confidence interval on SR should have the shape $k/\sqrt{\text{allele height}}$. We plot this curve with an assumed value for k in Figures 1.14 and 1.15.

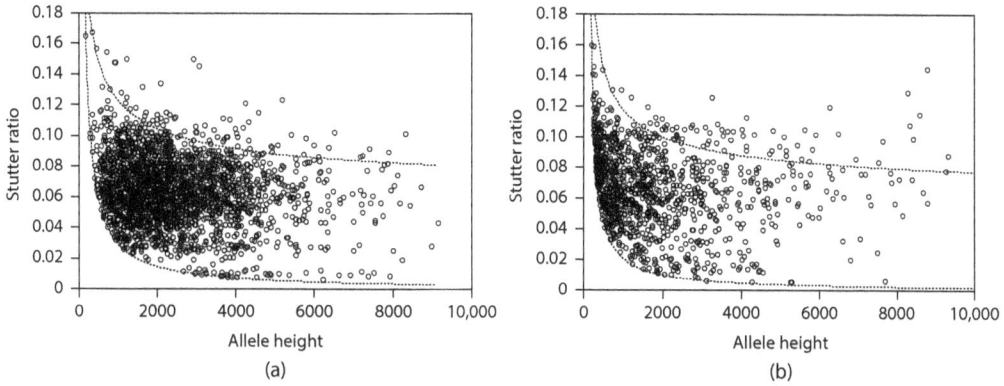

Figure 1.14 (a) Stutter ratio versus allele height for Identifiler data at 28 cycles of PCR on a 3130 capillary electrophoresis machine. (b) PowerPlex 21 data at 30 cycles of PCR on a 3130 capillary electrophoresis machine. The lower dotted line marks a void in the data caused by the analysis threshold. The upper dotted line is of the shape predicted by Weusten and Herbergs[135] for the upper 95% confidence interval on stutter ratio but we have simply guessed the proportionality constants.

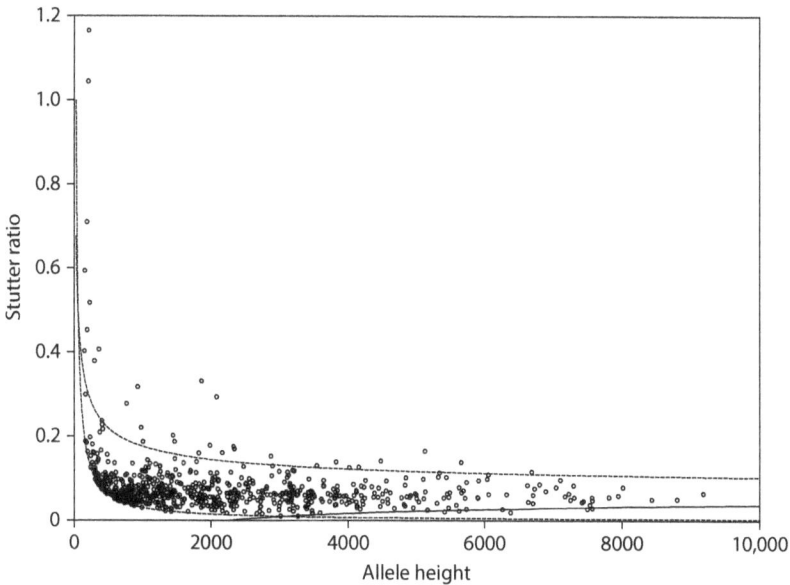

Figure 1.15 Stutter ratio versus allele height for SGMPlus data at 34 cycles of PCR on a 3130 capillary electrophoresis machine. The lower dotted line marks a void in the data caused by the analysis threshold. The upper dotted line is of the shape predicted by Weusten and Herbergs[135] for the upper 95% confidence interval on stutter ratio but we have simply guessed the proportionality constant.

The broad agreement of the shape, as opposed to the exact position, suggests that the empirical data does fit the WH model at least in this regard and approximately for the upper bound. The lower bound is a less good fit. To be fair to the WH model there is a large unmodelled systematic effect of SR. That is the effect of LUS. Alleles with high LUS stutter more. With this unaccounted for we expect a broadening on SR values irrespective of parent allele height.

Forward Stutter

Forward SR (FS) may be quantified using a ratio analogous to back stutter,

$$FS = \frac{O_{a+1}}{O_a}$$

where O_{a+1} refers to the observed height of the forward stutter peak and O_a the parent allele.

Forward stutter is a relatively rare event. In 2009 Gibb et al. reported an incidence rate of 4.51% (347 observations from 500 single source profiles) with a maximum recommended threshold for FS of 4.5% (for the D8S1179 locus) for AmpF*l*STR® SGM Plus™ data.[136]

More recently forward stutter observations within the AmpF*l*STR NGM™ kit[132] were reported. A threshold of 2.5% for most loci and 7.27% for the trinucleotide repeat D22S1045 was suggested. D22S1045 is a relatively new locus appearing in commercial kits. It is included in the extended European Standard Set of loci[46,137] and appears within the recently released commercial 24-locus multiplexes from Applied Biosystems (GlobalFiler) and Promega (PowerPlex Fusion). Higher rates of stutter[138] (including forward stutter) are expected for trinucleotide loci such as D22S1045 and in the presence of higher concentrations of magnesium, such as within the AmpF*l*STR Identifiler Plus™ multiplex compared with its predecessor Identifiler.

All of these reports of forward stutter observations in forensic profiles describe thresholds to manage their impact on profile interpretation. As with back stutter, the use of thresholds is an inefficient use of the profile data. A probabilistic treatment of forward stutter peaks is the best solution but at writing is not implemented in any software. An investigation into the explanatory variables for forward stutter is required to inform models.

Using standard casework and validation samples explanatory variables previously used to predict back stutter height such as parent allele height (O_a), locus and the LUS were found to be unsuitable for predicting the height of forward stutter peaks for all tetra- and pentanucleotide repeats.[139] This result was surprising given the known mechanism of stutter generation and the anecdotal observations of forward stutter being observed less rarely for parent peaks that had high peak heights.

It was hypothesized that forward stutter peak height does depend on parent peak height, however[139] only the highest few percent of all forward stutter peaks were seen and this caused dependencies to be masked. This was investigated by examining highly overloaded GlobaFiler™ samples which were read to the level of 10 rfu. This leads to observed forward stutter peaks in more than 50% of instances. In order to determine FS the height of the parent peak had to be estimated since it cannot be directly measured in overloaded samples. This was done using the observed height of the back stutter (O_{a-1}) and the SR for that allele and locus $\left(SR_a^l\right)$ to calculate the expected parent peak height (E_a) (see Equation 1.2). The expected parent peak height was used because the observed parent peak heights had reached saturation.

$$FS = \frac{O_{a+1}}{E_a} = \frac{SR_a^l \times O_{a+1}}{O_{a-1}} \tag{1.2}$$

Using this approach an effect of locus was discovered, although no effect of LUS or allele was found. This work also suggested that FS may fit a gamma distribution. However we need to recognize that we have introduced one extra level of uncertainly in the estimation process.

Given the lack of probabilistic systems to handle forward stutter, the modelling described above is excessive for laboratories at the time of writing. All that is required to handle these peaks is to set some sensible threshold above which a peak will be considered allelic. Below this value a lab has three options:

1. Treat the peak as ambiguous, either forward stutter or allelic

2. Leave the peak in and use a drop-in function to model the peak

3. Remove the peak

We are perfectly comfortable with removal of the peak. Any suggestion of bias should be ameliorated by the use of a preset threshold. We recognize this as an interim suggestion pending the implementation of effective forward stutter models.

Drop-In Alleles

The word *contamination* is a bit of a catch-all. Clearly DNA that got into the sample in the laboratory would be described, correctly, as *contamination*. However DNA could also be added by persons at the scene, such as attending officers, ambulance personnel or forensic scene investigators. This DNA could be their own, in which case it is a lesser evil. In principle, but rarely, the profiles of every investigator or medical attendant could be checked. Many jurisdictions have established databases of lab and scene staff to facilitate the identification of contamination. What must be guarded against is any possibility of transfer of DNA between crime scenes, or between items associated with the suspect and the crime scene. It is also possible that DNA may have been present on items before the crime occurred. This DNA is not strictly contamination but could more properly be called 'background'. We concentrate in this section on laboratory-based contamination but accept that this is only a part of the total.[140,141] In the Jama case in Victoria, Australia, it would appear that contamination of the complainant's intimate samples occurred at the medical examination office from sperm on the hair of a female complainant in a previous case.[142] James Fraser, while working on the Review of DNA Reporting Practices by Victoria Police Forensic Services Division (J. Fraser, J. Buckleton, and P. Gill),* emphasized that labs need to take ownership of standards pre-lab. This is a challenging but true statement. We are the ones with the motivation and knowledge to advise on procedures. Labs should establish outreach programmes designed to manage item handling pre-submission. Keeping to our own business and managing within-lab contamination is insufficient.

We recognize that this would be a significant extension of a laboratory's mandate. However if we consider, say, the European Network of Forensic Science Institutes[143] reporting guidelines, such an extension has clearly been envisaged:

> If there are concerns about contamination pre-submission: 'further enquiries will be made and if necessary discussions will take place with the mandating authority or party to agree a way forward. This may result in the items not being examined or, if they are, any limitation that affects the results and conclusions shall be stated in the report'.

Spurious alleles are observed in profiles even when DNA extractions have been carried out in facilities designed to minimize the chance of laboratory contamination at enhanced sensitivity. Most labs operating at 28 cycles report very little or no drop-in. Average drop-in rates of the order of 1%–4% per locus have been reported at 34 cycles on 3130 capillary electrophoresis instruments.[104,144,145] Contaminants were more often associated with the low molecular weight loci.[103,104]

Negative controls are designed to detect contamination within the reagents (such as distilled water) that are used for DNA extraction and PCR. Historically we have assumed that if contamination of a reagent occurs, then the same spurious alleles should be observed in every sample processed. However within the context of highly sensitive techniques it appears that the negative control does not act as an indicator of minor contamination within associated samples of the same batch. This is because some methods are sensitive enough to detect a single contaminant molecule of DNA. Single events such as this only affect one tube. Contaminants may be tube-specific and transfer could occur via minute dust particles, plasticware or other unknown processes. Hence the negative control cannot operate in the traditional sense. This has led to the drop-in concept that envisages single alleles from degraded or fragmented DNA that can randomly affect tubes, whether they contain casework samples or are negative controls.

---

* Issues in Gathering, Interpreting and Delivering DNA Evidence Judge Andrew Haesler. Available at: https://njca.com.au/wp-content/uploads/2013/07/Judge-Andrew-Haesler-SC-Issues-in-Gathering-Interpreting-and-Delivering-DNA-Evidence-paper.pdf

The consequence of this is that casework samples could be affected by laboratory-based contaminants that do not appear in the negative control and vice versa.

Nevertheless, the negative controls serve an important function as a 'health check' of the process. They indicate the rate of appearance of spurious alleles. This rate needs to be kept to a minimum. In the context of highly sensitive techniques replication of extraction negative controls is recommended in order to determine if laboratory-based contaminants are reproducibly amplified. If not, we suggest that there is no *a priori* reason to suppose that any alleles observed in the negatives have affected the associated extracted samples.

When working at markedly increased sensitivity it is necessary to accept that it is impossible to avoid laboratory-based contamination completely. This issue is ameliorated by replication. In high sensitivity casework it is typically not possible to carry out more than three separate tests of a DNA extract because of the limited size of the initial sample. If the sample were more generous, then a high sensitivity approach would not be needed. However if the contaminant events are truly random single events, then the chance of a contaminant appearing in each of two replicates is small. The risk that spurious alleles could be duplicated and reported in the consensus results has been estimated by pairwise comparisons of samples.[103] In this study four double-contaminant events out of 1225 comparisons were observed. Similarly it is useful to compare profiles against operator controls to guard against the possibility of gross contamination of a sample from an operator.

Tables 1.5 and 1.6 give examples of negative control data. We see that many negative controls do have an allele or alleles present. In order to determine the impact of contaminants on the evidential value, it is important that we understand the mechanism by which these alleles appear in the sample.

We have hypothesized that alleles appear singly using the drop-in model and that these 'fall' into samples independently of each other. We term this the 'alleles snowing from the ceiling' model. If this model is correct then the number of alleles in the negative controls should follow a Poisson distribution. Tables 1.5[146] and 1.6 illustrate the fit of a Poisson distribution with parameters equal to the sample mean. Subjectively the fit is poor for Table 1.5. We focus on the rows from five alleles onwards. There is a small (in absolute terms) excess of the observed probability over the expectation. This excess suggests that two processes are present. It seems necessary to treat the occurrence of multi-allele profiles as a separate

Table 1.5 A Comparison of the Observed Number of Contaminant Alleles in a Sample from the United Kingdom with the Predictions from a Poisson Model		
Number of Contaminant Alleles	Observed Probability of This Number of Contaminant Alleles	Expected Probability of This Number of Contaminant Alleles
0	0.44	0.23
1	0.24	0.34
2	0.15	0.25
3	0.07	0.12
4	0.04	0.05
5	0.02	0.01
6	0.01	0.0033
7	0.0087	0.0007
8	0.0065	0.00013
9+	0.0185	0.000025

Source: Buckleton, J.S. and Gill, P.D., personal communication.

Table 1.6   A Comparison of the Observed Number of Sporadic Contaminant Alleles in a Sample from New Zealand with the Predictions from a Poisson Model for the Period 2006–2013

Number of Contaminant Alleles	Observed Probability of This Number of Contaminant Alleles	Expected Probability of This Number of Contaminant Alleles
0	0.835	0.825
1	0.142	0.159
2	0.020	0.015
3	0.003	0.001
4	ESR defines four or more alleles as *gross contamination* and hence entries in these categories were impossible.	
5		

Source: J.S. Buckleton, personal communication, 2013.
Note: N = 4013 negative controls. ESR, Institute of Environmental Science and Research, New Zealand.

phenomenon to the drop-in model. We therefore propose to treat contamination as two different phenomena: first as drop-in and second as more complete partial profiles, i.e. multiple bands from a single source (termed *gross contamination*).

New Zealand has kept records of the sporadic drop-in events in their extraction and amplification negatives separately from the larger scale contamination since they began 34 cycle work in 2006.

Taken over the entire period of their operation it is possible to get the frequency of drop-in alleles and to compare it to that expected if drop-in events were independent (the Poisson model). This is given in Table 1.6 and suggests a good fit to the Poisson model also noted by others.[144] These data differ from those in Table 1.5 in that gross contamination events have been removed.

Interpretation models based around replication of alleles have been developed for these situations. They are termed *consensus models*. They appear to be remarkably robust to drop-in with the proviso that a few situations be taken into consideration. There is probably no statistical approach that can effectively militate against gross contamination. This therefore places a strong emphasis on reducing this type of contamination. Such contamination would be seen as an excess over Poisson expectations at a high number of alleles per profile. We do not imply by this that contamination by single alleles should be ignored but rather that it is a 'lesser evil'.

Models that have been suggested to deal with this situation include the following:

- Selecting one of two or more replicates (the selection model)
- The composite model
- The consensus model
- The semi-continuous model
- The continuous model

There are few published studies of the heights of drop-in alleles. Recently a published model for drop-in peak heights[147] suggested that the height of a drop-in peak should follow a gamma distribution. The gamma distribution can have a very wide range of shapes depending on the parameters and hence can be used to explain many observed distributions.

The experimental design used to inform the drop-in model should be matched to the use made of the drop-in function. This should consider any AT used and whether forward and double back stutter peaks will be removed manually. If forward and double back stutter peaks are to be dealt with using the drop-in function, then the data should be developed from positive samples with ground truth known. Allele and stutter peaks from the true contributor are ignored but others are included. What is required is data from a large number of samples, say 100. Positive samples, as described, if they will be used to cover forward and double backward stutter and either negative or positive samples if the drop-in function is not used to cover these peaks. These should be analyzed to very low heights, say 10 rfu, regardless of what value is used for the AT. The height of each peak should be recorded, as well as the number of peaks per control. In order for the peaks to be considered drop-in they should not be reproducible on subsequent PCR of the same DNA extract. If positive samples are used, a correction is made to the counts. Peaks in forward and double backward stutter positions are counted as 1. Peaks in other positions are counted as $1/S$, where S is the sum of the probabilities of all the allele and stutter positions occupied at this locus.

For the semi-continuous models it is the rate of drop-in that is required. However the continuous models require both the rate and the height. The same experimental design can be used for either SEP, but for the continuous models the data need to retain height information.

We demonstrated the gamma modelling using the MiniFiler amplification kit (Life Technologies, Carlsbad, California) performed at 30 PCR cycles to illustrate the approach. Negative control samples ($N = 467$) for the MiniFiler multiplex were read to 10 rfu using GeneMapper ID-X. Table 1.7 shows the observed counts of peaks per negative control.

The controls with high peak counts (to the right side of Table 1.7) would be considered contamination. Those to the left side would be described as *drop-in*. An arbitrary cut-off between these two mechanisms, ε, is often set.

For the data in Table 1.7, ε could be set at 2 or 3. That is, 1 and 2 or 1, 2 and 3 are designated as drop-in and above that the peaks are defined as contamination. This distinction is arbitrary but does have some scientific basis. We note that there is no 'conservative' side to Pr(C) for all cases. It will vary for different cases. Hence it is not safe to err deliberately upwards or downwards.

Figure 1.16 shows the observed number of peaks per profile (as a relative occurrence). This is overlaid with a Poisson distribution. The Poisson distribution is the expected distribution if the peaks appear independently as separate drop-in events. For the demonstration data, set the observed and Poisson lines separately at about $\varepsilon = 3$. This would suggest that we could define those samples with four or more peaks as contamination. Removing these lowers N to 458 and gives $x = 173$ drop-in events.

If it is assumed that each drop-in observation is an independent event, i.e. the probability of two drop-in events occurring is the product of each one occurring individually, then we need only a single drop-in probability, Pr(C). This probability can be calculated using data collated from the monitoring of negative control samples tested within the laboratory by

$$\Pr(C) = \frac{x}{N \times L}$$

where x is the number of observed drop-ins above the level to be used for the AT (amended by S if positive samples are used), N is the number of profiles examined and L is the number of loci. For the data in Table 1.3 and using AT = 10 rfu, and recalling that MiniFiler has eight loci, this is

$$\Pr(C) = \frac{173}{458 \times 8} = 0.046$$

Table 1.7	Count of Negative Controls with 0–10 Observed Alleles										
Number of peaks per control	0	1	2	3	4	5	6	7	8	9	10
Count of controls with this number of peaks	325	101	24	8	2	3	2	0	1	1	0

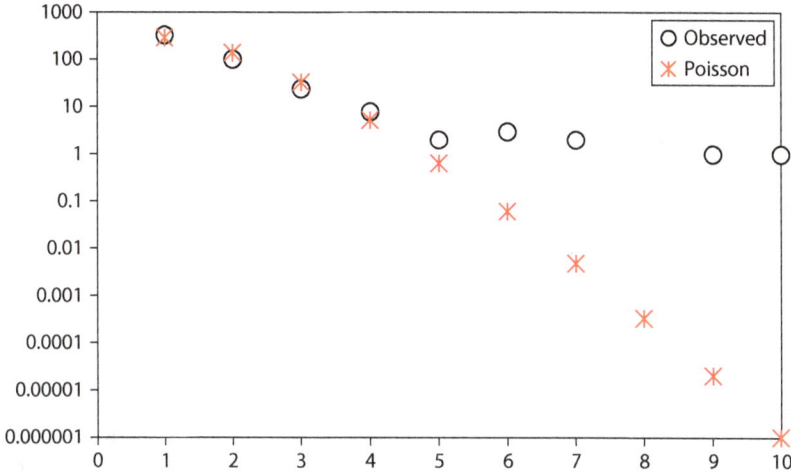

Figure 1.16 A plot of the observed and expected number of peaks per profile (as relative occurrence), the Poisson distribution fitted to this data and the contamination rate.

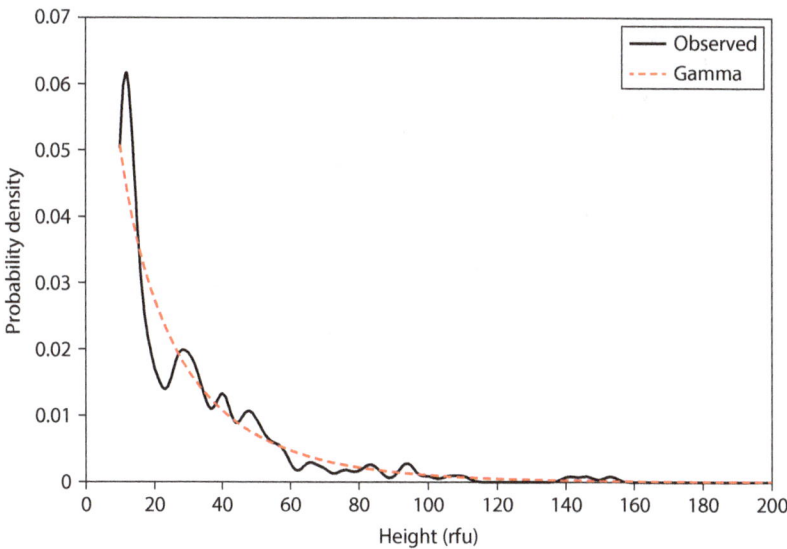

Figure 1.17 Gamma distribution fitted to the observed MiniFiler™ (30 cycles, AT = 10 rfu) drop-in data.

For the semi-continuous SEPs we suggest the following:

1. The counts per negative control should be recorded.

2. This should be plotted against a Poisson distribution and ε set.

3. x is then recalculated at the chosen AT and Pr(C) should be calculated.

For the continuous models it is necessary to consider the height of the drop-in peaks as well. Figure 1.17 gives the observed distribution of drop-in peak heights overlaid with a gamma distribution fitted by MLE and scaled for the probability 'missing' below 10 rfu.

Gill et al.[103] assumed that contaminant alleles appearing singly would occur in the frequency with which they appear in the population. Their origin is unknown but they may come from laboratory personnel or consumables, for example. It does not seem unreasonable that these alleles would appear in numbers close to their population frequency if they were sampled from a large number of people reasonably independently. However this assumption would benefit from experimental investigation.

A conclusion from this reasoning is that if an allele is found in a crime sample that does not match the suspect, it does not necessarily lead to an exclusion. The same confidence cannot be placed in the presence or absence of each allele in enhanced sensitivity work as in conventional work.

Additivity or Stacking

Additivity or *stacking* refers to the assumption that the contribution from different sources, either different donors or from stutter and allele, add.[148] This assumption is made almost unconsciously in most quantitative interpretations. Considering the PCR process, the primers and enzymes should not care what the original source of the template was as long as it has the correct sequence to bind. We would therefore have a strong expectation that the assumption should hold at least across the range where the peak is linearly related to the template. We have empirically investigated this assumption and found it to hold. It could be added that casework experience also supports this assumption.

Non-Specific Artefacts

Non-specific artefacts are generated as a result of the priming of DNA fragments during the PCR process, possibly from degraded human or bacterial DNA. The band shift test described by Gill et al.[70] is particularly useful to identify peaks as non-specific since they usually migrate atypically in the gel or polymer. This may be either because they have different sequences to STR alleles or because they are a partial renaturation of PCR products.

Other non-specific artefacts include the following:

- Spikes: where a small sharp peak is seen in the same position on all dye lanes. This is caused by crystallized salts passing across the detection area of an electrophoresis instrument, absorbing some light in all spectrums.

- Allele shadowing: where the denaturing of the double-stranded DNA is incomplete prior to loading on the electrophoresis instrument, the peaks of the DNA profile can be duplicated and shifted upstream, giving the appearance of a smaller second contributor 'shadow'.

- Dye blobs: where the fluorescent dye has separated from the primer. Dye blobs are typically broad and low and migrate at characteristically consistent rates.

Pull-Up

One problem commonly observed in STR profiles is pull-up. Pull-up is related to the spectral overlap of the different dye colours, which can cause the signal from one dye colour to produce artificial peaks in another. This typically occurs when a DNA profile is overloaded and a minor peak in one colour corresponds to a major allelic peak in another colour. Typically a blue peak may 'pull up' a green peak directly below it. This is only problematic if the minor peak coincides with the position of a potential allele. If such a possibility exists, options to consider include amplification of the locus under consideration by itself (singleplexing), re-PCR of the sample or reapplication of the matrix or spectral calibration.

Capillary Carryover

When using vertical acrylamide gels such as that used in the ABI Prism® 377 Gene Sequencer, leakage of a sample from one lane to another, commonly referred to as *lane-to-lane leakage*, was a problem. Modern electrophoresis instruments have replaced gel slabs with individual capillaries, eliminating lane leakage. However capillaries must be 'flushed' after each injection to reduce the risk of injection carryover. *Carryover* is where remnants of one injection are eluted along with the next sample run in the same capillary. This can present as a low-level additional profile.[149]

Suppression of Amplification Efficiency, Silent or Null Alleles

Peak-height asymmetry outside the normal range or the creation of a silent or null allele may occur because of a primer binding site mutation. This has the effect of altering annealing and melting temperatures, which changes the amplification efficiency and decreases the resulting signal. If a substitution mutation occurs at the 3′ end of the primer, a mismatch will result and amplification will fail completely, resulting in a silent allele. The closer the substitution is to the 5′ end of the primer, the lesser the effect will be on the amplification efficiency.[150–153] Butler and Reeder[66] and Whittle et al.[96] reported some silent allele frequencies.

Chang et al.[154] reported high occurrences of silent alleles at the amelogenin locus in some populations that interfered with the efficiency of the test. They found a rate of 3.6% in an Indian population and 0.9% in a Malay population. Clayton et al.[155] identified a set of silent alleles at the D18S51 locus associated with individuals of Middle Eastern descent. They confirmed the nature of these alleles using alternative primers. At this locus they found that the presumed primer binding site mutation was associated in 12 of 15 instances with an *18* allele. The remaining instances were one each of a *17, 19* and *20* allele. This supports the suggestion that the ancestral primer binding site mutation was associated with an *18* allele and that the *17, 19* and *20* alleles have subsequently arisen by mutation from this *18* allele. Other valuable reports continue to appear.[95,96,156–159]

Summary

The biological basis of contemporary forensic DNA profiling is linked to the processes of cell and human reproduction. From the many variations that subsequently exist on the human genome, STRs have emerged as the most suitable marker for current forensic identification. Standardizing on this polymorphism has led to further harmonization with regard to the specific loci that are targeted and analyzed in the international forensic community. As with any complex molecular technique however, the interpretation of data requires ongoing assessment and consideration.

2

A Framework for Interpreting Evidence

Tacha Hicks, John S. Buckleton, Jo-Anne Bright and Duncan Taylor[*]

Contents

[*] We acknowledge many valuable discussions over many years with Drs Chris Triggs, Christophe Champod, Ian Evett, Franco Taroni and Alex Biedermann who have contributed to the material presented in this chapter.

Introduction

This book is intended as a discussion of the interpretation of DNA evidence. However there is nothing inherently different about DNA evidence that sets it qualitatively aside from all other forensic disciplines or even all evidence.[160,161] We feel that it is important that DNA evidence be considered as one form of evidence, not as something completely separate. This opinion is not universally held. There is a view that the strength of the probabilistic models used in DNA sets it apart.[162] We cannot support this viewpoint and believe it originates from a false understanding of objectivity and subjectivity* in probabilistic reasoning.

We come to the issue of setting evidence into a framework that is appropriate for court. This topic has been the subject of entire books by more informed authors,[163] but it is by no means settled. The issue revolves around a basic contrast: the tools best fitted to interpret evidence coherently are also those that appear to be most problematic to explain to a jury or layperson. However the methods that can be easily explained have significant deficiencies. This is noticed most in the lack of power of such methods as Cumulative Probability of Inclusion (CPI) to express the true value of the evidence. We then face a dilemma: Do we assess results coherently, with the risk that they might be misunderstood? Or do we use an approach that is easily understood but less solidly founded?

Are there other solutions? One avenue could be to use different approaches to assess the results and to present them at court. Another could involve stronger collaboration between the judiciary and forensic scientists, as has been done in some countries such as Sweden, on how to assess and present results. Exploring this avenue would allow scientists to use a framework they believe adequate and to learn how to present it in an understandable way.

The interpretation of DNA results has been a key area for debate in the DNA field ever since the inception of this form of evidence.†

> The statistical interpretation of DNA typing results, specifically in the context of population genetics, has been the least understood and … the most hotly debated issue of many admissibility hearings.[3,4]

This statement is not only true but also very interesting. DNA evidence is actually much simpler and more extensively studied than most other forensic disciplines. Many evidence types, such as tool marks and handwriting comparison, are so complex that at present they defy presentation in a numerical form. On that aspect we have to underline that the essence of evaluation is not to give a precise number. Evaluation implies a use of expertise and reasoning, not just a calculus. What matters is to work within a framework that allows one to assess results logically, transparently and in a balanced way, and this can be done in all forensic disciplines. The development of good data allows the sharing of expertise, and where good data exist numerical assessment can be attempted. This is the case for glass and fibre evidence in New Zealand, Switzerland and the United Kingdom. The issues in both these fields are far more complex than in the DNA field. It is the very simplicity of DNA evidence that allows it to be presented numerically at all. And yet there is still much debate about how to present this evidence.

It could be argued that the presentation of scientific findings should bend to conform to the courts' requirements. Indeed a court can almost compel this. There have been several rulings‡ on this subject by courts that have been used to argue for or against particular approaches to the presentation of evidence. Instances of this include the Doheny and Adams[172] and the *R v T* rulings.[162]

---

* Some people think that probabilities derived from DNA results are not subjective, but they are. By *subjective*, we do not mean to say that probabilities are arbitrary or biased, but that they are based on personal knowledge (models, assumptions, data). One can also speak of *knowledge-based probabilities*. It is the same in other forensic disciplines.
† Parts of this section follow Triggs and Buckleton,[164] reproduced with the kind permission of Oxford University Press.
‡ For reviews of some court cases in Australia, New Zealand, the United Kingdom and the United States, see Refs. 161, 165–171.

These rulings have been, we believe erroneously, read as arguing against a Bayesian approach and for a frequentist approach (discussed later).* However a fairer and more impartial appraisal of the various methods offered for interpretation should proceed from a starting point of discussing the underlying logic of interpretation. Only as a second stage should it be considered how this logic may be presented in court or whether the court or jury have the tools to deal with this type of evidence. There is little advantage to the situation 'wrong but understood',[168,173] nor to the situation 'right but misunderstood'.

> To be effective in the courtroom, a statistician† must be able to think like a lawyer and present complex statistical concepts in terms a judge can understand. Thus, we present the principles of statistics and probability, not as a series of symbols, but in the words of jurists.[174]

In this chapter we propose to consider the underlying claims of three alternative approaches to the presentation of evidence. These will be termed the *frequentist approach*, the *likelihood ratio (LR) approach*, and the *full Bayesian approach*.[175] The first of these terms has been in common usage and may be familiar.[176] We have adopted a slightly different phrasing to that in common usage for the second and third approaches, which will require some explanation. This will be attempted in the following sections. The intention is to present the merits and shortcomings of each method in an impartial way, which hopefully will lead the reader to a position where it is possible to make an informed choice. However our hearts are firmly in the camp of the *LR* approach and it is likely our preference will show, so we are better disclosing it. At least two of the authors were not born Bayesian. They were convinced by the power of the logic, and we hope that a clear presentation may also convince the reader.

Juries may misunderstand any of the methods described, and care should be taken over the exact wording. In fact it is clear that care must be taken with all probabilistic work and presentation.[177-192] We would like to avoid situations such as the one where a famous statistician's evidence was described as 'like hearing evidence in Swahili, without the advantage of an interpreter'.[193]

Comparisons of the potential impact on juries of the different methods have been published.[194-197] It is necessary to countenance a situation in the future where the desirable methods for evaluation of, say, a mixture by simulation, are so complex that they cannot realistically be explained completely in court.

It is important that the following discussion be read without fear of the more mathematical approaches, as this fear wrongly pressures some commentators to advocate simpler approaches. It is probably fair for a jury to prefer a method for the reason of mathematical simplicity, but it would be a mistake for a scientist to do so. Would you like your aircraft designer to use the best engineering models available or one that you can understand without effort?

Uncertainty and Probability

At trial, and in life in general, we are surrounded with uncertainty. The language we use clearly reflects this, and expressions such as 'beyond reasonable doubt', 'probably' and 'likely' are only a few examples of some of the terms associated with uncertainty that can be heard in the courtroom. To reason in the face of uncertainty, we can rely on a framework or intuition. The latter has been shown to be quite deceptive. Probability, being a standard for uncertainty, is the obvious choice.[143]

---

* Robertson and Vignaux[161] give a more eloquently worded argument in support of this belief.
† Or a forensic scientist, in our case.

Examples of events of interest that are uncertain may be in the past, present or future. These events may be true or false and our uncertainty about the truth of these events (also called *propositions, hypotheses* or *allegations*) is influenced by our knowledge, the information that we are given and how effectively we use that knowledge.

It may intrigue the reader that it is possible to talk about the probability of a past or current event. Surely if an event is in the past, then it has 'happened' and therefore is either true of false. However if it is unknown to the assessor, then it is perfectly valid to speak of a probability. Here is an easy example: What is the probability the dinosaurs went extinct because of a meteor impact? Perhaps more subtly, at night one could ask, what is the probability it is raining? Plausibly the answer could be informed by the sound or absence of sound on a tin roof.

A distinction is often drawn between statistical and non-statistical probabilities. Statistical probabilities are those where exact repetition is possible. An overused example is throwing a die. The circumstances of each repetition must be exactly the same, and this condition can never quite be achieved. At least the time of the experiment must differ. However sometimes all meaningful variables may be the same. Non-statistical probabilities relate to those events where repetition is not possible.

> What is the probability that John F Kennedy was killed by a lone gunman compared with the probability that it was a conspiracy?

Some people would argue that probability has no place where at least the concept of repetition is absent. We will not subscribe to that approach. For nearly all forensic questions exact repetition, and often repetition at all, is impossible. The following could be examples of questions where it is not possible to repeat the event:

1. What is the probability of a second copy of this profile?
2. What is the probability that the deceased got DNA under her fingernails because the taxi driver drove her in his car?

To restrict ourselves strictly to statistical probabilities would rob us, and forensic science in general, of the use of the logical framework enabled by probability.

It is vital to recognize that all probabilities are *conditional*.[*] If we want to assign, for example, the probability that it is raining given that there is no sound of rain, then this will depend on our knowledge (we would expect to hear rain), the information that we are given (we are under a tin roof) and our assumptions.

Because this point is of great importance, we quote below a section of a key paper:[198]

> To assign a probability for the truth of a proposition, one needs information. Even if one considers something as simple as the toss of a coin, to assign a probability to the outcome one needs to know something about the physical nature of the coin and how it is to be tossed. In general the tossing mechanism (such as at the start of a sporting event between two teams) is chosen so as to maximise the uncertainty. Given such information, most would be content with the statement that a probability of a head is 0.5. In another kind of uncertain situation one might, as the Court was clearly aware, study an appropriate collection of data to condition a probability. The Court was content with the notion that this is properly and reliably done in the case of calculating a DNA match probability.[†]

However there are still further situations where the notion of using a database appears unrealistic. Consider, for example, the question: 'What is the probability that Mary, Queen of Scots, knew of the plot to murder her husband?'

---

[*] We acknowledge the teachings of Ian Evett.

[†] Reprinted from Berger, C.E.H., et al., Evidence evaluation: A response to the court of appeal judgment in *R v T*. *Science & Justice*, 2011. 51(2): 43–49, Copyright 2011, with permission from Elsevier.

Clearly, to address such a question it would be preferable to address historical sources. These may be extremely extensive, complicated and of varying degrees of veracity. It is not surprising, then, that different people would give different answers to the question. For the 'best' answer one would wish to look for the historian who is considered the most knowledgeable on the life of Mary. Similarly one would not be surprised to find that different historians have different views on the matter. It is this kind of example that makes it clear to us that probability is *personal* (but not arbitrary).

Probabilities such as that in the coin tossing example are described as *aleatory*; they arise in situations where the uncertainty derives solely from the randomness of the conditions that pertain. On the other hand the historical example above is of an *epistemic* probability; the uncertainty derives solely from limitations of knowledge.

All relevant knowledge improves the assignment of probability. Consider a question such as, 'Is the mountain pass open?.' Knowledge such as the time of the year and historic records of snowfall would greatly improve the assignment of a probability for this question. More directly a phone call to a store on the other side asking if anyone has come by who has traversed the pass may be very useful.

Information of no relevance should have no effect on the probability.

We hold that the scientist's evaluation should be governed by a set of logical principles. We outline two of these below and begin numbering principles for interpretation as P1, P2, etc. These principles have been supported by a varied group of scientific and legal scholars.[143,198,199]

P1: The interpretation of scientific results invokes reasoning in the face of uncertainty. Probability theory provides the only coherent logical foundation for such reasoning.

P2: All probabilities are conditional. To assign a probability for the truth of a proposition, one needs information. Interpretation must therefore be carried out within a framework of circumstances. It is necessary for the scientist to make clear any understanding of those aspects of the circumstances that are relevant to the evaluation.

We are not suggesting that irrelevant and potentially biasing information such as past offences should be disclosed to the scientist. However we are suggesting that relevant information is necessary.

Consider for example the information that a pair of underwear belongs to Ms X, who has one consensual partner, and that she had consensual sex the day before an alleged rape. Surely forensic scientists should have this information. The more (relevant) information we have, the more knowledge we can bring.

We are very strongly in support of the management of domain irrelevant information[200] whereby the information passed to the scientist is vetted by a person who understands the science but will not participate directly in this case.

Use of Notation

It can be convenient to use some notation in order to summarize a large number of words in a short mathematical formula. Events are often described in terms of symbols. For example, event A might be that the next card drawn from a pack is an ace and H_p the event that the DNA came from the person of interest (POI).

The probability of event A occurring is described as $\Pr(A)$. As we have seen, probabilities are conditional, so the probability of A given the information that we have can be summarized as $\Pr(A|I)$. The vertical bar (or conditional bar) stands for the word *given* and indicates that the probability of A is conditioned on the information. This information represents everything that we know, or assume, that is relevant to the truth of A.

Conversely the probability that event A is false can be noted $\Pr(\overline{A})$, where $P(\overline{A}) = 1 - \Pr(A)$.

The Frequentist Approach

At the outset it is necessary to make clear that the use of the frequentist approach in forensic science is related, but not identical, to the frequentist approach in probability theory.[201,202] The frequentist approach in forensic science has never been formalized and hence is quite hard to discuss. It appears to have grown as a framework by a set of intuitive steps. There are also a number of potential misconceptions regarding this approach that require discussion and this will be attempted. To begin, the approach will be subdivided into two parts: the coincidence probability and the exclusion probability. A discussion of 'natural frequencies' will follow.[203]

Coincidence Probabilities

For this discussion it is necessary to attempt to formalize this approach sufficiently. Use will be made of the following definition:

> The coincidence approach proceeds to offer evidence against a proposition by showing that the forensic findings are unlikely if this proposition is true. Hence it supports the alternative proposition. The less likely the findings are under the proposition, the more support that is given to the alternative.

This is called the *coincidence probability approach* because either the evidence came from, say, the suspect or a coincidence has occurred.

There are many examples of evidence presented in this way:

- Only* 1% of glass would match the glass on the clothing by chance.

- It is very unlikely to get this paint sequence match by chance alone.

- Approximately one in a million unrelated males would match the DNA at the scene by chance.

We are led to believe that the 'match by chance' event is unlikely and hence the findings support the alternative. At this stage let us proceed by assuming that if the evidence is unlikely under a particular proposition, then it supports the alternative.

This reasoning is strongly akin to formal hypothesis testing procedures in statistical theory. Formal hypothesis testing would proceed by setting up a hypothesis usually called the null, H_0. The probability of the evidence (or data) is calculated if H_0 is true. If this probability is small (say less than 5% or 1%), then the null is rejected. The evidence is taken to support the alternative hypothesis, H_1.[204-206]

To set up a DNA case in this framework we proceed as follows. Formulate the hypothesis, H_0: the DNA came from a male not related to the POI. We then calculate the probability of the evidence if this is true. We write the evidence as E, and in this context it will be something like the following:

E: The DNA at the scene is type α; the suspect (or POI) is also of type α.

We calculate the probability, Pr, of the evidence, E, if the null hypothesis H_0 is true, $\Pr(E|H_0)$. As before, the vertical line, or conditioning sign, stands for the word *if* or *given*.

Assuming that about one in a million unrelated males would have type α, we would assign $\Pr(E|H_0)$ as 1 in a million. Since this is a very small probability, we would assume that this result suggests that H_0 is not true and hence is support for H_1. In this context we might define the alternative hypothesis as follows:

H_1: The DNA came from the POI, Mr Smith.

Hence in this case the findings support the hypothesis that the DNA came from Mr Smith. Later we are going to need to be a lot more careful about how we define propositions.

---

* We would question the purpose of the word *only* in this sentence. Forensic scientists should avoid adding emotive words to their statements. *Only* is not quite emotive, but it adds an effect that goes beyond the number. We can leave the innuendo and posturing to others. There are plenty of sources of both in court.

Hypothesis testing is a well-known and largely accepted statistical approach. The similarity between the coincidence approach and hypothesis testing is the former's greatest claim to prominence. We will see, however, that it is not adequate, as the probability of the scientific findings (e.g. DNA profiles) given H_1 cannot always be assigned as 1. Typical examples where the coincidence approach is misleading would be paternity casework, cases with mixtures, trace DNA or relatedness cases.

Exclusion Probabilities

The exclusion probability approach calculates and reports the exclusion or inclusion probability. This can be defined as the probability that a random person would be excluded as the donor of the DNA, or the father of the child, or a contributor to the mixture. The details of these calculations will be discussed later. Again the formal logic has not been defined, so it will be attempted here.

> The suspect is not excluded. There is a probability that a random* person would be excluded. From this it is inferred that it is unlikely that the suspect is a random person. Hence the scientific findings (or the evidence) support the alternative proposition that the suspect is the donor of the DNA. The higher the exclusion probability, the more support that is given to the alternative.

Examples are again common. For instance, the three phrases given previously can be reworked into this framework:

- 99% of windows would be excluded as a source of this glass.
- It is very likely that a random paint sequence would be excluded as matching this sample.
- Approximately 99.9999% of unrelated males would be excluded as the source of this DNA.

An advantage of the exclusion probability approach is that it can be easily extended beyond these examples to more difficult types of evidence such as paternity and mixtures:

- Approximately 99% of random men would be excluded as the father of this child.
- Approximately 99% of random men would be excluded as a donor to this mixture.

It was stated previously that the use of the frequentist approach in forensic science is related, but not identical, to the frequentist approach in probability theory. There are two common definitions of probability.[207] These are called the *frequentist* and the *subjectivist* definitions. It is not necessary to discuss these differences in any length here, as they have long been the cause of deep discussion in both philosophy and the theory of probability. Briefly the frequentist approach treats probability as the expectation over a large number of events. The subjectivist definition accepts that probability is a measure of belief and that this measure will be conditional both on the information available and on the knowledge and assumptions of the person making the assessment.[†,209]

Let us consider a drawing pin (thumbtack). 👍📌 When one is tossed, it may fall point up (U) or point down (D). When tossed ten times, we obtain the result DUUDDDUDDD. What is the probability that the eleventh toss will result in a D? The frequency of D in the 10 tosses is 7/10, and we may feel that 0.7 is a reasonable assignment for the probability that the eleventh toss will be a D. Our probability is assigned based on the frequency of the event D. Because of this, we can say that we used a frequentist's approach to probability.

---

* Again we will come back later to the question of who this random person is.
† We follow the excellent book by D.V. Lindley, *Understanding Uncertainty*.[208]

BOX 2.1   FREQUENCY OR RELATIVE FREQUENCY

We misuse the word *frequency* in forensic science. We are not suggesting a change; in fact we suggest that we knowingly continue in this misuse. It is a pedantic point but we will define these just for general knowledge and so that a mathematician cannot make fun of us in court.

Consider a sample of 100. There are 32 yellows and 68 blacks. The frequency of yellows is 32; the relative frequency is 0.32 or 32%.

Next consider that the object was not a drawing pin but a coin that looks like a perfectly normal coin. When tossed it may land heads up (H) or tails up (T). The ten tosses result in THHTTTHTTT. What is the probability that the 11th toss will result in a T? The frequency of T in the 10 tosses is 7/10, but we may feel that a reasonable assignment for the 11th toss being a T is not 0.7 but 0.5. Indeed, based on our knowledge of coins in general, based on the supposition that this coin is fair and based on the model we have in our mind regarding fair coins, we may believe that it is more logical to assign our probability as 0.5. This makes explicit that a probability and a (relative) frequency may be different (Box 2.1).

Both the coincidence approach and the exclusion probability approach can be based on either frequentist or subjectivist probabilities. Proponents of the Bayesian or subjectivist school of probability criticize the frequentist definition. However it is unfair to transfer this criticism of a frequentist probability to the frequentist approach to forensic evidence.

The coincidence and exclusion probability approaches do appear to be simple and have an intuitive logic to them that may appeal to a jury. Their use was argued for in the OJ Simpson trial,[210] apparently on the basis that they were conservative* and more easily understood while accepting the greater power of *LR*s. The main issue with exclusion probabilities for the evaluation of DNA results is that only part of the results are being assessed (e.g. the DNA profile of stain or of a child); the profile of the POI (e.g. suspect, alleged father) is not taken into account. Therefore this approach robs the evidence of much of its probative power. The more (relevant) information we use, the more useful our evaluation will be to help discriminate the propositions of interest.

Both inclusion and exclusion probability can be dangerous for the evaluation of evidence. The pitfalls are to think that because the probability of the DNA profile given that the suspect is not the source of the DNA, i.e. $\Pr(E|H_0)$, is small then the probability that the suspect is not the source of the DNA given the findings, i.e. $\Pr(H_0|E)$, is also small, and that therefore the probability of the suspect being the source of the DNA is large. The second pitfall is to believe that, because the probability of the DNA profile given that the suspect is not the source of the DNA, i.e. $\Pr(E|H_0)$, is small, the probability of the DNA profile given that the suspect is the source of the DNA, i.e. $\Pr(E|H_1)$, is large.

Natural Frequencies†

Gigerenzer advanced the argument that 'to be good it must be understood'. He argued persuasively for the use of 'natural frequencies'. To introduce this concept it is easiest to follow an example.[203]

The expert witness testifies that there are about 10 million men who could have been the perpetrator. Approximately 10 of these men have a DNA profile that is identical‡ with the trace recovered from the crime scene. If a man has this profile, it is practically certain that a DNA analysis shows

---

* Some advocate that we use a conservative approach, but should this be our aim? Should we not try to adopt a fair and logical approach? If we really want to be conservative, then should we not always take the 'unknown twin' as an alternative?

† Our thanks to Michael Strutt for directing us to this work.

‡ It is worth mentioning that no two objects can be truly identical, as an object can only be identical to itself.

a match. Among the men who do not have this DNA profile, current DNA technology leads to a reported match in only 100 cases out of 10 million.[*]

The correct understanding was achieved by 1% of students and 10% of professionals when using conditional probabilities. This rose to 40% and 70%, respectively, when 'natural frequencies' were used.

Of course natural frequencies are nothing more than an example of the defence attorney's fallacy[†,191] or the recommendation of the Appeal Court regarding Doheny and Adams.[172,211]

We concede the seductive appeal of this approach. Let us accept at face value that they are more easily understood. We do, however, feel that this approach hides a lot of serious issues.

First consider the assumption that N men could have been the perpetrator. Who is to make this decision? One would feel that the only people qualified and with the responsibility of doing this are the judge and jury. They have heard the non-DNA evidence and they can decide whether or not this defines a pool of suspects. This approach has a tendency towards assigning equal priors to each of these men and to the suspect. This is a tenable assumption in some but not all circumstances. Essentially we have a partition of the population of the world into those in the pool of suspects and those out of it. Those in the pool are assigned a prior probability of $1/N$ (this means that before the DNA analysis, the probability of a person being the perpetrator is set as $1/N$). Those out are assigned a prior of 0.

What are we to do when the product of the match probability and the pool of possible suspects is very small? Let us take the case given above but reduce the match probability from one in a million to one in ten million. This change would lead to the following:

The expert witness testifies that there are about 10 million men who could have been the perpetrator. We can expect on average that approximately one of these men would have a DNA profile that is similar to the trace recovered from the crime scene.

The witness will have to take great care that the jury understand this statement. There is a risk that they may assume that the suspect is this one man. It is necessary to explain that this man is one man additional to the suspect and even then it is an expectation. On average we would expect one other person to have this DNA profile, but there may also be zero, two, three or more.

Let us take this case and reduce the match probability even further to 1 in a billion. This would lead to the following:

The expert witness testifies that there are about 10 million men who could have been the perpetrator. Approximately 0.01 of these men have a DNA profile that is identical with the trace recovered from the crime scene.

This will take some care to explain to the jury. Now suppose that the suspect has one brother in the set of 10 million men.

The expert witness testifies that there are about 10 million unrelated men and one brother who could have been the perpetrator. Approximately 0.01 of the unrelated men and 0.005 of the brother have a DNA profile that is identical with the trace recovered from the crime scene.

Taking the example further:

The expert witness testifies that there are about 10 million unrelated men and one brother who could have been the perpetrator. Approximately 0.002 of the unrelated white men of European descent, 0.004 of the unrelated black men, 0.004 of the unrelated Hispanic men and 0.005 of the brother have a DNA profile that is identical with the trace recovered from the crime scene.

---

[*] Gigerenzer is referring here to his estimate of error rates.

[†] Although the prosecutor's fallacy is indeed a real fallacy, the defence attorney's fallacy is less obviously so. The defence attorney's fallacy is equivalent to assuming that the POI has the average prior from among a group of possible perpetrators. This assumption is not really bad, and we do not want to unfairly critique Gigerenzer here.

If we accept the suggestion that it is more understandable, then it may have a use in those very simple cases where there is a definable pool of suspects, relatedness is not important, the evidence is 'certain' under the prosecution hypothesis and the product of the match probability times N is not small.

Outside this very restricted class of case, we would classify natural frequencies in the 'understood but wrong'* category. We really do doubt the usefulness of this approach. It is very difficult to see how to accommodate relatives, interpret mixtures or low-template DNA results and report paternity cases within this framework. The approach also subtly introduces the concept of 10 million replicate cases, all with the same probability of error. This may be an acceptable fiction to lure the jury into a balanced view, but it would take a lot of thinking to reconcile it with our view of probability. Even if we accept the statement that natural frequencies are more easily understood and we decide to use this presentation method in court, it is important that forensic scientists think more clearly and exactly about what a probability is, what constitutes replication and how probabilities may be assigned.

The Importance of Propositions

The methods to follow require the development of two propositions. This was the subject of a large-scale project at the Forensic Science Service (UK) called the Case Assessment Initiative.[212–215] One proposition should align with the prosecution position and this is often known. The defence are under no obligation to offer any proposition at all, and it would be wrong to demand that they do. They are permitted not one, but all propositions consistent with exoneration. If a position is developed on behalf of the defence, this should clearly be outlined in the statement. In addition, one ought to mention that should this alternative not reflect Defence's position then results will need to be reassessed (preferably not in Court).

The ENFSI guidelines[143] on evaluative reporting also treat this subject. They suggest that if the defence do not make known an alternative, as is often the case, then the analyst has three options available:

1. Adopt an alternative proposition that most likely and reasonably reflects the defence's position.

2. Explore a range of *explanations* for the findings.

3. State the findings, if needed, in a technical report and stress that in the absence of an alternative proposition it is impossible to evaluate the findings.

We are uncertain how anything other than the first option would play out. It would seem too easy for the defence to avoid, as is their right, giving a proposition. This would seem to prevent an evaluation of the findings. Some jurisdictions, quite rightly, do not allow testimony about corresponding DNA profiles without an interpretation. We suspect that only the first option is practical.

The concept of a hierarchy of propositions is essential: it helps the scientists to focus on the issue and identify the factors important for evidence evaluation. It can be seen as a tool for structuring our thinking and makes us consider what propositions are the most helpful, how we can add value and what findings we need to evaluate (this may seem trivial but it is not). It is therefore crucial that close attention is given to the formulation of propositions.

Propositions are classified into five levels: offence, activity, source, sub-source and sub-sub-source.[212,214] The top of the hierarchy is taken to be the offence level where the issue is one of guilt or innocence. An example of this could be 'Mr Smith raped Ms Doe' versus

---

* It is not the only error in this section by Gigerenzer. Professor Weir did not report *LR*s in the OJ Simpson case and most laboratories and all accredited ones do undertake external QA trials.

'Mr Smith has had consensual sex with Ms Doe'. It is often held that this level of proposition is for the courts to consider and above the level at which a forensic scientist would usually operate. This is not true because the scientist will always evaluate findings given the propositions and will not evaluate the propositions themselves. The court does not evaluate findings, and the scientist does not evaluate propositions, whatever the level. What is true is that it is more rare that the scientist can add value in order to go from activity-level propositions to offence-level propositions. In our example, at first, it is hard to see what forensic findings could help the court in discriminating the propositions 'Mr Smith raped Ms Doe as she described' versus 'Mr Smith has had consensual sex with Ms Doe, as he described'. We can imagine having different types of evidence (fibres, DNA location, wounds, etc.) given both propositions and information. A forensic scientist could therefore help in combining the different scientific findings, and in that case it would be perfectly adequate to evaluate the findings given offence-level propositions.

The next level is taken to be the activity level. Here we must say that sometimes the frontier between activity-level propositions and offence-level propositions can be blurry. An example would be 'Mr B shot the victim' versus 'he had nothing to do with the shooting'. Is shooting an activity? An offence? Or both? Another example could be (similarly to the Weller case[216]) 'Mr W inserted his fingers in the vagina of Ms V as she described' versus 'they had casual contact as he described'. Here the absence/presence of DNA on some of the fingers and on the hand as a whole can help in discriminating the two propositions. In one case we would expect DNA to be present mainly on the fingers used for the penetration, and in the other case we would expect to find DNA on the hand as a whole. Our findings would regard the distribution and quantity of the DNA and not the profile itself (as Mr W does not say it is not Ms V's DNA). We see again here that the information given by prosecution and defence is as important as the propositions themselves that are in fact a summary of the information given.

The next level in the hierarchy is the source level. At this level we consider propositions of the type 'the semen came from Mr Smith' versus 'it came from some unknown person'. Considerations at this level generally regard the origin of the DNA: scientists will evaluate the DNA profile (not the presence, absence of DNA or where it was found). Source-level propositions are easier to consider and do not involve as much expertise as activity-level propositions.

The level below the source level is termed the *sub-source-level*. This term has arisen because it is not always known from what body fluid the DNA may have come. For instance, if one has recovered 'trace DNA', a sub-source proposition could be 'the DNA came from the suspect'.

Sub-sub-source defines propositions that talk about part of a DNA profile, say the major. A sub-sub-source proposition could be 'the major component of the DNA came from the suspect'.

The further down the hierarchy the scientist operates, the more the responsibility for interpreting the evidence is transferred to the court.

This is a subject where there is persistent misunderstanding. Even experienced analysts seem to want to put part of the findings into the proposition. Consider the oft used 'the major comes from the POI'. We have heard sentences such as 'I think the court would want to know this'. What is misunderstood is that the observation that a component of the mixture is the major is a finding, not a proposition. We did not know that the POI would be the major before we looked at the profile. What we have done is to glance at the electropherogram, then form the proposition. It is important to avoid putting findings into the propositions. They are the part being assessed, the E in $Pr(E|H_p)$. By all means let us say that the POI corresponds with the major when describing the findings in the report, but we should avoid findings in the propositions. For a more convincing perspective, let us take it to an extreme: the major comes from someone who is unrelated to the POI and is a 7,9 at TH01, an 11,13 at D8, etc. All we have done is put all the findings about the major into the H_d proposition.

We do actually regularly transgress this rule at this time. Most modern mixture applications need an assignment of the number of contributors before proceeding. This is developed from the electropherogram. This is currently unavoidable, and in most cases there is no adverse effect on the interpretation (if this number is based on the trace and case information).

BOX 2.2   TRACE, LATENT, LOW TEMPLATE, CONTACT OR TOUCH

All of these terms have been used to describe essentially invisible traces analyzed for DNA. We discourage the use of the words *touch* and *contact*. These imply that it is known that the DNA was deposited by a touch. Touch is certainly one possibility and maybe the most plausible, but it is not the only option. We personally like *trace*.

It would be reasonable to leave the interpretation of such matters as the transition from sub-sub source upwards in the hierarchy to the court if that were the best body to undertake this interpretation. However if the matter requires expert knowledge regarding such matters as factors of 2 or transfer and persistence, it would seem wise for the scientist to attempt interpretation at a higher level in the hierarchy or, at least, to warn and equip the court to make such an attempt. The evidence must eventually be interpreted given offence propositions by the court. If the evidence cannot be put in the context of the offence, then it is in itself irrelevant to the court. Due attention must be paid to the position in the hierarchy of propositions that can be considered. This information must be effectively conveyed to the court to avoid the risk that a consideration at one level be interpreted at a higher level. We cannot emphasize the importance of this enough.

Evaluation of DNA given sub-source-level propositions can be problematic especially with trace DNA (Box 2.2).

In more and more cases the question of interest is not the source of the DNA, but how it was deposited. Cases such as Weller[216] or Kercher,[217] where the POIs did not contest that it might be their DNA but contested the activities alleged by the prosecution, show the limits of assessing DNA evidence given sub-source-level propositions. A recent case in the United Kingdom has shown how dangerous it can be to only consider sub-source-level propositions. The case involved David Butler, a former taxi driver from Wavertree, Liverpool, who was accused of murdering a local prostitute, Anne Marie Foy. The prosecution case was based in large part on traces of DNA (matching Mr Butler's) found on the victim's nails. Information on the case showed that the victim was wearing a glitter nail polish, which appeared to attract dirt or other extraneous material quite easily. In addition, Mr Butler suffered from a severe skin condition, which meant that he easily shed flakes of skin, leaving behind much larger amounts of DNA than an average person. Based on these elements, the defence successfully argued that secondary transfer could have occurred. Butler could have taken a passenger to the Red Light district, handed over some notes in change and passed on his DNA to the passenger who then met with Foy and later handed the notes, complete with Butler's DNA, to her. Newspapers reported this as DNA evidence in danger of being discredited.[218] However it is simply misplacement in the hierarchy. The forensic evidence was evaluated using sub-source-level propositions, i.e. the DNA came from Mr Butler or the DNA came from some unknown unrelated person. The newspaper – as would have the general public – has interpreted it at the crime or activity level, Mr Butler murdered/attacked Ms Foy.

Let us assume that the scientist can help in making the decision regarding at which level in the hierarchy the propositions should be formulated. The next step is to attempt to formulate one proposition for the prosecution and one for the defence. The defence are under no obligation to provide a proposition and, in fact, the defendant may have given a 'no comment' interview.*

Is it the role of the forensic scientist to formulate the defence proposition when 'no comment' is given?

If the scientist does formulate a proposition on behalf of the defence, how should the implications of this action be highlighted/exposed in the statement?

---

* McCrossan et al. (personal communication).

One issue here is consideration of the obvious alternatives:

H_d: The suspect had nothing to do with the … (activity associated with the crime).

H_d: An unknown person is the source of the DNA.

Such consideration tends to maximize the *LR* and hence has a tendency to maximize the apparent weight of the evidence.

There is an issue as to whether the defence must choose only one proposition or whether they can have many. In fact it is worthwhile considering what happens if the prosecution and defence propositions are not exhaustive. Let us assume that there could be three propositions H_1, H_2 and H_3. H_1 aligns with the prosecution view of the case, H_2 is the proposition chosen for the defence and H_3 is any proposition that has been ignored in the analysis but is also consistent with innocence.

This can be set hypothetically as follows:

Proposition H_i	$Pr(E\,|\,H_i,I)$
H_1	0.1
H_2	0.000001
H_3	1

Let us assume that we proceed with the *LR* approach and calculate

$$LR = \frac{Pr(E\,|\,H_1)}{Pr(E\,|\,H_2)} = \frac{0.1}{0.000001} = 100{,}000$$

which would be described as very strong support for H_1. Is this acceptable? Well, the answer is that it is only acceptable if the prior probability for H_3 is vanishingly small and if the three propositions exhaust all possible explanations. This is why it is so important to gather information that will help formulate the most useful propositions and to ensure that propositions are exhaustive *in the context* of the case.

Imagine a single sourced trace DNA profile that matches the reference DNA profile of a POI. H_1 is that the POI is the source of the DNA, H_2 is that an unknown person is the source of the DNA and H_3 is that the POI's identical twin is the source of the DNA. In most criminal cases H_1 and H_2 will both be considered as the two propositions. In such an instance H_3 has been discounted. It is necessary to check if this is reasonable, and we would suggest that this is the responsibility of the prosecution not the defence.

This approach to proposition formulation suggests that all propositions for which there is a reasonable prior probability should be considered, either directly by the scientist or after the defence have made the scientist aware of such a possibility. Under these circumstances there should be no risk of the *LR* being misleading. It is also important to outline in the statement why and how the alternative was chosen. It should be based on the case at hand. The future may entertain a more comprehensive solution based on the general form of Bayes' theorem.

The *LR* Framework

Bayes' theorem is a fundamental tool of inductive inference.[219]

Frustrations with the frequentist approach to forensic evidence have led many people to search for alternatives.[220,221] For many, these frustrations stem from discussing multiple stains or suspects or from trying to combine different evidence types.[202,222] The foremost alternative is the Bayesian approach.[223–228] This approach has been implemented routinely in paternity cases since the 1930s.[229] It was however only in the latter stages of the twentieth century that it made inroads into many other fields of forensic science.* It now dominates the forensic literature, but not necessarily forensic practice, as the method of choice for interpreting forensic evidence.[161,163,176,231–238]

Let

H_p: be the proposition advanced by the prosecution[†]

H_d: be a particular proposition suitable for the defence

E: represent the evidence (or more precisely, the scientific findings the scientist has to evaluate)

I: represent all the background information as well as everything that we know, or assume, that is relevant for assigning the probability of interest

The laws of probability lead to the following:

$$\frac{Pr(H_p|E,I)}{Pr(H_d|E,I)} = \frac{Pr(E|H_p,I)}{Pr(E|H_d,I)} \times \frac{Pr(H_p|I)}{Pr(H_d|I)} \qquad (2.1)$$

This theorem is known as Bayes' rule.[239] A derivation appears in Box 2.3. This theorem follows directly from the laws of probability. It can therefore be accepted as a logical framework for

---

BOX 2.3   A DERIVATION OF BAYES' THEOREM

The third law of probability states

$$Pr(a \text{ and } b|c) = Pr(a, b|c) = Pr(a|b, c)Pr(b|c) = Pr(b|a, c)Pr(a|c)$$

Rewriting this using H_p, H_d, E and I

$$Pr(H_p, E|I) = Pr(H_p|E, I)Pr(E|I) = Pr(E|H_p, I)Pr(H_p|I)$$

and

$$Pr(H_d, E|I) = Pr(H_d|E, I)Pr(E|I) = Pr(E|H_d, I)Pr(H_d|I)$$

hence

$$\frac{Pr(H_p, E|I)}{Pr(H_d, E|I)} = \frac{Pr(H_p|E,I)Pr(E|I)}{Pr(H_d|E,I)Pr(E|I)} = \frac{Pr(E|H_p,I)Pr(H_p|I)}{Pr(E|H_d,I)Pr(H_d|I)}$$

hence

$$\frac{Pr(H_p|E,I)Pr(E|I)}{Pr(H_d|E,I)Pr(E|I)} = \frac{Pr(E|H_p,I)Pr(H_p|I)}{Pr(E|H_d,I)Pr(H_d|I)}$$

cancelling $Pr(E|I)$

$$\frac{Pr(H_p|E,I)}{Pr(H_d|E,I)} = \frac{Pr(E|H_p,I)}{Pr(E|H_d,I)} \times \frac{Pr(H_p|I)}{Pr(H_d|I)} \qquad (2.1)$$

---

* We can note however that it has been applied in the nineteenth century; see Taroni F, Champod C, Margot P.[230]
† Rudin, Inman and Risinger criticize our use of H_p and H_d with some merit and suggest substituting H_1 and H_2. Recently we have been criticized for using H_1 and H_2. After back and forth editing we are currently at H_p and H_d.

interpreting evidence. The use of the term *framework* is a very important one; it means that this approach is not about applying a formula, but about principles that help scientists to assess their findings soundly. Three further principles of interpretation[240,257] can be inferred from this theorem:

P3: Scientific findings must be interpreted within a framework of relevant circumstances (*I*).

P4: Scientific evidence can only be interpreted by considering at least two propositions.

P5: Scientists ought to address questions of the kind 'What is the probability of the evidence given the proposition?' and it is the court that ought to address questions regarding the veracity of a proposition.

Equation 2.1 is often given verbally as follows:

$$posterior\ odds = likelihood\ ratio \times prior\ odds \qquad (2.2)$$

The prior odds are the odds on the propositions H_p before the DNA evidence. The posterior odds are these odds after the presentation of DNA evidence. The odds focus on the probability of the propositions, whereas the *LR* focuses on the probability of the findings (or on the likelihood of the propositions). At this point it is useful to define a 'likelihood'.

> We have written $\Pr(E|H)$ for your probability of *E*, given *H*. It is also referred to as your likelihood of *H*, given *E*.[208]

The *LR* (called the *Bayes factor* if there are only two propositions) also informs us how to relate prior odds and posterior odds. It would seem to be a very worthwhile thing to do, that is, to relate the odds before consideration of the evidence to those after the evidence. It informs us how to update our opinion in a logical manner having heard the evidence. It also helps in defining the role of the scientists and of the court; the former should be concerned with assigning their *LR* and the latter with assigning prior and posterior odds.

The prior odds, $\dfrac{\Pr(H_p|I)}{\Pr(H_d|I)}$, represent the view on the two competing propositions before the DNA evidence is presented.* This view is something that is formed in the minds of the judge and jury. The information imparted to the jury is carefully restricted to those facts that are considered admissible and relevant. It is very unlikely that prior odds are numerically expressed in the mind of the judge and jury and there is no need that they should be numerical.[161,170] Strictly it is not the business of the scientist to form a view on prior odds, and most scientists would strictly avoid this (for a differing opinion see Ref. 241 and the subsequent discussion in Ref. 242). These odds are based on the non-scientific evidence and it is the duty of judge and jury to assess this.[243,244] It has been suggested[245] that:

> In recent years, some examiners, particularly in the UK, have used what is known as the Bayesian approach.... Some also advocated the use of conditional information such as the suspect's motive, opportunity, past criminal record and the like.

We suspect that this is a misunderstanding of some statement about prior odds. Trying to approach such misunderstandings in a learning way, we think it is possible that the misunderstanding comes from the formulation of Bayes' theorem and how *I* is defined. We see in Equation 2.1 that the same letter *I* is used in the conditioning of the prior odds, of the *LR* and of the posterior odds.

However, in the definition of *I* we have noted that *I* is the information, assumptions and knowledge that are relevant for assigning the probability of interest. This means that some

---

* Our wording is wrongly implying an order to events such as the 'hearing of the DNA evidence'. In fact the evidence can be heard in any order. The mathematical treatment will give the same result regardless of the order in which the evidence is considered.[163]

information might be relevant for assigning prior odds and not for one's *LR* (and vice versa). It also means that some information might be relevant for assigning the probability of interest given H_p and other information might be relevant given the alternative H_d.

While it is true that in order to assign probabilities we will need to take into consideration the case information given to us, this information should not in any way concern past record, opportunity or motive. On the contrary we are trained in exactly the opposite approach: forensic scientists should only be given information that concerns the relevant alternative population (e.g. if the POI is not the source of the DNA, who is?), the alleged activities and how the offence was carried out (e.g. one or multiple offenders).[200]

We could therefore rewrite Equation 2.1 as follows:

$$\frac{Pr(H_p \mid E, I_1)}{Pr(H_d \mid E, I_2)} = \frac{Pr(E \mid H_p, I_{F1})}{Pr(E \mid H_d, I_{F2})} \times \frac{Pr(H_p \mid I_1)}{Pr(H_d \mid I_2)} \tag{2.3}$$

where *I*, the relevant information, might be different given the prosecution's or defence's propositions (I_{F1}, I_{F2}).[246] We assume that I_{F1} is some subset of I_1 and that I_{F2} is some subset of I_2. The subsets represent only that part of the background information required for the assessment of the *LR* and exclude that part that is unnecessary and potentially biasing. By formulating in this way we attempt to make explicit that the information that is relevant to prior and posterior odds is not similar to the forensic information that is relevant for assigning our *LR*.

This is not a fanciful concern. Representatives for the Innocence Project have also raised it with us. We need, as a community, to make it clear that I_{F1} and I_{F2} relate to matters such as whether a complainant in a sexual assault case has had consensual sex and the information may include the reference of her consensual partner. We do not need, and do not want to know, past record, motive, opportunity or the results of other unconnected forensic examinations. There is also no need for the examining scientist to know the name of the crime, the name of the accused, the name of the complainant or the rank of the submitting officer[200] until just before she writes the statement.

The *LR* approach typically reports only an *LR*. In taking this approach, the scientist reports the weight of the evidence (or findings) without transgressing on those areas reserved for the judge and jury. This is the reason that the term *logical approach** has been used to describe this method. The term that is being avoided is *Bayesian approach*, which is the term used in most papers on this subject including our own. This term is being avoided because, strictly, presenting a ratio of likelihoods does not necessarily imply the use of the Bayesian method. Most authors have intended the presentation of the *LR* alone without necessarily implying that a discussion of Bayes' theorem and prior odds would follow in court. The intent was to present the scientific evidence in the context of a logical framework without necessarily presenting that framework.

However the advantage of the logical approach is that the *LR* can be put into the context of the entire case and in a consistent and logical framework. This advantage is somewhat lost if judge, jury and scientist are reticent to use or even discuss Bayes' theorem in full.

Although likelihood ratios have appealing features, the academic community has yet fully to analyse and discuss their usefulness for characterising DNA evidence.[210]

Pfannkuch et al. describe their experiences teaching this material to undergraduate students:

Bayes' Theorem was the killer. There was an exodus of those mathematically unprepared and mathphobic students who were free to leave the course, supplemented by panic and agonised discussions with those who were trapped by their course requirements.[247]

---

* We first had this distinction explained by Christophe Champod.

These professional scientists and teachers persisted and found good methods for teaching even math-phobic students because of the 'wealth of socially important problems' that are best addressed by Bayes' theorem.

Fenton and Neil[248] argue forcefully that Bayes theorem is the method of choice for interpreting evidence while giving the fair criticism that Bayesians have failed in their duty of communication. They quote the fact that many lawyers and other educated professionals misunderstand the subject.

Is there a lesson here? Our own experience with practising forensic scientists is that they can achieve in-depth understanding of complex mathematical concepts and methods especially when placed in a good learning environment and supported by colleagues and management. In this regard we would like to commend the practice of the now closed UK Forensic Science Service (FSS) of secluding scientists during training (in England we used excellent hotels in Evesham and the 'Pudding Club' somewhere south of Birmingham). The FSS also undertook basic probability training and was considering putting in place a numerical competency in recruitment.

The Institute de Police Scientifique (University of Lausanne, Lausanne, Switzerland) offers e-learning courses on interpretation that are tailored for forensic practitioners.[249] These courses have been well received in the forensic community. Franco Taroni also teaches several courses on interpretation to students at the Faculty of Law, Criminal Justice and Public Administration at the University of Lausanne. His students (both in law and in forensic science) appreciate the usefulness and logic of the Bayesian framework.

To gain familiarity with Equation 2.2 it is useful to consider a few results. What would happen if our *LR* was 1? In this case posterior odds are unchanged by the forensic results. Another way of putting this is that the evidence is neutral: it does not help discriminate the propositions and therefore is irrelevant.

What would happen if our *LR* was greater than 1? In these cases posterior odds would be greater than prior odds. The evidence would have increased our belief in H_p relative to H_d. Another way of putting this is that the evidence supports H_p. The higher the *LR*, the greater the support for H_p.

If the *LR* is less than 1, the posterior odds would be smaller than the prior odds. The evidence would have decreased our belief in H_p relative to H_d. Another way of putting this is that the evidence supports H_d. The lower the *LR*, the greater the support for H_d. *LR* values less than 1 are sometimes called *negative LRs*, as a logarithm of their value would produce a negative number. The use of the logarithm of the *LR* has been suggested as the weight of evidence.[250] This allows the intuitive image of weighing evidence in the scales of justice with a likelihood ratio of a value greater than 1 increasing the odds in favour of the first proposition. A *LR* of less than 1 will decrease the odds in the favour of the first proposition and have a negative weight. An *LR* equal to 1 will leave the odds and the scales unchanged.

The allowable range for the *LR* is from 0 to infinity. A value of 0 indicates that H_p is impossible, and if H_p and H_d are the only two options, then H_d must be true. A *LR* value of infinity would indicate that H_p is infinitely more likely than H_d, and again if H_p and H_d are the only two options, then H_p must be true. Just to complete the set, if H_p and H_d are the only possibilities (exhaustive) and both $\Pr(E|H_p)$ and $\Pr(E|H_d)$ are 0, then the evidence we have just observed is impossible.

It has been suggested that a nomogram may be useful to help explain the use of this formulation. This follows from a well-known nomogram in clinical medicine. Riancho and Zarrabeitia[251] suggested the diagram that has been modified and presented in Tables 2.1 and 2.2. These tables are used by choosing prior odds and drawing a line through the centre of the *LR* value. The posterior odds may then be read directly. For example, assume that the prior odds are about 1 to 100,000 (against) and the *LR* is 10,000,000, then we read the posterior odds as 100 to 1 (on). We have never tried these in court and have never spoken with anyone who has.

Table 2.1   The Prosecutor's Nomogram

Prior		Likelihood Ratio	Posterior	
Probability	Odds		Odds	Probability
			100,000,000 to 1	99.999990%
0.001%	1 to 100,000		10,000,000 to 1	99.999989%
0.01%	1 to 10,000	10,000,000,000	1,000,000 to 1	99.9999%
		1,000,000,000		
0.1%	1 to 1,000	100,000,000	100,000 to 1	99.999%
		10,000,000		
1%	1 to 100	1,000,000	10,000 to 1	99.99%
		100,000		
9%	1 to 10	10,000	1,000 to 1	99.9%
		1,000		
50%	1 to 1	100	100 to 1	99%
		10		
91%	10 to 1	1	10 to 1	91%
99%	100 to 1		1 to 1	50%

Source: Reproduced and amended with kind permission from Springer Science+Business Media: *International Journal of Legal Medicine*, The prosecutor's and defendant's Bayesian nomograms, 116, 2002, 312–313, Riancho, J.A. and M.T. Zarrabeitia.

Note: The prior and posterior probabilities associated with these odds are given next to the odds.

The *LR* is a numerical scale. One point can be hinged to words without argument; an *LR* of 1 is neutral. Other words may be attached to this scale to give a subjective verbal impression of the weight of evidence.[252-256] This association of words with numbers is subjective and necessarily arbitrary. Evidence scales may have quite a deep history.[253] *LR*-based scales appear in the hallmark text by Evett and Weir[257,p. 225]. They also appear in Buckleton, Triggs and Walsh,[98] Butler,[258,p. 296] Aitken and Taroni[259,p. 107] and Evett et al.[240] and have received support from overview committees.[143,260] NRC II[176] does not specifically discuss verbal scales but does discuss *LR*s and juror comprehension extensively in Chapter 5.

Two scales are given in Tables 2.3 and 2.4. Our own efforts with similar scales have not been all success (Box 2.4). Standardization efforts between disciplines and between laboratories provoked heated and lengthy discussion.

For example, a scale very similar to the one given above was under discussion at the Institute of Environmental Science and Research (ESR) in New Zealand. Considerable discussion ensued on whether the numbers below 1 should be given as decimals or whether the propositions should be inverted and therefore only numbers greater than 1 produced. One read on the 'only numbers greater than 1' option from an independent analyst was that this was a symptom of prosecution bias, she having not noted the 'invert the

Table 2.2	The Defendant's Nomogram			
Prior		Likelihood Ratio	Posterior	
Probability	Odds		Odds	Probability
0.1%	1 to 1,000		100 to 1	99%
1%	1 to 100		10 to 1	91%
9%	1 to 10	10	1 to 1	50%
		1		
50%	1 to 1	1/10	1 to 10	9%
		1/100		
91%	10 to 1	1/1000	1 to 100	1%
		1/10,000		
99%	100 to 1	1/100,000	1 to 1,000	0.1%
		1/1,000,000		
99.9%	1,000 to 1	1/10,000,000	1 to 10,000	0.01%
		1/100,000,000		
99.99%	10,000 to 1	1/1,000,000,000	1 to 100,000	0.001%
			1 to 1,000,000	0.0001%

propositions' clause. This comment from an independent scientist highlights the dangers present in wordings.

Another comment that taxed us during attempts at standardization across Australasia was the suggestion that all *LR*s below 1 be reported as an exclusion. The most mathematically pure stance is to report the result 'as is' but what if we could live with some 'rounding of the edges'? For example, 1 is described as neutral, but what term should be used for 1.1? Is any damage done by calling very low *LR*s an exclusion? If we accepted this, we would next be asked what was meant by 'very low'.

The reader may note that exclusion and identification (or conclusive) do not appear on the scales. We treat these two, exclusion and identification, separately here although there should really have been some symmetry to them.[262]

The statement of exclusion has been useful for forensic science and the courts for many years. In an *LR* context it is an assertion that the evidence is impossible if H_p is true, and hence it is impossible that H_p is true. Forensic scientists have been comfortable making this assertion, and we see no pressing need to ask them to reconsider except in a specific situation we will consider below.

Identification, conclusive or individualizations, are more problematic to us. These are assertions that $Pr(H_p|E) = 1$. Where we have heard this stated and from the way it is given, we would write as $Pr(E|H_i) = 0$ for all $i \neq 1$.

Before proceeding, a small aside on Cromwell's rule. This rule was named by statistician Dennis Lindley in reference to Oliver Cromwell, who famously wrote to the synod of the Church

Table 2.3	Two Verbal Scales		
LR	**Verbal Wording[260]**	**LR**	**Verbal Wording[143]**
1,000,000+	Extremely strong	1,000,000+	...provide extremely strong support for the first proposition rather than the alternative ...are exceedingly more probable given... proposition ... than ... proposition...
100,000	Very strong	10,000–1,000,000	...provide very strong support for the first proposition rather than the alternative ...are far more probable given ... proposition ... than proposition...
10,000	Strong	1,000–10,000	...provide strong support for the first proposition rather than the alternative ...are much more probable given ... proposition ... than proposition...
1000	Moderately strong	100–1000	...provide moderately strong support for the first proposition rather than the alternative ...are appreciably more probable given ... proposition ... than proposition...
100	Moderate	10–100	...provide moderate support for the first proposition rather than the alternative ...are more probable given ... proposition ... than proposition...
10	Limited	2–10	...provide weak support[a] for the first proposition relative to the alternative ...are slightly more probable given one proposition relative to the other
1	Neutral	1	...do not support one proposition over the other ...provide no assistance in addressing the issue
0.1	Limited		
0.01	Moderate		
0.001	Moderately strong	*LR*s corresponding to the inverse (1/*X*) of these values (*X*) will express the degree of support for the specified alternative compared to the first proposition.	
0.0001	Strong		
0.00001	Very strong		
0.000001	Extremely strong		

LR, likelihood ratio.

[a] In providing a statement such as 'the forensic findings provide weak support for the first proposition compared to the alternative', forensic practitioners or their reports should avoid conveying the impression that the findings provide (strong) support for the stated alternative.

Table 2.4 The New Zealand (ESR) Verbal Scale			
Verbal Equivalent			
Provides extremely strong support		Over 1,000,000	
Provides very strong support		1000–1,000,000	
Provides strong support	For H	100–1000	LR
Provides moderate support		10–100	
Provides slight support		1–10	
Is neutral		1	
Provides slight support		1–10	
Provides moderate support		10–100	
Provides strong support	Against H	100–1000	1/LR
Provides very strong support		1000–1,000,000	
Provides extremely strong support		More than 1,000,000	

ESR, Institute of Environmental Science and Research, New Zealand; *LR*, likelihood ratio.

BOX 2.4   VERBAL SCALES

John Buckleton

The earliest attempt that I know of to establish a verbal scale based on likelihood ratios arose from the time that I was working with Ian Evett and Richard Pinchin at the Home Office Central Research Establishment in Aldermaston, England.[253] At this stage I was wildly enthusiastic about verbal scales and the positive effect that they could have on standardization across different evidence types. Over the years I have become very disillusioned. It is actually very hard to distort numbers. However words regularly become a plaything in court.

The most common criticisms are that the scale is arbitrary, which it is except for the word placed next to an *LR* of 1, and that it is subjective, which it is as evidenced by different people having different scales, and that it could add to confusion. This last criticism is probably unfair since there is evidence that no explanation of numerical evidence is any better.

My own experience involves such things as a single source case that had given an *LR* of 10^{10} for H_d: The DNA came from a person unrelated to the POI. The defence asked for a brother's calculation. Let us imagine that the brother's calculation returns *LR* approximately equals 10^3. The lawyer acting for the defence asks, 'So, you admit, do you not, that the evidence might not be extremely strong but instead merely strong. Do you not admit this?'*

Let us take up the idea of calling the region around 1 inconclusive and a region of low *LRs* an exclusion for complex low template four-person mixtures. Our reasoning might be that there is considerable uncertainty in the development of an *LR* for such mixtures, and we 'feel' that this is a more fair expression of the evidence. Further let me say that I'm going to call 1000–0.001 inconclusive and 0.001 downwards an exclusion. Next let us imagine that someone is in court with an *LR* of 1001. The almost inevitable question is, 'Is this nearly inconclusive?'

---

* Of course I am making a point about my experience of the misphrasing of questions in court. I have taken to answering such questions 'no'.

Let us imagine that I describe 1000–0.0001 as *inconclusive* and my colleague testifies to a Y chromosome case with an *LR* of 100. Is her *LR* inconclusive because I described mine as *inconclusive*?

I've started to wonder if the verbal scale is doing any good at all.

A recent publication measuring the effectiveness of verbal scales[261] gives a telling comment: 'If the intention of verbal conclusion scales is to facilitate effective and accurate communication of opinions regarding evidential weight, then that aim has not been achieved. Across all three examinations results indicated a tendency to undervalue all but the lowest strength evidence'.

I saw the New York State subcommittee on DNA evidence debate this topic on 13 March 2015. They spent probably 30 minutes of the available three hours on this one topic. This one act, early in the proceedings, doomed the meeting to run out of time. However it did show that the attempt to assist a court in understanding the number attracts extreme attention and strong opinion even in midst of a packed agenda. The initial discussion was entirely negative. It included perfectly rational comment such as, is an *LR* in the range 1–10 correctly described as *slight support*? This was discussed, reasonably, noting that if there is uncertainty in the assignment, it may indeed be inconclusive. There was also a very reasonable wish to emphasize the continuous nature of the *LR*. Indeed success in emphasizing this would greatly improve the scale. Amanda Sozer asked, 'Where is the validation?'

Are we now going to 'validate' the phrases in our guidelines for statement writing? What would a validation of a verbal scale look like? What is a 'pass' result? Do we demand that a jury understand the statement? If so, this is a new requirement and one never yet achieved. Will it be applied to the number as well? Is this an exercise such as those already undertaken and published on the verbal scale and which largely show that it has deficiencies? This latter is the only possible validation of which I can think has been done, plausibly the verbal scale failed the test, and this emeritus committee had not read about it. 'It affects people's lives', stated Allison Eastman.

It is important that oversight committees such as this move from accepted but dramatic statements to thinking about how evidence could be improved. It is far too easy to be a critic but offer no way forward.

Interestingly the discussion about the verbal scale ended positively. This happened when it was pointed out that one of the main purposes was that weak DNA evidence be effectively portrayed as weak and not falsely assumed to be much more by a 'CSI'* educated public.

---

* CSI, 'Crime Scene Investigation' (TV series).

of Scotland on 5 August 1650, saying 'I beseech you, in the bowels of Christ, think it possible that you may be mistaken'.

What the rule suggests is that prior probabilities of 0 or 1 should be avoided. Such a statement would challenge many forensic scientists, so it is worthwhile reprising Lindley's argument, which we support. Any statement of a probability of 0 or 1 is a statement that no amount of evidence could ever persuade you otherwise. This is a barely tenable position for a scientist.

Recall all the people who said that heavier-than-air flight or travel to the moon were impossible.

Lindley was referring to prior probabilities. This differs a little from the context needed for a statement of 'conclusive'. What is needed there is a statement that the evidence is impossible under all other possible causes. This is quite a statement and it would be quite hard to see how it could ever be substantiated.

To quieten the inevitable outcry, we accept that there is a pragmatic usefulness to the word *exclusion* when that benefits the defendant. However exclusion does not always have this effect[263]. One instance, highlighted in a US case,[108] is that the exclusion of person A may be quite inculpatory for person B. It is unfortunate that many prominent commentators encourage the notion that lower *LR*s are always conservative.[264]

Returning to verbal scales, the Australian case *R v Meyboom* is an excellent source of useful examples of misinterpretation. Here is one such example from CJ Higgins, the judge in Meyboom, that argues rather elegantly for the usefulness of the verbal scale: 'Even on the assumption made, a 127 times likelihood is an extremely weak correlation'. How would one feel about increasing the odds by a factor of 127 of living a healthy life until age 90? Of course a factor of 127 is actually quite large in many contexts.

Discussion of scales is not unexpected (choosing scales is usually the topic of debates, see for example the metric scale or the temperature scales), and discussion between scientists and judiciary is necessary but unlikely (Box 2.5). A successful consensus regarding the scale used in Sweden[265] has been reported. This approach is very useful, as discrepancies between scales appear to give good exercise for critics, of which there are many.

The discrepancies in scales has been assigned to the *LR* approach.[245] This overlooks the discrepancy between scales which do not use an *LR* approach. An example is the Bodziak and ENFSI 2 scales for footwear analysis in Table 2.5.*

BOX 2.5   WHICH WAY UP?

When we introduced Bayes' theorem, we wrote it as follows:

$$\frac{Pr(H_p|E,I)}{Pr(H_d|E,I)} = \frac{Pr(E|H_p,I)}{Pr(E|H_d,I)} \times \frac{Pr(H_p|I)}{Pr(H_d|I)} \tag{2.1}$$

Why did we write it this way up? What was wrong with the following way?

$$\frac{Pr(H_d|E,I)}{Pr(H_p|E,I)} = \frac{Pr(E|H_d,I)Pr(H_d|I)}{Pr(E|H_p,I)Pr(H_p|I)}$$

This approach would work just as well. High numbers would be support for H_d, typically aligned to the defence hypothesis. Is the reason we defined it with H_p on top an indication of subconscious bias? Is this the reason Balding, Donnelly and Nichols[270] wrote their *LR*s up the other way? Were they trying to help us to see something?

David Balding has informed us that the reason was not this deep. It simply led to simpler expressions. However the deeper question remains.

Because most people deal better with high numbers (1,000,000) than small numbers (0.000001), it is also possible to reverse the *LR* in order to have a number that is easier to communicate. For instance, instead of saying that the results are 0.000001 more probable given the proposition that the blood came from Mr A than given the proposition that it came from an unknown person, we would say that the results are a million times more probable given the proposition that the blood came from an unknown person than given the proposition that it came from Mr A.

---

* The Bodziak and ENFSI 2 scales regard the probability of the propositions themselves and not the value of the findings. They give posterior probabilities that need to be based on factors other than inference alone and that should be left to the court. We therefore strongly disapprove the use of the Bodziak and ENFSI 2 scales or any scale based on posterior probabilities.

Table 2.5 Three of the Published Shoeprint Conclusion Scales Showing the Two Primary Styles		
ENFSI 1[a]	**Bodziak**[268,pp. 372–374]	**ENFSI 2**[a]
Identification	Positive identification	Identification
Very strong support for proposition A	Probably made	Very probably
Strong support		
Moderately strong support		Probably
Moderate support	Possibly made	
Limited support		
Inconclusive		Inconclusive
Limited support for proposition B	Possibly did not make	Likely not
Moderate support		
Moderately strong support		
Strong support		
Very strong support		
Elimination	Non-identification	Elimination

[a] Part of the ENFSI marks working group conclusion scale.[266,267]

The verbal scale can become a legal plaything. A taste of this is given below:

Mr Gill (to Dr Simon Walsh, Australian Federal Police, in R v Meyboom[269]*):* So doctor, those are terms of art, those phrases? (In Australia you can turn a statement into a question by a raised inflection at the end of the sentence. Obviously this does not show in transcript.)

Dr Walsh: Yes, they are. Certainly they've been picked to try to reflect the actual mathematical value. We use them in a table so that we're consistent with the terminology that we use and obviously we attempt to reflect the strength of the evidence using those terms.

Mr Gill: But in reality they have no meaning independent from the numbers from which they're derived?

Dr Walsh: No. They themselves follow on from the number that's been calculated.

If the objective of the verbal scale was to obtain some standardization between laboratories and across evidence types, this has proven remarkably difficult to achieve.

The Full Bayesian Approach

The analysis given under the title of 'the logical approach' works well if there are two clear propositions aligned with the prosecution and defence positions. However regularly it is difficult to simplify a real casework problem down to two propositions.

To put this in context consider a relatively simple short tandem repeat case. We have a stain at the scene of a crime. Call this stain c and the genotype of this stain G_c.[257] A person comes to the attention of the police. Call this person s and his genotype G_s. The genotype of the person and the crime stain are found to be the same. We will write this as $G_s = G_c$.

Under the coincidence approach this would be the match that is caused by the suspected person being the donor of the crime stain or by a coincidence. To make the comparison with hypothesis testing we would formulate

H_0: The DNA came from a male not related to the suspect.

H_1: The DNA came from the suspect.

We then calculate the probability of the findings if this is true and given the information at hand. Let us write this as $\Pr(G_c|G_s, H_0, I)$, which can be read as the probability of the DNA profile of the crime stain if the crime stain came from a male unrelated to the suspect (and the suspect's genotype is G_s) and given the information at hand (for example, the offender is Eurasian). This is often written as p and taken to be the occurrence of the crime stain genotype (or the suspect's genotype since they are the same) in the relevant population. We assume that this occurrence is small and hence there is evidence against H_0 and for H_1.

Under the 'logical approach' we simply rename these propositions:

H_p: The DNA came from the suspect.

H_d: The DNA came from a male not related to the suspect.

We then assign the probability of the DNA results under each of these proposi-tions.[226,231,236,257,271–275] $\Pr(G_c|G_s, H_p, I) = 1$ since the crime genotype will be G_c if it came from the person who is G_s. Again we take $\Pr(G_c|G_s, H_d, I) = p$. Hence

$$LR = \frac{1}{\Pr(G_c \mid G_s, H_d)} = \frac{1}{p} \tag{2.4}$$

which is (typically) very much larger than 1 and hence there is evidence against H_d and for H_p.

However note that the two following propositions are not exhaustive:

H_p: The DNA came from the suspect.

H_d: The DNA came from a male not related to the suspect.

What about those people who *are* related to the suspect? Should they be considered? Genetic theory would suggest that these are the most important people to consider and that they should not be omitted from the analysis. What we need is a number of propositions. These could be as follows:

H_p: The DNA came from the suspect.

H_{d1}: The DNA came from a male related to the suspect.

H_{d2}: The DNA came from a male not related to the suspect.

Now consider H_{d1}. What do we mean by *related*? Obviously there are many different degrees of relatedness. Suppose that the suspect has one father and one mother, several brothers, numer-ous cousins and second cousins, etc. We may need a multiplicity of propositions. In fact we could envisage the situation where there is a specific proposition for every person on Earth:

H_p: The DNA came from the suspect.

H_{d1}: The DNA came from person 2, the brother of the suspect.

H_{d2}: The DNA came from person 3, the father of the suspect.

...

H_{di}: The DNA came from person i, a member of the subpopulation of the suspect.

...

H_{dj}: The DNA came from person j, so distantly related that we consider him effectively unrelated to the suspect.

What we need is a formulation that can handle from three to many propositions. Considering the enumeration given above there would be almost 7,000,000,000 propositions, one for each person on Earth (given that the entire Earth is the relevant population).

This is provided by the general form of Bayes' theorem (derived in Box 2.6).[270,275,276] This states as follows:

$$\Pr(H_1 \mid G_c, G_s, I) = \frac{\Pr(H_1 \mid I)}{\sum_{i=1}^{N} \Pr(G_c \mid G_s, H_i, I)\Pr(H_i, I)} \tag{2.5}$$

This equation is very instructive for our thinking but is unlikely to be directly useful in court, at least in the current environment. This is because the terms $\Pr(H_i|I)$ relate to the prior probability that the ith person is the source of the DNA. This approach was advanced and strongly advocated by Balding in his outstanding book,[277] although he revised his view by the time he was advising the UK regulator.[59]

BOX 2.6   GENERAL FORM OF BAYES' THEOREM

A comprehensive equation has been proposed[275] based on the general formulation of Bayes' rule. Following Evett and Weir[257]: for a population of size N we index the suspect as person 1 and the remaining members of the population as 2, ..., N. We will call the proposition that person i is the source of the DNA H_i. Since the suspect is indexed as person 1, the proposition that the suspect is, in fact, the source of the DNA is H_1. The remaining propositions, H_2, ..., H_N, are those propositions where the true offender is some other person. Before we examine the DNA profiles, each person has some probability of being the offender $\Pr(H_i|I) = \pi_i$. Many factors may affect this probability, one of these being geography. Those closest to the scene may have higher prior probabilities while people in remote countries have very low prior probabilities. Most of the people other than the suspect or suspects will not have been investigated. Therefore there may be little specific evidence to inform this prior other than general aspects such as sex, age, etc. The POI is genotyped and we will call his genotype G_s. The stain from the scene is typed and found to have the genetic profile G_c, which matches the suspect. The remaining 2, ..., N members of the population have genotypes G_2, ..., G_N. These 2, ..., N people have not been genotyped. We require the probability $\Pr(H_1|G_c, G_s, I)$. This is given by Bayes' rule as

$$\Pr(H_1 \mid G_c, G_s, I) = \frac{\Pr(G_c \mid G_s, H_1, I)\Pr(G_s \mid H_1, I)\Pr(H_1 \mid I)}{\sum_{i=1}^{N} \Pr(G_c \mid G_s, H_i, I)\Pr(G_s \mid H_i, I)\Pr(H_i \mid I)}$$

Assuming that $\Pr(G_s|H_1, I) = \Pr(G_s|H_i, I)$ for all i, we obtain

$$\Pr(H_1 \mid G_s, G_c, I) = \frac{\Pr(G_c \mid G_s, H_1, I)\Pr(H_1 \mid I)}{\sum_{i=1}^{N} \Pr(G_c \mid G_s, H_i, I)\Pr(H_i \mid I)}$$

We assume that the probability that the scene stain will be type G_c given that the suspect is G_s and he contributed the stain is 1. Hence

$$\Pr(H_1 \mid G_s, G_c, I) = \frac{\Pr(H_1 \mid I)}{\displaystyle\sum_{i=1}^{N} \Pr(G_c \mid G_s, H_i, I)\Pr(H_i \mid I)} \tag{2.6}$$

$$= \frac{1}{1 + \displaystyle\sum_{i=2}^{N} \dfrac{\Pr(G_c \mid G_s, H_i, I)\Pr(H_i \mid I)}{\Pr(H_1 \mid I)}} = \frac{1}{1 + \displaystyle\sum_{i=2}^{N} \dfrac{\Pr(G_c \mid G_s, H_i, I)\pi_i}{\pi_1}}$$

Writing $\dfrac{\pi_i}{\pi_1} = w_i$, we obtain $\Pr(H_1 \mid G_c, G_s, I) = \dfrac{1}{1 + \displaystyle\sum_{i=2}^{N} \Pr(G_c \mid G_s, H_i, I)w_i}$, which is the

equation given on p. 41 of Evett and Weir. Here w_i can be regarded as a weighting function that expresses how much more or less probable the ith person is than the suspect to have left the crime stain based on only the non-DNA evidence.

The introduction of such considerations by a forensic scientist is unlikely to be permitted in court.[*] However such an approach may be possible in the unlikely event that the court supplies its view of prior odds. This has never happened to our knowledge. The terms *forensically relevant populations*[278] and *relevant subgroup*[172] provide inadvertent references to such a prior. The time will come when courts countenance this type of consideration. We could envisage the situation where a court instructs the witness to consider only the sub-group 'Caucasian sexually active males in the Manchester area', which is in effect setting a prior of 0 outside this group.

In the likely absence of courts providing such priors, it is suggested that this unifying equation should be used to explore various forensic approaches and to instruct our thinking. However there is so much benefit in the use of this equation that research into how it could be used in court would be very welcome.

Bayesian networks have been shown to be a valuable tool that help forensic scientists to assess results given multiple propositions. Since specialist books exist on this subject,[279] we do not discuss them further here.

A Possible Solution

There is a 'halfway house' between the *LR* approach and the unifying equation that has some considerable merit.[280] Using the same nomenclature as above we rewrite the *LR* as

$$LR = \frac{\Pr(G_c \mid G_s, H_p)}{\displaystyle\sum_{i=2}^{N} \Pr(G_c \mid G_s, H_i, H_d)\Pr(H_i \mid H_d)} \tag{2.7}$$

where $H_2, \ldots, H_N$ is an exclusive and exhaustive partition of H_d (termed *sub-propositions*[281]). The advantage of this approach is that it only requires priors that partition the probability under H_d. There is no requirement for the relative priors on H_p and H_d. This may be more acceptable to a court. This approach is studied in further detail in Chapter 4.

---

[*] Meester and Sjerps[241] argue elegantly to the contrary.

A Comparison of the Different Approaches

The very brief summary of the alternative approaches given above does not do full justice to any of them. It is possible, however, to compare them. In the most simplistic overview we would state as follows:

- The frequentist approach considers the probability of the evidence under one hypothesis.

- The *LR* approach considers the probability of the evidence under at least two mutually exclusive propositions (and exhaustive in the context of the case).

- The full Bayesian approach implies the use of prior odds. It is used, for example, in Switzerland or Germany in paternity cases. To differentiate the use of the *LR* only from the full Bayesian approach, the use of the term *evaluation* for the former and *interpretation* for the latter has been suggested.[273]

If we turn first to a critique of the frequentist approach, the most damning criticisms are a lack of logical rigor and of balance. In the description given above you will see that we struggled to define the frequentist approach and its line of logic with any accuracy. This is not because of laziness but rather that the definition and line of logic has never been given explicitly, and indeed it may not be possible to do so.

Consider the probability that is calculated. We calculate $\Pr(E|H_0)$. If it is small we support H_1.

First note that because $\Pr(E|H_0)$ is small, this does not mean that $\Pr(H_0|E)$ is small. This is called the *fallacy of the transposed conditional*.[191]

Second note that simply because $\Pr(E|H_0)$ is small, it does not mean that $\Pr(E|H_1)$ is large. What if it was also small?

Consider a child abuse case*: Evidence is given that this child rocks (back and forth) and that only 3% of non-abused children rock. It might be tempting to assume that this child is abused since the findings (R: rocking) are unlikely under the proposition (H_0: this child is non-abused). However we may be wrong to do so. Imagine that we now hear that only 3% of abused children rock. This would crucially alter our view of the value of the evidence. We see that we cannot evaluate our findings by considering its probability under only one hypothesis. As mentioned previously, this has been given as a basic principle of evidence interpretation.[240,257]

The logical flaws in the frequentist approach are what have driven many people to seek alternatives. Fortunately for justice and unfortunately for the advance of logic in forensic science, this flaw does not manifest itself in most simple short tandem repeat cases where the propositions are 'the blood came from Mr A' versus 'it came from an unrelated person'. This is because the evidence is often considered as certain under H_1. In such cases the frequentist approach reports the probability of the unknown profile in the population of interest and the logical approach reports the *LR* (i.e. 1 divided by the probability of the unknown profile in the population of interest or $1/p$). Critics of the logical approach understandably ask what all the fuss is about when all that is done in simple cases is to calculate 1 divided by the *p*. Other criticisms have been offered. Effectively these relate to reasonable criticisms of the difficulty of implementation and less reasonable criticisms arising largely from a lack of understanding of the underlying logic.[282,283] This brings us to a critique of the logical approach.

If we start with difficulty of implementation, one reasonable criticism of the logical approach is the ponderous nature of a statement involving an *LR*. Contrast the following:

A: The frequency of this profile among unrelated males in the population is less than 1 in a billion.

B: These findings are more than a billion times more probable given the proposition that the DNA came from the suspect than given the proposition that it came from an unrelated male.

---

* Adapted from Robertson and Vignaux.[163]

Many people would prefer A over B, and in fact studies have demonstrated that there are serious problems with understanding statements like B.[195,196] Some respondents described B type statements as 'patently wrong'. This is not to imply that there is no prospect of misunderstanding a frequentist statement because there clearly is, but rather to suggest that the *LR* wording is more ponderous and will take more skill and explanation to present.

This is not a fatal flaw as *LR*s have been presented in paternity evidence since the mid-1900s. In this context they are typically termed *paternity indices* and are the method of choice in paternity work.[*]

Inman and Rudin[175] note, 'While we are convinced that these ideas are both legitimate and useful, they have not been generally embraced by the practising community of criminalists, nor have they undergone the refinement that only comes with use over time'. This was at the time a fair comment from a US viewpoint, but practice is changing, partly by the tuition of Inman and Rudin themselves. The considerations given above are real issues when applying the *LR* approach. There are a few more objections that arise largely from a misunderstanding of the underlying logic. These would include criticisms of conditioning on *I* and H_p and the arbitrariness of the verbal scale.[202]

Forensic scientists are raised in a culture that demands that they avoid any bias that may arise from ideas seeded into their mind by the prosecution (or anyone else). We fully agree, but one should not throw out the baby with the bathwater. This view has led to the interpretation that scientists should consider the evidence in isolation from the background facts or the prosecution proposition. This idea is a misconception or misreading of the use of the conditioning in the probability assessment. As we have discussed, in essence all probabilities are conditional and the more relevant information that is used in the conditioning the more relevant the resulting probability assignment will be. Failure to consider relevant background information would be a disservice to the court.

Consider the question[†]: What is the probability that Sarah is over 5 feet 8 inches? We could try to assign this probability but our view would change markedly if we were told that Sarah is a giraffe. Ignoring the background information (Sarah is a giraffe) will lead to a much poorer assignment of probability. This is certainly not intended to sanction inappropriate information and conditioning.

The second argument is a verbal trick undertaken in the legal context. Consider the numerator of the *LR*. This is $\Pr(E|H_p, I)$, which can be read as 'the probability of the evidence given that the prosecution proposition is correct and given the background information'. The (false legal) argument would be that it is inconsistent with the presumption of innocence to 'assume that the prosecution proposition is true'. This again is a misconception or a misreading of the conditioning. When calculating the *LR* we are not assuming that the prosecution proposition is true, which indeed would be bias. What we are doing is weighing the prosecution and defence propositions against each other by assigning the probability of the findings *if* these propositions were true. This is an instance where the verbal rendering of Bayes' rule can be misconstrued (possibly deliberately) to give a false impression never intended in the logical framework.

Regarding the arbitrariness of the verbal scale, this point must be conceded except with reference to the point labelled neutral. However any verbal scale, Bayesian or otherwise, is arbitrary. The problem really relates to aligning words that are fuzzy and have different meanings to different people to a numerical scale that possesses all the beauty that is associated with numbers. This problem will be alleviated in those rare cases where the logic and numbers are themselves presented and understood in court.

---

[*] The Bayesian approach is used in numerous scientific disciplines, for example medicine, physics, environmental sciences, finance and astronomy. For more, see *The Theory That Would Not Die: How Bayes' Rule Cracked the Enigma Code, Hunted Down Russian Submarines, and Emerged Triumphant from Two Centuries of Controversy*, Sharon Bertsch McGrayne, Yale University Press, reprint edition 2012.

[†] An example given by Dr Ian Evett.

There is an accepted barrier to adopting this approach. This plausibly stems from unfamiliarity and complexity. More recently a prominent US commentator (and two of us) have attempted to move matters forward by developing halfway steps.[284] We await the results of these attempts.

This brings us to the full Bayesian approach. Its advantage is that the *LR* can be placed in the context of a logical framework. This logical framework requires application of Bayes' rule and hence some assessment of priors. However the legal system of many countries relies on the 'common sense' of jurors and would hesitate to tell jurors how to think.[168,211] Forcing jurors to consider Bayes' theorem would be unacceptable in most legal systems. It is likely that application of common sense will lead to logical errors, and it has been shown that jurors do not handle probabilistic evidence well. However there is no reason to believe that these logical errors would be removed by application of a partially understood logical system, which is the most likely outcome of trying to introduce Bayes' theorem into court. If we recoil from introducing Bayes' theorem in court, then the *LR* approach forfeits one of its principal advantages, although it certainly retains many others in assisting the thinking of the scientists.

There is little doubt that this approach is the most mathematically useful. Most importantly it can accommodate any number of propositions, which allows us to phrase the problem in more realistic ways. It is the underlying basis of Bayesian networks, which play a prominent part in helping scientists evaluate their findings. The use of Bayesian networks will probably continue to expand in the future.[279,285]

When weighing these approaches against each other the reader should also consider that the vast majority of the modern published literature on evidence evaluation advocates the logical or full Bayesian approaches. There is very little published literature advocating a frequentist approach, possibly because the lack of formal rigor in this approach makes publication difficult.

Throughout this book we will attempt to present the evidence in both a frequentist and an *LR* method where possible, even if we are of the opinion that is easier to use just one metric. There are some situations, such as missing persons' casework, paternity, low template level DNA and mixtures, where only the *LR* approach is logically defensible.

Evidence Interpretation in Court
The Fallacy of the Transposed Conditional

Much has been written about the fallacy of the transposed conditional (see Refs. 163,168,169,172,173,187,191,211,237,248,257,286–301), which is also known as the *prosecution fallacy* or the *inversion fallacy*.

It is a fallacy very difficult to avoid even for experienced scientists, and in the press, at conferences or in court transcripts it is common to encounter 'a transposed conditional'.

What can we add to a debate that is already well written about but does not go away? We will again explain it here for those readers for whom the fallacies are new. We have expanded a section that attempts to assess the mathematical consequences of this error and gives some tips on how to avoid making a transposition. Many of these tips come from our experiences working with colleagues at the Interpretation Research Group of the FSS in the United Kingdom.* Few forensic caseworkers have written on the subject, although most have faced it.

The fallacy of the transposed conditional is not peculiar to the *LR* approach. It can occur with a frequentist approach as well. In essence it comes from confusing the probability of the evidence given a specific proposition with the probability of the proposition itself. In the terms given above this would be confusing $\Pr(E|H_p)$ with $\Pr(H_p)$, $\Pr(H_p|E)$, or $\Pr(H_p|E,I)$.

---

* Champod, McCrossan, Jackson, Pope, Foreman and most particularly Ian Evett.

We introduce the subject[302] by asking, 'What is the probability of having four legs *if* you are an elephant?'

Let us write this as $\Pr(4|E)$ and we assign it a high value, say 0.999.

Next we consider, 'What is the probability of being an elephant *if* you have four legs?' Write this as $\Pr(E|4)$ and note that it is a very different probability and not likely to be equal to 0.999. This example seems very easy to understand both verbally and in the symbolic language of probability. However this fallacy seems to be quite tricky to avoid in court.

Imagine that we have testified in court along the lines of one of the statements given below:

- The probability of obtaining this profile from an unrelated male member of the New Zealand population is one in a billion.

- The calculated probability of this profile among members of the population of New Zealand unrelated to Mr Smith is one in a billion.

- This profile is one billion times more likely if it came from Mr Smith than if it came from an unrelated male member of the New Zealand population.

The first two are frequentist statements and the last is a statement of the *LR*.

Let us work with the first. We are quite likely in court to face a question along the following lines: 'In lay terms do you mean that the probability that this blood came from someone else is one in a billion?'

This is the fallacy of the transposed conditional. It has led to appeals and retrials. It appears to be very natural to make this transposition, however incorrect. Every newspaper report of a trial that we have read is transposed, and we suspect that many jurors and indeed judges make it.

How can a scientist who is testifying avoid this error?

The answer involves training and thinking on one's feet and most importantly judgement. We report here Stella's spotting trick (named after Stella McCrossan) and Ian's coping trick (named after Ian Evett).

1. *Stella's spotting trick*: The key that Stella taught was to ask oneself whether the statement given is a question about the findings or the proposition. Probabilistic statements about the proposition will be transpositions. Those about the findings are likely to be correct. The moment that you notice the statement does *not* contain an *if* or a *given* you should be cautious. Consider the sentence given above: 'In lay terms do you mean that the probability that this blood came from someone else is one in a billion?' Is this a statement about a proposition or the findings? First it has no *if* or *given*. The proposition here is that the blood came from someone else. And indeed the statement is a question about the probability of the proposition. Hence it is a transposition.

2. *Ian's coping trick*: The essence of this trick is to identify those statements that you are confident are correct and those that you are confident are incorrect. This is best done by memory. There will be a few standard statements that you know to be correct and a few transpositions that you know to be incorrect. Memorize these. Then there is the huge range of statements in between. These may be correct or incorrect. Prosecutors may have transposed in their head and may be trying to get you to say what they think is a more simple statement. That is their fault not yours (if you are a forensic scientist reading this). They should have read and studied more. In this circumstance we suggest you say something like the following:

   I have been taught to be very careful with probabilistic statements. Subtle misstatements have led to appeals in the past. I am unsure whether your phrasing is correct or incorrect. However I can give some statements that I know are correct.

These will include the numerical statement of type given above or the verbal statements given in Tables 2.3 and 2.4.

Of course care by the scientist is no guarantee that the jury, judge or press will not make the transposition themselves. For instance, Bruce Weir had gone to great trouble with the wording in the report for his testimony in the OJ Simpson case. Weir was careful and correct in his verbal testimony as well. As an example he reported that there was a 1 in 1400 chance that the profile on the Bronco centre console would have this DNA profile *if* it had come from two people other than Mr Simpson and Mr Goldman. This was transposed by the recently retired Linda Deutsch of the Associated Press (26 June 1995) to 'a chance of 1 in 1,400 that any two people in the population could be responsible for such a stain'. To quote Weir: 'It is incumbent on both the prosecution and defence to explain the meaning of a conditional probability of a DNA profile'.[303]

We found another transposition in an interesting place. Horgan[304] was warning about errors in the Simpson case and went on to commit the prosecutor's fallacy while explaining the error of the defender's fallacy! 'Given odds of 1 in 100,000 that a blood sample came from someone other than Simpson, a lawyer could point out that Los Angeles contains 10 million people and therefore 100 other potential suspects. That argument is obviously specious...'

More recently, in the judgement of the Court of Appeal for *R v T* a number of transposition errors were made.[301]

US National Institute of Justice DNA initiative[305] publication "DNA for the Defense Bar" gives us an exemplar *LR* statement: 'The DNA mixture profile obtained from [the item of evidence] is: 4.73 quadrillion times more likely to have originated from [suspect] and [victim/complainant] than from an unknown individual in the U.S. Caucasian population and [victim/complainant]'. Again quite simply a transposition.

Dr Anna Sandiford fluently transposes: 'Mr Sheep had probably been in contact with breaking or broken glass that originated from the Mini and the Toyota'. This is simply a statement about the proposition not the findings.[306]

Based on this evidence we table the following proposition: However likely a person is to transpose the conditional, they are less likely to do so after they have studied probability. Our view is therefore that it is important to educate scientists and help the readers understand what our results mean and what they do not. A first step is for the scientists to think rationally. A second step is to find useful ways so that conclusions are understood by laypersons. Some of our colleagues in document examination attach to their reports a short article describing how to understand an *LR*. Others write in their reports that an *LR* of a billion does not mean that the proposition is a billion times more likely. It does not mean that Mr A is the source of the trace. This later probability depends not only on DNA, but also on the other elements of the case, for example motive and alibi. It is for the court to weigh all these elements and then to decide, based on the whole case, whether Mr A is the source of the DNA or not.

3. *The Mathematical Consequences of Transposition*: The transposition is of no consequence if the prior odds are in fact 1. This is because the answer arrived at by transposition and the 'correct' answers are the same in this circumstance. The issue only occurs if the prior odds differ from 1. If the odds are greater than 1, then the transposition is conservative. For a high *LR* the practical consequences are negligible if the prior odds are not extremely small. Examples showing the impact of an *LR* of one billion (or respectively 10,000) on posterior odds are given thereafter.

Propositions (POI vs Unknown Unrelated)			
Prior Odds	LR	Posterior Odds	Posterior Probabilities
1:7,000,000,000		0.14	0.125000
1:1,000,000,000		1	0.500000
1:8,000,000		125	0.992063
1:1,000,000	1.0×10^9	1000	0.999001
1:500,000		2000	0.999500
1:100,000		10,000	0.999900
1:10,000		100,000	0.999990
1:1000		1,000,000	0.999999

Propositions (POI vs Unavailable Sibling)			
Prior Odds	LR	Posterior Odds	Posterior Probabilities
1:7,000,000,000		1.4E–05	0.000014
1:1,000,000,000		0.0001	0.000100
1:8,000,000		0.0125	0.012346
1:1,000,000		0.1	0.090909
1:500,000		0.2	0.166667
1:100,000	1.0×10^5	1	0.500000
1:10,000		10	0.909091
1:1000		100	0.990099
1:100		1000	0.999001
1:10		10,000	0.999900
1:1		100,000	0.999990

The practical consequences are for lower *LR*s and where there is little other evidence against the defendant or where there is evidence for the defendant.[307,308] However we are of the opinion that good scientific practice should involve not transposing the conditional. The role of forensic scientists is to evaluate their findings given propositions. The role of the court is to decide whether a proposition is true or not. Moreover let us remind the reader that very large *LR*s are generally obtained when propositions are at the source level. However with trace DNA the issue will concern the activities or the offence. Moreover very large *LR*s do not take into account the possibility of errors. This topic will be discussed below.

4. *The Defence Attorney's Fallacy*: This concept is also attributable to the hallmark paper by Thompson and Schumann.[191] It is rather misunderstood. Consider that the POI matches the crime stain. Let us imagine that the match probability is p. We describe some population of size $N + 1$, of which the POI is one, leaving N others. The expected number of matching persons is $Np + 1$. The Np are the people expected to match from N persons and the 1 is the POI. This part is fine and there is no fallacy. The defence

attorney's fallacy occurs not when the expected number is created, for example the $Np + 1$ given above, but when it is asserted that the POI is one of the $Np + 1$ and hence the probability that he is the donor is 1 in $Np + 1$. This latter statement, 'the probability that he is the donor is 1 in $Np + 1$' makes an additional assumption. This additional assumption is that the POI has an average chance of being the donor compared with all the others given the non-DNA evidence.

The courts have been rather enamoured in creating the expected number, and there is no fallacy in this. For example, in *R v Doheny* and *R v Adams*:

> If one person in a million has a DNA profile which matches that obtained from the crime stain, then the suspect will be one of perhaps 26 men in the United Kingdom who share that characteristic. If no fact is known about the Defendant, other than that he was in the United Kingdom at the time of the crime the DNA evidence tells us no more than that there is a statistical probability that he was the criminal of 1 in 26.
>
> He will properly explain to the Jury the nature of the match ('the matching DNA characteristics') between the DNA in the crime stain and the DNA in the blood sample taken from the Defendant. He will properly, on the basis of empirical statistical data, give the Jury the random occurrence ratio - the frequency with which the matching DNA characteristics are likely to be found in the population at large. Provided that he has the necessary data, and the statistical expertise, it may be appropriate for him then to say how many people with the matching characteristics are likely to be found in the United Kingdom – or perhaps in a more limited relevant sub-group, such as, for instance, the Caucasian sexually active males in the Manchester area. This will often be the limit of the evidence which he can properly and usefully give. It will then be for the Jury to decide, having regard to all the relevant evidence, whether they are sure that it was the Defendant who left the crime stain, or whether it is possible that it was left by someone else with the same matching DNA characteristics.[172,211]

And also in *R v Adams DJ*:

> Suppose the match probability is 1 in 20 million. That means that in Britain (population about 60 million) there will be on average about 2 or 3 people, and certainly no more than 6 or 7, whose DNA matches that found at the crime scene, in addition to the accused. Now your job, as a member of the jury, is to decide on the basis of the other evidence, whether or not you are satisfied that it is the person on trial who is guilty, rather than one of the few other people with matching DNA. We don't know anything about the other matching people. They are likely to be distributed all across the country and may have been nowhere near the crime scene at the time of the crime. Others may be ruled out as being the wrong sex or the wrong age group.[309]

Errors in Analysis

There have been justified complaints that most discussions, including our own, start from the premise that the typing has been completed in an error-free way.[172,210,211,310–315] Other than this brief section we will also assume that the analysis is error free.

However there is clear evidence that errors do occur.* The occurrence of such errors is probably low and quality assurance goes some way to reassuring the court and public that the error rate is not high. Nonetheless it must be admitted that there is little knowledge available that would help us to assign the probability of an error (exceptions exist[321]). Nor could one value be applied fairly to different cases, different laboratories or even different operators. The community is understandably but unconstructively resistant to embracing the concept of error.

The question arises as to what constitutes an error; for example, is a typographical error in a court report, calculation or sub-optimal extraction an error, or is an error only when contamination has occurred? Additionally, is the error still an error if it is picked up by a laboratory's quality

---

* For a brief review see Thompson et al.[316] and the following correspondence.[317–320]

system? Many laboratories would be inclined to say that it is not an error if detected before the report is issued. An error is defined here as any misinformation that is not detected by a laboratory's quality system and is unknowingly reported. This is a phenomenon that is very difficult to measure.

There have been calls for monitoring how often errors do occur.[*] The probability of an error would be very hard to assign, and there are clear practical difficulties. This may have forestalled any large scale effort that could help scientists assign the probability of an error in their case. A more likely explanation is the quite legitimate wish of forensic scientists that whenever an error is found they do not want to count it; rather they want to eliminate the possibility of its future reoccurrence. However we endorse efforts to investigate the occurrence of errors, and this was also called for by the US National Academy of Science report.[323] One reason for such investigation is that all forensic scientists we know are honest, dedicated persons, and any investigation such as this will be used primarily to improve methods.

Despite these barriers there are modern collaborative exercises that take a very responsible approach to assessing the occurrence and source of errors and that make suggestions for their reduction. Parson et al.[324] give the outcome of a very large mitochondrial DNA collaborative exercise. They report 16 errors. Ten of these errors were clerical, two were sample 'mix-ups', one was assigned as contamination and the remainder were assigned as arising from interpretational issues.

The Definition of *Error*

As mentioned earlier, errors can be of several types. Clearly false exclusions (i.e. false negatives) and false inclusions (i.e. false positives) have different consequences.

If we consider false inclusions, there is a small chance that the genotype of a non-donor actually is not excluded. This is the limit of the system, not a laboratory error. A lawyer would rightly call this an error of DNA typing but a laboratory might equally rightly argue that they have done everything correctly and even reported correctly that there is a small chance of an adventitious match.

Errors can also happen anywhere along the process: on the crime scene, in the laboratory (recovery of the material, extraction of the DNA, analysis), when analyzing data or when assessing the results.

The most serious errors would be sample swapping or contamination of the trace. Examples of cases have been reported in the United Kingdom (e.g. the Adam Scott case) and in Australia (e.g. the Jama case[142]). In the Jama case a woman, M, was found unconscious in a toilet cubicle locked from the inside at a nightclub in Doncaster. She had no clear recollection of what had happened. There was no evidence that the accused Mr Jama had been anywhere near this event. Ms M was examined in a crisis care unit and vaginal swabs taken. The doctor had examined a different woman ('B') about 28 hours previously in the same location. B had engaged in sexual activity with Mr Jama. No charges were laid with respect to Ms B. It seems certain that contamination occurred at this crisis care unit.

With eloquent directness,[142] '... DNA evidence was perceived as so powerful ... that none of the filters upon which our system of criminal justice depends to minimize the risk of miscarriage of justice, operated effectively at any stage until a matter of weeks, before Mr Jama's appeal was expected to be heard'.

Indeed, if a scene sample is contaminated with suspect DNA, then the suspect is at great risk. Forensic scientists are aware of these risks and treat them very seriously but complacency, which we have never detected, should be rigorously opposed.

During the Review of DNA Reporting Practices by Victoria Police Forensic Services Division (J. Fraser, J. Buckleton, and P. Gill)[†] directly in the aftermath of the Jama case and other events in

---

[*] Reviewed again in Thompson et al.; see also Chakraborty.[322]

[†] Issues in Gathering, Interpreting and Delivering DNA Evidence Judge Andrew Haesler. Available at: https://njca.com.au/wp-content/uploads/2013/07/Judge-Andrew-Haesler-SC-Issues-in-Gathering-Interpreting-and-Delivering-DNA-Evidence-paper.pdf

Victoria, James Fraser emphasized a continuum of responsibility from crime to court. His view, which we support, is that forensic scientists must operate outside of the bounds of their own laboratories to motivate and ensure high standards of crime examination and sample collection. This applies to cases not directly under the control of the lab. This is a big responsibility and one which labs are not empowered to undertake. However it is the correct solution for the simple reason that the labs are the ones with the correct knowledge to advance standards. We would go further. Lab accreditation should start to extend its remit backward to the scene.

The presence of completely random contamination, from, say, plasticware, in a normal corroborative case is unlikely to lead to a false identification implicating the suspect. This type of contamination may be identified by the negative controls if the contamination is repeated. The same contamination in a database search case, if missed by the controls, could have far more serious consequences, for example implicating a worker in a plastic factory who is on the database or losing considerable manpower on false investigative leads (for example, the so-called phantom of Heilbronn).[325]

The risks of contamination from mortuary or hospital surfaces,[326,327] medical staff,* laboratory consumables,[328,329] scene officers,[330,331] as well as the presence of third party DNA, for example after simulated strangulation,[332] have been discussed. One can put in place strategies to try and limit contamination. However it is not possible to eliminate background DNA. Thus for trace DNA it is of the upmost importance to try and help address activity-level propositions.

Other risks are run whenever judgement is involved. The first steps in DNA interpretation involve examination of an electropherogram. A number of judgments are often made at this stage. There is a valid concern that these judgments may be affected by knowledge of the genotypes of the persons of interest.[333,†] These are errors in observation, recording or decision making that are affected by the state of mind of even the most honest and diligent observer. Observers have been making this warning for some time:

> When you employ the microscope, shake off all prejudice, nor harbour any favourite opinions; for, if you do, 'tis not unlikely fancy will betray you into error, and make you see what you wish to see.[337]

A famous example is the count of human chromosomes. Early visualization techniques were rudimentary and counting was very difficult. In 1912 Hans von Winiwater reported 47 chromosomes in men and 48 in women (the Y chromosome is very small). In 1923 Theophilus Painter confirmed the count of 48 after months of indecision. This was despite his clearest views only showing 46. Despite improvements in the preparation and dyeing of chromosomes in the intervening 30 years, it was not until 1956 that Levan gave the correct count of 46. Levan was a plant biologist and did not 'know' that humans had 48 chromosomes.[13] 'Men generally believe quite freely that which they want to be true'.[338]

Such effects are widely considered in other fields of science, and protocols to deal with them are in place.[316,334,335,339] These protocols include well-known experimental methods such as the double-blind testing mechanism in much medical research. Why not, then, in forensic science? We recommend these subjects as necessary reading for all forensic scientists and recommend they be included in their basic training, as well as the relevant sections on bias, over-interpretation and 'how much should the analyst know' in Inman and Rudin.[175,‡] We therefore strongly recommend that DNA profiles from stains should be assessed blindly (i.e. without looking at the DNA profile of the persons whose DNA is contested).

---

* Lukis Anderson was charged in the death of Monte Sereno millionaire Raveesh Kumra after his DNA was found on the victim's fingernails. This case is the first in the United States where contamination from the paramedics was reported. It is believed that Anderson's DNA was transferred to the crime scene by the paramedics that had picked up Anderson and were at the murder scene a short time later.

† Risinger et al.,[334] Saks et al.[335] and Dror and Hampikian[336] also give a very well-argued examination of the risks of observer effects in forensic science.

‡ For additional comment see also *USA Today*[340] and King.[341]

The American Society of Crime Laboratory Directors/Laboratory Accreditation Board (ASCLD/LAB) have issued Guiding Principles of Professional Responsibility for crime laboratories and forensic scientists.[342] These guidelines are one of many professional codes describing the ethical and professional responsibilities of the forensic scientist. They include the requirement to be independent, impartial, detached and objective.

However knowledge that we are susceptible to observer effects or contextual bias does not guard against them. They appear to be a fundamental feature of the human mind. 'Knowing that you are colour blind does not make you see in colour'. For some years Bryan Found has been successfully experimenting with context management in the document section of the Victorian Police Forensic Services Department in Australia.[200] This is an example we could all emulate.

Other possibilities for error include deliberate or accidental tampering from external persons. The FSS reported 156 security breaches in the year ending June 2002, a 37% decrease from the previous year. The report outlined two of these as examples. They involved theft of property such as computers and credit cards rather than evidence tampering.[343] In our own laboratories the honest boxes with charity sales of, say, chocolate often come up short.

Returning to DNA the most common 'error' of which we are aware is the assumption that a heterozygote is a homozygote because an allele is undetected. We discuss this aspect in Chapter 8, but let us note here that there are models that allow management of this aspect.

Without more data on the occurrence of errors we are left with speculation. The probability of an error is clearly greater than 0. No forensic scientist would claim that it is 0. This is obviously a legitimate avenue for defence examination, and we would recommend that all prosecution witnesses should treat it as a legitimate form of examination and should not react in a hostile or defensive manner.

Combining the Probability of Error with the Conditional Genotype Probability

We come now to the issue of combining the probability of an error and the 'match' probability, p_m. Various models* have been presented that are based on different assumptions and different definitions of errors. If similar assumptions are made, then formulae agree. If the probability of an error (denoted 'e') is larger than the profile probability in the relevant population, it will dominate the equation. In that case, given source level propositions, the LR formula will be approximately equal to 1 divided by the probability of a false positive, denoted 'k' ($LR \approx 1/ke$).

	LR Formula
Buckleton and Triggs	$\dfrac{1-(1-k)e}{p_m(1-e)+ke}$
Thompson et al.	$\dfrac{1}{p_m+ke(1-p_m)}$
Weir	$\dfrac{1-ke}{p_m(1-2ke)+ke}$

We note that the above-mentioned work has been done considering source-level propositions. Because this will not generally be the real issue for the court, we would like to explore what would be the effect of errors if one considers activity-level propositions. We will illustrate our approach with a simple example but fully acknowledge that situations can become more complex depending on the circumstances and on the propositions. In that instance we recommend the analysis of the given case with Bayesian networks as advocated in Taroni et al.[346]

---

* Hagermann,[344] Weir,[345] Thompson et al. (see Ref. 316 for a review), Balding,[277] as well as Triggs and Buckleton[98].

Model from Buckleton and Hicks

We believe that laypersons will have difficulties going from source-level propositions to activity-level propositions, except in very simple cases where a large amount of blood or semen from a single source is recovered. In these situations there is generally no need for specialized knowledge regarding transfer of DNA. However, with trace DNA, transfer mechanisms, persistence and background levels of the material may have a significant impact on the understanding of the alleged activities and require expert knowledge. Clearly this is an expert matter and should be tackled by forensic scientists.

Let us imagine a scenario where a car is stolen in order to commit a crime. Shortly after the crime, the car is recovered and DNA is found on the rear vision mirror. Mr A is arrested; he says he has nothing to do with the incident and that he has never been in this car. The propositions in that case would be 'Mr A stole/drove the car' versus 'he had nothing to do with the incident'.[*] The DNA results are that the single profile recovered from the rear vision mirror corresponds to Mr A's profile.

In its most brutal form, and ignoring some small terms, we need the following:

F: The event that the same source DNA is falsely excluded by, say, false exclusionary allele calls or heterozygote balance calls

C: The event that DNA came from Mr A by error, say, contamination (by the police or the real offender)

D: The event that DNA came from someone other than Mr A by error, say, contamination

f: The probability that the same source DNA is falsely excluded by, say, false exclusionary allele calls or heterozygote balance calls

c: The probability that DNA came from Mr A by error, say, contamination (by the police or the real offender)

d: The probability that DNA came from someone other than Mr A by error, say, contamination

p_m: The probability that different source DNA match adventitiously

B_0: The event that there was no DNA present as background

b_0: The probability of no background DNA on the item

B_1: The event that there was one background DNA source present on the item

b_1: The probability of one background DNA source on the item

T: The event that DNA was transferred during the offence

t: The probability that DNA was transferred from the true offender

Given the prosecution's proposition and the information at hand, there is one possibility that dominates the *LR*:

- DNA from Mr A was transferred to the rear mirror (T), there was no false exclusion (not F), there was no DNA present as background (B_0) and there was no contamination from someone else (not D).

- Here we discard the possibility that there is no transfer while stealing the car (not T) and that either there was no contamination at all (not C and not D) but background (B_1) that happened to match (p_m) or that there was a contamination from Mr A (C)

---

[*] Note that here offence and activity level propositions are very close.

that matched, no contamination from someone else (not D) and no background (B$_0$) or there was no contamination from Mr A (not C), contamination from someone else (D) that happened to match adventitiously and no background (B$_0$).

If Mr A has not stolen the car and we observe a match, then this means that there was no false exclusion (not F). There are then three possibilities:

1. There was no transfer of DNA from the real offender (not T), there was no background (B$_0$) and there was a contamination (C, either from the laboratory or by secondary/tertiary transfer from the offender or the owner of the car) and it is a true positive with a probability of approximately 1.

2. There was transfer from the real offender (T), the true unknown offender happened to have to have the same profile as Mr A adventitiously (p_m) and there was no background (B$_0$).

3. There was no transfer from the real offender (not T), there was no background (B$_0$), there was contamination from someone else (D) who happened to have the same profile (p_m) or there was background that happened to have the same profile (p_m) and there was no transfer from the real offender (not T).

These different possibilities are illustrated in Figure 2.1, and the LR formula can be written as follows:

$$LR \approx \frac{tb_0(1-d)(1-f)}{\left[(1-t)b_0c+tb_0p_m+(1-t)(b_0d+b_1)p_m\right](1-f)}$$

$$\approx \frac{1-D}{p_m+\dfrac{(1-t)}{t}\left(c+p_m\left[d+\dfrac{b_1}{b_0}\right]\right)}$$

$$\approx \frac{1}{p_m+e}$$

where $e = \dfrac{(1-t)}{t}\left(c+p_m\left[d+\dfrac{b_1}{b_0}\right]\right)$. It is easy to note that $p_m + e$ must be greater than p_m. If the conditional profile probability is small (e.g. one in a billion), we see that we need to acquire data on transfer and on the possibility of contamination/transfer from Mr A both after the crime (from the laboratory or the police for example) and from the alternative offender during the crime or from the car owner.[347]

In conclusion the probability of an error and the probability of the DNA profile in the relevant population can be mathematically combined, and it is likely that Bayesian networks constructed on a case-specific basis are the most viable option. Depending on the assumptions made and on the model chosen, we will have different LR formulae. However all models show that the probability of an error and the probability of the DNA profile in the relevant population can be mathematically combined. The question is, should they be? The arguments for and against have occurred in the literature (reviewed in Thompson[186] and indeed in court, e.g. *Regina v Galli*[296]). Those making the 'for' argument would comment, correctly, that the jury may not be able to weigh the respective contributions of error and rarity of the profile.[181] Those supporting the 'against' argument would argue that a probability of error cannot be assigned and hence the equation is not implementable. The concept of error relates to many things. The arguments given above are phrased largely in the context of a single reference sample and a single stain. In many cases there are multiple traces collected and perhaps typed at differing times.

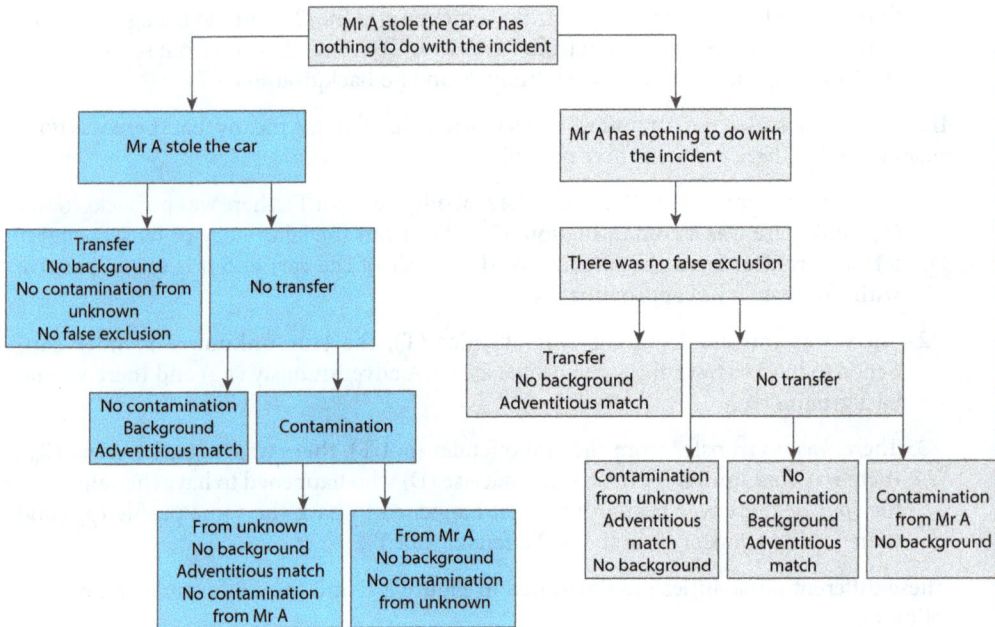

Figure 2.1   The different possibilities for explaining the findings given both activity propositions taking into account errors. Given the prosecution's proposition, in our formula we have omitted the situation where there is no transfer.

All of this would affect the probability of an error and that subset of errors that represent false inclusions. Lynch[348] makes the interesting point that eyewitness evidence is known to be fallible. Juries have been asked to evaluate this 'eye witness' risk on a case-by-case basis for a long time, and no explicit combination is made of the probability of error with the weight of evidence. Of course eyewitness evidence is not presented numerically at all, and this may be a fundamental difference.

Our view is that the possibility of error should be examined on a per-case basis and is always a legitimate defence explanation for the DNA result. The two possible propositions that are consistent with innocence should be explored. Depending on the case, this can be done by the court or jury. However, because the jury may be unable to weigh the two propositions consistent with innocence (one information presented numerically and the other not) and may give undue weight to the match probability, it is important that professional help be available to combine these elements.

Let us assume that we intend to develop a case-specific assignment of the probability of an error as Thompson suggests:

> … it makes little sense to present a single number derived from proficiency tests as *the* error rate in every case, … I suggest that it be evaluated case-by-case according to the adequacy of its scientific foundation and its helpfulness to the jury.[186]

The innocent person who has been implicated by an error or indeed by a coincidental match is at great risk of a false conviction. The Thompson et al. formula or any of the other options, if applied, may very occasionally help such a person. In effect the formula reduces the *LR*, and it may do so to the point where a jury will not convict depending on the other elements of the case. The reality, in our view, is that most often the wrongly implicated persons will almost have to prove their innocence by establishing that an error *has* happened or to produce very strong alibi evidence. Unless the wrongly accused can produce considerable evidence in their favour, it is possible or even likely that they will be convicted. However there is very little that statistics can do to help. The reduction of the *LR* affects both the correctly accused and the wrongly accused equally. We suspect that it is of some but probably inadequate help to the wrongly accused persons and a false benefit to the correctly accused. The answer lies, in our mind, in a rational examination of errors and the constant search to eliminate them. The forensic community would almost universally agree with this.

Findlay and Grix[197] make the reasonable point that the very respect given to DNA evidence by juries places an obligation on scientists to maintain the highest standards and to honestly explain the limitations of the science in court.

Language

In this section we take a lead from the article 'The biasing influence of linguistic variations in DNA profiling evidence'.[349] These authors use the *R v Aytugrul* case as an example. Without drowning the reader in detail, assume that the match probability for a mitochondrial match* for this case was assigned as 1 in 1680. This value was contrasted with a 99.9% exclusion rate. The authors also mention that this statistic could be given as 10 in 16,800. They make the reasonable case that these three versions could produce very different impressions.

We take this on board. Factually equivalent statements can have different impacts and hence are not equivalent in that sense.

We have also often heard phrases along the lines of 'the suspect's alleles are in the mixture' or even still when referring to a mixture 'my man is in there'. These are not appropriate phrases.

We would like to end this section with an appeal for higher standards of the already considerable impartiality in forensic laboratories. We recommend that all forensic scientists read the account by the father of the victim of a miscarriage caused by wrongful fingerprint evidence[350] or the call for standards by Forrest in his review of the Sally Clark case.[351] Most forensic scientists aspire to a position of impartiality, but unconscious effects must be constantly opposed. The most obvious way, as demonstrated by Found, is to remove all contextual information unnecessary for the case. In our view language is one tool that can be utilized. The words *suspect* and *offender* have specific meanings but are often used interchangeably. Both should be avoided as they have too many emotional associations: Would you buy a *suspect* car? The preferable term is *Mr* or *Ms*. We also object to the placing of the *suspect's* name in capitals as required by the procedures in some laboratories. Why is it *Detective Smith* but the suspect is termed *Mr JONES*? All emotive terms or terms with unnecessary implications should be avoided, and we are in the process of excising *suspect* from our writing and using POI. Further, we encourage the use of the term *complainant* as opposed to *victim*, the use of which implies a crime has been committed.

The matter is one of culture. Everyone in a laboratory needs to cooperate in developing and supporting the culture of impartiality. This effort should involve practical steps in context management. People lose their life or liberty based on our testimony, and this is a considerable responsibility. In the same line of context we believe that when there is need for specialized knowledge regarding transfer mechanisms, persistence and background, then forensic scientists ought to help the justice system assess the findings given activity-level propositions, taking into account the possibility of the presence of the DNA of the POI for some other reason than the alleged activities.

Omagh

Omagh is a market and administrative town in County Tyrone, Northern Ireland. It is mixed Catholic and Protestant, with a small Catholic majority. On Saturday, 15 August 1998, a car bomb exploded in the town centre, killing 29 people and injuring over 200 others, many seriously and permanently disabled as a result.

---

* There is a small difference between the hair at the scene and the mitochondrial DNA sequence of Mr Aytugrul's buccal swab. This occurs in a c-stretch. Hence the word *match* hides a number of considerations.

The homemade explosive device was based on a commercial fertilizer with the detonator being Semtex. The car was a red Vauxhall Cavalier saloon that had been stolen in Carrick, from across the border in County Louth in the Republic of Ireland. It had been fitted with ringer plates, false plates that tallied with a real car of similar description. The stolen car was stored in a secluded lock-up garage until being driven over the border by two men. The two drivers rendezvoused with a local guide. The plan was to park the car outside the courthouse. Half an hour prior to the planned time of the explosion a warning was to be given to allow evacuation of the area.

However for unknown reasons, possibly panic on the part of the drivers, the car was parked on Market Street some distance from the courthouse.

The first of three warnings was received by Ulster TV, 'Bomb Courthouse Omagh Main Street, 500 lbs explosion 30 minutes', and the code words 'Martha Pope' were given. The police proceeded to clear the area around the courthouse and, by an unfortunate chance, directed many of the evacuees down Market Street. A large number of the diverted people were surrounding the car containing the bomb, actually leaning against the car, or huddled closely around it.

The detonation left a hole 3 feet deep in the road and sent molten shrapnel up to 80 metres away in all directions.[352,353]

Sean Hoey was charged with 58 counts arising from 13 bomb and mortar attacks, attempted attacks or unexploded devices. The prosecution case was based on similarity of construction of the devices, some fibre evidence and DNA evidence in four of the 13 incidents: Lisburn, Armagh and Blackwatertown Road in the 1998 series of events and from the single 1999 incident at Altmore. We concentrate here on the DNA evidence.

DNA profiles matching each other were recovered from unexploded devices recovered from the main street in Lisburn and Altmore Forest. These profiles were obtained in 1999 and 2001 from the underside of tape used in the construction of the devices. The unknown profile obtained was matched to Mr Hoey in September 2003. Although a POI earlier, his sample could not be taken until he crossed the border to Northern Ireland from the south. A further examination of the device planted at Newry Road Barracks was examined in November 2003 and also shown to match Mr Hoey.

Despite being developed at 34 cycles, these profiles are clean and unambiguous requiring neither dropout nor drop-in if they arise from Mr Hoey. The peaks are large and the balance between apparent heterozygotes is not extreme. The profiles appear to be from a single source. This is a useful example that not all 34 cycle work is low template DNA (LTDNA) and not all LTDNA is 34 cycle.

The Omagh bombing itself was not linked by DNA but by similarities in the devices. In 2007 Mr Hoey was acquitted.

In his ruling Mr Justice Weir commented, understandably, on his concerns about sample handling and storage. For example, a scene of crime officer (SOCO) and a Detective Chief Inspector gave evidence of wearing protective clothing at this scene. Photographs taken at the scene suggested this was untrue.*

An email from the Director of Forensic Northern Ireland read, *inter alia*: 'I don't remember touching anything but who knows'.

We are aware of a suggestion that the profile of Mr Hoey, if indeed it was from him at all, had got under the tape because he was an electrician and someone must have used his tape to make the devices.

This case is quite useful to highlight the provenance aspects of LTDNA analysis. Since LTDNA is often latent and it may be difficult or impossible to state what body fluid it is from and when and how it was deposited, there are a number of potential ways that a profile could appear on a given item. We examine this case using a Bayesian approach.

---

* This suggestion was disproved in a subsequent report by the Northern Ireland police ombudsman.[354]

We define the following events:

H_p: Mr Hoey stuck the tape on the device.

H_{d1}: An unknown person stuck the tape on the device; Mr Hoey has never been near the tape.

H_{d2}: An unknown person stuck the tape on the device; Mr Hoey handled the roll of tape previously.

E: There is a single unmixed profile matching Mr Hoey from the underside of the tape.

T: The person who made the device transferred DNA to the underside of the tape, which occurs with probability t.

C: There was contamination of the underside of the tape at the scene or in the lab by DNA from an unknown person (not Mr Hoey), occurring with probability c.

L: There was contamination of the underside of the tape at the scene or in the lab by DNA from Mr Hoey.

A: Mr Hoey transferred DNA to the underside of the tape when he handled the roll of tape previously (action unconnected with manufacture of the device), occurring with probability a.

B_0: There is no background DNA on the underside of the tape, b_0.

B_1: There is one background DNA source on the underside of the tape, b_1.

P: The event that a profile matches Mr Hoey if the DNA is not from him, occurring with probability p.

We assign the probability of the event L as 0 because Mr Hoey's DNA was not present in the lab at the time of the examination.

With three propositions we need to use the general form of Bayes' theorem.

$$\Pr(H_p \mid E) = \frac{\Pr(E \mid H_p)\Pr(H_p)}{\Pr(E \mid H_p)\Pr(H_p) + \Pr(E \mid H_{d1})\Pr(H_{d1}) + \Pr(E \mid H_{d2})\Pr(H_{d2})}$$

Inserting probabilities and ignoring small terms

$$\Pr(H_p \mid E) = \frac{b_0 t(1-c)\Pr(H_p)}{b_0 t(1-c)\Pr(H_p) + \begin{bmatrix} b_0 t p(1-c) \\ +b_0(1-t)cp \\ +b_1(1-t)p(1-c) \end{bmatrix} \Pr(H_{d1}) + b_0(1-t)(1-c)a\Pr(H_{d2})}$$

Assuming $a = 0.05$, $t = 0.5$, $p = 10^{-9}$, $20c = 1 - c$, $b_0 = 20b_1$

$$\Pr(H_p \mid E) = \frac{20\Pr(H_p)}{20\Pr(H_p) + 22\times10^{-9}\Pr(H_{d1}) + \Pr(H_{d2})}$$

Assuming that 22×10^{-9} is sufficient to overwhelm any prior on H_{d1}, we can recover $LR = 20$.

The final LR may be quite surprising, and it has taken us some time to discern why. In brief it is quite hard to get a single unmixed profile corresponding to Mr Hoey under H_{d1}. This suggests that H_{d2} will dominate the consideration given our postulated values and it is the plausibility of this proposition that is crucial.

The Absence of Evidence: Evaluating DNA Findings Given Activity-Level Propositions

Special attention is given in this section to interpreting the 'absence' of evidence. This is necessary largely because of a widespread misunderstanding of the subject despite excellent writing on the matter (see for instance Inman and Rudin[175]). This misunderstanding has been fostered by the clever but false saying, 'The absence of evidence is not evidence of absence'.

One of us, in his youthful folly, used this sentence, which he had been taught, in court. He can recall the impressed look on the lawyers' faces.

In most of this book we will help address sub-source-level propositions, but in order to assess the absence of DNA or any other trace, one needs propositions that are at least at the activity level. Source (or sub-source) propositions do not allow us to assess the absence of findings.

Let us first take an example where the presence of DNA would be very probable given one proposition and its absence very probable given the alternative. Imagine that there is a case where DNA is searched on the POI, Mr Smith, arrested 20 minutes after the alleged event. The prosecution states that he attacked Ms Johnson, who spat several times in the direction of his face and on his t-shirt. Mr Smith says that he has never met Ms Johnson. From the case information, it is known that Mr Smith was arrested in a bar, which he entered a few minutes after the incident and that he has not changed his t-shirt all day. The t-shirt is searched for DNA, and there is only one single profile that corresponds to its owner. Let us call the event of absence of any other profile $\bar{E}$. Bayes' theorem gives us a correct way to interpret this finding.

$$LR = \frac{\Pr(\bar{E} \mid H_p, I)}{\Pr(\bar{E} \mid H_d, I)}$$

The issue then is one of assessing whether the finding of no extraneous DNA was more or less probable given that Ms Johnson spat on Mr Smith than given that Mr Smith and Ms Johnson never met.[*] Unless some very special circumstances pertain, the finding of no DNA will be more probable given the defence's proposition (H_d) than given the prosecution's proposition (H_p), and hence the absence of DNA matching the complainant supports H_d. Often, in real casework, this is only limited support for the defence's proposition. If we take our example, before searching for the DNA, one should assess the probability of finding DNA corresponding to the complainant if she spat on Mr Smith's t-shirt and if they have never met. It is important to think about those transfer probabilities before knowing the results, in order to avoid post hoc rationalization (a term coined by Ian Evett) or so-called bias. One would typically expect to have a table similar to the following:

Event	Probability	Ms Johnson Spat on Mr Smith	Mr Smith Has Never Met Ms Johnson
No transfer	t_0	0.1	NA
Transfer of DNA	t	0.9	NA

These probabilities need to be based on published data, knowledge or/and data experiments. Let us imagine here that experiments have been done simulating the actions alleged and that the expert has assigned the above probabilities before looking at the garments.

---

[*] In the case information in our statement, we would describe what the alleged activities are and give the relevant information, such as timing. In the context of the case the two propositions are mutually exclusive and exhaustive.

In order to evaluate the absence of DNA corresponding to the complainant, one needs to assign the probability of this finding given the two propositions. If Ms Johnson spat on Mr Smith, then there was no transfer of DNA or/and it was not recovered. We can denote this probability by t_0. If Mr Smith has never met Ms Johnson, then what is the probability of recovering no extraneous DNA or no DNA present as background? We expect that the probability is high, but it is not 1.

In that case our LR would simply be t_0 (denoting the probability of transfer given the prosecution's proposition). Indeed the factor b_0 (denoting the probability of recovering background DNA or DNA present for unknown reasons) appears both in the numerator and denominator and thus is cancelled.

In that fictitious case our LR would be as follows:

$$LR = \frac{Pr(\bar{E}\,|\,H_p,I)}{Pr(\bar{E}\,|\,H_d,I)}$$

$$= \frac{t_0 b_0}{b_0}$$

$$= 0.1$$

Our findings (no DNA other than DNA corresponding to the profile of the t-shirt owner) would therefore be about 10 times more probable given the information and the proposition that Mr Smith never met Ms Johnson than given the proposition that Ms Johnson spat on Mr Smith. Therefore the findings provide limited support for the defence proposition compared to the defence's.

This (correct) mathematical argument is not accepted by many forensic scientists and lawyers but is universally accepted by interpretation specialists. The counter argument is that one can often think of an explanation for the absence of evidence. However we can also think of explanations for a DNA correspondence (as an explanation we could say that the DNA came from the unknown twin of the POI). One should remember that in order to assess our findings we need propositions, not explanations (as the probability of the results given an explanation is always 1; see for example Ref. 355).

Another example we can imagine is that that a fight has occurred where one person was stabbed and bled extensively. A suspect is found and no blood is found on his clothing. How is this to be interpreted? Many forensic scientists will observe that the suspect may have changed or washed his clothes or that contact may have been slight in the first place. These observations are correct but are more along the lines of explanations of the (lack of) evidence. As evaluators, we should look at this problem from the point of view of propositions. What is the probability that the suspect would have blood on him *if* he were the offender? Let us imagine that we do not know whether or not the suspect has changed or washed his clothes. Further let us imagine that we have some information about the fight but that it is inexact or unreliable. From this we must accept that it is uncertain whether we expect to find blood on the clothing or not, even if the suspect is, indeed, the offender. However we must feel that this probability is not 0. There must have been some probability that we would find blood on the clothing; why else were we searching for it? Only if this probability is 0 is the evidence neutral (if the probability of recovering blood is 0, then the probability of not recovering blood is 1, and our LR is 1). Otherwise the absence of blood will support the defence proposition.

Clearly this area is not well understood, nor is there widespread agreement. Further discussion in the literature would be most welcome on how to assign the value of DNA findings given activity-level propositions.[356,357] Research on transfer and persistence of DNA as well as presence of extraneous DNA is also seen to be of great importance.

Why Did We Ever Decide to Be Conservative?

Throughout this book we will occasionally use the word *conservative*. This is a word in very common usage in forensic DNA interpretation. It is used in a tone that gives the impression of approval. Its most common usage is to describe a numerical statistic or action that lowers the expression of the weight of evidence. One usage of the word *conservative* describes a method as being more conservative than another if it, for example, gives a lower *LR*.

We cannot remember how the use of this word started. It may predate DNA. The early usages of the word were often describing workarounds where we could not assign some value or probability well but felt we could at the least give some sort of lower bound. Over time it has been elevated from describing an often inefficient but pragmatic choice to a principle. It is sometimes taught as the principle of conservatism. The word *principle*, in science, usually relates to a theory that has been very thoroughly established.

We feel that this concept has become endowed with a respect that it does not deserve and that it needs to be put back in its place.

When thinking about how this situation has developed, we can identify a number of causative factors. These could start from the very power of DNA. Because DNA evidence is so powerful, no one objects if the assignment of weight is lowered a little. The next factor we would add is that lowering the expression of the weight of evidence is usually, but not always, in favour of the defendant. However this is not the end of the matter. We add the following factors:

1. There are genuine uncertainties in the interpretation process.

2. There is a reasonable aversion to very complex solutions.

3. There are limited resources for training and research.

Taken collectively these factors lead to a force along the lines of 'if in doubt go to the lowest option'.

Consider a relatively simple form of evidence such as a single source profile of good template matching a POI. If this is interpreted using the equations of Balding and Nichols,[358] then we believe that there will be a strong tendency to underestimate the match probability. It is likely we have used a value for the co-ancestry coefficient at the top end of the plausible range. We may have added two copies of the POI's profile to the database, a minimum allele probability or an estimate of sampling uncertainty. We have no very firm idea how far under the median estimate this number might be.

This is only part of the story. In a more complex case a few or many loci may not have been used in the interpretation. Consider the portion of a profile shown in Figure 2.2. Under common CPI practice in the United States, the locus D21S11 cannot be used in the calculation since the 31 peak at height 102 rfu is between the analytical threshold (100 in this case) and the stochastic threshold (ST) (250 in this case). This is accepted because 'it is conservative'. In this case the known ground truth contributor to the minor is 28,31. Indeed omitting this locus is probably conservative in this case, although the 28 peak is rather small.

Now please change the POI from 28,31 to 30,31 or 31,31 or 31,32. Are you still sure omitting this locus is conservative? Please change the POI again to 32,33. Now we can be confident of an exclusion, and indeed most labs would use this locus now for exclusionary purposes.

The result of such behaviours is that the statistic we offer in court may have only a distant relationship to a reasonable assignment of the weight of evidence.

We feel that conservatism could be used when there is genuine doubt. However it is not a principle. It is often a rather shoddy action to avoid up-skilling or investment. There are much higher and better goals than conservatism to which we should subscribe.

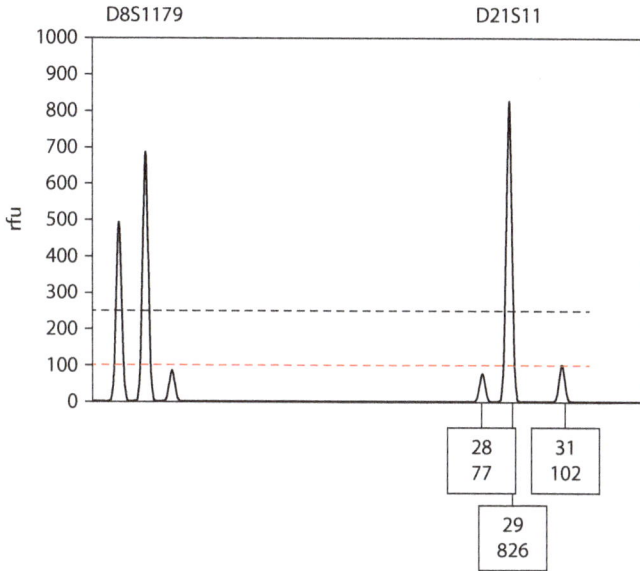

Figure 2.2   Stylized electropherogram showing two loci.

Summary

This chapter has reviewed options for a framework for interpretation. The subsequent chapters will focus on details of DNA interpretation. It is, however, very important to understand this fundamental structure for interpretation before proceeding to detailed analysis. In particular a number of principles for the interpretation of forensic evidence have been advanced and largely accepted.[257] An extension of the earlier work by Evett and Weir, Berger et al.[198] offered principles for interpretation that have appeared scattered about the text. We gather them together in Appendix 2.1.

Additional Reading

Inman and Rudin[175] give an elegant discussion of many aspects of evidence interpretation. This book would serve very well as part of all training courses in forensic science.

Robertson and Vignaux[222,359] consider both the legal concerns regarding this type of analysis and more specifically the situation where the evidence itself is both multiple and uncertain. This is a level of complexity above and beyond anything considered in this chapter. They also introduce the useful concept of Bayesian networks that are being extensively researched as a tool for forensic interpretation.

Appendix 2.1: Principles and Standards of Forensic Interpretation

We label principles P_1 ... and standards S_1 ...

Personnel
Qualifications

All personnel shall have a relevant tertiary qualification.

Training

1. The training requirements shall be documented.

2. The training shall include the following:

   a. The laws of probability

   b. The different expectations of the investigative and evaluative stages; understanding the different forms of opinion, their strengths and limitations

   c. The hierarchy of propositions

   d. The concept of pre-assessment

   e. Evaluation of findings and reporting of conclusions

      i. Development of likelihood ratio (LR) formulae given at source- and activity-level propositions

      ii. An understanding of how to take into account case circumstances when assessing the results

      iii. Use and relevance of databases

      iv. Conclusion scales used and their justification

      v. A critical appraisal of other conclusion scales reported in the literature

      vi. An understanding of the transposed conditional and how to avoid it

      vii. Legal issues relevant to jurisdiction

3. Each area of instruction shall have documented objective(s) and a formal assessment of the trainee's competency (e.g. written test, practical test and/or oral test).

4. A training record shall be kept for each trainee.

5. Access to relevant texts, journals and other professional literature is required for training.

6. The effectiveness of the training shall be evaluated.

7. It is recommended that professional development/continuing education is available to fully trained examiners.

Requirements for the Trainers

1. The principal trainer shall have been qualified in the relevant field for three years and have received training in teaching.

2. The principal trainer may establish objectives for each module of the training programme and have overall responsibility for the quality of the training delivered.

3. The suitability of other trainers shall be approved by the principal trainer.

S1: To help address investigative issues, an examiner generally offers opinions in the form of explanations or, if prior information and expert knowledge are taken into account, in the form of posterior probabilities for explanations.[215]

S2: To help address evaluative issues, an examiner would have a pair of clearly stated propositions and consider the probability of the findings given each of the propositions. The opinion expressed would reflect the ratio of those two probabilities (the LR).

There are limitations to both investigative and evaluative opinions, and these should be made clear at the outset:

1. Explanations are not necessarily exhaustive.

2. Posterior probabilities for explanations depend crucially on the examiner generating, prior to making observations, all feasible hypotheses and assigning to them realistic, reliable prior probabilities. Robust assignment of probabilities for the observations is a further prerequisite for such opinions.

3. *LRs* require, first, consideration of propositions that are based on the case circumstances and the competing allegations and, second, reliable and valid assignment of probabilities for the observations.

There is a further type of opinion, that of an 'exclusion'. This type of opinion, if deductive in nature, is acceptable.

All efforts should be made to ensure the following:

1. The issues in the case have been clearly identified.

2. The potential contribution of DNA examination has been assessed.

3. There is an understanding of the limitations of the opinions that may be offered.

This process should be documented on the case file or, if a general approach is more appropriate for some elements of the process, in the overall service-level agreement.

Reaching a Conclusion for DNA Comparisons

Conclusions can take various forms but, for the purposes of this document, only those conclusions that are in the form of opinions will be considered here. It has already been noted the opinions fall generally into three different types: explanations, posterior probabilities and *LRs*.

S3: Whichever type of opinion is offered, there should be full documentation of how the examiner arrived at that opinion, including references to any data that may have been used in arriving at the opinion.

Opinions and Interpretations

S4: The conclusions in the report that are opinions shall be clearly identified as such.

S5: The process by which examiners reach an opinion for an examination and the factors taken into account shall be clearly documented.

S6: The opinions that are offered shall flow from the issues previously identified and agreed.

When opinions in the form of *LRs* are given, the following requirements shall apply:

P1: The interpretation of scientific findings invokes reasoning in the face of uncertainty. Probability theory provides the only coherent logical foundation for such reasoning.

P2: All probabilities are *conditional*. To assign a probability for the truth of a proposition, one needs information. Interpretation must therefore be carried out within a framework of circumstances. It is necessary for the scientist to make clear any understanding of those aspects of the circumstances that are relevant to the evaluation.

P3: Scientific findings must be interpreted within a framework of relevant circumstances (I).

S7: Any information used to form the propositions or assess probabilities shall be stated in the report.

S8: Information not required for the formation of propositions or the assessment of probabilities shall not be made available to anyone forming or checking an evaluative opinion.

P4: Scientific evidence can only be interpreted by considering at least two propositions.

S9: The propositions shall be clearly stated in the report.

P5: Scientists ought to address questions of the kind 'what is the probability of the results given the proposition?' and it is the court that ought to address questions regarding the veracity of a proposition.

It is likely that the prosecution have formed their hypothesis and this is often known to the forensic scientist. It is unlikely that the defence will have formed their hypothesis and there is no requirement for them to do so. Under these circumstances we would offer the following as guiding principles:

P5: The prosecution are entitled to set their hypothesis.

P6: There is no requirement for the defence to set or disclose their hypothesis. From the case information, the forensic scientist should select a reasonable proposition consistent with exoneration. If this proves to be a poor choice subsequently, the analysis should be redone. In the report it will be made clear why and how the alternative was chosen.

The probability of the findings under each of the propositions should be assigned through the expert, intelligent use of relevant data, experience and knowledge.

S10: The information used to form the probabilities shall appear in the report. Those probabilities formed from data and those formed from judgement or experience shall be outlined.

a. The report shall explain the competing propositions considered and justification for the expert's assignment of probabilities.

b. The interpretation scale used to report LRs shall be documented.

c. The conclusion(s) should be carefully worded to convey the appropriate evidential value of the comparison.

d. Any conclusion scale chosen should be based on logical principles and avoid the fallacy of the transposed conditional.

   i. If opinions in the form of explanations are given, there shall be documentation of why those, and only those, explanations have been offered.

   ii. If opinions in the form of posterior probabilities for explanations are given, there shall be explicit justification of the choice of initial propositions, their prior probabilities and the probabilities for obtaining the evidence (the outcome of the comparison process).

   iii. The report shall document the basis upon which the opinion is made. If data have been used to assist in reaching a conclusion regarding the significance of a comparison, then reference to these data shall be made in the report.

   iv. The examiner shall be able to explain clearly the interpretation framework used, for example when presenting evidence in court.

   v. In the statement it will be noted that the evaluation is valid given the information at hand and that should this information change the conclusions will need to be re-evaluated.

3

Population Genetic Models

John S. Buckleton, Duncan Taylor,
James M. Curran and Jo-Anne Bright

Contents

Introduction

This section will discuss those population genetic models used for assigning a profile or preferably a match probability. Three models – the product rule and two variants of the subpopulation correction – will be discussed.

The interpretation of DNA evidence often requires the assignment of a probability to the event of observing a second copy of a particular genotype in a certain population, termed the *match probability*. Implicit in this apparently simple statement are many questions about what this probability should be, how it should be assessed and upon what other information, if any, it should be conditioned.

In common usage the word *frequency* is often substituted for *probability*. This usage is sufficiently common that there has come to exist a frequentist view of probability. Using an example we have already discussed consider a drawing pin (thumbtack). When tossed it may end up point up (U) or point down (D). Suppose we toss it 10 times and obtain UUDUDUUUUU, which we denote as *x*. Note that there are 8 Us and 2 Ds. You are about to throw it the 11th time. What is your probability for U? The frequency of U in the 10 tosses was 0.8, so that may inform your probability for a U on the 11th toss. This example can be used to define a frequency in a series of 10 known outcomes and a probability, which is a statement about an uncertain event. Let us imagine that you feel that the probability of a U on the 11th toss given the data on the 10 tosses is 0.8. Is it reasonable to pass from a frequency to a probability in this way? The matter is not quite that straightforward.

First consider what we would do if there had only been one toss of the drawing pin in our database, *x*. This was a U. Would we feel comfortable assigning a probability for U of 1? Presumably we do feel that there is some probability of the drawing pin landing point downwards. If 10 is enough and 1 is not, then where do we pass from insufficient to sufficient?

Next please substitute the drawing pin for a coin that appears to be a perfectly normal coin. Again we have tossed it 10 times and obtained eight heads and two tails. What is the probability that the 11th toss will result in a head? We would say 0.5. Why? In fact it would take a rather immense amount of data to move us from our belief in 0.5.

These two thought experiments help us conceptualize that a match probability is a statement made about an uncertain event that may in part be informed by the frequency of certain things, usually alleles in a database. However, this match probability is not a match frequency.

We take the following hypotheses:

H_p: The DNA came from the suspect.

H_d: The DNA came from a male not related to the suspect.

Taking the logical approach for these hypotheses, the likelihood ratio (*LR*) can be determined as follows:

$$LR = \frac{1}{\Pr(G_c \mid G_s, H_d)} = \frac{1}{f} \tag{3.1}$$

In the equation above we have substituted $\Pr(G_c \mid G_s, H_p) = 1$ in the numerator of the *LR* as we are assuming G_c is a complete and unambiguous profile that matches G_s.

Modern DNA multiplexes are capable of developing a profile of human DNA at more than 20 loci. Forensic evidence associated with a match of DNA from a scene and a person of interest is usually presented with an associated assessment of the weight of evidence. This weight of evidence may be expressed using the assigned match probability in the simplest of scenarios.

Match probabilities for single source matches at 20 loci are often very small, often smaller than 10^{-12} and may be described as *microprobabilities*, although that might have implied 10^{-6}. As a rough rule of thumb each additional short tandem repeat (STR) locus will provide an order of magnitude in the discriminating power of a profile.

The reader may have noted the use of the word *assigned* associated with the match probability. It is not currently possible to directly estimate multilocus match probabilities by direct sampling. In any sample of practical size it is likely that a genotype at multiple loci will be unobserved.

Probabilities such as 1 in 10^{21} are assigned (as opposed to estimated) using a population genetic model and empirical allele frequencies. The word *assigned* refers to the subjectivity associated with the choice of model, the choice of certain parameters in the model and the choice of sample to provide the allele probability estimates. Most notably the inbreeding coefficient, θ, is not typically an input at its most likely value but at some value believed to be at the upper end of its plausible distribution. This is necessary because, if we were truly attempting to estimate the probability, we would integrate over a distribution of values for θ. The result of this integration is difficult to predict, but using the most likely value for θ will result in an underestimate. To avoid the mechanics of this integration a plug-in value at the upper tail of plausible values is assigned.

DNA microprobabilities produced by these models are currently untestable. We have some confidence in them in that portions of the modelling process can be, and have been, tested. In the early days of forensic modelling the core assumptions were Hardy–Weinberg and linkage equilibrium, collectively termed the *product rule*. These were examined by independence testing.[360,361] However, it was soon realized that independence testing on the datasets available did not have the power to find departures from independence of the size that was plausible for human populations.[362-364] The product rule itself has largely been replaced by a model based on the *Second National Research Council report on forensic DNA evidence* (NRC II) Recommendation 4.1 in the United States and *NRC II* Recommendation 4.2 in Europe and Australasia.[176]

The next phase of testing involved simulating plausible population genetic effects and assessing their impact.[365,366]

Following the development of substantial databases, Weir[367] suggested testing the observed number of near matches against their expectations under the population genetic models. This allowed direct empirical testing of probability assignments out to approximately 1 in 10^{10}. This testing has found the assignments using *NRC II* Recommendation 4.2 to be reasonable[368-371] or unreasonable,[372] depending on the author. *Reasonable* is the correct conclusion.

However most commentators would agree that the inputs into the assignment process have some uncertainty associated with them and that although there may be a body of work that suggests that they are reasonable, it would be improper to suggest that they were exact in some way.

A probability depends on the question being asked. If we seek to model the probability that an unrelated person would have a matching profile, we would obtain one answer. If we seek to model the probability that a sibling would have a matching profile, we would obtain a different answer. In real casework, relatives will be alternative suspects to greater or lesser extents. There is no need for there to be any direct evidence pointing towards a relative for them to be a plausible alternative donor. Their mere existence in a pool of approximately equally likely alternatives has a very considerable effect.[373]

We are left with the situation where an analyst testifying in court may have in his or her file one or a few probability assignments for, say, unrelated persons, siblings and various ethnic databases. These assignments may have been produced using one population model in the United States and Canada and another in Europe and Australasia. Sampling uncertainty may or may not have been estimated. These probability assignments, at least for the unrelated hypothesis, may be a microprobability.

The assignment of a probability to a multilocus genotype is an unusual activity. Few other fields of science require such a probability assignment. The field of genetics is well established but largely concerns itself with things such as allele probabilities or genotype probabilities at one or a very few loci. Therefore the attempt by forensic scientists to assign probabilities to a second copy of a multilocus genotype is a relatively novel experiment peculiar to forensic science. It may be based on genetics and statistics, but it is a new extension of previous methods.

These probabilities cannot be directly measured by any mechanism that we can envisage. Ian Evett has discussed his view of whether these probabilities can be considered estimates at all:

> Probability is a personal statement of uncertainty. In the DNA context, I take some numbers (that are estimates of things like allele proportions and F_{ST}) and stick them into a formula. Out comes a number and on the basis of that I assign … a probability. That is a personal, subjective probability,

which incorporates a set of beliefs with regard to the reliability/robustness of the underlying model. So, whenever you talk about estimating a probability, I would talk about assigning a probability.

Thus I would not say, as you do … that the probabilities are 'untestable estimates'. I would ask – 'is it rational for me to assign such a small match probability?'

Evett

In this chapter the options currently in use to assign these genotype probabilities are discussed.

Product Rule

This is the simplest of the available population genetic models. It is deterministic as opposed to stochastic.[374] This means that it assumes that the populations are large enough that random effects can be ignored. It was the first model implemented in forensic DNA analysis, having previously been used for a number of years in blood group analysis. It is based on the Hardy–Weinberg law and the concept of linkage equilibrium.[375,376] Both of these concepts have been extensively discussed. However it is worthwhile making a few comments that are specifically relevant to forensic science.

Hardy–Weinberg Law

This concept was first published in 1908 by Hardy and Weinberg, not Dr Hardy-Weinberg as put by an independent analyst in Australia.[377,378] Simpler versions had been published previously.[379-381] This thinking developed naturally following the rediscovery of Mendel's work.[382] It concerns the relationship between allele probabilities and genotype probabilities at one locus. In essence the Hardy–Weinberg law is a statement of independence between alleles at one locus.

The Hardy–Weinberg law states that the single locus genotype frequency may be assigned as the product of allele probabilities

$$P_i = \begin{cases} p_{i1}^2, & A_{i1} = A_{i2} \\ 2p_{i1}p_{i2}, & A_{i1} \neq A_{i2} \end{cases} \tag{3.2}$$

for alleles A_{i1}, A_{i2} at locus i.

This will be familiar to most in the form

$$\begin{cases} p^2 & \text{homozygotes} \\ 2pq & \text{heterozygotes} \end{cases}$$

This law will be exactly true in all generations after the first if a number of assumptions are met. It may also be true or approximately true under some circumstances if these assumptions are not met. The fact that the equilibrium genotype frequencies are obtained after one generation of random mating means that we do not need to inquire into the deep history of a population to describe the genotype frequencies at one locus[374] if these requirements are met. It also means that any perturbation from equilibrium is likely to be rectified rapidly. The assumptions are not exactly true for populations with overlapping generations, such as humans, where equilibrium is achieved asymptotically as the parental population dies. A few other exceptions to the rule that equilibrium is achieved in one generation are given in standard population genetic texts such as Crow and Kimura.[374]

The assumptions that make the Hardy–Weinberg law true are that the population is infinite and randomly mating and that there are no disturbing forces. Inherent in this law is the assumption of independence between genotypes. Specifically the knowledge of the genotype of one member of a mating pair gives no information about the genotype of the other. The assumption of random mating assumes that the method of selection of mates does not induce dependence between genotypes. This is often translated comically and falsely along the lines 'I did not ask my spouse his/her genotype before I proposed'. When the assumption of random mating is questioned, no one is suggesting that people who are genotype *ab* deliberately go and seek partners who are type *cd*. What is suggested is that geography, religion or some other socio-economic factors induce dependence. This subject will be discussed later but the most obvious potential factor is that the population is, or more importantly has been in the past, divided into groups that breed more within themselves than with other groups.

A consequence of the assumption of an infinite population and random mating is that the allele proportions are expected to remain constant from one generation to the next. If the population is infinite and randomly mating and the allele proportions do not change, then the Hardy–Weinberg law will hold in all generations after the first. This is true whether or not the Hardy–Weinberg law holds in the first generation, the parental one. It therefore describes an equilibrium situation that is maintained indefinitely after the first generation. Note that it does take one generation of random mating to achieve this state. Such a stable state would describe an equilibrium situation and hence this state is often called *Hardy–Weinberg equilibrium* (HWE).

There are, however, a number of factors that can change allele proportions. These are referred to as *disturbing forces*. The term is derived from the fact that they change genotype proportions from those postulated by HWE. These factors include selection, migration and mutation. There are comprehensive texts available describing the effect of these forces on both allele proportions and on HWE, and they will not be discussed at length here. In this chapter we will simply consider how close the Hardy–Weinberg assumptions are to being fulfilled and what the probable consequences of any failure of these assumptions may be. Remember a model may be useful even though it is not an exact description of the real world.

Linkage and Linkage Equilibrium

HWE describes a state of independence between alleles at one locus. *Linkage equilibrium* describes a state of independence between alleles at different loci.

The same set of assumptions that gives rise to HWE plus an additional requirement that an infinite number of generations has elapsed also lead to linkage equilibrium. This result was generalized to three loci by Geiringer[383] and more generally to any number of loci by Bennett.[384]

However, recall that HWE is achieved in one generation of random mating. Linkage equilibrium is not achieved as quickly. Strictly the state of equilibrium is approached asymptotically but is not achieved until an infinite number of generations have elapsed. However, the distance from equilibrium is halved with every generation of random mating for unlinked loci, or by a factor of $1 - r$, where r is the recombination fraction for linked loci. Population subdivision slows this process.[385]

It is worthwhile discussing the difference between linkage equilibrium and linkage, as there is an element of confusion about this subject among forensic scientists. Linkage is a genetic phenomenon and describes the situation where one of Mendel's laws breaks down. It was discovered in 1911 by Morgan,[386,387] working on *Drosophila*. The discovery was a by-product of his team's studies of inheritance that had largely led to the confirmation of the chromosomal theory of inheritance. The first paper on gene mapping appeared in 1913.[388]

Specifically the phenomenon of linkage describes when alleles are not passed independently to the next generation. The physical reason for this phenomenon had been identified by 1911 and related to the non-independent segregation of alleles that are sufficiently close on the same chromosome.[389]

The state of linkage can be described by the recombination fraction or by the distance between two loci. Typical data for distance may be expressed in centiMorgans (cM) or in physical distance in bases. It is a commonly held belief that a distance of 50 cM is sufficient to assure independence. However, the relationship between physical distance and recombination is not linear and a distance of 50 cM does not equate to a recombination fraction of 50%.[52,53] The physical distance may be converted to a recombination fraction by standard formulae (see Chapter 1). Recombination fractions tend to be different for each sex. Distances may be given separately or sex-averaged.

It seems likely that linkage disequilibrium varies among populations and across the genome. A range of 10–30 kb for linkage disequilibrium that is useful for association mapping has been suggested[390] for the extensively studied northern European populations and less in African populations. Of course linkage disequilibrium does not end abruptly at some distance but tends to fade away with distance. The ability to detect it is also, obviously, dependent on the sample size.

Table 1.1 contains a list of linked loci found within common multiplexes and their genetic and physical distance. These loci are orders of magnitude more separated than those typically found in linkage disequilibrium caused by linkage.

Linkage disequilibrium is a state describing the relationship between alleles at different loci. It is worthwhile pointing out that linkage disequilibrium can be caused by linkage or by other population genetic effects such as population subdivision. These two causes for linkage disequilibrium need to be considered and dealt with statistically, in different ways. This will be demonstrated later.

It is therefore incorrect to advance the following line of logic:

A. The loci are on different chromosomes or are well separated on the same chromosome.

Statement A implies the following:

B. There is no linkage.

Statement B in turn implies the following:

C. There is no linkage disequilibrium.

Modern genetic understanding would state that the progression from statement A to statement B is logical and grounded on experimental observation. However, the progression from statement B to statement C is not supportable without additional data.

We actually meet the argument most often in reverse. That is, these loci are linked; therefore it is not possible to calculate any statistic in the case we are discussing. This is also false.

The most likely causes of linkage disequilibrium for unlinked or loosely linked loci are population genetic effects such as population subdivision or admixture.[385,391] These effects will be discussed in some detail later.

If the population is in linkage equilibrium, then a multilocus genotype probability (P) may be assigned by the product of single locus genotype probabilities (P_i).

$$P = \prod_i P_i \qquad (3.3)$$

Consideration of the Hardy–Weinberg and Linkage Equilibrium Assumptions

There are five assumptions for the Hardy–Weinberg law to hold and one additional assumption for linkage equilibrium to hold. In this section each of these assumptions will be considered with regard to whether or not they are true and in particular to how far from true they may be.

Infinite Population

This assumption is clearly violated to greater or lesser extents depending on the size of the population. In addition there is ample evidence for the existence of population bottlenecks in the past. The effect on disturbing the equilibrium in the present is likely to be very limited for most realistic populations unless a relatively recent bottleneck is suspected. Recall that one generation of random mating is sufficient to restore HWE. A finite population size is going to have the greatest effect on the frequencies of rare alleles.

Crow and Kimura[374] give the following:

$$\Pr(A_i A_i) = p_i^2 - p_i(1 - p_i)f$$

$$\Pr(A_i A_j) = 2 p_i p_j (1 + f)$$

where N is the number of individuals and $f = \dfrac{1}{2N - 1}$. We see that any departure from equilibrium is expected to be very small for most realistic values of N.

No Mutation

One of the assumptions for Hardy–Weinberg and linkage equilibrium is that there is no mutation at the loci in question. With regard to the commonly used STR loci this assumption is clearly violated. In fact we believe that the STR loci are mutational 'hot spots' with mutation rates above much of the coding DNA but probably less than the VNTR loci or mitochondrial DNA.

Various treatments have been offered that deal with change in allele frequencies due to mutation or to the effects of mutation and selection.[258] If, however, we accept that these loci are selectively neutral, then the most realistic situation that we need to consider is the situation of mutation and genetic drift. The effect of mutation, of the type observed at STR loci, on a divided population is that it tends to oppose the effect of drift. If drift is tending to remove genetic variation from separated subpopulations, mutation tends to reintroduce it. When a mutation occurs at a STR locus, it tends to add or subtract a single repeat, with mutational losses or gains of multiple repeats being much rarer (see Chapter 1 for a summary of mutation references). The simplest description of the STR mutational process, whereby only mutations that result in a single repeat unit difference are allowed, the stepwise mutation model, was first proposed by Kimura and Ohta.[392] The other extreme is the infinite alleles model (IAM) proposed by Kimura and Crow[393] in which a mutation to any allele occurs and gives rise to a state not previously seen in the population. Intermediate models exist (such as the K-allele model[374]) but one which fits well with a theoretical model is the two-phase model proposed by DiRienzo et al.,[394] where mutations which result in a single repeat unit difference occur with probability p and those that result in a multiple repeat unit difference occur with a probability $1 - p$, where the repeat unit difference follows a geometric distribution.[395]

If we consider two populations that have become separated or isolated, we note that they then begin to evolve separately and their respective allelic frequencies tend to drift apart. This process will be associated with an increase in relatedness within the separated subpopulations and can be quantified by an increase in the inbreeding coefficient θ. The effect of stepwise mutation to alleles already present is to lower relatedness and hence θ.[396–398] This effect may seem odd. The people are still related, but their alleles can no longer be identical by descent as they are no longer identical. The equilibrium situation that may result is given by Evett and Weir.[258] Whether drift or mutation is the dominant factor depends on the product $N\mu$, where N is the population size and μ the mutation rate. If $N\mu \ll 1$, the population will typically be moving towards fixation for one allele, which means that genetic drift forces are dominant. If $N\mu \gg 1$, then mutation is the dominant force and multiple alleles will be present.[399]

This effect can be elegantly demonstrated using simulation software. Two programs have been offered by forensic programmers: Gendrift (Steve Knight and Richard Pinchin, FSS*) and Popgen (James Curran, University of Auckland) and there are others in the population genetics community.

---

* FSS, UK Forensic Science Service.

It would be unwise, however, to assume that mutation is a completely benign phenomenon from the perspective of decreasing associations between individuals. The exact nature of the mutational process does have a serious effect on the departures that may be observed and the validity of models to correct for them. This is discussed briefly later.

No Migration into or Away from the Population

Allele probabilities will change if migration occurs into or away from the population. Emigration from a moderately sized population has very little effect since the subtraction of a few alleles from the gene pool alters the allele probabilities very little. Immigration of alleles into the population from a different population can have a much more marked effect. Such gene migration is often accompanied by physical migration of people but this is not necessarily a requirement.

To consider this issue it is critical to consider the interaction of migration and our definition of population. Most of our current definitions of population have both an ethnic and a geographical basis. Consider the New Zealand population. We currently subdivide this arbitrarily into Caucasian, Eastern Polynesian (Maori and Cook Island Maori), Western Polynesians (Samoans and Tongans) and Asians. The physical migration of a British person to New Zealand would represent migration of alleles into the New Zealand Caucasian gene pool. The intermarriage of Caucasians and Maori would represent migration of Caucasian genes into the Eastern Polynesian gene pool without necessarily involving any physical migration of people. The fact that this is treated as a migration of genes *into* the Eastern Polynesian gene pool is dependent on how we intend to (arbitrarily) define the ethnicity of the resulting progeny.

The effect of migration on equilibrium is dependent on the difference in allele frequencies between the donor and recipient populations.[258] Hence the physical migration of British people to New Zealand is likely to have a very small effect on the equilibrium situation of New Zealand Caucasians since the allele frequencies in the two populations are similar. However the migration of Caucasian genes into the Eastern Polynesian gene pool is much more likely to disturb the equilibrium since the populations have more differing allele probabilities.

No Selection

At this stage most of the argument in favour of there being little or no selection at STR loci relates to the fact that these loci are non-coding and hence do not produce any gene products. Theoretically, then, any mechanism for selection would have to operate by an indirect route, say by hitchhiking on other advantageous or disadvantageous genes or by affecting DNA packing, replication or repair.

The observation of greater microsatellite diversity amongst Africans[400] is consistent with the out-of-Africa event and a selectively neutral model. However greater diversity among Africans is certainly not proof of selective neutrality. Mitochondrial DNA also shows a deviation from selective neutrality; however this is postulated to be the result of a selective sweep in modern humans outside Africa.

When first studied, these DNA sections were thought to be non-functional and were termed *junk DNA*.[401] Makalowski[402] discusses the origin of the phrase *junk DNA* and reinforces the modern conception that this DNA may have important functions. The editors of *Science* ranked the discovery of the relevance of junk DNA as the fifth most important discovery of 2004. Some STR loci are intronic. Introns are thought to have 'invaded eukaryotic genes late in evolution, after the separation of transcription and translation'.[22,23] Mattick[22,23] argues convincingly for a role for at least some intronic products in gene expression and postulates that they were a crucial step in the development of multicellular organisms. Among the 13 CODIS* loci, 5 lie in introns.[403] The first official results of the Encyclopaedia of DNA Elements Consortium were released on 5 September 2012. The results showed that approximately 20% of non-coding human DNA is functional and an additional 60% is transcribed with no known function.[404]

---

* CODIS, Combined DNA Index System.

Some opponents of the forensic use of DNA have used these findings to argue that collecting DNA for arrestee databases is unconstitutional.[405] The question arises as to whether there is a function for the specific intronic segments used in forensic work.[406] Wagner summarizes the debate in a recent plea for scientists to drop the term *junk DNA*.[407]

Selection is a proven phenomenon in some blood group systems such as ABO and rhesus.[408] A mechanism has been proposed for the selective interaction between ABO and haptoglobin.[409] However these genes are clearly coding and produce important gene products. Hence direct selective mechanisms are expected.

Selection by association with disease loci is a mechanism that may possibly affect STR loci. Such associations at other loci are known.[410] Several core STR loci have been putatively linked to genetic diseases. The forensic vWA locus lies within intron 40 of the von Willebrand factor (vWF) gene, a gene associated with von Willebrand's disease (vWD), a clotting disorder. However no evidence of linkage disequilibrium (LD) blocks was found around the forensic vWA intronic locus. In addition there was evidence for recombination within 3 kb of intron 40.[403]

In a recent paper Katsanis and Wagner characterized the genomic regions and phenotypic associations of the 13 US core STRs and the proposed additional 11 STRs.[411] All loci were associated within 1 kb of at least one phenotype. TH01 has been associated with 18 phenotypes including schizophrenia[412] (disputed in Ref. 413), alcoholism, bipolar disorder (disputed in Ref. 413) and heart disease[414] (disputed in Refs. 415, 416). The authors conclude that 'association with these traits does not imply necessarily that individual CODIS marker genotypes are predictive or causative of any trait'.[411] This comment by the authors is only partially sustainable. There is certainly no suggestion, as yet, that any forensic allele is causative of a phenotypic trait. However any association of traits will lead to a predictive power. This may be quite weak but it will exist. Equally any association with a physical trait that is under selection will lead to selection at the STR. This may also be quite mild selection if the trait is rare or has only slightly reduced fitness or the association is weak.

Phillips et al.[417] report an active recombination landscape around many STR markers. This would suggest that the range of LD may be quite short and associations mild.

The effect of a selective sweep affecting the CODIS forensic loci was considered using the Phase I Hapmap data. This identified that the genomic regions in which vWA and D13S317 reside may be affected by selection.

Neuhauser[399] compares random drift and selection and notes that if $Ns \ll 1$, where N is the population size and s is the selective advantage of one allele over another, for a two-allele locus, then selection does not have much effect and the locus acts almost as if it were neutral.

A theoretical model for estimating mutation rates at di-, tri-, and tetranucleotides from the distributions of their allele sizes was given by Chakraborty et al.,[418] who noted the departure of the predictions of the model from directly observed values. This led Chakraborty et al. to an interesting discussion of whether there is any evidence of constraints in the number of DNA repeats at a locus, which may be evidence for the existence of selection. They concluded that the shape of modern allele distributions is inconsistent with the existence of constraints.

In summary there are reasonable theoretical reasons to believe that these loci are selectively neutral or nearly so, and no direct evidence for strong selection at forensic loci has been reported in a number of studies designed to look for it.

Random Mating

Of the various assumptions given in this section, this is the one that has deservedly attracted the most attention. It is clear that we do not select our mates on the basis of their DNA genotypes at the STR loci. Most of us do not even know our own genotype at these loci. We also believe that these genotypes have no physical manifestation, which is to say that they do not affect the phenotype of an individual. Hence we should be unable to detect these genotypes by looking at a person. This should preclude some inadvertent selection of genotypes. However it would be wrong to assume from this that random mating is a fair assumption.

Crow and Kimura[374] discuss the two main types of non-random mating: inbreeding and assortative mating. Assortative mating is not discussed here. There is considerable evidence that it does occur in humans. For instance, an intelligent person is more likely to marry another intelligent person. Jared Diamond discusses this in some detail in his popular science book *The Rise and Fall of the Third Chimpanzee*.[419] In the STR context we believe that the issue of importance is inbreeding.

What is alleged is that the population is made up of subpopulations,[420,421] whose members preferentially mate within their subpopulation, possibly for religious, language or other reasons, but more probably just because of geographical proximity (for an excellent review see Excoffier[422]). This is termed *inbreeding*. In the past people travelled a lot less than they do now. The notion of marrying the 'girl or boy next door' is not universal nor is it totally unknown. It is important to note that there is no suggestion that the subpopulations are completely isolated from each other. All that is required is any departure from a completely random choice of mates. The more isolated the subpopulations, the larger is the effect, but partial isolation will also lead to some subpopulation effects.

In lectures on DNA around the world, a trial with the various classes has been performed. Unfortunately the results have not been retained, which would make an interesting section. However the general flavour of them can be reported. What was asked was for people to give the 'ethnicity' of their four grandparents. Table 3.1 gives the results for the area around John's desk at the laboratory at the former Forensic Science Service at Trident Court in Birmingham, UK. Each cell represents one individual's self-declared ethnicity for their four grandparents.

This experiment would not meet minimum survey standards; however let us treat it as a demonstration rather than as evidence. First let us note that this arrangement does not look random. Too many ethnicities occur together. For instance there are four Chinese entries and four Indian entries together. Let us assume that we separated these two individuals out as being of a different 'race'. What we are left with still does not look like a random arrangement. For instance there are four Greek Cypriots and two Iraqis together. Let us assume further that we take these out and put them into different categories. Still what we are left with does not look random. There are too many Irish and Swiss together. If we could peer deeper into the past, we might find that the people reporting *English* have differing amounts of Celtic, Scandinavian or Saxon heritage.

This experiment has worked wherever tried, in New Zealand, Australia, the United States and the United Kingdom. We, personally, do not believe that the modern human population is the result of random mating. We do believe that we are the result of an evolutionary process whereby our ancestors mated in groups to a greater or lesser extent. This is breaking down in modern times but the process is far from complete.

Table 3.1 The Self-Declared Ethnicity of Some Staff at the Former Forensic Science Service Laboratory, Trident Court, in 2002	
Irish, Irish, Irish, Irish	Swiss, Swiss, Swiss, Swiss
English, English, English, Irish	English, English, English, English
English, English, English, English	Chinese, Chinese, Chinese, Chinese
Welsh, English, English, Scottish	English, English, English, English
Scottish, Scottish, English, English	English, English, Irish, Scottish
English, English, English, English	English, English, English, Scottish
Hungarian, Scottish, Scottish, English	English, English, English, Scottish
English, English, English, English	Greek Cypriot, Greek Cypriot, Greek Cypriot, Greek Cypriot
English, English, English, English	Irish, Irish, Iraqi, Iraqi
English, English, English, Scottish	Indian, Indian, Indian, Indian

This leads us to the classical consideration of the Wahlund principle.[423] Assume that a certain area is made up of two or more sub-groups that breed within each group but not to any large extent between the two groups. Further assume that there are some allele probability differences between these groups. Then even if the subpopulations themselves are in HWE, the full population will not be. An example is given in Table 3.2.

First we note that the mixed population is not in HWE even though each subpopulation is. Next we note the classical Wahlund effect that all the probabilities for homozygotes are increased above Hardy–Weinberg expectation. The total heterozygote probabilities are generally decreased, although individual heterozygotes may be above or below expectation. Note that in this example two of the heterozygotes are below expectation, whereas one is above. The total for all the heterozygotes will always be down (which is really the same as saying the total of the homozygotes is always up).[258,424] Memory cue:

Too many homs and not enough hets,
That's what we call the Wahlund effect.

The same subpopulation phenomenon will induce between-locus dependence, that is, it will induce linkage disequilibrium. This is more complex but not harder to demonstrate. In Table 3.3 we give a numerical demonstration. This table shows the 'correct' genotype proportions and two incorrect calculations. The first incorrect calculation proceeds by combining the two sub-populations and then using the population allele probabilities – this incorrectly assumes Hardy–Weinberg and linkage equilibrium in the population. This is the type of error (although greatly exaggerated) that would occur if we assumed that a structured population was homogeneous. The second incorrect calculation (again carried out on the combined population) proceeds as if we had performed some sort of testing and had abandoned the assumption of HWE but instead had used observed genotype proportions and then multiplied across loci. This approach is a better method to assign probabilities as it corrects for Hardy–Weinberg disequilibrium; however it fails to account for linkage disequilibrium.

The third approach was adopted, incorrectly, by Buckleton and Weir in some of their early recommendations but is now abandoned. It was described as the 'Cellmark wrinkle' in the descriptions of the OJ Simpson case in the first edition of this book.* It persists in recommendations by other authors but should be superseded.

Table 3.2	Example of the Wahlund Effect			
Allele		*a*	*b*	*c*
Subpopulation 1		0.7	0.2	0.1
Subpopulation 2		0.2	0.1	0.7
Genotype	**Subpopulation 1**	**Subpopulation 2**	**1:1 Mix**	**Hardy–Weinberg Expectation**
aa	0.49	0.04	0.2650	0.2025
bb	0.04	0.01	0.0250	0.0225
cc	0.01	0.49	0.2500	0.1600
ab	0.28	0.04	0.1600	0.1350
ac	0.14	0.28	0.2100	0.3600
bc	0.04	0.14	0.0900	0.1200

---

* John S. Buckleton. Population genetic models. In *Forensic DNA Evidence Interpretation*, John S. Buckleton, Christopher M. Triggs, and Simon J. Walsh, Eds. Boca Raton, FL: CRC Press; 2005.

Table 3.3   Two Locus Genotype Probabilities for a Population Consisting of Two Subpopulations in Equal Proportions

	Allele	Subpopulation 1	Subpopulation 2
Locus 1	a	0.7	0.2
	b	0.2	0.1
	c	0.1	0.7
Locus 2	d	0.5	0.2
	e	0.2	0.4
	f	0.3	0.4

1:1 Mix Correct					
	dd	ee	ff	De	df	ef
aa	0.062	0.013	0.025	0.052	0.077	0.036
bb	0.005	0.002	0.003	0.005	0.007	0.004
cc	0.011	0.039	0.040	0.040	0.041	0.079
ab	0.036	0.009	0.016	0.031	0.045	0.023
ac	0.023	0.025	0.029	0.036	0.043	0.053
bc	0.008	0.012	0.013	0.015	0.017	0.025

1:1 Mix from Alleles					
	dd	ee	ff	De	df	ef
aa	0.025	0.018	0.025	0.043	0.050	0.043
bb	0.003	0.002	0.003	0.005	0.006	0.005
cc	0.020	0.014	0.020	0.034	0.039	0.034
ab	0.017	0.012	0.017	0.028	0.033	0.028
ac	0.044	0.032	0.044	0.076	0.088	0.076
bc	0.015	0.011	0.015	0.025	0.029	0.025

1:1 Mix from Genotypes					
	dd	ee	ff	De	df	ef
aa	0.038	0.027	0.033	0.048	0.061	0.058
bb	0.004	0.003	0.003	0.005	0.006	0.006
cc	0.036	0.025	0.031	0.045	0.058	0.055
ab	0.023	0.016	0.020	0.029	0.037	0.035
ac	0.030	0.021	0.026	0.038	0.048	0.046
bc	0.013	0.009	0.011	0.016	0.021	0.020

Note: Genotype probabilities are calculated in three ways.

Inspection of these numbers shows that the 'correct' probabilities for two loci cannot be determined if the population structure is ignored. Proceeding from either the population allele probabilities or the population genotype probabilities will give incorrect answers.

The demonstration that the multiplication of population genotype probabilities gives an incorrect answer shows that linkage disequilibrium can be induced by population substructure whether or not the loci are physically linked. Loci that are on different chromosomes may, therefore, be in disequilibrium[425-428] and expressions have been derived to estimate the magnitude of the disequilibrium.[258,424] In fact almost any instance of disequilibrium in the forensic literature involves loci that are on different chromosomes. Some of the most common causes of disequilibrium are population genetic effects, such as the existence of subpopulations, and such disequilibria occur for the same reasons as the Wahlund effect.[429,430]

This disequilibrium phenomenon is sufficiently understood that decay rates for linkage disequilibrium for non-linked loci have been calculated and appear in standard texts.[258,385,424] The dependency effects are not expected to be large for loci with low mutation rates. There is a slight tendency for the dependencies to rise with the number of loci.[431,432]

We give examples later using the ESR[*] data for Eastern Polynesians. Analysis of this data suggests disequilibrium regardless of the chromosomal position of the loci. In this particular case the most likely explanation is not population subdivision but the effects of admixture with Caucasians. The population in the United States described as *Hispanics* may be showing the same admixture effects or this may be the result of subpopulations, or both. The Hispanic population is often subdivided into south-eastern and south-western Hispanic.

Conversely, loci that are closely linked on the same chromosome may be in equilibrium (or near it). In fact there is no absolute relationship between the position on a chromosome and the state of independence between loci. However, as a generalization, Hudson[385] notes 'loosely linked loci are typically observed to be near linkage equilibrium in natural populations ... In contrast ... very tightly linked loci often show some signs of linkage disequilibrium'.

There is growing evidence of a block-like structure to linkage disequilibrium. This implies that some regions of the genome are closely linked and others are unlinked. This structure can, obviously, be produced by recombination hotspots but interestingly can also be produced without such hotspots.[433]

In summary, a lack of random mating, in particular the existence of subpopulations with different allele probabilities, will cause Hardy–Weinberg and linkage disequilibrium. The proportions of the different subpopulations and the differences in their allele probabilities will affect the magnitude of this disequilibrium. The larger the differences in the allele probabilities between the differing subpopulations, the larger will be the resulting disequilibria. Excoffier[422] notes that population subdivision will also produce a larger number of observed alleles, with an excess of rare alleles.

The first human populations that came under intense scrutiny by the forensic community were the Caucasian populations of the United Kingdom and the United States. These populations comprise subpopulations arising from different areas of the United Kingdom and Europe. Studies have suggested that there are only minor differences between these Caucasian subpopulations in Europe or the United Kingdom, per se. Although these differences are real,[408,434,435] they are small and hence they give rise to very small disequilibrium effects. The effect of these disequilibria is a very mild bias in the product rule towards the assignment of a genotype probability that is too low.

An Infinite Number of Generations

Loci that are on different chromosomes or well separated on the same chromosome will assort in a Mendelian manner. The linkage disequilibrium associated with such loci is expected to halve with every generation[258] and hence will approach equilibrium asymptotically, but never

---

[*] Institute of Environmental Science and Research, Porirua, New Zealand.

quite get there if the disturbing force is removed. Linked loci will also approach equilibrium but more slowly, depending on the rate of recombination between the loci. An example of very tightly linked loci that are near equilibrium is given by Mourant, when he discusses the rhesus blood group (a set of three linked loci) in Australian Aborigines.[434]

Summary

It was a pity that the first population extensively studied by the forensic community was the Caucasian population. This population is probably one of those nearest to Hardy–Weinberg and linkage equilibrium of the large modern human populations. Hence it was the least likely to educate us on departures from equilibrium and how to manage these. At that time we did not understand the weakness of our independence tests and this contributed to our misunderstandings. We return to this subject in Chapter 5. However we note here that there is now considerable evidence of departure from independence in many populations (for example, see Refs. 436–444).

We close this section with a quote from Wild and Seber: 'What often happens is that, in the absence of knowledge of the appropriate conditional probabilities, people assume independence ... this can lead to answers that are grossly too small or grossly too large – and we won't know!'[445] The situation in DNA is probably not this bad, but the warning is real nonetheless.

How Big Is the Potential Departure If We Use the Product Rule?

Early efforts to answer this question compared estimates made in different ways and led to the plausibly unsustainable conclusion that the error induced by ignoring subpopulation effects may be of the order of a factor of 10.[446–450]

The comparison of an estimate with an estimate is interesting and would give us some confidence that the effect of changing estimation methods is minor. However it does not show that either estimate is close to the true value. It is the latter question, how far our estimate is from the true value, that is of forensic interest.

This may be the correct time to ask 'What is the true value?'* Our suspicion is that this is a concept that is held by many forensic scientists and participants in the judicial process. They would claim, fairly, that it is desirable that the assigned match probability be close to the true value. We suspect that the most plausible interpretation of the concept of a true value is the actual count of genotype G in population p at time t. At the risk of inciting the ire of our valued Bayesian colleagues[198] we will work with this for the time being, but only to show the problems. First imagine that, by some method, we knew that x out of N persons in population p at time t had genotype G. The first thing we note is that x is likely to be 0 or 1 for most multilocus genotypes. Since our assignments will be microprobabilities, they will all differ from 0 or 1 out of N. Since every single estimate will be wrong in some sense of the word, no matter how performed, we need some concept of calibrating an estimation process. There are two viable concepts of which we are aware. One is based on Tippett testing, first pioneered in the DNA field by Evett but now used quite extensively for this purpose. The second concept is simulation testing, whereby a computer may actually know the values for x and N in some infinite population. We discuss both later in this chapter.

It is often assumed that cosmopolitan populations do not exhibit subdivision. While this may be true, there are many instances where it may not. If the population is old and well mixed, there should be very little, if any, population subdivision. However a cosmopolitan population may be something like that of London or New York, which consist of people with very different genetic backgrounds who live in the same area. This is exactly the situation where we expect subpopulation effects.

---

* This follows a set of concepts discussed between Justice Mulligan and John during *R v Karger*.[451] We are indebted to Justice Mulligan for sharing his insight in this matter, which is often hard to convey in a court situation.

Populations Separated by Genetic Drift

If we accept that the loci that we consider in forensic applications are selectively neutral, then we expect the main evolutionary force producing differences between separated populations to be the random drift of allele probabilities. This is an extensively researched subject and is only covered very superficially here. A visual representation of the structure of the model is given in Figure 3.1.

Even if all other evolutionary forces were absent, the allele probabilities in one generation would still differ slightly from the previous one. This difference is caused by the random transmission of alleles to the new generation. For large populations this effect is very small and takes a long time to be observable. However for smaller populations the effect may be quite rapid.

The difference between populations that are diverging by drift is often characterized by a parameter, θ or F_{ST}, which may be treated as synonyms for the purposes of this text. This parameter is often termed the *between-person co-ancestry coefficient*. It is a very useful parameter for characterizing the subpopulation effect; however it is both difficult to visualize and to measure. For the purposes of this section it will be adequate to consider it as a measure of the genetic distance between subpopulations. The larger the distance between subpopulations, the longer we assume that they have been separated and the higher θ will be.

It turns out that θ may also be considered as a measure of the relatedness between people in the subpopulation. If this subpopulation has been separate from others for some time, then people in this subpopulation will be more related to each other than they would be to a person taken from a different subpopulation. To help give a feel for the size of θ values, consider that first cousins would have $\theta = 0.0625$.

A formula relating θ to the time since separation is given in many standard texts:[424]

$$\theta_t = 1 - \left(1 - \frac{1}{2N}\right)^t$$

where t is the time since separation in generations and N is the effective size of the population (strictly a monoecious population in which selfing is allowed). Evett and Weir[257] discuss

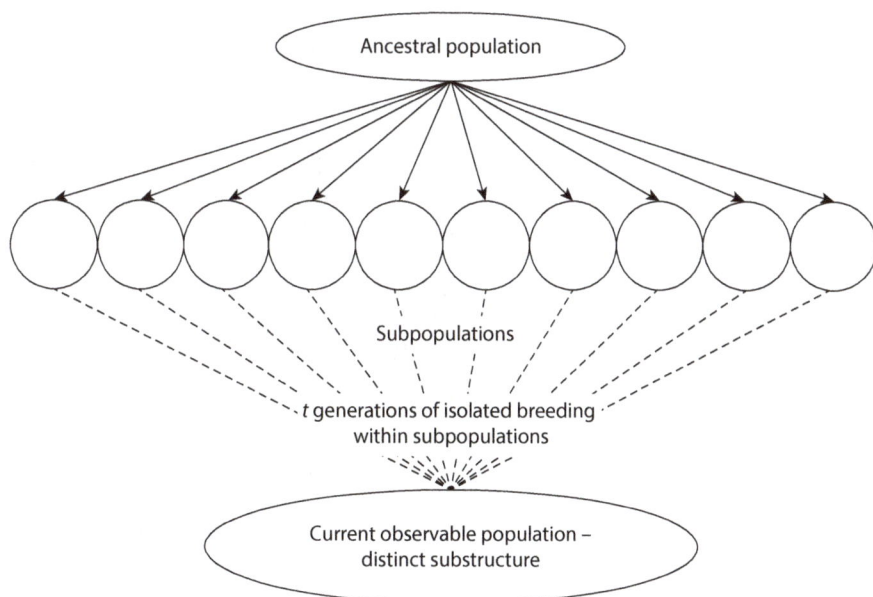

Figure 3.1 A simplified population model. (Reproduced in amended form from *Forensic Science International*, 135(1), Curran, J.M., et al., What is the magnitude of the subpopulation effect? 1–8, Copyright 2003, with permission from Elsevier.)

the avoidance of selfing and show that the above model is a close approximation. Crow and Kimura[374] give $\dfrac{1}{N_e} = \dfrac{1}{4N_m} + \dfrac{1}{4N_f}$ for the effective size of the population (N_e) when separate sexes of number N_m and N_f are present. When the sexes are present in equal numbers $N_m = N_f = \dfrac{N}{2}$ and hence $N_e = N$. Crow and Kimura discuss the effect of differing numbers of progeny on N_e.

If mutation of the infinite alleles type is added to the model, then the opposing forces of drift and mutation may form an equilibrium state, given in several texts:[258,424] $\hat{F} \approx \dfrac{1}{1+4N\mu}$ where $\hat{F}$ is the equilibrium value of the between-person inbreeding coefficient and μ is the mutation rate.

NRC II Recommendation 4.1

NRC II Recommendation 4.1 offered a correction for Hardy–Weinberg disequilibrium caused by the Wahlund effect. It was suggested that a correction upwards in frequency be applied to correct for the expected upward bias produced by population subdivision. It was further suggested that this correction should be applied only to homozygotes. No correction was recommended for heterozygotes since, on average, these should have a downward bias (recall that individual heterozygotes may be displaced from expectation in either direction). This comment is generally true for the event of population subdivision but would be untrue for populations undergoing admixture. In admixing populations the number of heterozygotes is likely to be elevated.

The recommendation suggests

$$P_i = \begin{cases} p_{i1}^2 + p_{i1}(1 - p_{i1})F & A_{i1} = A_{i2} \\ 2p_{i1}p_{i2}, & A_{i1} \neq A_{i2} \end{cases} \tag{3.4}$$

where F is the within-person inbreeding coefficient, not the between-person inbreeding coefficient, θ, as written in NRC II.

Curran et al. tested Recommendation 4.1 by comparing this assignment with the Gold Standard Profile Frequency for a population with a true inbreeding coefficient $\theta = 0.03$ created by simulation. This is reproduced in the section 'Simulation Testing', below. In this simulation 54.4% of values are less than 1 (reduced from 64.7% for no correction). We see that this estimator still has a small prosecution bias and some undesirable variance properties.

This recommendation is a logical way of correcting for Hardy–Weinberg disequilibrium but makes no attempt to correct for linkage disequilibrium. It will suffer from the same approximations that are revealed in Table 3.3 for the 1:1 mix from genotypes. Hence it will still have a very mild tendency to underestimate multilocus genotype probabilities. This is discussed further in the following section.

The Subpopulation Formulae NRC II Recommendation 4.2

If it is difficult to calculate the genotype probability in the population due to the effects of population subdivision, can we calculate it in the subpopulation of the suspect? We note that the subpopulation of the suspect may not be known, may not be easily defined and almost certainly has not been sampled.

A potential solution has been offered by Balding and Nichols and has found widespread acceptance both in the forensic and the legal communities. These formulae[176,258,358,452,453] calculate the conditional probability of a second profile matching the stain from the subpopulation of the suspect given the profile of the suspect.

These formulae follow from a formal logic given initially by Balding and Nichols and appearing as Equations 4.10 in *NRC II* and 4.20 in Evett and Weir, but they date back to the work of Sewall Wright[454] in the 1940s. A reasonably gentle derivation appears in Balding and Nichols.[455]

$$P_i = \begin{cases} \dfrac{\left[3\theta+(1-\theta)p_{i1}\right]\left[2\theta+(1-\theta)p_{i1}\right]}{(1+\theta)(1+2\theta)}, & A_{i1}=A_{i2} \\[3mm] \dfrac{2\left[\theta+(1-\theta)p_{i1}\right]\left[\theta+(1-\theta)p_{i2}\right]}{(1+\theta)(1+2\theta)}, & A_{i1}\neq A_{i2} \end{cases}$$

$$P = \prod_i P_i \tag{3.5}$$

Let us call the profile found at the scene of a crime profile C with genotype G_c. We will write the probability that the offender has this profile as $\Pr(G_c)$. Such a probability is called a profile probability, as the probability is not conditioned on any other information. Recommendation 4.1 is an attempt to calculate this probability.

However let us consider whether the probability of a second copy of a certain genotype is raised slightly if one other person is known to have this genotype. There are many reasons why this may be true. Initially we will merely assume that it is true. If we had no knowledge as to whether or not this genotype had ever been found previously in an individual then, indeed, we would be required to resort to a profile probability and Recommendation 4.1 may be an appropriate method. The 'true' value of most of these profile probabilities would be 0, as discussed in Chapter 2.

We invariably have the information that at least one copy of the profile exists. We have seen it in the suspect. In other words we are not talking about the vast majority of profiles that do not exist; we are talking about one of the few that do, indeed, exist in the real world.[456] Let us call the genotype of the suspect G_s, and we note that G_s and G_c are the same. In other words the suspect could be the source of the stain at the scene. We are interested, however, in calculating the probability that a second person has this profile given that the suspect has it. This probability is written $\Pr(G_c|G_s)$ and is called a match probability. It will be the same as the profile probability $\Pr(G_c)$ only if the knowledge that one person has the profile has no impact on our assessment that a second person has the profile. This is the assumption of independence discussed in product rule.

For the various population genetic reasons given above, we expect the assumption of independence to nearly hold, but to be violated in a minor way, in real populations. The main reason for this is population subdivision and relatedness. The fact that one person has the profile slightly increases the probability that his relatives or other members of his subpopulation have the profile. We are therefore led to the consideration of match probabilities.

It has been assumed that application of these formulae requires an assumption of independence between loci.[457,458] This follows from the way that the single locus probability assignments are assembled into a multilocus probability assignment. Indeed these are multiplied and this gives the impression of an assumption of independence.

However this is not true and was explicitly stated in Balding and Nichols: 'Further, we have restricted attention to the suspect's sub-population and hence concerns about the Wahlund effect and correlations among loci can be ignored. Therefore the whole profile match probability is, to a close approximation, the product of the single-locus probabilities'.[358] For those who prefer to investigate this statement in an algebraic way, some formative thoughts are given in Box 3.1.

The subpopulation formulae of Balding and Nichols were designed to give an estimate of the match probability in the same subpopulation as the suspect. Most implementations of this approach apply this correction (in an overly conservative manner) to the whole racial group to

---

BOX 3.1   LINKAGE EQUILIBRIUM AND CONDITIONAL PROBABILITIES

JS Buckleton and CM Triggs

Consider two loci (loci 1 and 2). The crime stain has genotype G_C^i at locus i. The suspect matches and hence has genotype G_S^i at this locus. We note that $G_C^i = G_S^i$ for each of the loci, i, examined. We require $\Pr\left(G_C^1, G_C^2 \mid G_S^1, G_S^2\right)$. Using the third law of probability:

$$\Pr\left(G_C^1, G_C^2 \mid G_S^1, G_S^2\right) = \Pr\left(G_C^1 \mid G_C^2, G_S^1, G_S^2\right)\Pr\left(G_C^2 \mid G_S^1, G_S^2\right)$$

Balding and Nichols's equation (Equation 3.5) approximates this as

$$\cong \Pr\left(G_C^1 \mid G_S^1\right)\Pr\left(G_C^2 \mid G_S^2\right)$$

This is not an assumption of independence between G_C^1 and G_C^2. One condition that will make this true is if

$$\Pr\left(G_C^1 \mid G_C^2, G_S^1, G_S^2\right) = \Pr\left(G_C^1 \mid G_S^1\right) \text{ and } \Pr\left(G_C^2 \mid G_S^1, G_S^2\right) = \Pr\left(G_C^2 \mid G_S^2\right)$$

Looking at the first equality we note that this does not imply independence between G_C^1 and G_C^2 unconditionally but rather implies that G_C^1 is independent of G_C^2 and G_S^2 in the presence of G_S^1. In other words G_C^2 and G_S^2 provide no further information about G_C^1 given G_S^1. The truth of this assumption depends on our belief in the population genetic model.

The second equality requires that G_C^2 be independent of G_S^1 in the presence of G_S^2. The Balding and Nichols equations are not a simple assumption of independence between loci.

The model upon which the Balding and Nichols equations (Equation 3.5) are based assumes Hardy–Weinberg and linkage equilibrium at the subpopulation level (as well as some other assumptions). This is an explicit assumption of disequilibrium both within a locus and between loci at the population level. It is therefore seen that Balding and Nichols formulae correct for that component of linkage disequilibrium that is caused by population subdivision.

---

which the suspect belongs, rather than simply applying it to the subpopulation of the suspect. This is an understandable response to the difficulties in defining the subpopulation of the suspect, which most often is unknown and not definable even if known. Equally the proportion of this subpopulation in the population is likely to be unknown. However the approach of applying the correction to the whole race usually results in the correction becoming an overcorrection and hence gives rise to considerable conservativeness (or even performs in an overly conservative manner[*]) in the probability assignments.

Over the years we have received a lot of adverse criticism to the use of this correction regarding the difficulties in defining the subpopulation of the suspect. The difficulties can be demonstrated by taking almost any person and considering the question, 'To what subpopulation does he belong?' Consider a Caucasian resident of New Zealand, born in London to New Zealand parents. He has Irish, Scottish, Norwegian and English ancestors. It is almost impossible to define a subpopulation for him. This would be true of most people. This is termed a *population-centred approach* and it can be depicted graphically (see Figure 3.2). In this arbitrary graphic are

---

[*] Clearly the term *overly conservative* used here has no objective definition. Rather it is a subjective term used to imply a very strong bias in favour of the defendant.

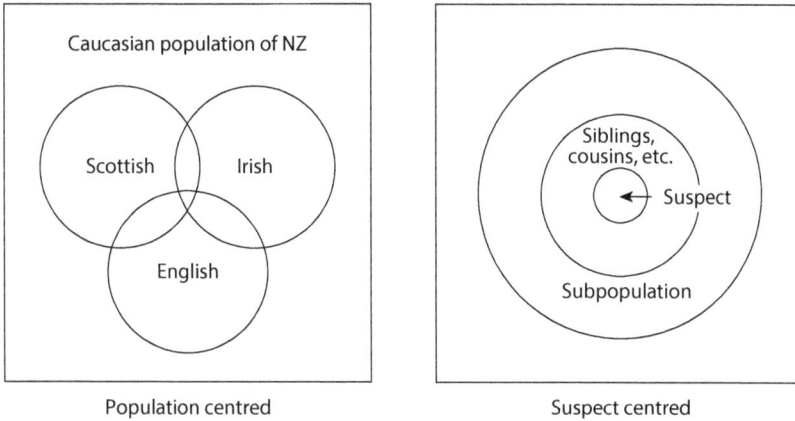

Figure 3.2   Diagrams depicting the population-centred and suspect-centred views of defining a subpopulation.

placed circles depicting the Irish, Scottish and English subpopulations. These all overlap in differing ways. Where should we now place Norwegian? Nor have we really been specific enough. Should we have said *Graham* rather than Scottish? Hence the argument goes: subpopulations are indefinable.

However the problem is illusionary. This can be shown by a similar graphic. Consider the same population but from a suspect-centred approach. The suspect has a number of close relatives: siblings, parents and children. He also has more distant relatives: uncles, cousins. Further out he has second cousins and so forth. Beyond this there are a number of people to whom he is related more remotely. He may not know these people and there is probably no collective name for them. These are his subpopulation.[*,459]

Simulation Testing

By simulating populations[365] with different effects we can 'know' the true value (termed *gold standard*) and compare it with the estimate. We present the ratio of the estimate and the gold standard in Figure 3.3. If the estimate is exactly correct, then this ratio is 1. The simulations are set up so that there is no sampling effect. So a 'perfect' answer has all points on the line $y = 1$. The conservative side is above the line and the non-conservative side below. This defines *conservative* as overestimating the match probability. In certain case circumstances the conservative and non-conservative sides may swap. Accepting that perfection is difficult to achieve we might accept a series of points just on the conservative side of the $y = 1$ line, but we would not want to be too far above the line as that is overly conservative.

It can be seen from these experiments that the product rule estimator has a very small bias in favour of the prosecution in most cases where the population is subdivided. The magnitude of this bias is not large and it is important not to overemphasize it. However it is real and is not

---

* Subpopulations do not end, they fade out. We could envisage persons who are progressively more and more remotely related to the suspect. This could be approximated, if necessary, by bands of persons with differing θ values or better by the use of the general formulation whereby each pair of persons has a θ appropriate for their relationship. For this diagram we take an arbitrary boundary to the subpopulation. The further out we push the boundary, the more people who are included in the subpopulation but the smaller the average value of θ. The correct approach is given by Balding[277] and involves the concept of a certain θ for every person. Balding suggests, and we agree, that this should be approximated by the bands of relatedness approximation described above.

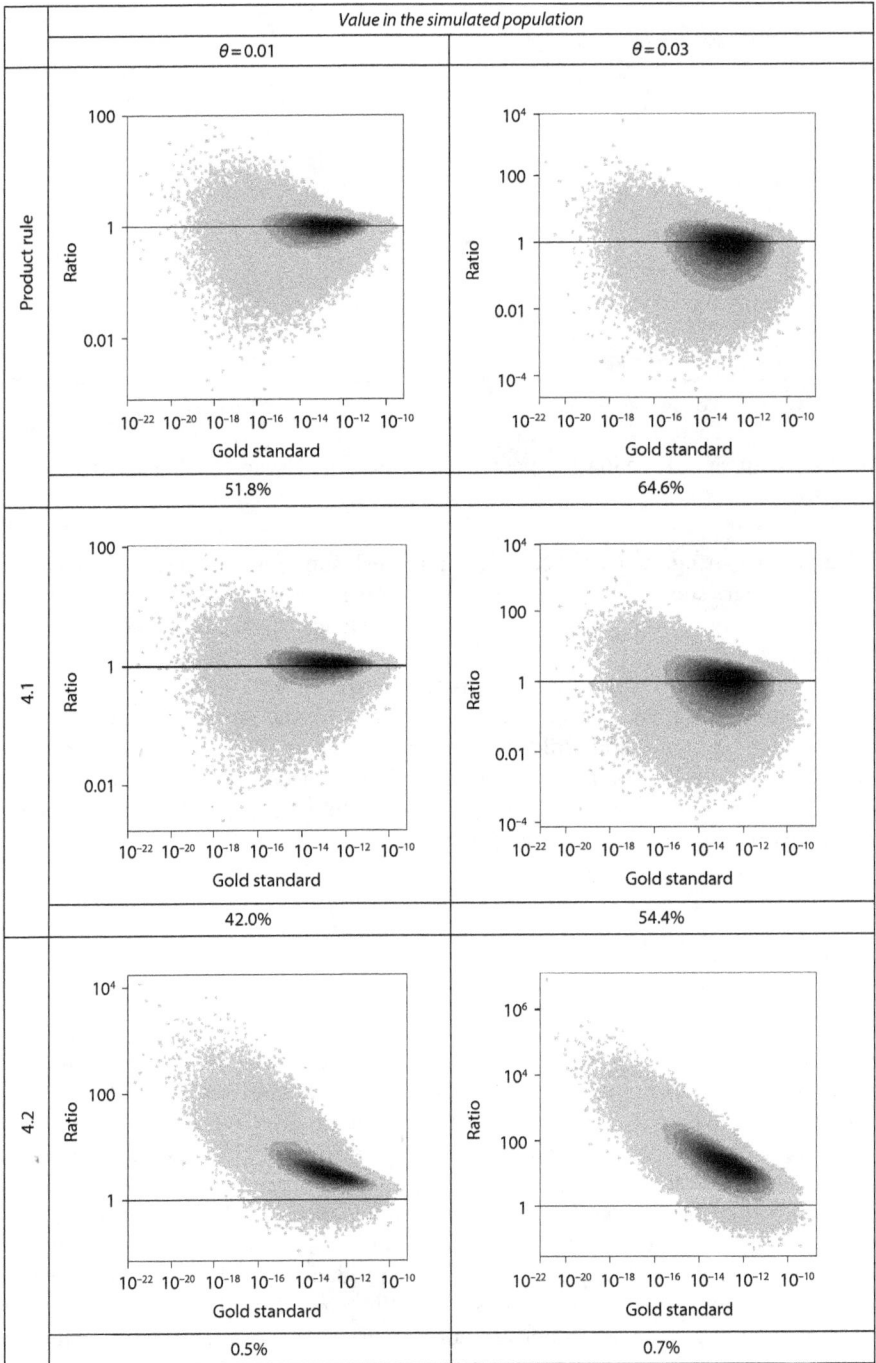

Figure 3.3   The ratio of the estimate to the gold standard value for populations with true θ values of 0.01 and 0.03 and using the product rule and Recommendation 4.1 or 4.2. The percentages below each figure are the fraction of points on the non-conservative side. For Recommendation 4.1 or 4.2 the true θ values of 0.01 and 0.03 are used.

the result of sampling uncertainty. It will be larger for strongly subdivided populations and smaller for less subdivided populations. The effect may be more than a factor of 10. This finding adds an important verification relative to a true match probability.* It does put into perspective comments such as 'implementation of the product rule is a reasonable best estimate',[313,460,461] which must be qualified with our current understanding that the product rule is unlikely to be an unbiased estimator.

We come to 'scoring' the plots for performance. If we went for least total bias, then the product rule or 4.1 would be a perfectly acceptable choice. If we scored data that erred in favour of the prosecution as 'bad' and those that erred in favour of the defendant as 'acceptable', then we would choose 4.2. However it is logically much worse than it might appear. It stems from a significant misunderstanding of the question. Recommendation 4.1 attempts to correct for within-person correlation. How can this be of any interest? The question is, given that the person of interest has this profile, what is the chance that someone else has this profile? This clearly requires a consideration of between-person correlations. It is a pity that Recommendation 4.1 has become normal practice in the United States and that reconsideration does not appear to be on the agenda. This has been fostered by calling this the *subpopulation correction* or the *theta correction*.

> In US forensic practice, owing to a long-standing misunderstanding introduced by the NRC2 report (Natl. Res. Counc. 1996), FST (also called θ) is usually used to model only within-individual genetic correlations (i.e., excess homozygosity). However, these correlations are of little relevance to evidential weight. Only between-individual correlations matter in practice, and failing to model them results in *LR* values that are biased against defendants. Modelling only excess homozygosity, as proposed in the NRC2 report Recommendation 4.1, is essentially irrelevant and gives a false impression of having adjusted for coancestry.[462]

The Curran et al. simulations do not include a specific consideration of mutation. Consideration of an infinite allele mutational process has suggested that this may have a significant effect on the estimation process:

> The product rule probability always underestimates the two-locus match probability. For highly mutable minisatellite loci, these probabilities can differ by an order of magnitude or more ... the degree of underestimation worsens for more loci.[432]

This statement is for an infinite allele mutation model and may not be appropriate for a stepwise mutation model. However it does suggest that further research is warranted if the product rule is to be used.

Tippett Testing

A method for investigating the magnitude and consequence of random matches has been championed by Evett and is colloquially called *Tippett testing*. Examples of Tippett plots appear on pages 213–215 of Evett and Weir[258] and large-scale Tippett-type experiments are reported by Weir.[431] The tests originate from an experiment by Tippett et al.[463] on paint. Evett has applied the same technique to data from both glass and DNA.

In the DNA context we imagine that we have a database of N profiles. We compare each person in the database with every other person. There are $\dfrac{N(N-1)}{2}$ possible comparisons.

---

* Of course this is not a 'true match probability' either but it is the true match probability under THIS model.

For each comparison the result is either a correspondence of profile (a match) or a difference (a non-match). We can therefore directly obtain the average match probability.

For demonstration consider the comparison of 1401 Caucasian FSS Quadruplex genotypes undertaken by Evett et al.[464] For this set there are 980,700 pairwise comparisons. (Note also that not all these comparisons are independent, although the consequences of this are probably negligible.) In almost all of these comparisons the profiles will be different. In such cases the LR is 0. On 118 occasions there was a four-locus match, and for such occasions an LR was calculated. This is as close to a direct measurement of the average match probability as we are going to get. We can say that in $\frac{118}{980,700} = 1$ in 8311 comparisons we will obtain a match between different people for this multiplex. If the database was constructed from unrelated Caucasians, then we have the estimate that 1 in 8311 unrelated pairs of Caucasians will match at these four loci.

Several things need to be noted about the general Tippett approach. First it makes very few assumptions and hence does not rely to any large extent on models. It is therefore our best approach to directly measuring average match probabilities. However match probabilities are usually quoted for the profile in question in court. This approach yields an average match probability across all N profiles that exist in the database.

The next thing that may be done with this data is to shuffle the alleles in the database. This action effectively imposes Hardy–Weinberg and linkage equilibrium on the data by breaking any possible association between alleles, whether or not it was there originally. We can then perform the experiment over and over again and obtain the distribution of the number and magnitude of matches expected if independence was true. What we typically note is that this distribution contains the number of matches that we observed in the unshuffled data. Does this method test the assumption of independence? Are we entitled to a statement such as, the number of matches observed is consistent with the assumption of independence?

It turns out that this would be a misleading conclusion. Making databases with known amounts of disequilibrium, possibly by simulation, and performing the experiment can show this. Often enough the databases with deliberately made disequilibrium also pass this test, that is, the number of observed matched and their relative magnitude is also consistent with the assumption of dependence. Hence the Tippett-type tests cannot really distinguish between databases that are in equilibrium and those that are not (there is no current method to do this of databases of realistic size), and consequently they cannot measure the extent of departure. What they do show is that the presence of relatively large amounts of disequilibrium has very little effect on the number and magnitude of matches.

To demonstrate this method Curran and Buckleton (unpublished results) considered an example given by Foreman et al.[465] They investigated the performance of this concept under two genetic models. One population is in Hardy–Weinberg and linkage equilibrium; the second is a sub-structured population characterized by an inbreeding coefficient $\theta = 0.03$ created by simulation. Databases were simulated many times from these populations and the number of matches counted. Figure 3.4 shows the distribution of the number of matches under each model. It is immediately apparent that the inclusion of a relatively large amount of disequilibrium has very little effect on the number of matches in each simulation. A direct consequence of this is that the number of matches is a very poor tool to use to distinguish between the independence model ($\theta = 0.00$) and the model with a value of $\theta = 0.03$. This had been previously shown algebraically by Weir.[466]

As databases have grown it has become difficult to know whether the match originates from the same or different people. Databases now contain profiles from the same person sampled twice under the same, similar or different names, twins, close relatives or unrelated people. It may be very difficult to ascertain the true state.

This challenge was solved by Weir who focussed on the partially matching profiles.[367] Consider a nine locus profile. When we compare this profile with another, it is possible that

Number of matches

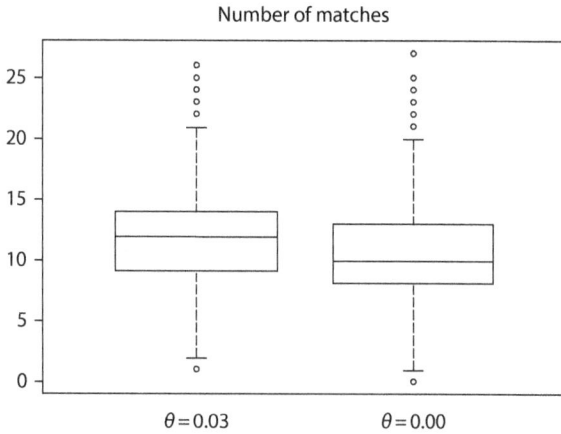

Figure 3.4   Number of pairwise matches per database.

all nine loci match. This is termed a *9/0 match*. It is also possible that eight loci match and one allele of the last locus matches. This is termed an *8/1 match*. Hence we could have 8/0, 7/2, 7/1, 7/0 matches and so on.

The Weir advance was not in determining the observed number of matches which is obtained empirically but in estimating the expected number of matches under certain values for θ.

It became apparent that the high-end partial matches, those nearest to a full match, would be dominated by pairs of relatives in the database. The Weir approach was extended to include an allowance for pairs of siblings, parents, children and cousins.[368–371] The algebra is probably at its tidiest in Tvedebrink et al.[368] (Box 3.2).

These experiments show a very good correspondence between the observed and expected partial matches when substructure and close relatives are modelled. This is the best empirical support currently available for the population genetic model of Balding and Nichols. The largest of these studies is Tvedebrink et al.,[368] who undertook 1.3×10^9 comparisons. We reproduce part of their table (Table 3.4).

The 10 locus matches have been edited and it is unsurprising to note none of these. However there are no 9 locus matches, either with or without the 10th locus partially matching. There are 1.3×10^{10} pairs of nine locus comparisons. It is important not to overinterpret such results.[468] Studies of approximately one billion partially dependent comparisons (10^9) in a Danish dataset should not be taken as proof that match probabilities are completely accurate, either in a Danish population or more importantly in a different population. More subtly the level of relatedness in the database is obtained from the data, not from some external source. In doing this the fit of the model to the data is optimized and not verified by external data.

However, on balance, these experiments give considerable support to the robustness of a properly formed population genetic model (Balding and Nichols) that incorporates substructure and relatedness.

In Figure 3.5 we present a summary of some of these experiments.

Inspection of the graphs concentrating on the high match end, the right hand end shows a very good correspondence between the observed and expected partial matches often with expected being above (conservative) observed. This is the best empirical support currently available for the population genetic model of Balding and Nichols.

The decisions in North America and the United Kingdom were made long before these simulation experiments were done and positions become entrenched.

BOX 3.2 ALGEBRA FOR MATCHING/PARTIALLY MATCHING LOCI

Let G_{i_1} and G_{i_2} be any two DNA profiles from different individuals in the dataset. Let $\pi = \mathbb{E}[M(G_{i_1}, G_{i_2})]$ be a matrix of match/partially match probabilities. That is, $\pi = \{\pi_{m/p}\}_{m,p}$ is the matrix of probabilities for the match/partially match events (m,p), where $m = 0, ..., L$ and $p = 0, ..., L - m$.

The elements of π may be computed using recursion over loci. Let π^ℓ denote the probability based on l loci, i.e. using only a subset of size l of the L loci such that $m = 0, ..., l$ and $p = 0, ..., l - m$. Furthermore, let $P_{m/p}^\ell$ refer to the $P_{m/p}$ probabilities for the lth added locus. We set $\pi_{1/0}^1 = P_{1/0}^1$, $\pi_{0/1}^1 = P_{0/1}^1$ and $\pi_{0/0}^1 = P_{0/0}^1$. Given these definitions and the initial values, then the following equation denotes how to compute $\pi_{m/p}^{\ell+1}$ by recursion:

$$\text{for } l = 1, \ldots L-1: \ \pi_{m/p}^{\ell+1} = \begin{cases} P_{0/0}^{\ell+1}\pi_{m/p}^\ell + P_{0/1}^{\ell+1}\pi_{m/p-1}^\ell + P_{1/0}^{\ell+1}\pi_{m-1/p}^\ell & m > 0 \text{ and } p > 0 \\ P_{0/0}^{\ell+1}\pi_{0/p}^\ell + P_{0/1}^{\ell+1}\pi_{0/p-1}^\ell & m = 0 \text{ and } p > 0 \\ P_{0/0}^{\ell+1}\pi_{m/0}^\ell + P_{1/0}^{\ell+1}\pi_{m-1/0}^\ell & m > 0 \text{ and } p = 0 \\ P_{0/0}^{\ell+1}\pi_{0/0}^\ell & m = 0 \text{ and } p = 0 \end{cases} \qquad (3.6)$$

where the 'sum' of the subscripts for each term on the right-hand side equals the subscript on the left-hand side, e.g. the subscripts of the last term in the first equation gives $1/0 + m - 1/p = m/p$.

The probabilities, $P_{m/p}$, depend on the co-ancestry coefficient, θ, through the match probability equations of Balding and Nichols.[358] These were given by Weir[367]

$$P_{0/0} = \frac{\theta^2(1-\theta)(1-S_2) + 2\theta(1-\theta)^2(1-2S_2+S_3) + (1-\theta)^3\left[1-4S_2+4S_3+2S_2^2-3S_4\right]}{(1+\theta)(1+2\theta)}$$

$$P_{0/1} = \frac{8\theta^2(1-\theta)(1-S_2) + 4\theta(1-\theta)^2(1-S_3) + 4(1-\theta)^3\left[S_2-S_3-S_2^2+S_4\right]}{(1+\theta)(1+2\theta)}$$

$$P_{1/0} = \frac{6\theta^3 + \theta^2(1-\theta)(2+9S_2) + 2\theta(1-\theta)^2(2S_2+S_3) + (1-\theta)^3\left[2S_2^2-S_4\right]}{(1+\theta)(1+2\theta)}$$

where $S_2 = \sum_i p_i^2$, $S_3 = \sum_i p_i^3$, $S_4 = \sum_i p_i^4$ are the sums of squared, cubed and 4th power of the allele probabilities at a given locus.

Weir[467] showed that for a specified family relationship of a pair of profiles, $P_{m/p}$ is updated using the probabilities, k_1, that the two individuals share I alleles identical by descent (IBD):

$$\tilde{P}_{0/0} = k_0 P_{0/0} \quad \tilde{P}_{0/1} = k_1(1-\theta)(1-S_2) + k_0 P_{0/1}$$

and

$$\tilde{P}_{1/0} = k_2 + k_1[\theta + (1-\theta)S_2] + k_0 P_{1/0}$$

and $\tilde{P}_{m/p}$ denotes the probability that two individuals with the specified family relationship will match as m/p at a given locus. From $\tilde{P}_{m/p}$, it is clear that close relatives have an increased probability of sharing alleles due to alleles being IBD.

For a pair of R-relatives (close relatives of type R), the expected numbers of matching/partially matching loci, $\tilde{\pi}_R$, are calculated by replacing $P_{m/p}$ with $\tilde{P}_{m/p}$ in Equation 3.6.

Table 3.4   Number Partially Matching Loci After 1.3 × 10⁹ Comparisons

Number of Matching Pairs		Partially Matching Loci (p)				
		0	1	2	3	4
Fully matching loci (m)	6	470	1685	2272	1414	378
	7	26	96	91	64	
	8	3	6	21		
	9	0	0			
	10	0				

Source: Reprinted from *Forensic Science International: Genetics*, 6(3), Tvedebrink, T., et al., Analysis of matches and partial-matches in a Danish STR data set, 387–392, Copyright 2012, with permission from Elsevier.

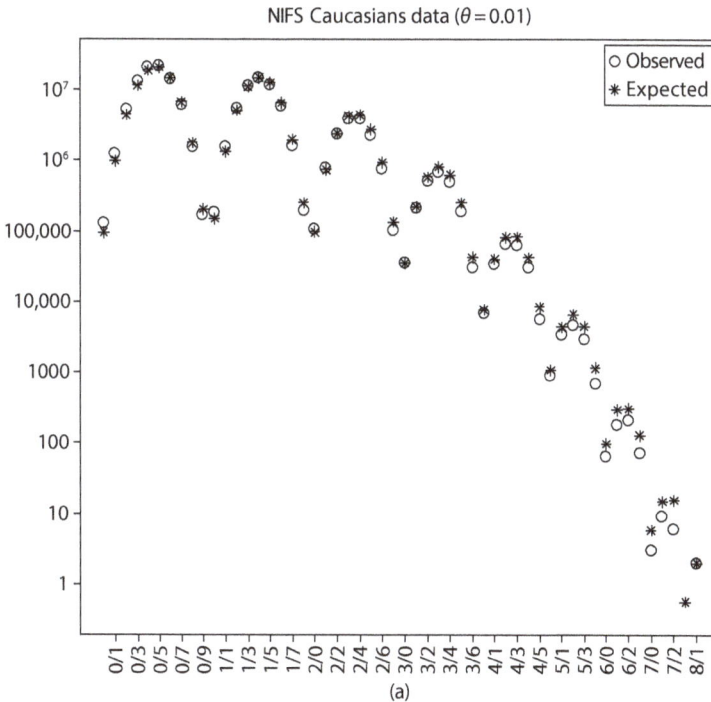

Figure 3.5   A sample of published Tippett test results. (a) NIFS (National Institute of Forensic Science, Australia) Caucasian. (From Tvedebrink, T., et al., *Forensic Science International: Genetics*, 6(3), 387–392, 2012; Curran, J., et al., *Australian Journal of Forensic Sciences*, 40(2), 99–108, 2008; Curran, J.M., et al., *Forensic Science International: Genetics*, 1(3–4), 267–272, 2007.)

(Continued)

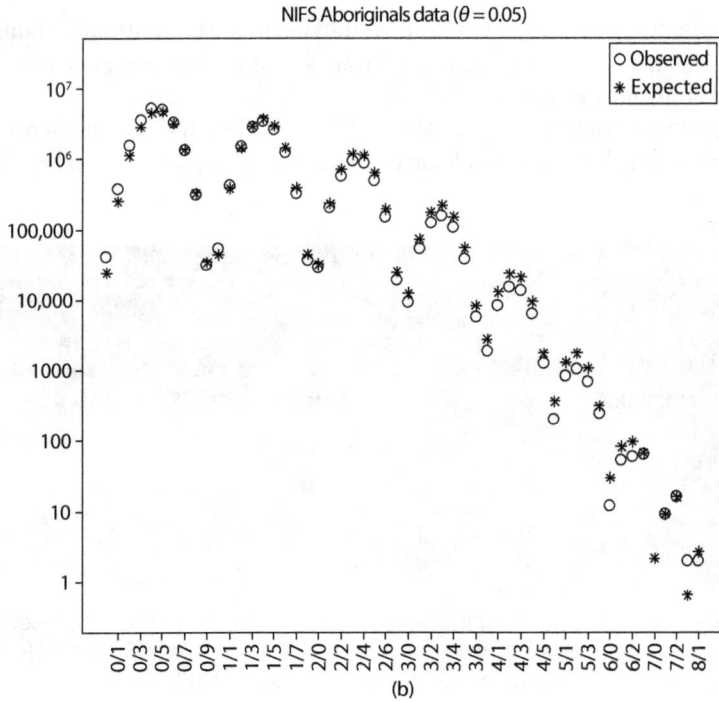

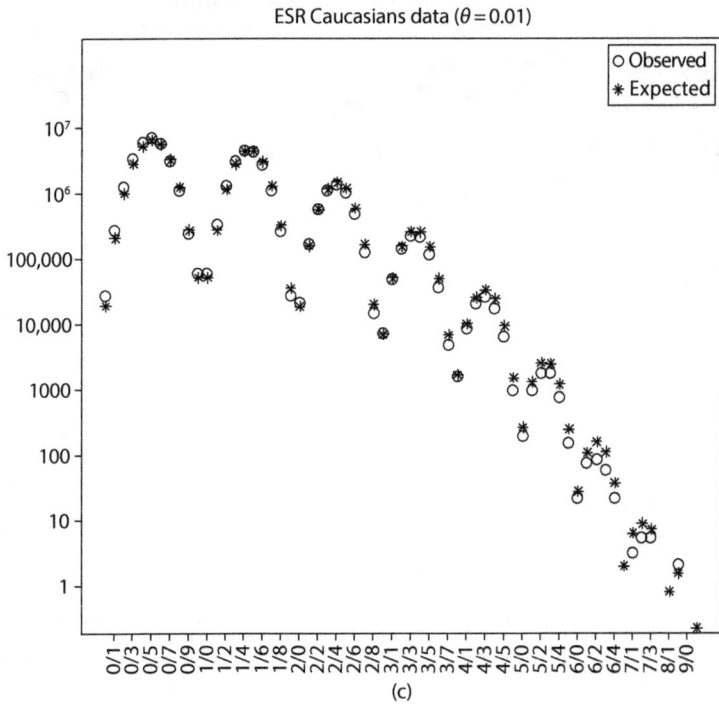

Figure 3.5 (Continued)   A sample of published Tippett test results. (b) NIFS Aboriginal (c) ESR Caucasian. (From Tvedebrink, T., et al., *Forensic Science International: Genetics*, 6(3), 387–392, 2012; Curran, J., et al., *Australian Journal of Forensic Sciences*, 40(2), 99–108, 2008; Curran, J.M., et al., *Forensic Science International: Genetics*, 1(3–4), 267–272, 2007.)   *(Continued)*

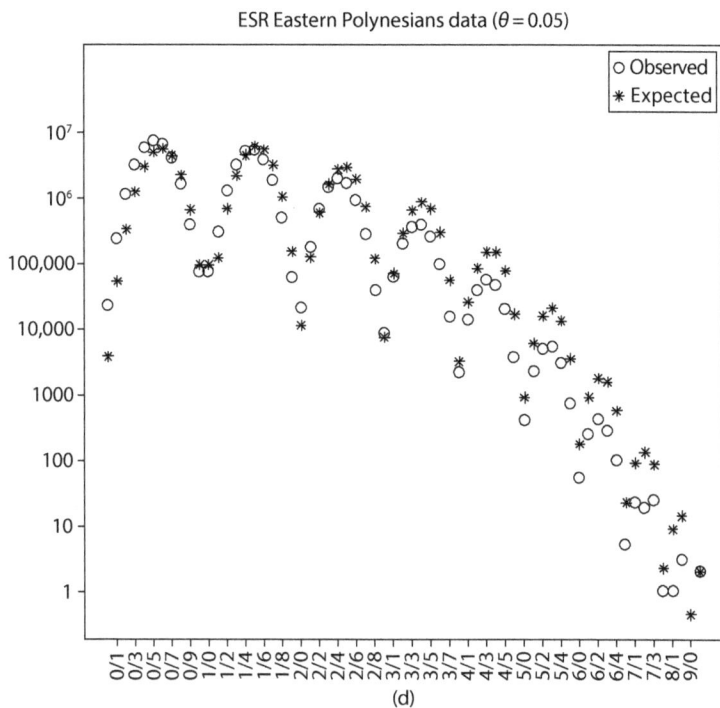

ESR Eastern Polynesians data ($\theta = 0.05$)

(d)

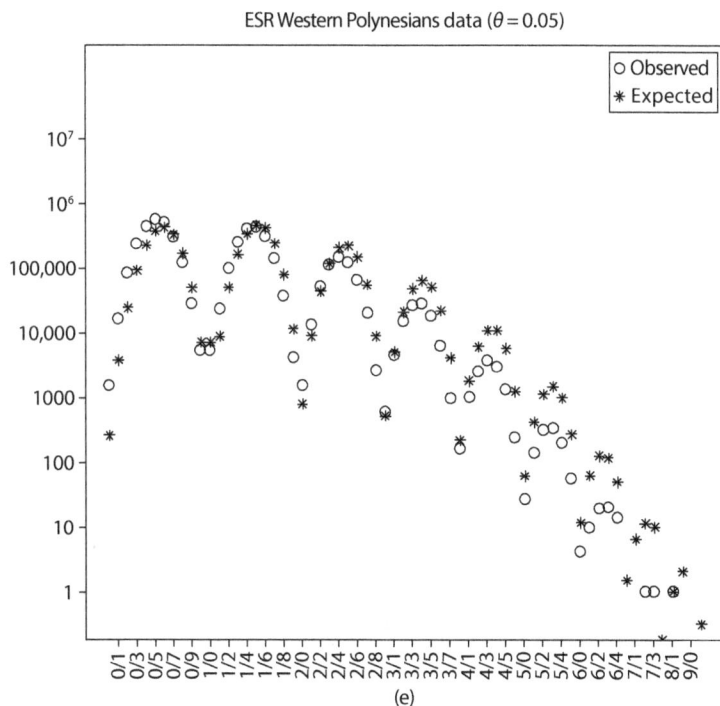

ESR Western Polynesians data ($\theta = 0.05$)

(e)

Figure 3.5 (Continued)   A sample of published Tippett test results. (d) ESR Eastern Polynesian (e) ESR Western Polynesian. (From Tvedebrink, T., et al., *Forensic Science International: Genetics*, 6(3), 387–392, 2012; Curran, J., et al., *Australian Journal of Forensic Sciences*, 40(2), 99–108, 2008; Curran, J.M., et al., *Forensic Science International: Genetics*, 1(3–4), 267–272, 2007.)   *(Continued)*

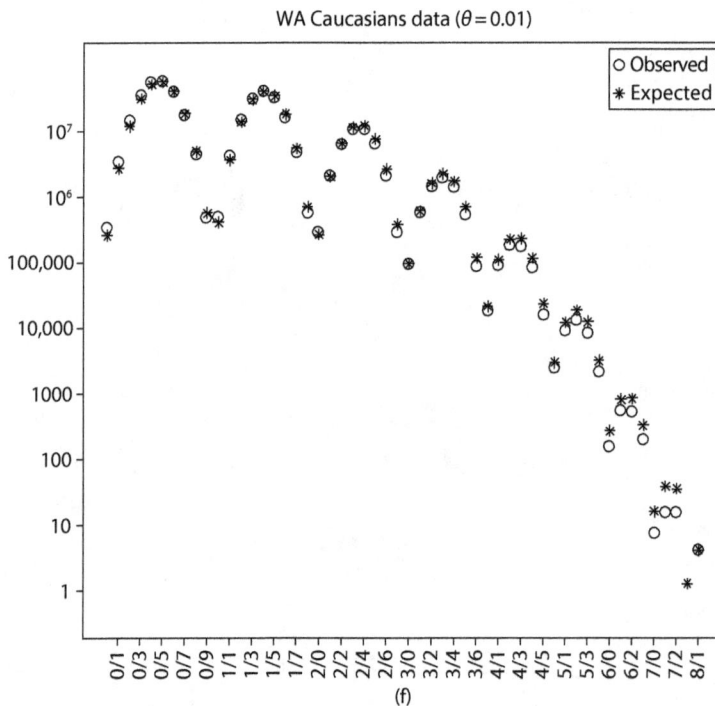

WA Caucasians data ($\theta = 0.01$)

(f)

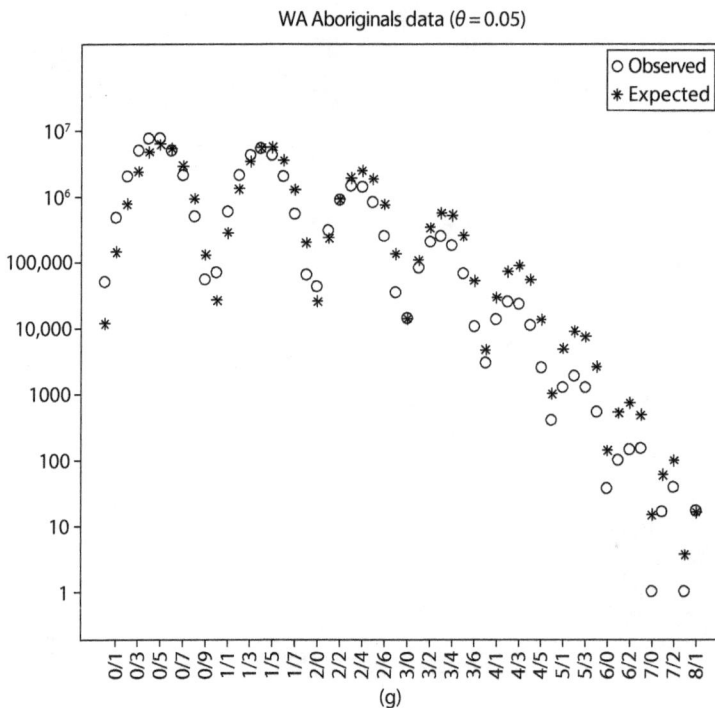

WA Aboriginals data ($\theta = 0.05$)

(g)

Figure 3.5 (Continued) A sample of published Tippett test results. (f) Western Australian (WA) Caucasian (g) WA Aboriginal. (From Tvedebrink, T., et al., *Forensic Science International: Genetics*, 6(3), 387–392, 2012; Curran, J., et al., *Australian Journal of Forensic Sciences*, 40(2), 99–108, 2008; Curran, J.M., et al., *Forensic Science International: Genetics*, 1(3–4), 267–272, 2007.)   *(Continued)*

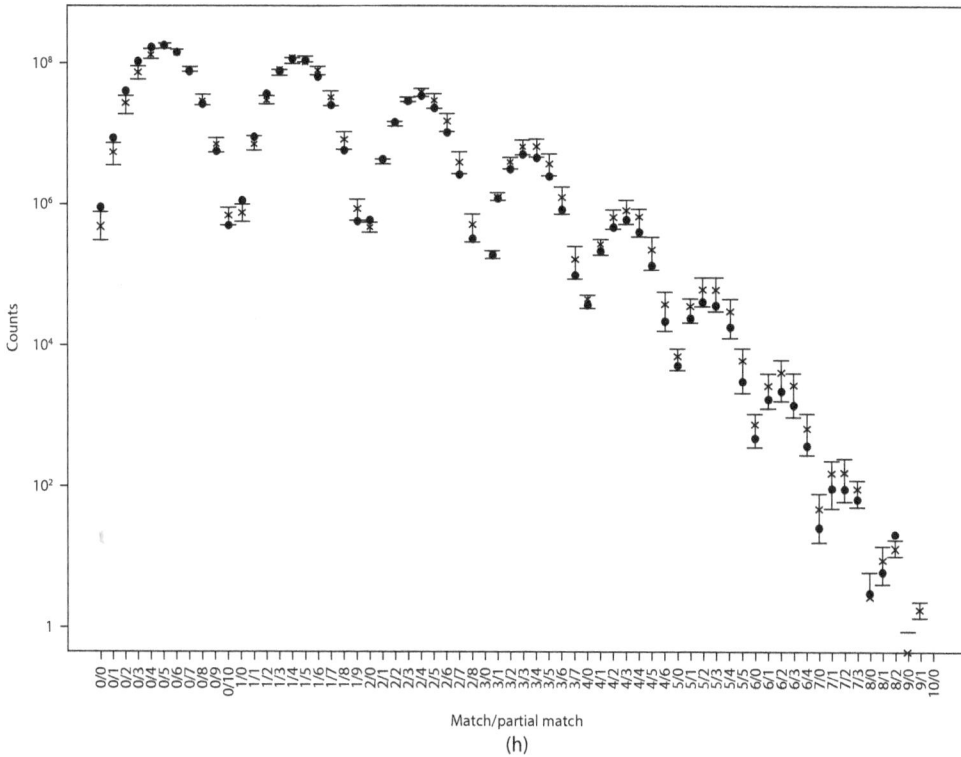

Figure 3.5 (Continued)   A sample of published Tippett test results. (h) WA Aboriginal. (From Tvedebrink, T., et al., *Forensic Science International: Genetics*, 6(3), 387–392, 2012; Curran, J., et al., *Australian Journal of Forensic Sciences*, 40(2), 99–108, 2008; Curran, J.M., et al., *Forensic Science International: Genetics*, 1(3–4), 267–272, 2007.)

Discussion of the Product Rule and the Subpopulation Model

If we are able to show by population genetic studies that the effects of population subdivision are so minor that we are prepared to ignore them, then it is permissible to use the product rule as a first-order approximation provided that it is understood that it is probably slightly biased in favour of the prosecution. A useful review of various approaches is made by Gill et al.[450]

The belief on which the use of the product rule or use of Recommendation 4.1 is based can arise only from well-constructed population genetic examinations[469] that assess the population genetic subdivision at the genetic level. It is vital that this examination be at the genetic rather than the geographical level especially in countries settled largely by recent colonization. This is because geographic samples in, say, the United States taken from Caucasians from different states or cities are unlikely to express the underlying genetic diversity. Suppose that we took two samples each of, say, 33% Scottish, 33% English and 33% Italian. The allele frequencies demonstrated by these two samples would probably be very similar. Whereas if we compared comparable samples drawn separately from the Scottish, English and Italian populations, we would find small but real differences between them.

A common and reasonable response is that the difference between the product rule estimate and a fair and reasonable assignment of the evidential value is not forensically significant.[446,447] This is probably true in many instances; however there is divergent evidence. For instance in the identification of war victims from the 1991–1995 war in Croatia, Birus et al.[470] found an unexpectedly high number of false matches between skeletal remains and the relatives of missing persons. They attribute this to substructure in Croatia and warn:

> Although genetically and statistically sound and widely accepted, calculations that we perform today produce numbers that might not be fully applicable in all situations. One of the factors not included in these calculations (the product rule) is the effect of local inbreeding.

It remains important to understand that the commonly applied approach of independence testing in no way measures the extent of departure from equilibrium. It cannot be used to estimate the difference between the product rule assignment and a fair and reasonable assignment (for early discussions see Refs. 177,312,421,471–473).

Therefore the statement that the potential error is not forensically significant, if true at all, cannot be based on independence testing. Again it can only be investigated at all, and certainly not proved, by a population genetic model or perhaps by experiments of the type pioneered by Tippett in the case of less vanishingly small probabilities.

It may be interesting to note the expected behaviour of these two approaches, if indeed the requirement of independence is not fulfilled. If we pick a genotype at random, irrespective of whether it is known to exist or not, then Recommendation 4.1 is likely to provide a fair and reasonable probability assignment (note that although it is fair and reasonable it is not necessarily the true value). However if we now add the additional information that one person, the suspect, has this profile then we have two options:

> First we could ignore this additional information and still proceed with Recommendation 4.1. This is no longer an unbiased approach. In fact using Recommendation 4.1 the probability assignment is likely to have a small bias in favour of the prosecution because the knowledge that we have ignored increases the probability that a second copy of this genotype exists. The extent of this bias is dependent on how large or small are the dependence effects.

> Second we could follow the Bayesian approach, which does, in fact, lead to consideration of the conditional probabilities such as $\Pr(G_c|G_s)$ discussed above. These have a remarkable robustness to deviations both from Hardy–Weinberg and linkage equilibrium and as such, we believe, represent a more fair and reasonable probability assignment. However we accept that, as implemented, they appear to represent an overcorrection. For a discussion on implementation in the United Kingdom see Foreman et al.[474] (unfortunately not generally available).

This difference between these two approaches is as fundamental as the difference between unconditional probabilities and conditional ones.[258,475] An approach based on mathematical logic leads us to the conditional probabilities. In fact it would appear that some former major proponents of the validity of the product rule have now modified their position in the face of increasing data.[391,476–480]

There is only just emerging a possibility of experimentally verifying probability assignments this small. They represent, in multilocus cases, extrapolation way beyond anything that can be experimentally examined.

It must be accepted that, like the product rule, the subpopulation formulae rely on a population genetic model, albeit one that is more robust and concedes doubt correctly to the defendant. Whereas it is possible to say that the product rule is mildly biased towards the prosecution, it is not possible to state whether or not the subpopulation formulae are also biased. It is at least theoretically possible that they are conservative, and the experimental evidence given here suggests that this is so.

A discussion of the ethics of this debate is given by Beyleveld,[481] who also discusses some of the pressures that have been brought to bear on independent bodies when considering these issues.

The Effect of Mutation

The effect of mutation on the assessment of multilocus genotype probabilities has recently been considered. Laurie and Weir[432] warn of the consequences of mutation of the infinite allele type on the estimation process. This model may be a reasonable model for minisatellites although a consensus has not yet been developed.

Laurie and Weir suggest that the assumption of independence understates the two locus match probabilities for such loci. The effect increases with increasing mutation rate. For loci with high mutation rates the two locus probabilities may differ substantially from the product of single locus probabilities. They show that these dependency effects accumulate across loci. 'These results indicate a potential concern with using the product rule to compute genotypic match probabilities for highly mutable loci'.[432]

In loci with high mutation rates, alleles stand an increased chance of being recent and rare. 'Hence, if two individuals share alleles at one locus, they are more likely to be related through recent pedigree, and hence more likely to share alleles at a second locus'.[432]

This conclusion may hold for the IAM. This model is unlikely to be applicable to STRs and the effect of mutation on between locus dependencies at these loci has yet to be settled.

We consider the question, do the Balding and Nichols formulae give an adequate assignment of the match probability in the subpopulation of the suspect? If we restrict ourselves to this question, we again must accept the impossibility of experimentally testing such multilocus estimates.

We are left with examining the validity of the assumptions of the model and simulation results. This matter is elegantly considered by Graham, Curran and Weir,[482] who point out that the assumptions of the Balding and Nichols model include a steady-state population and a mutation model in which the allelic state after mutation is independent of the state prior to mutation. Both of these assumptions are untenable. Graham et al. investigate the consequences of a generalized stepwise model and conclude '[the Balding and Nichols] theory can still overstate the evidence against a suspect with a common minisatellite genotype. However Dirichlet-based estimators [the Balding and Nichols formulae] were less biased than the product rule estimator, which ignores coancestry'.

Laurie and Weir finish with the following conclusion:

The method of adjusting single-locus match probabilities for population structure [the Balding and Nichols equations] when multiplied across loci has been shown empirically to accommodate the dependencies we have found for multiple loci.

4

Relatedness

John S. Buckleton, Jo-Anne Bright and Duncan Taylor[*]

Contents

Introduction

In this chapter we discuss the evaluation of the joint and conditional probabilities of obtaining various genotypes for two people who are related and the effect of this relatedness on the interpretation process. Formulae are given for some common relationships. Most of this work has appeared elsewhere, for instance in Evett and Weir.[257] Elegant algorithms have been published[483-485] that perform these and far more complex analyses. Such probabilities have many uses outside the specific forensic context.

In our forensic work we will often need to consider relatedness. This need can occur because of a specific defence such as 'my brother committed the crime'[486] but is becoming increasingly relevant even in the absence of such a specific defence. There are several probabilities that we may be interested in regarding relatives. These probabilities would include answers to questions such as the following:

1. What is the probability that a brother would 'match'?

2. Given that these two individuals match, what is the probability that they are brothers?

In fact the probabilities that forensic scientists would be providing when addressing these two questions would be

1. The probability of obtaining a profile from person 1 if person 2, his brother, had the same profile

2. The probability of obtaining two matching profiles given they are brothers

---

[*] Based on an earlier edition by John Buckleton and Christopher Triggs.

These scenarios appear quite similar and the same methods can be used to evaluate the probabilities associated with these two questions although they are applied slightly differently. Note that we are discussing probabilities and not likelihood ratios (*LRs*). To answer the questions above we need only to calculate a single probability rather than considering the probability of the evidence given two competing hypotheses. The latter style of calculation, which is commonly used for addressing the 'brother's defence', produces an *LR*.

There are at least three methods we are aware of that are used to calculate these probabilities. All give the same result. We will discuss two methods, both of which utilize the concept of identity by descent (IBD) initially introduced in 1940 by Cotterman[487] and extended by Malecot,[488] Li and Sacks[489] and Jacquard[490] (see also Refs. 488, 491–494). Two alleles are said to be IBD if they are the same *because* they are copies of the same ancestral allele.

Consider two people X and Y (termed a *dyadic relationship*).[495] We can label the alleles at a specific locus for person X as ab and person Y as cd. This does not imply that person X has genotype *ab* but rather that we have labelled his two alleles a and b. In such a case the labels a, b, c and d are referred to as *placeholders*. The actual allele in place a is denoted by an italicized label. See Box 4.1.

The sign ≡ is often used to signify that two alleles are IBD. Hence a ≡ b means that the alleles with labels a and b are IBD. Consider the relationship of a parent and a child (Figure 4.1).

BOX 4.1   BUCKLETON'S BUCKETS

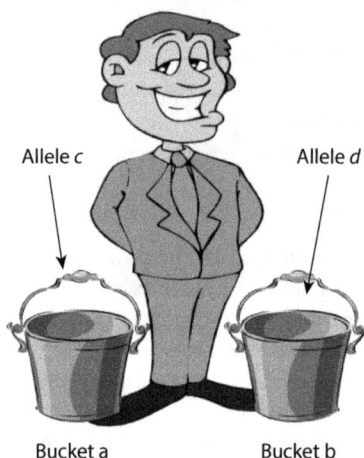

Allele *c*   Allele *d*

Bucket a   Bucket b

This term was coined by Weir. The distinction between the actual allele and the label of the allele, or placeholder, is one that in our experience many readers, students and teachers find difficult to either understand or communicate. However it is vitally important to clearly understand the distinction. We may illustrate the concept of placeholders using the following figure. A useful visual metaphor for the label or placeholder is that of a bucket.

A person has two buckets, a and b; they contain the alleles *c* and *d*.

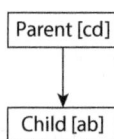

Parent [cd]

Child [ab]

Figure 4.1   A pedigree for a parent and child.

We have labelled the alleles in the parent c and d and those in the child a and b. The laws of Mendelian inheritance state that one of the alleles labelled a or b must be a copy of one of the alleles labelled c or d. The actual allele that is a copy of the parental allele is IBD.

Conditional Probabilities

These are the probabilities that an untyped relative will have a certain genotype, G_2, given that a typed relative has genotype G_1. Such probabilities can be used to answer most questions of forensic interest, such as 'What is the probability that a brother of the matching suspect will also match?' Such conditional probabilities may be developed in two ways, either directly or via the joint probability and the definition of a conditional probability, $\Pr(G_2 | G_1) = \dfrac{\Pr(G_2, G_1)}{\Pr(G_1)}$. Either method has its merits and drawbacks. Both the method of Balding and Nichols[358] and that due to Weir[257] can be used to evaluate the conditional probabilities.

The Method of Balding and Nichols

Any two people possess four alleles at a specific locus. If we consider one of these people, then they may have zero, one or two alleles IBD with the other person.* Following Balding and Nichols we consider the following events:

Z_0: Zero alleles are IBD, with probability $\Pr(Z_0)$.

Z_1: One allele is IBD, with probability $\Pr(Z_1)$.

Z_2: Two alleles are IBD, with probability $\Pr(Z_2)$.

Consider the relationship between a parent and child (Figure 4.1).

The child has two alleles which we have labelled a and b (completely arbitrarily). By the principle of Mendelian inheritance we can see that we expect one of these alleles to be IBD with one of the alleles from the parent. Thus we can see that for a parent/child relationship $\Pr(Z_1) = 1$ and $\Pr(Z_0) = \Pr(Z_2) = 0$.

Consider now a pair of siblings (Figure 4.2).

Each sibling will receive an allele from his or her father. With probability 1/2 these will be copies of same allele, and thus IBD. Thus with probability 1/2 they will not be IBD. Similarly the probability that the two copies of the maternal allele will be IBD will also be 1/2. Therefore both will be IBD with probability $\Pr(Z_2) = \Pr(\text{IBD}_{\text{Maternal}}) \times \Pr(\text{IBD}_{\text{Paternal}}) = \frac{1}{2} \times \frac{1}{2} = \frac{1}{4}$.

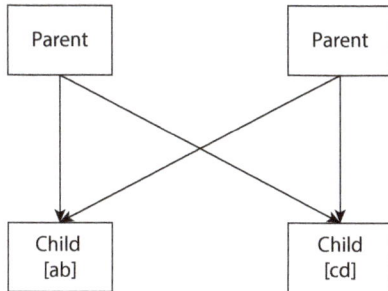

Figure 4.2   A pedigree for siblings.

---

* Of course the relationship is reflexive. Balding and Nichols also make the assumption that the two alleles within an individual are not IBD. Thus their method can only be applied to dyadic relationships and hence cannot handle those situations where one or more of the founders are inbred.

There are two ways in which a pair of siblings can have one pair of IBD alleles. They may share only the maternal or only the paternal allele and hence

$$\Pr(Z_1) = \Pr(\mathrm{IBD_M}) \times \Pr(\overline{\mathrm{IMD_P}}) + \Pr(\overline{\mathrm{IBD_M}}) \times \Pr(\mathrm{IBD_P}) = \tfrac{1}{2} \times \tfrac{1}{2} + \tfrac{1}{2} \times \tfrac{1}{2} = \tfrac{1}{2}$$

Similarly it follows that the probability that they have zero IBD alleles, $\Pr(Z_0) = \tfrac{1}{4}$. Similar arguments lead to Table 4.1, which gives the values of $\Pr(Z_0)$, $\Pr(Z_1)$ and $\Pr(Z_2)$ for some of the forensically important relationships between two individuals.

To demonstrate the use of this table we calculate the conditional probability that a person has genotype aa given that his sibling has genotype ab. We will write this as $\Pr[aa|ab,\text{siblings}]$. We will omit the conditioning on siblings for simplicity except where the omission may cause ambiguity.

Using the law of total probability* this can be written as follows:

$$\Pr[aa|ab] = \Pr[aa|ab, Z_2]\Pr(Z_2) + \Pr[aa|ab, Z_1]\Pr(Z_1) + \Pr[aa|ab, Z_0]\Pr(Z_0)$$

This can be further broken down by considering that under Z_1 the a allele or the b allele could be IBD:

$$\Pr[aa|ab] = \Pr[aa|ab, Z_2] + \tfrac{1}{2}\left(\Pr[aa|ab, Z_1^{a=IBD}] + \Pr[aa|ab, Z_1^{b=IBD}]\right)\Pr(Z_1)$$
$$+ \Pr[aa|ab, Z_0]\Pr(Z_0)$$

If the two siblings share two pairs of IBD alleles, then they must have the same genotype. Since it is not possible to obtain the aa genotype from an ab genotype with two alleles IBD, then $\Pr[aa|ab, Z_2] = 0$.

If the two siblings share one pair of IBD alleles, then with probability $\tfrac{1}{2}\Pr(Z_1)$ the a allele in the conditioning genotype is IBD, and we need the other bucket to be filled with the a allele by chance. Hence we assign $\Pr[aa|ab, Z_1] = p_a/2$. With probability $\tfrac{1}{2}\Pr(Z_1)$ the b allele in the conditioning genotype is IBD, but here we have $\Pr[aa|ab, Z_1] = 0$ since it is not possible to obtain the aa genotype if the b allele is IBD.

If the two siblings share zero pairs of IBD alleles, then $\Pr[aa|ab, Z_0] = p_a^2$ since both buckets in the individual whose genotype is in front of the conditioning bar are unconstrained – that is,

Table 4.1 Probabilities That Two Individuals with a Given Relationship Share Zero, One or Two Pairs of IBD Alleles

Relationship	$\Pr(Z_0)$	$\Pr(Z_1)$	$\Pr(Z_2)$
Parent/child	0	1	0
Full siblings	¼	½	¼
Half-siblings	½	½	0
Grandparent/ grandchild	½	½	0
Uncle/nephew	½	½	0
First cousins	¾	¼	0

IBD, identity by descent.

---

* We assume that the IBD state and the genotype of the conditioning individual are independent $\Pr[Z_i|ab] = \Pr[Z_i]$.

not determined by any IBD state – and each bucket must be filled with separate copies of the allele a.

This calculation can be set down in a general stepwise process.

Table 4.2 illustrates the general algorithm to evaluate $\Pr[G_1|G_2]$, which can easily be implemented in a spreadsheet by following these six steps.

1. First lay out a table with four rows, one for each of the cases of two or zero pairs of IBD alleles and two for the case of one pair of IBD alleles.

2. In a column write the probabilities for the events Z_2, $\tfrac{1}{2}Z_1$, $\tfrac{1}{2}Z_1$ and Z_0 with the corresponding values for the relationship from Table 4.1.

3. In the next column write the probabilities of observing genotype G_1 given genotype G_2 and the corresponding IBD state.

4. For the next column:

   a. The probability in the Z_2 row will have either a 0 or a 1 in it, depending on whether or not the persons before and after the conditioning bar have the same genotype.

   b. When the genotype G_2 behind the conditioning bar is a heterozygote, we use two rows for the Z_1 event to account for each allele in G_2 being the allele involved in the IBD pair. When G_2 is homozygous, these two rows will contain the same value.

   c. The Z_0 row describes the event when the two genotypes have no IBD alleles. Initially we use the product rule to evaluate $\Pr[G_1|G_2, Z_0]$.

5. In the final column of the table, form the product of the previous two columns.

6. Sum the final column to give required probability.

To drop the assumption of independence in the calculation of $\Pr[G_1|G_1, Z_i]$ we can introduce the conditional probability[358] at Step 3. The example above, evaluating $\Pr[G_1 = aa|G_2 = ab]$ for a pair of siblings and involving the subpopulation correction, is given in Table 4.3.

This method of calculation leads to the formulae given in Table 4.4.

Table 4.2	The Calculation of $\Pr[aa|ab]$ for Siblings				
Pairs of IBD Alleles	$\Pr[Z_i]$	$\Pr[Z_i]$ Siblings	$\Pr(ab|aa, Z_i)$	Product	
2	$\Pr(Z_2)$	¼	0	0	
1	$\tfrac{1}{2}\Pr\left(Z_1^{a=IBD}\right)$	¼	p_a	$\dfrac{p_a}{4}$	
	$\tfrac{1}{2}\Pr\left(Z_1^{b=IBD}\right)$	¼	0	0	
0	$\Pr(Z_0)$	¼	p_a^2	$\dfrac{p_a^2}{4}$	
			Sum =	$\dfrac{p_a(1+p_a)}{4}$	

IBD, identity by descent.

Table 4.3 The Conditional Calculation for $\Pr[aa|ab]$ for Brothers Including the Subpopulation Correction

Pairs of IBD Alleles	$\Pr[Z_i]$	$\Pr[Z_i]$ Siblings	$\Pr(ab|aa, Z_i)$	Product
2	Z_2	¼	0	0
1	$\frac{1}{2}Z_1^{a=IBD}$	¼	$\dfrac{\theta+(1-\theta)p_a}{1+\theta}$	$\dfrac{\theta+(1-\theta)p_a}{4(1+\theta)}$
	$\frac{1}{2}Z_1^{b=IBD}$	¼	0	0
0	Z_0	¼	$\dfrac{\left(\theta+(1-\theta)p_a\right)\times\left(2\theta+(1-\theta)p_a\right)}{(1+\theta)(1+2\theta)}$	$\dfrac{\left(\theta+(1-\theta)p_a\right)\times\left(2\theta+(1-\theta)p_a\right)}{4(1+\theta)(1+2\theta)}$

$$\text{Sum}=\frac{\theta+(1-\theta)p_a}{4(1+\theta)}\times\left(1+\frac{\left(2\theta+(1-\theta)p_a\right)}{(1+2\theta)}\right)$$

IBD, identity by descent.

Table 4.4 Conditional Probabilities for Some Relatives (R) Including the Subpopulation Correction

Genotype of Typed Person, G_2	Genotype for the Untyped Relative, G_1	$\Pr(G_1|G_2,R)$
aa	aa	$Z_2+Z_1\dfrac{\left(2\theta+(1-\theta)p_a\right)}{1+\theta}+Z_0\dfrac{\left(2\theta+(1-\theta)p_a\right)\left(3\theta+(1-\theta)p_a\right)}{(1+\theta)(1+2\theta)}$
	bb	$Z_0\dfrac{(1-\theta)p_b\left(\theta+(1-\theta)p_b\right)}{(1+\theta)(1+2\theta)}$
	ab	$Z_1\dfrac{(1-\theta)p_b}{1+\theta}+Z_0\dfrac{\left(2\theta+(1-\theta)p_a\right)(1-\theta)p_b}{(1+\theta)(1+2\theta)}$
	bc	$Z_0\dfrac{2(1-\theta)^2 p_b p_c}{(1+\theta)(1+2\theta)}$
ab	aa	$\dfrac{Z_1}{2}\dfrac{\left(\theta+(1-\theta)p_a\right)}{1+\theta}+Z_0\dfrac{\left(\theta+(1-\theta)p_a\right)\left(2\theta+(1-\theta)p_a\right)}{(1+\theta)(1+2\theta)}$
	ab	$Z_2+\dfrac{Z_1}{2}\dfrac{\left(2\theta+(1-\theta)(p_a+p_b)\right)}{1+\theta}+Z_0\dfrac{2\left(\theta+(1-\theta)p_a\right)\left(\theta+(1-\theta)p_b\right)}{(1+\theta)(1+2\theta)}$
	ac	$\dfrac{Z_1}{2}\dfrac{\left((1-\theta)p_c\right)}{1+\theta}+Z_0\dfrac{2\left(\theta+(1-\theta)p_a\right)(1-\theta)p_c}{(1+\theta)(1+2\theta)}$
	cc	$Z_0\dfrac{\left((1-\theta)p_c\right)\left(\theta+(1-\theta)p_c\right)}{(1+\theta)(1+2\theta)}$
	cd	$Z_0\dfrac{2(1-\theta)^2 p_c p_d}{(1+\theta)(1+2\theta)}$

The Method of Weir

A more precise nomenclature was given by Weir.[257,424,497] It was based on four-allele descent measures. This requires a labelling of the alleles in each person. We name the alleles in Person 1 as ab and in Person 2 as cd (Table 4.5), where the a, b, c and d are placeholders (buckets). These allele designations must be tied to the pedigree to give the values given by Weir. Consider, for example, the case of half-siblings (Figure 4.3). In this figure we assign allele a as coming from Person G, allele b as coming from Person H, c from H and d from I as indicated.

If we assume that H is the father and G and I mothers, then we are labelling b and c as paternal alleles and a and d as maternal alleles. This labelling of the alleles is arbitrary and troubles many people. However any other arrangement can be used and produces the same result.

We need to consider 14 possible IBD states for the four alleles. For example, the term δ_{abcd} represents the probability that all the alleles a, b, c and d are IBD. The expression $a \equiv b$ implies that alleles a and b are IBD but not IBD with alleles c or d, nor is c IBD with d.

Table 4.5 Four-Allele Descent Measures Following Weir

Alleles IBD[a]	Term	Probabilities		
		Full Siblings	Cousins	Half-Siblings
None	δ_0	¼	¾	½
$a \equiv b$	δ_{ab}			
$c \equiv d$	δ_{cd}			
$a \equiv c$	δ_{ac}	¼		
$a \equiv d$	δ_{ad}			
$b \equiv c$	δ_{bc}		¼	½
$b \equiv d$	δ_{bd}	¼		
$a \equiv b \equiv c$	δ_{abc}			
$a \equiv b \equiv d$	δ_{abd}			
$a \equiv c \equiv d$	δ_{acd}			
$a \equiv b, c \equiv d$	$\delta_{ab,cd}$			
$a \equiv c, b \equiv d$	$\delta_{ac,bd}$	¼		
$a \equiv d, b \equiv c$	$\delta_{ad,bc}$			
$a \equiv b \equiv c \equiv d$	δ_{abcd}			

IBD, identical by descent.
[a] If the alleles are not mentioned they are not IBD.

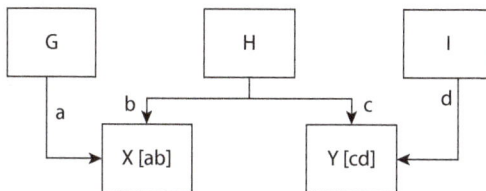

Figure 4.3 A pedigree for half-siblings (X and Y).

125

The same procedure for developing the conditional probability directly as given under Balding and Nichol's method also applies here except that part of the ambiguity regarding Z_1 is resolved using the Weir approach. In Table 4.6 we reproduce the calculation for $\Pr(aa|aa)$ for full siblings. The method is analogous to the approach given by Balding and Nichols but is more versatile.

Even using the Weir nomenclature there is a wrinkle that one needs to be aware of when only one pair of alleles is IBD. This occurs if we try to write down the conditional probability directly but does not occur if we proceed via joint probabilities (see later) and only when the conditioning profile is heterozygotic. This wrinkle can be demonstrated using an example involving cousins. Consider the probability $\Pr(ac|ab)$ for cousins (Table 4.7).

Following Weir[254,287,497] we describe the process: it is necessary to consider the cell marked with the question mark (?). For this cell we know that the alleles marked by the b and d placeholders are IBD. However this does not inform us whether the a allele is the one involved in this IBD state. If the b allele is involved then we cannot obtain an ac genotype. The a allele is the one involved 1/2 of the time. This results in a value of $\dfrac{\Pr(c|ab,\text{unrelated})}{2}=\dfrac{(1-\theta)p_c}{2(1+\theta)}$ for the question mark cell. By multiplying across the rows and adding downwards, $\Pr(ac|ab)$ for cousins is

Table 4.6 The Calculation of Pr($aa|aa$, Siblings) Following the Weir Methodology

Alleles IBD	Term	Full Siblings	Probabilities
None	δ_0	¼	$\Pr(aa|aa, \text{unrelated}^a)$
$a \equiv c$	δ_{ac}	¼	$\Pr(a|aa, \text{unrelated})$
$b \equiv d$	δ_{bd}	¼	$\Pr(a|aa, \text{unrelated})$
$a \equiv c, b \equiv d$	$\delta_{ac,bd}$	¼	1
Sum of the products $= \dfrac{1}{4}\left(1+\dfrac{2\left(2\theta+(1-\theta)p_a\right)}{1+\theta}+\dfrac{\left(2\theta+(1-\theta)p_a\right)\left(3\theta+(1-\theta)p_a\right)}{(1+\theta)(1+2\theta)}\right)$			

IBD, identical by descent.
[a] *Unrelated* is shorthand for 'unrelated members of the same subpopulation'.

Table 4.7 The Calculation of Pr($ac|ab$, Cousins) for Cousins Following the Weir Methodology

Alleles IBD	Term	Cousins	Probabilities
None	δ_0	¾	$\Pr(ac|ab, \text{unrelated})^a$
$b \equiv d$	δ_{bd}	¼	?
Sum of the products			

IBD, identical by descent.
[a] This is $\Pr(ac|ab)$ for unrelated members of the same subpopulation.
This is written as $\dfrac{2(1-\theta)p_c\left[\theta+(1-\theta)p_a\right]}{(1+\theta)(1+2\theta)}$.

$$\Pr(ac \mid ab, \text{cousins}) = \frac{3\Pr(ac \mid ab, \text{unrelated})}{4} + \frac{1}{4} \times \frac{\Pr(c \mid ab, \text{unrelated})}{2}$$

$$= \frac{3 \times 2(1-\theta) p_c [\theta + (1-\theta) p_a]}{4(1+\theta)(1+2\theta)} + \frac{(1-\theta) p_c}{8(1+\theta)}$$

$$= \frac{(1-\theta) p_c}{8(1+\theta)} \left(1 + \frac{12(\theta + (1-\theta) p_a)}{(1+2\theta)} \right)$$

We do not pursue this approach in depth here as it is much more extensively and better described in Evett and Weir.[257] The use of such descent measures permits us to consider much more complex pedigrees than merely dyadic relationships. However it leads to the same results as the Balding and Nichols method for the simple pedigrees considered here.

Joint Probabilities

In this section we consider the probability that a pair of individuals would have genotypes G_1 and G_2. These joint probabilities are useful for answering questions of the type, 'We have a match on the database between two males, what is the support for the suggestion that they are brothers?'

We can approach the problem by calculating the set of joint probabilities under the related conditions. Li et al. describe a similarity index approach, which is not discussed here since an LR approach is almost universally preferred.[498]

Tables of joint probabilities have been produced[258,424] that typically give the joint probability for 'unordered' pairs. Hence the genotype pairs aa, ab and ab, aa are equivalent. However care must be taken when progressing to multilocus genotypes and it is our opinion that working with ordered pairs is safer.

If we think of G_1 and G_2 as an unordered pair of multilocus genotypes, we note that $\Pr(G_1, G_2) = 2 \prod_l \Pr(G_1^l, G_2^l)$, where $\Pr(G_1^l, G_2^l)$ is the probability of the ordered pair of geno-

types. If the formulae for the unordered pairs at each locus are used such as given on p. 206 of Weir[424] or on p. 116 of Evett and Weir[257] there are likely to be too many factors of 2. This typically does not affect any LR calculated from these terms, as the same excess of 2s appears in the numerator and denominator. Table 4.4 gives the probability that may be assembled into the joint probability of ordered pairs of genotypes.

Remembering that $\Pr(G_1, G_2 \mid R) = \Pr(G_1 \mid G_2, R) \times \Pr(G_2)$, to produce the joint probabilities take the probability in the column $\Pr(G_1 \mid G_2 R)$ in Table 4.4 and multiply it by either $p_a[\theta + (1 - \theta) p_a]$ if the genotype of G_2 is aa or $2p_a p_b(1 - \theta)$ if the genotype of G_2 is ab.

This gives the probability of the ordered set $\Pr(G_1, G_2 \mid R)$. Thus, for example, if we were interested in the joint probability of two people with genotypes $G_1 = [a, c]$ and $G_2 = [a, b]$ if they are cousins, from Table 4.3:

$$\Pr(G_1 \mid G_2, \text{cousins}) = \frac{Z_1}{2} \frac{((1-\theta) p_c)}{1+\theta} + Z_0 \frac{2(\theta + (1-\theta) p_a)(1-\theta) p_c}{(1+\theta)(1+2\theta)}$$

And we obtain from Table 4.1 for cousins $\Pr(Z_0) = \tfrac{3}{4}$, $\Pr(Z_1) = \tfrac{1}{4}$ and $\Pr(Z_2) = 0$:

$$\Pr(G_1 \mid G_2, \text{cousins}) = \frac{(1-\theta) p_c}{8(1+\theta)} + \frac{3(\theta + (1-\theta) p_a)(1-\theta) p_c}{2(1+\theta)(1+2\theta)}$$

Finally multiplying $\Pr(G_1|G_2, R)$ by $\Pr(G_2)$ gives

$$\Pr\left(G_1, G_2 \mid \text{cousins}\right) = \frac{(1-\theta)^2 \, p_a p_b p_c}{4(1+\theta)} + \frac{3\left(\theta + (1-\theta) p_a\right)(1-\theta)^2 \, p_a p_b p_c}{(1+\theta)(1+2\theta)}$$

$$= \frac{(1-\theta)^2 \, p_a p_b p_c}{1+\theta} \left[\frac{1}{4} + \frac{3\left(\theta + (1-\theta) p_a\right)}{1+2\theta} \right]$$

If the unordered pairs from Evett and Weir are used, it is likely that both terms will be larger by a factor of 2.

The correct LR is obtained using the formulae for unordered pairs of genotypes because both the numerator and denominator will be incorrect by the same factor.

Rather than using 'joint probabilities' the brother's defence problem can be solved by using an LR, noting

$$LR = \frac{\Pr\left(G_1, G_2 \mid B\right)}{\Pr\left(G_1, G_2 \mid U\right)} = \frac{\Pr\left(G_1 \mid G_2, B\right)}{\Pr\left(G_1 \mid U\right)} = \frac{\Pr\left(G_2 \mid G_1, B\right)}{\Pr\left(G_2 \mid U\right)}$$

and utilizing the conditional probabilities.

The Effect of Linkage

We consider here the effect of linkage on the joint and conditional probabilities for relatives. Because of the expansion in size of modern STR multiplexes, more linked loci are involved. A list of linked loci, their genetic distances and the multiplexes they appear in is given in Chapter 1. These distances are sufficiently large that we would not expect linkage disequilibrium at the population level but are sufficiently small that they will affect match probabilities for some close relatives. Buckleton and Triggs have previously given formulae for both joint and conditional match probabilities for siblings and half-siblings with no account of subpopulation effects.[499] In this section we extend the work of Buckleton and Triggs to include a subpopulation correction of the form first suggested by Balding and Nichols[358] and to a wider set of relationships as published by Bright et al.[55]

Table 4.8 is a summary of the nomenclature used in this section. In Table 4.9 we repeat the two locus identity by descent (IBD) states for a number of common relationships. These formulae assume that the two people have no relationship other than the one specified, that is their parents are not related nor are they inbred. In Table 4.10 we give the probabilities for various genotypes of Person 1 (G_1) and Person 2 (G_2) that will be used to form the joint probability. The multiplications inherent in these formulae assume that there is no linkage disequilibrium at the population level for these loci. The joint probability of G_1 and G_2, given a relationship state, is assigned as follows:

$$\Pr\left(G_1, G_2 \mid \text{Relationship}\right) = \begin{bmatrix} A_0 & A_1 & A_2 \end{bmatrix} \begin{bmatrix} Z_{00} & Z_{01} & Z_{02} \\ Z_{10} & Z_{11} & Z_{12} \\ Z_{20} & Z_{21} & Z_{22} \end{bmatrix} \begin{bmatrix} B_0 \\ B_1 \\ B_2 \end{bmatrix}$$

$$= A_0 B_0 Z_{00} + A_0 B_1 Z_{01} + A_0 B_2 Z_{02}$$

$$+ A_1 B_0 Z_{10} + A_1 B_1 Z_{11} + A_1 B_2 Z_{12}$$

$$+ A_2 B_0 Z_{20} + A_2 B_1 Z_{21} + A_2 B_2 Z_{22}$$

Term	Formula
	Table 4.8 A Summary of the Nomenclature Used in This Section
A_i	The probability of the second genotype given the first genotype and the IBD state at Locus 1 is i
B_i	The probability of the second genotype given the first genotype and the IBD state at Locus 2 is i
C	$2(1-\theta)\mathrm{Pr}_p\,\mathrm{Pr}_q$
D	$\mathrm{Pr}_p\,(\theta+(1-\theta)\mathrm{Pr}_p)$
E	$\left(\theta+(1-\theta)\mathrm{Pr}_p\right)/2(1+\theta)$
F	$\left(2\theta+(1-\theta)(\mathrm{Pr}_p+\mathrm{Pr}_q)\right)/2(1+\theta)$
H	$\left(\theta+(1-\theta)\mathrm{Pr}_p\right)\left(2\theta+(1-\theta)\mathrm{Pr}_p\right)/(1+\theta)(1+2\theta)$
I^a	$(1-\theta)\mathrm{Pr}_r\left(\theta+(1-\theta)\mathrm{Pr}_r\right)/(1+\theta)(1+2\theta)$
J	$2(1-\theta)^2\mathrm{Pr}_r\,\mathrm{Pr}_s/(1+\theta)(1+2\theta)$
K	$2\left(\theta+(1-\theta)\mathrm{Pr}_p\right)\left(\theta+(1-\theta)\mathrm{Pr}_q\right)/(1+\theta)(1+2\theta)$
L	$\left(2\theta+(1-\theta)\mathrm{Pr}_p\right)/(1+\theta)$
M	$(1-\theta)\mathrm{Pr}_q/(1+\theta)$
N	$\left(3\theta+(1-\theta)\mathrm{Pr}_p\right)/(1+2\theta)$
O	$2(1-\theta)\mathrm{Pr}_q/(1+2\theta)$
R	Recombination fraction
$\bar{R}$	$1-R$
S	$(1-\theta)\mathrm{Pr}_r/(1+\theta)$
T	$(1-\theta)\mathrm{Pr}_r/(1+2\theta)$
V	$\dfrac{1}{4}\left(R^2+\bar{R}^2\right)\bar{R}^2+\dfrac{1}{8}R^2$
W	$\dfrac{1}{2}\left(R^2+\bar{R}^2\right)\bar{R}+\dfrac{1}{4}R$
X	$R^2+\bar{R}^2$
Y	$2R\bar{R}$
Z_{ij}	The probability of i IBD alleles at Locus 1 and j IBD alleles at Locus 2
θ	Co-ancestry coefficient

IBD, identity by descent.

[a] This corrects the typographical error in Bright et al.[55] This was brought to our attention by the careful work of Tacha Hicks-Champod.

Table 4.9 Probability of Two Locus IBD States for Some Common Relationships Accounting for Linkage

Relationship	IBD State								
	Z_{22}	Z_{21}	Z_{20}	Z_{12}	Z_{11}	Z_{10}	Z_{02}	Z_{01}	Z_{00}
Siblings	$\frac{1}{4}X^2$	$\frac{1}{2}XY$	$\frac{1}{4}Y^2$	$\frac{1}{2}XY$	$\frac{1}{2}(X^2+Y^2)$	$\frac{1}{2}XY$	$\frac{1}{4}Y^2$	$\frac{1}{2}XY$	$\frac{1}{4}X^2$
Parent/child					**No effect**				
Uncle/nephew	0	0	0	0	W	$\frac{1}{2}-W$	0	$\frac{1}{2}-W$	W
Half-uncle/nephew	0	0	0	0	$\frac{X\bar{R}}{4}$	$\frac{1-X\bar{R}}{4}$	0	$\frac{1-X\bar{R}}{4}$	$\frac{2+X\bar{R}}{4}$
Cousins	0	0	0	0	V	$\frac{1}{4}-V$	0	$\frac{1}{4}-V$	$\frac{1}{2}+V$
Grandparent/grandchild	0	0	0	0	$\frac{\bar{R}}{2}$	$\frac{R}{2}$	0	$\frac{R}{2}$	$\frac{\bar{R}}{2}$
Half-siblings	0	0	0	0	$\frac{X}{2}$	$\frac{Y}{2}$	0	$\frac{Y}{2}$	$\frac{X}{2}$

IBD, identity by descent.
Note: We correct errors in the sibling's formulae in Buckleton and Triggs.[499]

Table 4.10 Probabilities for the A_i and B_i Terms Used to Form the Joint Probability of G_1 and G_2

G_1	G_2	A_2 or B_2	A_1 or B_1	A_0 or B_0
pq	pq	C	CF	CK
	pp	0	CE	CH
	pr	0	$CS/2$	$4CET$
	rr	0	0	CI
	rs	0	0	CJ
pp	pp	D	DL	DLN
	pq	0	DM	DLO
	pr	0	DS	$2DLT$
	rr	0	0	DI
	rs	0	0	DJ

Conditional probabilities $\Pr(G_1|G_2)$ can be obtained by dividing the joint probabilities by $\Pr(G_2)$. In the forensic context the situation where G_1 is equal to G_2 is of interest (the top row for each G_1). Table 4.10 provides other examples, for example with one or no shared alleles, which may be useful for other scenarios.

The match probabilities for parent/child are unaffected by linkage. However those for siblings, half-siblings, uncle/nephew, cousins and grandparent/grandchild are affected. The effect is typically not large. It is smallest for common alleles and largest for rare alleles.[55,56] In Table 4.11 we repeat the percentage overstatement of the *LR* for the most common profile in the New Zealand Caucasian and Asian subpopulations given in Bright et al.[55] Generally the difference in match probabilities decreases as the genetic distance increases between the individuals under consideration.

In Table 4.12 we give the maximum effects for various pairs of loci calculated for simple pedigrees. These maxima occur for half-uncle/half-nephew relationships and a clearly resolved profile matching the person of interest, where allele probabilities = 0 and θ = 0. As an example, GlobalFiler™ has three sets of linked loci. The combined maximum effects when considering

Table 4.11 Overstatement of Match Probabilities When Linkage Is Not Considered for Different Relationships for the Most Common Profile in the New Zealand Caucasian and Asian Subpopulations

Relationship	Caucasian (%)	Asian (%)
Full siblings	12.6	14.8
Grandparent/grandchild	6.3	15.1
Half-siblings	2.0	7.0
Uncle/nephew	1.5	5.3
Half-uncle/nephew	3.7	3.9
First cousins	1.6	2.1

Table 4.12 Maximum Effect of Linkage on the Match Probability for Different Linked Loci Appearing in Commercial Multiplexes

Locus Pairs		vWA/D12S391	D5S818/CSF1PO	D21S11/Penta D	TPOX/D2S441
Distance cM		11.94	27.76	44.73	88.81
Recombination fraction (Kosambi function)		0.117	0.252	0.357	0.472
Match probability with linkage/Match probability without	Siblings	2.518	1.553	1.170	1.006
	Uncle/nephew	1.518	1.184	1.053	1.002
	Half-uncle/half-nephew	**2.802**	**1.864**	**1.391**	**1.059**
	Cousins	1.518	1.184	1.053	1.002
	Grandparent/grandchild	1.766	1.496	1.286	1.056
	Half-siblings	1.587	1.246	1.082	1.003

LR, likelihood ratio.
Notes: The largest effect for each locus pairs is indicated in bold. Numbers greater than 1 indicate that the match probability is greater with linkage considered.

a sibling as an alternative source of DNA would be a 3.95 times increase in the *LR* if linkage were ignored. In all other circumstances the effect is less, excluding complicated pedigrees as described in Kling et al.[500]

Because of the complexity of the analysis and the relatively small differences, there may be temptation to avoid making any correction. The Bright et al. paper could usefully produce data that could inform judgements by forensic organizations or policy-making bodies. Match probabilities are always non-conservative if linkage is ignored, but typically by a small amount. However any approximate analysis that runs any risk of overstatement of the *LR* must come under court scrutiny and we feel that the provision of software could be most useful.

5

Validating Databases

John S. Buckleton, Jo-Anne Bright, James M. Curran
and Duncan Taylor

Contents

Introduction

This chapter is concerned with the issue of validating population databases for forensic work. The issue of independence testing is discussed. It is worthwhile considering here a quote from Weir,[345] reproduced with permission: 'Arguments have arisen that could have been avoided if the deliberate pace with which scientific investigation proceeds had been applied to the forensic uses of DNA evidence.' The situation has improved since 1992, but there is an unfortunate reluctance in some areas to adopt continuous improvement due to entrenched views, fear of complexity and fear of retrospective review of past cases.

Open publication of data and analysis and the open debate on the conclusions that may be drawn from this data represent a sound scientific approach to alleviating this type of problem. In 1995 Strom[501] complained that 'the refusal by the FBI laboratory of outside inspection and data verification is troubling, especially when I have been called upon to testify in support of its findings. Regardless of the reasons for this policy, I believe that the FBI laboratory should be held to the same standards and requirements as other laboratories.' (Reproduced with the kind permission of *Nature* and Dr Strom.) This situation appears to have been remedied in part by the placement of the FBI population data into the public domain,[502] which is an admirable policy that should be widely implemented. That is, let's have the arguments out of court – not in it. This involves openness by the government agencies responsible for the majority of forensic work. In fact it involves actively supporting independent or defence reanalysis whether this support is reciprocated or not.

In this call for openness we are ourselves currently aspirational. We have managed to place our population data and validation studies in the public domain, but we have been restricted by IP considerations in placing our manuals in the public domain.[31,32,34,35] These are made available for view by independent analysts in casework but are not copied or disclosed under other circumstances.

Which Is the Relevant Population?

As discussed in Chapter 3 profile or match probabilities are estimated with reference to a population. This raises the question 'What is a population?' or 'Which population?'[177,179,311,312,420,503–507] Two options briefly discussed here are the race to which the suspect belongs and the 'general population'. A brief discussion is provided here, as on balance the use of the 'unifying formula' discussed in Chapter 3 is preferred, which does not require the definition of a relevant population. Nonetheless there has been much debate on the appropriateness of one or other of the two options outlined above.[508]

Consider the question, 'Why are we doing a calculation?' Typically the answer would be to assess the evidence if the suspect is not the contributor, or under the Bayesian framework to assess the evidence under H_d.[160] It is clear then that the race of the suspect does not define the relevant population. That is defined more by the circumstances of the crime or other evidence such as eyewitness evidence.[376,503,505,509,510] The circumstances or evidence may point to one ethnic

---

BOX 5.1   CHOICE OF DATABASE

1. The database of interest is one which defines the race of the offender.
2. We typically don't know the race of the offender but can sometimes use eyewitness accounts to guide us.
3. If the investigators are acting on valid information there is a small increase over random chance that the suspect and offender are from the same racial group.
4. If the reported statistical weighting is the smallest produced from calculations using a suspect-oriented database and a geography-oriented database, then this practice can only be conservative compared to a geography-oriented database alone.

---

group wholly or partially, or the location of the crime may suggest which set of persons had opportunity.[243,244] Using the race of the suspect is typically conservative; however it is not necessarily a reasonable representation of the relevant population. Hence it is more appropriate to attempt to model a population defined by the crime. This is typically multiracial. In a later section we discuss how to combine estimates from separate races into one for a multiracial population. Even given the above reasoning, many labs will still typically calculate a statistical weighting using a population database that corresponds to the race of the suspect. The reasoning for this decision is given in Box 5.1.

The valid question has arisen as to whether the ethnicity of the person of interest plays any part in the determination of weight of evidence. The National Research Council second report in 1996[176] stated that the sub-group to which the person of interest belongs is irrelevant. Although their logic is correct, we cannot quite agree in one rather small detail. This is also best covered in the section on combining estimates for a multiracial population.

Population Databases

Population databases are distinct from intelligence databases. They are used to estimate the rarity of a profile in a population in order to give an indication to a court of the strength of the DNA evidence.

Consider the highly stylized diagram of the human population given in Figure 5.1. This figure is not intended to imply that there is some objective definition of the term *race*. This term has come to be viewed as increasingly arbitrary as our understanding of human population genetics and evolution has improved. Rather it simply implies that there is some structure to the human population. This is more properly viewed as a continuum, but most models treat it as a hierarchy of partitions. For reasons that were discussed in Chapter 3, the estimation process will have a small error if we ignore the structure in the human population. This and other issues relating to the validation of population databases are discussed in this chapter.

Validating Population Databases

It is general practice for a laboratory to validate the population database it intends to use before proceeding to court with estimates of evidential weight. This is a desirable feature as is publication or deposition of the details in the public domain. Typically there may be a challenge to the use of a database in the first few court cases undertaken by a particular laboratory. The challenges may include issues about the size of the database, the method of selection of the samples and dependence effects. The process of validating databases was thrown into a particular light by a case in South Australia; *R v Karger*, before the Honourable Justice Mulligan.[451] The effect of this case and questions from the judge have led us to believe that it is not the database that should be validated but rather a system of interpretation. There is an inherent interplay

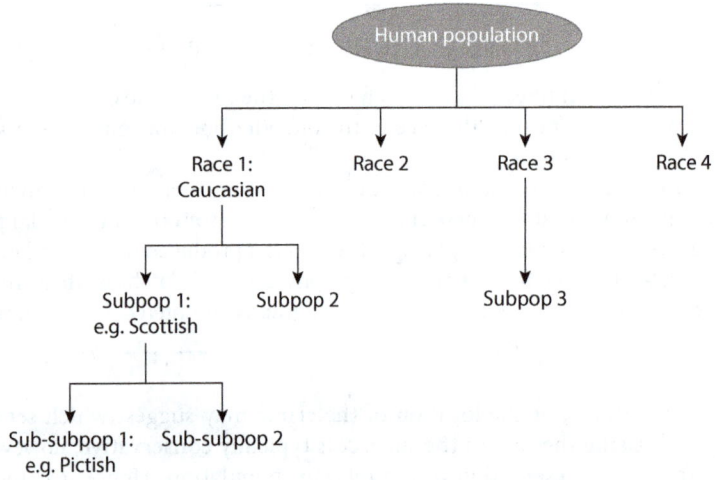

Figure 5.1   A highly simplified and stylized diagram of the structure of the human population.

between what is expected of a database and the mode by which the testimony will be developed. The concept of 'fitness for purpose' is closely akin to this process. The key questions are, What are you going to do with the database? Is it fit for this purpose?

In this regard noted authors such as Brinkmann[511] write: 'For their application in forensic casework, extensive studies have to be carried out. This would include population studies … A minimum of 200 unrelated individuals and/or 500 meioses have to be investigated for each STR system to study allele frequencies, the Mendelian inheritance, and whether significant numbers of mutations exist.'

The number 200 has become the *de facto* standard for the size of the database. This size certainly suffices for estimation of allele probabilities especially if sampling error is considered. Smaller samples may also suffice, again especially if sampling error is considered. This is discussed further in Chapter 6. However a sample of 200 profiles will not inform us much with regard to 'population studies' if our plan is to investigate deviations from Hardy–Weinberg and linkage equilibrium by hypothesis testing. Other population genetic studies, such as comparisons with other populations, appear to be more informative in this regard.

Sampling Races or Populations?

Let us begin with the question: Should we survey general populations, say the population of the state of Victoria, Australia, or should we divide this population according to some partition, which for the purposes of this section we will call *race*? Both approaches are currently used. It is normal practice in the United States, United Kingdom, Australia and New Zealand to divide according to race.

Consider, again, the highly simplified model of the human population given in Figure 5.1. There has already been considerable argument over the question 'How many races are there?' or even 'What is a race?' Many studies suggest that there is little evidence of a clear subdivision of humans into races, but rather that variation is essentially continuous.[512] From the genetic point of view 'race' is simply an arbitrary partition of the total human diversity.

However these somewhat arbitrary partitions of the human population do correspond in some way to our view of recent human evolution. The more we clump groups together (that is, the higher we go in this hierarchy) the higher will be the resulting dependence effects within and between loci. The examples illustrating the Wahlund effect (Tables 3.2 and 3.3) showed that the bigger the effects were, the more the allele frequencies differed between the groups. If we mix 'races' to create a 'general' population, we create larger dependence effects. Conversely the more we subdivide the population into genetic groups, the lower the remaining dependence effects should be, since the remaining subdivisions of these groups should be more similar to each other.[375,376]

A common compromise implemented in many laboratories is to subdivide the population as far as races but not further. It is possible to recombine these estimates into a general population estimate if required and the preferred option is stratification (see Box 5.2).[510,513]

The second report of the National Research Council in 1996[176] stated that the sub-group to which the suspect belongs is irrelevant. The logic followed the line that we desire to estimate the probability of the evidence if the suspect is innocent and that instead a random individual committed the crime. This is substantially correct but overlooks the issue that the presence of some members of the subpopulation among the group of potential offenders may have a significant impact on the total weight of the evidence (see Chapter 4).

To answer the question of the magnitude of the diversity between subpopulations, fairly extensive studies have been carried out estimating the genetic differences between different groups of people. These are reviewed later in this chapter. In general these studies support the notion that differences between subpopulations are modest.

Variation between subpopulations can be accommodated by the use of a correction factor (F_{ST} or θ),[358,453] discussed in Chapter 3. Since differences between subpopulations are typically minor, inferences for a subpopulation for which a database is not available can be accommodated by using a general database so long as the θ correction is incorporated.

The choice of sampling method also has implications for the way in which sampling variation is calculated. The difference lies with the amount of information we have about a subpopulation from increased database size. If a subpopulation-specific sampling scheme is used, then additional sampling will lead to more precise allele frequency estimates and the intervals produced by accounting for sampling variation will contract around the point estimate. These intervals will also contract around the point estimate when a general sampling scheme is used; however they asymptotically reach a minimum level of contraction, as additional sampling of the general population will not provide further information about the specific subpopulations.

Practically this is taken into account by including an additional F_{ST} term in the variance or covariance components of a confidence interval calculation when a general sampling scheme is used (see Chapter 6).

BOX 5.2   STRATIFICATION

Consider an area with races R_1, R_2, ..., R_N resident. We consider the prior probability that a person from each race is the donor of the stain. As a first approximation we take these priors to be simply the fraction of the population that these races represent. Suppose these are in the proportions $\Pr(R_1)$, $\Pr(R_2)$, ..., $\Pr(R_N)$ in the population that we consider relevant. Suppose that the probability of the evidence (E) depends on which race is the donor. We could then write $\Pr(E|R_1)$, $\Pr(E|R_2)$, ..., $\Pr(E|R_N)$ if these partitions are exclusive and exhaustive, then

$$\Pr(E)=\sum_{i=1}^{N}\Pr\left(E|R_i\right)\Pr\left(R_i\right),$$

which suggests a fairly easy way to combine different estimates. However use of the general form of Bayes' theorem is superior (see Chapters 2 and 4; under the full Bayesian approach to interpretation).

The above calculation of $\Pr(E)$ leads to the requirement for stratification separately under each hypothesis if ambiguities exist in the genotypes of contributors; i.e. the hypotheses contain unknowns.

Source of Samples

There has been considerable discussion in the courts along the lines that the samples used in forensic work are not collected by random sampling methods.[506] The accusation stems from standard statistical theory. Randomly selected data has much less chance of being affected by various types of bias in the sampling.

Most forensic samples are convenience samples. This means that they have come to the laboratory by some 'convenient' way, such as from blood donors, staff or offender databases. As such they do not comprise random samples. An incorrect response is to say that they were not selected on the basis of their genotypes and hence no bias is expected. Indeed they are not selected on the basis of their genotypes, but the accusation is that the bias is inadvertent.

We argue that this is not a major issue. However to set the scene let us postulate some extreme examples. Imagine that we use as our sample the staff of the Informatics Department of North Carolina State University. This consists, on this day, of two New Zealanders, a Canadian, three Chinese and a few US nationals. The US nationals come from many states, but none come from North Carolina. If this sample were to be used to model the North Carolina population, it would be very unrepresentative. This is not because we have deliberately made an unrepresentative sample by knowing the genotypes of the candidates, but rather that our sampling strategy has an in-built bias (in this case to people who have relocated).

Real situations are likely to show a much less pronounced bias. We could imagine that blood donors and staff over-represent some groups and under-represent others. It is harder to argue that offender databases are unrepresentative, as they certainly seem close to a representative sample of 'alternate offenders'.[509] To summarize the statistical argument: only random sampling can guarantee a representative sample.

To turn now to the counterargument, it is wise to admit that we cannot guarantee that our samples are representative. This is for two reasons: first we do not undertake random sampling, and second we do not always know what group we are trying to represent.

Consider crimes in one of the US states. In some cases we may want to represent small rural populations; in others large cosmopolitan populations. In other cases there may be evidence from, say, eyewitnesses which directs us towards a particular group. The very act of defining a population of alternate offenders is very difficult (and unnecessary and unhelpful if we use the unifying formula of Balding).[503,505]

Consider then our surveying requirements if we wished to meet the strictest statistical standards: first we must define our population of offenders, next we need to randomly sample from these and last we need to do this for every crime.

If we concede that we cannot guarantee databases that are truly random samples, where does this lead us? Many defence analysts would argue that it leaves us nowhere and that all future arguments are built on an insecure foundation. However there really is quite a body of population genetic evidence that suggests that, although we might have slightly unrepresentative samples, the effect is likely to be minor. Fung[514] provides important experimental support for this. There is also a theory, the subpopulation theory, available to attempt to accommodate this unrepresentativeness.

How bad could our sample be? Let us imagine that we intend to sample race x in a specific locality. We take samples by self-declaration of that race at, say, a blood donation clinic. We could imagine the following biases:

- A bias caused by the self-declaration process. This will be dealt with separately.

- A bias caused because one subpopulation over donates and others under donate.

- Systematic typing bias. This will also be dealt with separately.

We are left, in this section, with the task of assessing the possible effect of the bias caused by one subpopulation over-donating and others under-donating. The pertinent questions are as follows:

- How much do subpopulations differ?

- How much could one subpopulation over-donate?

- Do we intend to make any compensation for non-representativeness in our testimony?

Thus we come to the first task when validating a database: How much bias could the sampling process have induced, *and* will we compensate for it?

Self-Declaration

Most laboratories obtain samples for their DNA database from volunteers or from offender databases. These are typically separated into races by self-declaration. Self-declaration is taken to be the process by which people nominate their own race. More occasionally other methods are used such as surname. The issue has been raised often in court as to whether the self-declaration (or surname) process introduces any unacceptable bias.[303]

There are many instances of possible self-declaration bias. Wild and Seber[445] note, 'In recent US censuses there has been a big upsurge in the census counts of American Indians that could not be explained by birth and death statistics.'

From our own experience we can confirm that there are, at least, errors in the self-declaration process. In the New Zealand subpopulation databases all 'matches' (incidence of duplicate STR profiles) were, for many years, investigated. Most often these matches occurred because the same person has been sampled twice. There have also been instances of identical twins on the database. It is not uncommon for the declaration to be different for the different occasions an individual is sampled or for each member of the pair of twins. This is typically a difference of detail, such as a claim of one-half Maori on one occasion and one-quarter Maori at another.

Does this render the process useless? The evidence suggests not. For New Zealand the Maori and Samoan data was further divided into subsets of varying levels of ethnicity, representing the dilution of the selected ethnic subpopulation largely by Caucasians. For example, New Zealand Maori samples were distributed into six subsets – full-blood, ¾, ½, ¼, ⅛ and ¹⁄₁₆. Similarly Samoan samples from the database were distributed into four sub-groups – full-blood, ¾, ½ and ¼. An estimate has been made of the pairwise genetic distance between the self-declared ethnicity for the New Zealand STR data. This was possible through a self-declaration process based on ancestral information over four generations.[515]

The results of the genetic distance estimates (Tables 5.1 and 5.2) show that the genetic distance, θ, from the Caucasian population increases as the level of self-declared Maori or Samoan ethnicity increase.[516] This matrix of genetic distances was also represented using principal coordinates (Figure 5.2) and the same pattern can be seen. This provides significant support for the effectiveness of self-declaration as a means of segregating reference samples by ethnicity. There is no claim that it is error-free, yet it cannot be totally random or we would not get this logical pattern.

The points corresponding to small reported fractions of Maori and Samoan ancestry are closer to each other than they are to the point representing the Caucasian population. Walsh et al.[515] suggested that this is because the admixture is complex, and a person reporting a small fraction of, say, Samoan ancestry may also have some Maori as well as Caucasian ancestors.

Rosenberg et al.[396] typed 377 autosomal microsatellite loci in 1056 individuals from 52 populations. Without using any prior information they identified six main genetic clusters, five of which corresponded to major geographical regions, and sub-clusters that often corresponded to individual populations. There was a general agreement of this 'genetically determined' origin with self-reported ancestry. This is, again, important confirmation of the

Table 5.1 Distance for New Zealand Maori from Caucasian

Self-Declared Ethnicity Level	Distance from Caucasian
Full Maori	0.037
¾ Maori	0.030
½ Maori	0.023
¼ Maori	0.014
⅛ Maori	0.010
≤¹⁄₁₆ Maori	0.003

Source: Walsh, S.J., et al., *Journal of Forensic Science*, 48(5), 1091–1093, 2003. With permission.

Table 5.2 Distance for Samoans from Caucasian

Self-Declared Ethnicity Level	Distance from Caucasian
Full Samoan	0.038
¾ Samoan	0.021
½ Samoan	0.014
≤¼ Samoan	0.001

Source: Walsh, S.J., et al., *Journal of Forensic Science*, 48(5), 1091–1093, 2003. With permission.

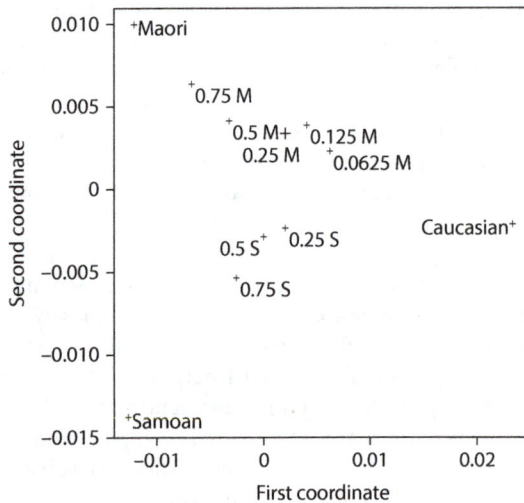

Figure 5.2 Principal coordinate representation of the interpopulation genetic distances. (From Walsh, S.J., et al., *Journal of Forensic Science*, 48(5), 1091–1093, 2003. With permission.)

usefulness of self-reported ancestry (the subsequent discussions[397,398] relate to mathematical treatments of the data and do not affect this conclusion).

Systematic Mistyping or Systematic Non-Typing

These are the two potential sources of bias in any population survey. The first is far more dangerous than the second although both may be important.

Systematic mistyping describes the situation where one or more genotypes are systematically mistyped as a different genotype. An instance could be that some heterozygotes are systematically mistyped as homozygotes because of allelic dropout or severe heterozygote imbalance. The result will be the appearance of slightly too many homozygotes that may be detected during the statistical analysis. Experience suggests that this does occur and some anomalies that have been highlighted during statistical analysis are a consequence of this effect.

Another possible mistyping is to designate a common homozygote or heterozygote as a nearby rare option because of band shift.[74] For instance, analysis of the New Zealand subpopulation data detected one instance of a 10,10 genotype at the TH01 locus for Caucasians that, when re-examined, was found to be the common 9.3,9.3. This datum was noticed because 10,10 should be rare. Mistyping between common genotypes is unlikely to be detected during statistical analysis.

Hence the validation of the database by statistical analysis may lead to the detection of some mistyping. It would be unwise, however, to assume that all instances of mistyping would be found, as it is likely that statistical analysis will fail to detect all but the most obvious. The integrity of the remaining samples does not rely on statistical testing but on the quality standards of the laboratory doing the typing.

> Statistical examination cannot, in any meaningful way, guarantee the correctness of the data. That relies principally on the quality standards of the laboratory.

Systematic non-typing refers to a situation where certain alleles or genotypes are less likely to 'type' or 'be called'. This is realistic if, say, the larger alleles are harder to amplify. Another possibility is that low peak area homozygotes are classed as, say, '11,?'. The operator means by this that the genotype has the 11 allele but he or she is uncertain whether or not another allele may be present. It is difficult to process and as such it is often omitted. Thus some homozygotes could systematically be removed from the data.

This effect is akin to a 'non-response' bias in classical sampling terminology. It could lower the apparent frequency of those alleles or genotypes that are hard to type and hence raise the relative frequency of the others. The check for this is to see how many genotypes are classified as 'missing', e.g. '11,?'. Obviously, if there is little or no missing data, then there can be no bias from systematic non-typing.

What should be done if there is a substantial amount of missing data? Let us say that at a locus there is of the order of 10% of the data missing due to non-typing. This opens the possibility of systematic non-typing bias, but it does not prove that such a bias exists. If the non-typing is random, that is if it is evenly spread among all the alleles, then this will have no effect. The only clues as to whether the non-typing has affected one allele predominantly would be a comparison with a closely related population.

Many laboratories, understandably, perform their statistical survey at the implementation phase of new technology. This is the time when they are most prone to mistyping and non-typing. This leads us to another possible task when validating databases:

> Check for the possibility of non-typing bias.

Size of Database

How big should a database be to be valid? This must be the most prevalent question asked of the statistician either by laboratories or in court. It is an entirely reasonable question because in statistical sampling size does matter. However it is surprisingly difficult to answer in a logical way.

Once again, the answer comes down to 'fitness for purpose'. The two key factors in this assessment of fitness are as follows:

- Whether or not the database is meant to inform choice of population genetic model
- Whether or not the testimony will include sampling error estimates

Most published attempts at validation of databases suggest that they in some way inform the choice of population genetic model, in particular that they somehow validate the product rule or some other population genetic model. If we intend to validate the use of the product rule on the basis of *this* database rather than base the validation on all the literature on the subject, then the database has to be enormous. In essence, to set this size of the database to 'validate' the product rule we need some 'acceptance' criteria for the product rule. In particular we need to answer the question, 'How wrong are we prepared to be?' Do not assume from this statement that we will be able to produce the correct answer from our pocket, but we do need to think about tolerable limits for error. To date the question, 'How wrong are we prepared to be?' has never been answered. In fact it may actually never have been asked in this way. We could further discuss whether this is a decision for a scientist or a court.

Let us assume that we intend to tackle the question, 'How wrong are we prepared to be?' Do we want these limits to be phrased as a ratio, for instance 'this estimate could be high or low by a factor of 10'? The scientist (or court) may be more tolerant of an estimate that is likely to err in favour of the defendant than one that may err in favour of the prosecution. This may result in them being inclined to give limits for 'acceptance' that are asymmetric. Do we become more tolerant of error as the estimates get smaller? For instance, do we need a higher level of accuracy for estimates in the area of one in a million, but after one in a billion can we tolerate more uncertainty? This suggests some sort of sliding scale that may be definable on a logarithmic scale. For instance, do we want the log of the estimate to be within a factor of, say, ±17%?

Embedded in the argument above is a concept of defining *wrong*. The obvious answer is to use the concept of a true answer that we unfortunately do not know the 'truth'. This approach to defining an acceptance criterion is set up to fail.

What would suit us best would be if we could define something like 'I will use the product rule if I can be reasonably certain that θ is less than 1%'. This would allow us to do power studies and determine how big a database would need to be so that we can be 90% sure of finding dependence if $\theta = 0.01$.

Clearly most databases are not of this size, and hence they could not validate the population genetic model under this criterion. It is argued below that no database per se can realistically validate the population genetic model. Any validation must rely on population genetic studies.

> Examination of one database of the order of hundreds or a few thousand samples cannot validate the product rule, nor can it validate any other population genetic model. If advice is to be given on the choice of population genetic model it should be based on an understanding of the population genetics of the populations in question.

If we are not going to validate the population genetic model, then all we are going to use the database for is to determine allele probabilities. As long as we make a consideration of sampling error, then almost any size database will do.

> If a sampling error correction is used then there are almost no restrictions on how large or small a database needs to be.

What if no consideration of sampling error is to be made? Then we are back to the question, 'How wrong are we prepared to be?' Fortunately this time we have a body of statistical theory that allows us to estimate the expected sampling error for a given database size. Thus, if we are informed how wrong the analyst is prepared to be, we can give him or her an approximate estimate of how big the database needs to be. This is necessarily approximate as it depends on the number of loci and the separate allele probabilities for each particular genotype. A sample of size 200 has become the *de facto* standard, but this is more by common acceptance rather than by forceful scientific argument that this is the correct number.

If no consideration of sampling error is to be made for each case, then it is wise to assess the probable uncertainty arising from sampling during validation.

Validating the Population Genetic Model

Let us assume that the act of validating a database also includes the necessity to validate the population genetic model that is to be used in court. The proof of the validity of a population genetic model can proceed from population genetic considerations completely independently of the existence of a genetic database. It is at least theoretically feasible that the laboratory could study mating patterns with their population and the other requirements for Hardy–Weinberg and linkage equilibrium and conclude that the product rule or some other model was a valid approximation without ever typing a DNA sample. However the assumptions for Hardy–Weinberg and linkage equilibrium are never *exactly* fulfilled in real human populations, and hence it will not be possible to conclude *exact* correspondence to the product rule from a purely population genetic argument. In fact the reality of population genetics would lead us to doubt the validity of *exact* adherence to Hardy–Weinberg and linkage equilibrium in the first place.

Can the existence of a database save us from this dilemma by its examination by independence testing? The answer is no. We now turn to a discussion of independence testing.

Independence Testing

There are a number of tests that may be undertaken to investigate departures from genetic equilibrium.[361] The recommended test for STR data is Fisher's exact test and it is used in most situations. This and a number of other options are discussed. This section follows Law[517] extensively.

The Exact Test

Genotype counts are expected to follow a multinomial distribution and hence depend on the unknown true allele frequencies. To avoid the requirement for the unknown allele frequencies, the exact test for the hypothesis of allelic independence is conditioned on the observed allelic counts.[518] The exact test has been reported to have better power when compared to alternative testing strategies.[456,519]

Following Law et al.[363] we write

P_c: The conditional probability of the genotype counts

n: The total number of genotypes

n_g: The genotype counts

n_{lj}: The allelic counts of allele j at locus l

$H = \sum_l \sum_g H_{gl}$: The total number of heterozygotic loci in the sample

Then

$$P_c = \frac{n!2^H}{\prod_g n_g!} \prod_l \frac{\prod_j n_{lj}!}{(2n)!} \tag{5.1}$$

The exact test compares P_c calculated from the observed sample with the values in all genotype arrays with the same allele counts as the observed sample. The *p*-value of the test is the proportion of arrays with a probability no more than that for the observed sample. Box 5.3 shows an example of Fisher's exact test being applied.

It is typically impossible to enumerate all possible genotype arrays, as there are too many of them. An approach attributed to Felsenstein (in Guo and Thompson[518] who proposed a Markov Chain approach) is to take a sample of all possible genotype arrays. The alleles at each locus are

---

BOX 5.3 FISHER'S EXACT TEST

Imagine a single locus with two possible alleles *a* and *b* each with a frequency of 0.5. Hardy–Weinberg equilibrium (HWE) would suggest that we expect to see genotypes in the following proportions:

[A,A] – 0.25
[A,B] – 0.50
[B,B] – 0.25

We have a sample of 50 individuals with the following genotype counts:

[A,A] – 24
[A,B] – 2
[B,B] – 24

(note that $f_A = f_B = 0.5$) and we want to know whether this population deviates from HWE based on the Fisher's exact test at the 5% significance level. Using the formula above the conditional probability of the observed genotype counts is

$$P_c = \left(\frac{50!2^2}{24!2!24!} \right) \frac{50!50!}{(2 \times 50)!} = 1.57 \times 10^{-12}$$

We now calculate the conditional probability for all combinations of 50 counts of [A] and 50 counts of [B]:

[A,A]	[A,B]	[B,B]	P_c
12	26	12	0.219
13	24	13	0.210
11	28	11	0.167
14	22	14	0.148
10	30	10	0.093
15	20	15	0.076
9	32	9	0.037
16	18	16	0.028
8	34	8	0.011
17	16	17	0.007
7	36	7	0.002

Continued

[A,A]	[A,B]	[B,B]	P_c
18	14	18	0.001
6	38	6	3.10E–04
19	12	19	1.74E–04
5	40	5	2.80E–05
20	10	20	1.44E–05
4	42	4	1.60E–06
21	8	21	7.33E–07
3	44	3	5.50E–08
22	6	22	2.12E–08
2	46	2	9.60E–10
23	4	23	3.01E–10
1	48	1	6.80E–12
24	2	24	1.57E–12
0	50	0	1.10E–14
25	0	25	1.25E–15

To obtain the *p*-value we sum all combinations with a probability equal to or less than this one. There are three (the lowest three rows), hence the *p*-value is 1.58×10^{-12}; i.e. Fisher's exact test shows a significant deviation from equilibrium for our observed dataset. We can also see that the combination with the highest conditional probability is

[A,A] – 12
[A,B] – 26
[B,B] – 12

which is the closest possible arrangement to the HWE expectation.

permuted separately to form new multilocus genotypes. The proportion of permuted datasets that give rise to a smaller P_c value than the original data is noted and serves as the empirical *p*-value of the test.

When a permutation approach is used, a portion of the statistic is invariant and can be omitted. Hence instead of calculating

$$P_c = \frac{n!2^H}{\prod_g n_g!} \prod_l \frac{\prod_j n_{lj}!}{(2n)!}$$

as in Equation 5.1 the simpler quantity

$$\frac{2^H}{\prod_g n_g!}$$

can be used. This is no longer the conditional probability of the genotype counts, but it is proportional to that probability.

Zaykin et al.[360] showed that the power of the exact test increases when more loci are used in the testing procedure. However Law et al.[363] show that this is only true for certain population genetic events such as substructure but not for, say, admixture.

Total Heterozygosity Test

Total heterozygosity may be used as a test for some types of disequilibrium. It should be noted however that this is not a test for independence per se as there are types of dependency that do not affect total heterozygosity. Under allelic independence the total heterozygosity is

$$H^e = L - \sum_l \sum_j p_{slj}^2 \tag{5.2}$$

This allows reduction of the genotype array to two categories – the heterozygous and homozygous genotypes.

This gives the total heterozygosity test statistic

$$X^2 = \frac{(H - H^e)^2}{H^e} + \frac{(H - H^e)^2}{nL - H^e} = \frac{nL(H - H^e)^2}{H^e(nL - H^e)} \tag{5.3}$$

where nL is the total count (where n is the sample size and L is the number of loci).

The statistic X^2 has a chi-square distribution with one degree of freedom under the hypothesis of within-locus allelic independence. This is a two-sided test and rejects the hypothesis of allelic independence for both large and small values of H in the data. However the true allele frequencies in the population are generally unknown and need to be estimated from the data when H^e is calculated. Consequently X^2 will no longer have a chi-square distribution under the null hypothesis due to the use of estimated allele frequencies. Hence there is expected to be a loss of power for the test.

Alternatively permutation methods may be used instead of the chi-square test to estimate the distribution of the test statistic, H, under the null. The empirical p-value of the test is calculated from the proportion of permuted genotype arrays with fewer (H^- test) or more (H^+ test) heterozygous genotypes than the original data.

Variance of Heterozygosity Test

Brown and Feldman[520] and Chakraborty[521] suggested that the variance of the number of heterozygous loci for each genotype in the sample could be used as a test for between-locus associations. They give the variance of the heterozygosity test statistic as follows:

$$V = \frac{\sum_g H_g^2 n_g}{n-1} - \frac{H^2}{n(n-1)}$$

where H_g is the number of heterozygous loci in genotype G_g. The test statistic V is the variance of the number of heterozygous loci for each genotype in the population.

Performance of the Tests

Power of the Tests

Fisher's exact test is the method of choice for investigating departures from independence. The power of the test depends to a considerable extent on the size of the sample. For samples of size 200 it has limited power to find realistic departures and it is wrong to infer much about the validity of any particular population genetic model from independence tests on such samples.

Table 5.3	Power Estimates for the Exact Test	
	Sample Size	
θ	80	200
0.00	4.8%	4.9%
0.01	5.8%	5.6%
0.03	8.1%	10.7%

Source: Buckleton et al., *Journal of Forensic Sciences*, 46(1), 198–202, 2001. Reprinted with permission.

Table 5.3 can be read as, '10.7% of datasets of size 200 with a level of inbreeding equivalent to $F_{ST} = 0.03$ will demonstrate a departure from HWE when assessed using Fisher's exact test'.[522]

It is not likely that Hardy–Weinberg disequilibrium, at the level thought to exist in human populations, will be detected with samples of 1000 or less.[456]

Some samples available now are in the tens of thousands. We reproduce some results in the section on a typical report on database validation reproduced below. Our own experience largely in New Zealand and Australia is that Caucasian datasets are close to equilibrium while Aboriginal, Eastern and Western Polynesian datasets show overwhelming evidence of departure. Our own conclusion is that the recent event of admixture largely with Caucasians has caused considerable disequilibrium in the populations and that the samples are large enough to detect it.

We conclude this section with a quote from Bruce Weir[1] that may lighten this dour narrative and contextualize it against the realities of the adversarial legal system: 'My own involvement in the US courts ended after a case in Colorado when the defence objected that my use of Fisher's exact test for independence was hearsay and that the prosecution needed to call Mr Fisher to the stand. It was clear that the public defender was not at all interested in independence testing and had no idea that [Sir] Ronald Fisher had died in 1962. He was simply interrupting my testimony. I was wasting my time.'

Multi-Testing
Another problem arises from the multi-testing nature of the problem. If we examine, say, 13 loci there will be 13 Hardy–Weinberg tests and $\frac{N(N-1)}{2} = 78$ tests between pairs of loci. A significance test at the 5% level would be expected to give a few significant results even if the null hypothesis were true. Weir[456] discusses what should be done, or what should not be done, when a test does cause rejection. 'To ignore single rejections on that (the multitesting) basis calls into question the logic of performing the test in the first place.' Weir points out the shortcomings of the Bonferonni correction, which requires each of x tests to meet a $\frac{0.05}{x}$ significance level in order to declare rejection, describing it as 'unduly conservative'. Note that the word *conservative* in this sense does not have the desirable properties that it has in much of the rest of DNA work.

An elegant way to deal with multiple tests like this is described by Zaykin et al.,[360] who follow Fisher. This involves forming the sum of $-2\ln(p)$ across, say, x independent tests.* This is expected to have a chi-square distribution with $2x$ degrees of freedom and is known as the *truncated product method*. An example is given in Box 5.4.

---

* The tests in a DNA database analysis are not all independent. For example, if we have tested the pairs D3–D8 and D3–D5, then we have some information about the pair D8–D5. However the approach is useful nonetheless.

BOX 5.4   AN EXAMPLE USING THE TRUNCATED PRODUCT METHOD FOR HARDY–WEINBERG TESTS ON NINE LOCI

This approach could also be used on the 36 (or any number) linkage equilibrium tests for nine loci (not shown). It is set up in Excel but any equivalent package should suffice.

$$= -2*\ln(p)$$

Locus	p-value	
D3	0.115915	4.3
D8	0.613721	1.0
D	0.566165	1.1
vWA	0.521490	1.3
D21	0.760857	0.5
D13	0.589834	1.1
FGA	0.973626	0.1
D7	0.188993	3.3
D18	0.312987	2.3
Sum	**15.0**	0.66

= 2*loci

= chidist(15.0,18)

This is the p-value for the null that all nine loci are in HWE

This approach assumes that the tests are independent, which they are not. It is a useful approach nonetheless.

Another useful way is treat the multiple comparison problems by examination using a $p–p$ plot (Figure 5.3 and Box 5.5).[523] In this examination the p-values are expected to be uniformly distributed between 0 and 1 if the null hypothesis (independence between alleles) is true and therefore should lie along the diagonal. The envelopes of values that would be expected to enclose 99% of the points in the null case are superimposed.

Figure 5.3 provides clear evidence for an excess of low p-values for the Eastern and Western Polynesian populations.[*,†] There is no indication of deviation from linkage equilibrium in the Caucasian[‡] or Asian datasets.[§] Due to the smaller size of the Asian dataset we would not expect to find disequilibria whether or not they were present.[515]

Example 5.1: A Standard Report from Our Group

We analysed 20,352 Identifiler™ profiles with self-declared ethnicity data. The profiles originated from the four major New Zealand subpopulation groups: Asian, Caucasian, Eastern Polynesian and Western Polynesian. All DNA profiles were fully designated at all loci (there were

---

* $N = 8730$ and 2644 Identifiler™ profiles, respectively.
† $p < 0.001$ on omnibus tests using the truncated product method.[361]
‡ $N = 8248$ Identifiler profiles.
§ $N = 377$ Identifiler profiles.

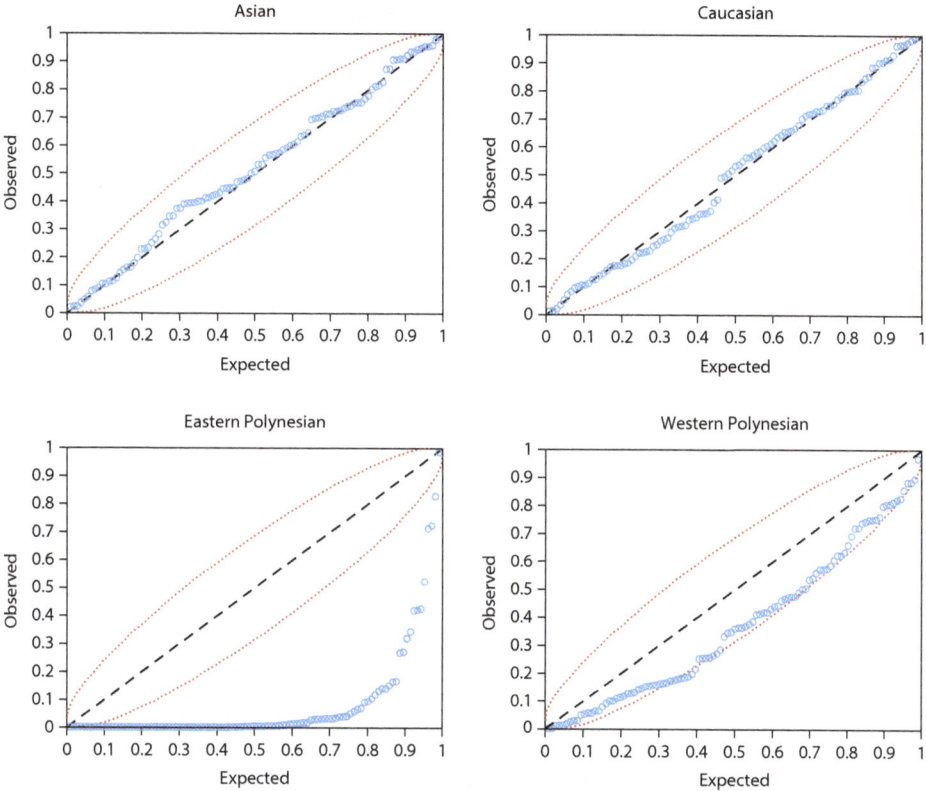

Figure 5.3   p–p plots investigating deviations from Hardy–Weinberg and linkage for each of the four major subpopulations in New Zealand. (From Triggs, C.M., personal communication, unpublished results, 2002.)

BOX 5.5   HYPOTHETICAL EXAMPLE SHOWING THE CREATION OF A *P–P* PLOT FOR THE 36 LINKAGE EQUILIBRIUM TESTS FOR NINE LOCI

Again it is set up in Excel.

	A	B	C	D	E
			p-value	=rank(C1,C1:C35)	=D1/37
1	D3	D8	0.437	14	0.378
2	D3	D5	0.835	32	0.865
3	D3	vWA	0.820	30	0.811
4	D3	D21	0.756	27	0.730
5	D3	D3	0.428	12	0.324

This table continues for the 36 values.

Plot column C on the y-axis and column E on the x-axis. It helps to add the line of Slope 1. A deviation from equilibrium is shown by a deviation from the diagonal line.

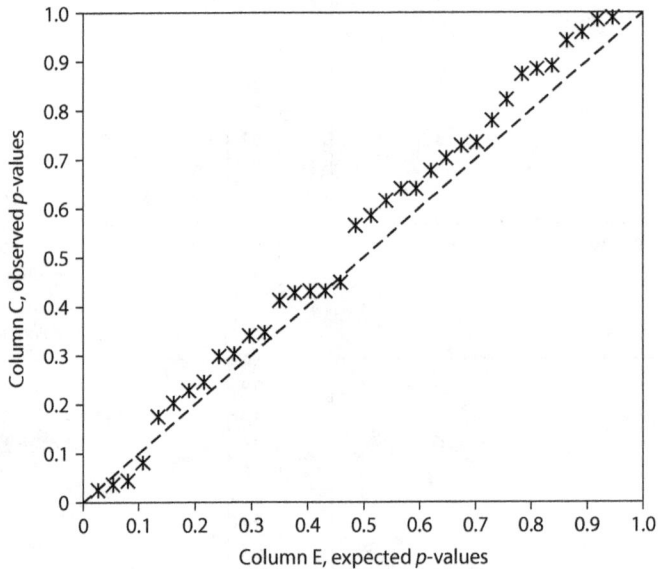

More sophisticated packages can place the 95% or 99% confidence interval on the p–p line.

The envelope as seen in Figure 5.3 is created based on the behaviour of Fisher's exact text on data that is in Hardy–Weinberg equilibrium (HWE). For such datasets we would expect the Fisher's exact test to produce independence test values uniformly between 0 and 1. Therefore to generate envelopes we generate x arrays containing n elements (where x is the number of tests that have been performed and n is an arbitrary number) and fill them with numbers drawn from U[0,1].

The nth element of each array are sorted in ascending order and then each of the x arrays is sorted in ascending order. The envelopes are then created by selecting the elements in each of the x arrays that correspond to the interval of interest and graphing them against each other.

no partial profiles). All rare alleles were retained within the dataset. Ambiguous alleles such as those falling between two loci ranges were labelled R (standing for *rare allele*). Both alleles in a triallelic pattern were designated R,R.

The profiling data was checked for duplicate entries. A duplicate entry occurs when the same DNA profile is represented in the dataset more than once. This can occur for a number of reasons:

- Multiple entries of the same sample.
- More than one sample from the same person has been submitted.
- The samples originate from twins or siblings.
- The samples originate from unrelated individuals. The DNA profiles appear the same due to an adventitious match.

We removed 329 duplicate entries. The majority of these were the same individual represented in multiple ethnicity clusters as judged by the same surname and date of birth or by information from the police. We acknowledge that identical twins also have the same surname and date of birth. A summary of the number of samples per subpopulation is provided in Table 5.4.

For each locus in the sample an exact test of allelic association was conducted. Significance levels (p-values) were generated empirically by the permutation procedure, with 10,000 permutations (Table 5.5). This number is expected to give a 95% confidence interval of ±0.0043 for a p-value around 0.05.

Graphical representations of the linkage-equilibrium data are presented in Figure 5.4. As an example, the $x = y$ line in the p–p plots represents equilibrium. The 95% confidence limit is also

Table 5.4 Summary of Subpopulations Tested and Number of Samples

Subpopulation	Number
Asian	377
Caucasian	8248
Eastern Polynesian	8730
Western Polynesian	2644

Table 5.5 Results of Fisher's Exact Test for Allelic Association for Each Locus Hardy–Weinberg Equilibrium (HWE) for the New Zealand Identifiler™ Dataset

Locus	Asian		Caucasian		Eastern Polynesian		Western Polynesian	
	p-Value	−2ln(p)	p-Value	−2ln(p)	p-Value	−2ln(p)	p-Value	−2ln(p)
CSF	0.64	0.89	0.32	2.27	0.09	4.75	0.76	0.54
D13	0.78	0.51	0.62	0.94	0.09	4.79	0.89	0.24
D16	0.81	0.42	0.61	0.98	0.73	0.64	0.17	3.54
D18	0.20	3.24	0.18	3.48	0.32	2.27	0.17	3.50
D19	**0.01**	8.57	0.48	1.46	**0.00**	13.82	**0.01**	9.00
D2	0.18	3.48	0.44	1.64	0.11	4.49	0.24	2.83
D21	**0.00**	16.22	0.52	1.30	0.68	0.78	0.20	3.20
D3	0.35	2.10	0.69	0.73	0.13	4.11	0.13	4.09
D5	0.46	1.57	0.48	1.49	**0.02**	7.72	0.36	2.05
D7	0.31	2.36	0.38	1.93	0.05	6.05	0.40	1.84
D8	0.97	0.07	0.17	3.49	0.71	0.68	0.20	3.19
FGA	0.97	0.07	**0.02**	8.21	**0.04**	6.59	0.23	2.91
THO1	**0.00**	12.24	0.16	3.63	0.92	0.16	0.17	3.58
TPOX	0.99	0.02	0.74	0.59	0.28	2.54	0.09	4.72
vWA	0.95	0.11	0.14	3.97	0.21	3.15	0.06	5.75
Sum[−2ln(p)]	51.85		36.13		62.53		50.97	
p-Value	0.01		0.20		0.00		0.01	

Note: Values below 0.05 are shown in bold.

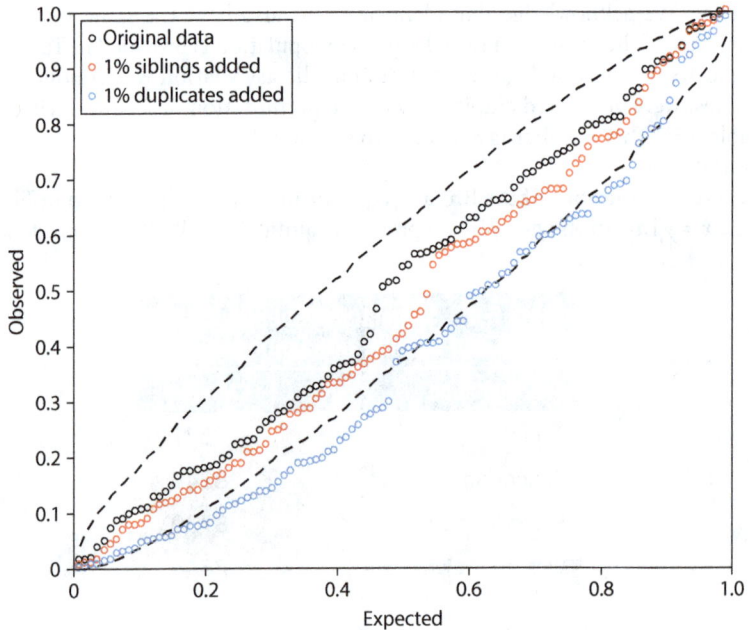

Figure 5.4   *p–p* plots for a dataset of several thousand individuals (black); the same dataset with the addition of 1% siblings (red) and 1% duplicates (blue).

displayed on the *p–p* plots as the region within the two curved lines. In the *p–p* plots for the Asian, Caucasian and Western Polynesian subpopulations, the data remains within the boundaries of this envelope. The data is outside the boundaries for the Eastern Polynesian subpopulation group. As with the last population data statistical analysis the Eastern Polynesians exhibit clear departures from expected *p*-values.

The dataset analysed here is large by international standards and the Eastern Polynesian subpopulation does appear to indicate departures from equilibrium. Regardless of the results of independence testing, our knowledge of the history of human populations leads us to expect that some level of admixture or substructure exists in all populations. With this in mind it is advised that balanced conclusions should be drawn from the testing of these datasets. An example may be, 'These tests cannot differentiate between the model of independence and the model of mild departure, therefore it is in the interests of balanced testimony to concede that mild departure may exist.'

Example 5.2: *R v Bropho*: A Discussion of Independence Testing[*]

In 2004 Mr Robert Bropho, a prominent Western Australian of Aboriginal descent, was tried for the historic rapes of a then-teenage girl in his care. Of five charges the prosecution offered no evidence on three and they were dismissed. Mr Bropho had elected trial by judge alone and Judge Mazza presided. At issue was, *inter alia*, the parentage of the complainant's oldest child, ACS. The prosecution sought to bolster the credibility of the complainant and diminish that of

---

[*] This section is adapted from an article[524] that was first published by Thomson Reuters in the Australian Law Journal. The original article should be cited as Buckleton, J.S., J.M. Curran, and S.J. Walsh, R v Bropho: Careful interpretation of DNA evidence required for courtroom decision making, 2005. 79: 709–721. For all subscription inquiries please phone, from Australia: 1300 304 195, from overseas: +61 2 8587 7980 or online at www.thomsonreuters.com.au/ catalogue. Reproduced with permission of Thomson Reuters (Professional) Australia Limited, www.thomsonreuters. com.au

the accused by the presentation of DNA evidence supporting the suggestion that Mr Bropho was indeed the father of ACS. It was thought that ACS was conceived between 7 March and 11 April 1977 and was born on 21 December 1977.

The complainant was born in 1962 and was 42 at the time of the trial. She stated that Mr Bropho was her uncle by marriage and that at the times of the rapes she was living with him and his now-deceased wife, Edna, her aunt. Two of five initial allegations were eventually taken to trial. The complainant alleged that Mr Bropho had intercourse with her without her consent in the bush on Saunders Street and under a bridge in Guildford. Mr Bropho denied ever having intercourse with the complainant. The defence therefore denied that intercourse had occurred; however, Judge Mazza correctly insisted that the Crown should prove both that intercourse had occurred and that it was not consensual.* The DNA evidence to be discussed later only bears on the parentage of the eldest child and hence on the question of whether or not intercourse had occurred. Forensic parentage analysis of this type is never conclusive but can be expressed in a probabilistic manner, in this case as a paternity index. It could not show that conception was a result of one or other of the two incidents representing these allegations. It would be possible for Mr Bropho to be the father but for conception to have occurred at some other time. In addition the DNA evidence did not, to any extent; bear on the question of consent.

The complainant went to live with her aunt and Mr Bropho when she was 13 or 14 (1975–1976), reportedly because of the drinking of her mother. Mr Bropho and Edna had 10 children, two of whom were close to the complainant in age. She lived with Mr Bropho and Edna at two locations: at a house at Dixon Street and in tents at the Saunders Street camp. At this latter address everyone lived in tents and the complainant recalled that she was happy there. It was at this time that she alleges the rapes occurred.

In the first complaint she related an incident where she, aged approximately 13, and the accused went for a walk to a shop. On the way the accused walked into some bushes at the side of the road not far from the camp and she walked over to him. Mr Bropho asked her to lie on the ground and the first alleged rape occurred. She did not relate the incident to anyone at the time, stating subsequently that she was frightened to do so.

The second complaint that was taken to trial also related to events that occurred when the complainant was 13 or 14. The complainant related that she; her aunt, her cousins and Mr Bropho went to a park in Guildford. The complainant and Mr Bropho walked to a nearby bridge where Mr Bropho was to give her some money. It was underneath this bridge that the second rape was alleged to have occurred. The complainant described taking her own pants off and lying down because she knew what was expected of her. Again she told nobody.

The last time that the complainant lived with Mr Bropho was when she was 15. At that time she was pregnant with her eldest child, subsequently alleged to be the child of Mr Bropho. The first time that the matters comprising these complaints surfaced was in 1999 when the complainant related these alleged matters to her mother at the funeral of one of the complainant's children.

It was agreed by both defence and prosecution that the complainant had been admitted to Graylands Hospital with a diagnosis of schizophreniform psychosis in 1985. By 1991, she was suffering paranoid schizophrenia and by 1999 she was dealing with paranoid schizophrenia, alcoholic hallucinosis and cognitive/frontal lobe impairment and impaired impulse control. From mid-2002, she related concerns that Robert Bropho would come into prison disguised as a prison warder and harm her. Concerns that 'cultural lawmen' would come to kill her and her family were voiced after she was released from prison. In October 2002, she was involuntarily admitted to a psychiatric ward.

The complainant nominated during cross-examination another man PRJ, now deceased, as the father of her eldest child.

Mr Robert Charles Bropho was 74 at the time of the trial. His wife, Edna, had died four years previously.

---

* Mr Utting for the defence did not concede the issue of consent, nor should he have.

DNA evidence was offered at trial in support of the suggestion that the accused was the father of a child (ACS). At no point did the prosecution suggest that the DNA evidence was sufficiently powerful as to constitute proof that Mr Bropho was the father of ACS.

Mr Bropho was acquitted and the judgement expressed concerns about the DNA evidence. The guilt or innocence of Mr Bropho and the verdict per se are not the subject of this example, nor should these ever be a matter of any professional interest to a forensic scientist. It is those aspects of this ruling with implications for the wider forensic use of DNA that we discuss. Those aspects relate to the evaluation of the weight of evidence and in particular the interpretation of the results of hypothesis testing and the use of population genetic models.

All parties agreed that Mr Bropho could not be excluded as the father of the complainant's eldest child, ACS. Once the accused is not excluded, DNA evidence is usually reported with a measure of the weight of evidence and is virtually useless or even dangerous without this. In this case it was agreed by all parties that the appropriate measure should be the paternity index. The prosecution offered evidence that the paternity index was of the order of 3100. It was the basis for assigning this number or indeed any number that was argued.

The simplest model for assigning a weight of evidence assumes that the occurrence of alleles at each locus and across loci is independent. The assumption of independence of alleles at one locus is called *Hardy–Weinberg equilibrium* and departure from independence is termed *Hardy–Weinberg disequilibrium*. Independence across loci is termed *linkage equilibrium* and departure from it *linkage disequilibrium*.

The concept of independence is central to this discussion and has occurred in legal argument frequently in the past, both in DNA and non-DNA testimony. It dominated argument in DNA testimony in the United States in the early 1990s and was termed the *DNA wars*. These arguments led the US National Research Council to commission two reports. The second report largely, but not completely, settled matters in the United States. This discussion never reached the same intensity in the United Kingdom as the main forensic provider in that country, the Forensic Science Service, moved to accommodate the criticisms early and adapted their approach. However the subject of independence still occasionally occupies a time-consuming and more rarely a pivotal position in court proceedings in Australia.

The ruling appeared to assume that we have effective mechanisms that can assign pairs of loci as 'in' or 'out' of linkage equilibrium. This matter is usually examined using statistical testing called hypothesis testing. During the database validation stage of the Western Australian data, Walsh and Buckleton applied a hypothesis test to each locus and each pair of loci. Each hypothesis test returns a number called the p-value. In a 13-locus set, such as used in *Bropho*, each locus is examined and is also involved in 12 pairs, one with each of the other loci.

In classical hypothesis testing a low p-value is typically taken as evidence against the hypothesis. Sometimes an arbitrary level of 0.05 is assigned as a decision threshold below which the hypothesis is taken to be 'rejected'. Above this threshold the hypothesis is accepted or more pedantically 'non-rejected'.

However this approach is really quite simplistic and has come under increasing scrutiny. It is largely abandoned or was never used by leading forensic statisticians. It does, unfortunately, still persist extensively in the forensic literature. The shortcomings of this approach were noted in the Walsh and Buckleton report on the Western Australian data.

First note that if the hypothesis of linkage equilibrium were true, then the p-values would be expected to scatter evenly from 0.00 to 1.00. Hence about 5% of these would give p-values less than 0.05 and hence give false indications of departure – a false positive. Accordingly the false positive rate is about 5% and the true negative rate about 95%.

If the hypothesis of linkage equilibrium were false, we do not know how the p-values should spread. They are likely to cluster at the low p-value end, but we do not know how much they should cluster in this direction. The extent of this clustering depends on the amount of disequilibrium, the size of the database, other factors such as the number of alleles at this locus and a very significant random element. For most realistic datasets and realistic disequilibria the clustering in this direction is mild. Hence, if we accept the hypothesis of linkage equilibrium every time the p-value is greater than 0.05, then we stand a significant chance of making incorrect decisions. This is the unknown false negative rate.

Hence our hypothesis tests have a 5% false positive rate and an unknown but probably large false negative rate.

To further illustrate this we assembled a database of 15 loci with substantial disequilibrium at each locus and between each pair. Since all loci and all pairs have disequilibrium, the correct answer from every test is 'rejection'. Hence we desire all the p-values to be less than 0.05. Since the true state is one of significant disequilibrium, values less than 0.05 represent true positives and values above 0.05 represent false negatives. We took samples from this database of varying sizes and conducted independence testing on them. In Figure 5.5 we present the p-values plotted against sample size. From this plot we can see the effect of sample size on the false negative rate.

Looking at the small sample size end of Figure 5.5 (expanded view given in Figure 5.6), it is possible to see that the p-values are nearly evenly spread between 0 and 1 and hence the false negative rate is close to 95%. Recall the population has disequilibrium; hence all negative findings are false.

By the time that the sample is of the order of 5000, there is a clustering towards lower p-values, but still not all values are in the very low range. It would take samples much larger than 5000 to guarantee that the false negative rate was low.

The false positive rate of 5% may seem tolerable, but a false negative rate of the order of 95% is clearly worrying. It transpires that the false negative rate is the one that is directly involved in decision making in the DNA context. This is because, for population genetic reasons, we expect the true state in any real population to be one of mild disequilibrium. Hence there can only be true positives and false negatives. For moderate sized databases there will be mainly false negatives.

Hence, it is very wrong to sort loci or pairs of loci into those that are in and out of equilibrium on the basis of independence testing. Regretfully there is still evidence of this practice in the forensic literature and in court.

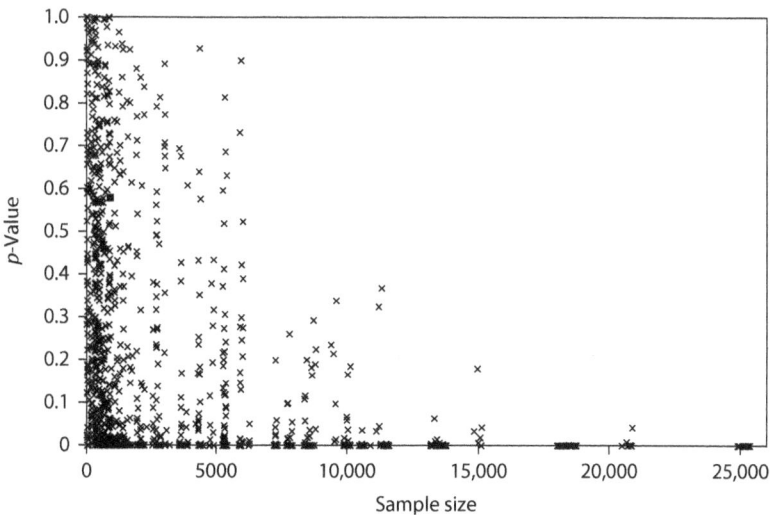

Figure 5.5   A plot of p-value versus sample size (number of individuals).

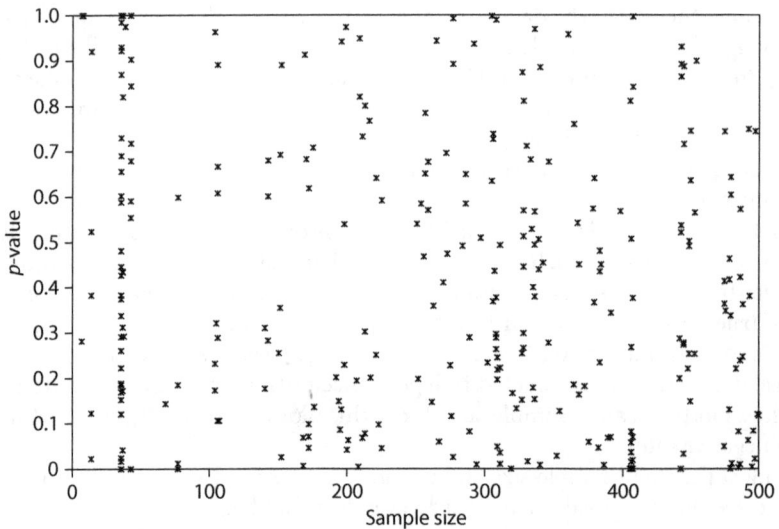

Figure 5.6   Expanded view of the low sample size end of the plot displayed in Figure 5.5.

We also point out that the Balding and Nichols model (NRC II Recommendation 4.2) does not assume linkage equilibrium in the population. It does assume it in the subpopulation.

Recently *Nature* published an article titled 'Scientific method: statistical errors'[525] that shows that overinterpretation of *p*-values is still an issue in 2014. Regina Nuzzo gives some valuable quotes about *p*-values, comparing them to the following:

1. Like mosquitoes (annoying and impossible to swat away)

2. The emperor's new clothes (fraught with obvious problems everyone ignores)

3. The tool of a sterile intellectual rake who ravishes science but leaves it with no progeny

4. Rechristened as 'statistical hypothesis inference testing' for the acronym

The Effect of Silent Alleles
Despite our reserved comments about the usefulness of significance tests, they do appear useful to detect genetic phenomena that lead to excess homozygosity, especially primer binding site mutations. If there is a mutation at the 3′ flanking region of the primer binding site, then polymerase chain reaction can be completely inhibited. The result is that the genotype will appear to be a homozygote. An excellent example is given by Budowle et al.,[526] who observe that binding site induced allelic drop-out was present at D8S1179 in Chamorros ($n = 68$) and Filipinos ($n = 74$). Thirteen individuals typed with the PowerPlex 16 kit were heterozygotes, whereas only single alleles were observed with the Profiler Plus kit. The observation of a deviation from Hardy–Weinberg proportions at this locus in these two populations suggested that further investigation was merited and indeed led to the discovery of the silent alleles.

Such silent alleles would be expected at low frequency at all loci. This will increase counts of homozygotes, albeit mildly.

Investigating Allelic Dependencies
If dependencies are found by the Fisher's exact tests, it is possible to delve further into this finding by examining the genotypic makeup at a locus. Table 5.6 shows the observed and expected

156

Table 5.6	D13S317 Observed and Expected Genotype Counts						
	7	**8**	**9**	**10**	**11**	**12**	**13**	**14**
7	0/0	0/0	0/0	0/0	1/0	0/0	0/0	0/0
8		23/19	11/8	3/6	52/53	37/39	7/11	2/3
9			**3/1**	0/1	6/10	4/8	4/2	0/1
10				0/0	12/8	4/6	0/2	**4/0**
11					37/37	48/54	21/15	4/5
12						28/20	7/11	4/3
13							3/2	0/1
14								0/0

genotype counts for the data at locus D13S317. If in equilibrium, these values should adhere to a chi-square distribution with 1 degree of freedom. A chi-squared value of 3.84 returns a *p*-value of 0.05. This means that if we calculate the test statistic

$$X^2 = \frac{\left(Observed - Expected\right)^2}{Expected}$$

any values greater than 3.84 are an indication of departure. If significant values are on the diagonal (indicating an excess of homozygotes), then this can indicate the database has sub-structure. Excess heterozygotes may be indicative of a Wahlund effect (see Chapter 3 for more on this). Table 5.6 shows support for departures from Hardy–Weinberg equilibrium in the two genotypes outlined in bold.

A disadvantage of this approach is that it is sensitive to genotypes with low expected counts. The low numbers of genotypic combinations that support departures from Hardy–Weinberg equilibrium indicate that the overall departure from Hardy–Weinberg equilibrium at locus D13S317 may be driven by a few rare genotypes.

The Effect of Relatives or Duplicate Profiles on the Database
The preferred method of sampling is random. Random sampling will include some relatives. However truly random sampling is not possible and databases are often convenience samples. There is some evidence for the over-representation of relatives.

There are two aspects to consider with over-representation of relatives or duplicates on the database:

1. What effect will they have on tests for dependencies?

2. What effect will they have on allele frequencies?

This point has been brought up in a case in South Australia (*R v Cannell*) where the discussion was lead to the effect that a few pairs of siblings would have on allele frequencies:

Defence council: … an ideal database that would be truly representative of the random population, would that database not include sibling profiles?

Scientist: I suppose in an ideal world it wouldn't, although inclusion of relatives on a database isn't enough to make much difference.

…

His Honour: ... the exclusion of those individuals, why does that mean the database would be more random? These relationships exist.

Scientist: It's not so much the randomness of the database that including relatives on the database would effect, it's more the allele frequencies. If you have a group of relatives on a database they're going to have the same alleles more commonly than the population at large because, obviously, within a family you have similar DNA. But in a practical sense the inclusion of a few relatives on a database, especially one of hundreds or thousands, makes negligible difference....

We end this section by pointing out that the preferred sampling is random. Random sampling will include some relatives and this is the correct result. The presence of some relatives may cause some dependencies in the data and this is the correct result. The presence of some relatives will have a very minor effect on the allele probabilities and there is likely to be no bias to this effect.

Misuse of Genetics

In Chapter 3 we discussed the assumptions that underlie the Hardy–Weinberg law and the state of linkage equilibrium. Often validation of the use of the product rule contains an amalgam of statistical and genetic logic. In principle this approach is perfectly reasonable, but the practice is often wayward. For instance, it would be wrong to point out that some genetic conditions leading to equilibrium are present but not to point out that others are not.

It is misleading to suggest that validation of the product rule has much of anything to do with allelic segregation. In particular it would be wrong to suggest that linkage implies linkage disequilibrium and that a lack of linkage implies linkage equilibrium. The most likely causes of linkage disequilibrium are not genetic linkage but population genetic effects such as population substructure.

The linkage state of two loci will suggest the rate at which equilibrium will be established after a disturbing event if all the disturbing forces are removed. For example, allelic associations decay by a factor of $1 - R$ each generation, where R is the recombination fraction. For unlinked loci $R = \frac{1}{2}$ and hence any allelic associations halve every generation, but only in the absence of any disturbing forces. Where disturbing forces, such as selection or continuing population subdivision and admixture, continue they will maintain the disequilibrium even for unlinked loci. In this context Thompson[496] terms them *maintaining forces*.

Linkage

Emerging STR multiplexes have loci physically close on the same chromosome. This leads to justifiable concerns about the possibility of allelic association. Tests for the hypothesis of no disequilibrium do exist but tend to have limited power to detect realistic levels of disequilibrium. Data requirements to identify realistic levels of disequilibrium are likely to be very large[258,424] and well beyond the studies already presented or are confounded by the effects of subdivision or admixture.

Physical linkage does not directly imply allelic association. Linked loci may show little or no allelic association.

Equally allelic association often results from an evolutionary event such as genetic drift in finite populations,[428] founder effects, natural selection, population admixture and the associated Wahlund effect. These events affect both linked and unlinked loci. Linked and unlinked loci do however differ in the rate at which independence is re-established. The difference is therefore quantitative rather than qualitative.

Recently O'Connor et al.[527,528] and Budowle et al.[529] investigated allelic association between two STR loci, both sited on the *p*-arm of Chromosome 12, namely vWA and D12S391. These loci are components of the new generation multiplex systems, including AmpF*l*STR® NGM™ and GlobalFiler™ and Promega PowerPlex ESI 17® and Fusion. Both sets of authors recommended multiplication of the single locus probabilities for loci D12S391 and vWA to estimate combined allelic probabilities for both single source and mixture casework[529] (hereafter *multiplication*). The sample sizes for both studies are relatively small and are unlikely to detect realistic levels of allelic association. Hence these studies support, but fall short of, proof that multiplication will provide a robust estimate.

The lack of allelic association observed in one study[529] was ascribed to mutation. Mutation at either of two linked loci may reduce or increase linkage disequilibrium – if it is to a novel allele it will increase; if it is to a pre-existing allele it will decrease. In STRs most mutations are to pre-existing alleles. However mutation rates are of the order of 10^{-3}; hence even the combined chance of mutation at two loci is likely to be at least an order of magnitude less than the recombination rate, even for these linked loci. Recombination is therefore the most plausible explanation for the observed lack of allelic association.

By simulating admixing populations it is possible to observe the match probability as generations of admixture occur.[530] Weir[367] gave a formula to predict the match probability for various θ values assuming no linkage (hereafter the *Weir estimate*). By comparing the observed match probability in simulated populations with the theoretical estimate for unlinked populations, Gill et al. concluded[530] that for realistic populations it seems likely that the application of a θ correction factor of the magnitude typically applied and the use of the Balding and Nichols[358] equations (Equations 3.5) would be effective in preventing overestimates of the *LR*, especially if a few generations have passed. We are unaware of experiments that test Recommendation 4.1 (Equations 3.4).

Estimating θ
Historic and Modern Consanguineous Marriage

A summary of historic consanguinity does not have any direct implication for modern θ values; however it may imply that there was a high level of inbreeding in historic human populations. The question of whether or not this has been erased in modern times is unanswered. However the prevalence of consanguinity in ancient times and its considerable persistence into modern times is worthy of discussion in the context of forensic DNA interpretation. This is because the mating patterns of humans in the past are likely to impact on modern θ values. In particular, we do not need to consider simply consanguineous marriage, which is a relatively extreme form of inbreeding; we also need to consider any restriction of the mating choice. The most obvious non-cultural restriction is geographical availability.

It is worth noting that there are several cultural forces driving consanguinity. These include maintenance of family property and bride wealth. In societies where inheritance is divided among progeny, there is a considerable incentive to consanguineous marriage. In addition the economic burden of bride wealth is an important driver of consanguinity. Under these circumstances consanguineous marriage is economically the most feasible option where culturally permissible.

Bittles and Neel[531] present a review specifically with the intent of assessing the load of lethal recessives in the population and their impact on modern consanguineous marriages. 'As the great religions emerged (Buddhism, Confucianism, Islam, Hinduism, Judaism, Christianity) only one – Christianity – had specific proscriptions against non-incestuous consanguineous marriage, and even those were not enunciated until the Council of Trent in the mid-sixteenth century.'[531] These authors conclude that the relatively low modern load of lethal recessives is strong evidence for ancient inbreeding.

Much of the subsequent discussion follows Bittles.[532] '"Western" opinion tends to be that whether or not consanguineous marriage was present in the past it has largely disappeared in modern society. This is untrue and it is worthwhile reviewing the evidence for both the relatively recent prohibition of consanguinity and the persistence of it into our generation.'

Prohibition on second- and third-cousin marriages was formally rescinded by the Roman Catholic Church in 1917. Specific dispensation remains a prerequisite for Roman Catholic marriages between first cousins who wish to have their marriage recognized by the church.[532] First cousin marriages are criminal offences in 8 of the 50 United States and are subject to civil sanction in a further 31 states[533] under statutes introduced from the mid-nineteenth century onwards. Exceptions have been incorporated for specific communities. For instance, uncle/niece marriage is permissible for Jews in Rhode Island. It may be of interest to the reader to note that Charles Darwin was married to his cousin Emma Wedgewood.

In North America and Western Europe the rates of first cousin marriage are about 0.6%,[534,535] with Japan at about 3.9%.[536,537] Bittles et al. gave estimates in the range of 20%–50% for marriages between second cousins or closer in the Muslim countries of North Africa, Central and West Asia and in most parts of South Asia.[538] The preferred type of marriage in Muslim society is for a male to marry his father's brother's daughter. Uncle/niece marriage is prohibited by the *Koran*. In the primarily Hindu states of southern India, 20%–45% of marriages are consanguineous, with uncle/niece and mother's brother's daughter especially popular.

Information from modern China is not available. However before the Second World War first cousin marriage of the type mother's brother's daughter was the accepted custom among the Han, who make up approximately 90% of the population.

Bittles draws the conclusion that consanguinity is not an unusual or rare phenomenon but rather was and is the preferred or prescribed form of marriage in much of the world. The expected reduction in consanguineous marriage in the latter half of the twentieth century does not appear to be happening universally. Bittles also points out that many immigrant groups maintain these cultural norms when they move to Europe or North America and the inbreeding may even be enhanced by the reduction of choice in smaller communities.

A Practical Estimation of θ

(*B.S. Weir, Jerome Goudet, Duncan Taylor, James Curran, Alexandre Thiery, and John Buckleton*)
Data were obtained from published population reports in forensic journals. Not all of the data collated in this study was originally collected for forensic purposes. A proportion was collected more probably for anthropological reasons than validation of forensic multiplexes for casework. The net effect of this fact is that we have some issues regarding non-standard loci and non-standard allele designations, as well as small samples.

Errors in the data were apparent in a significant number of cases. Most of these errors were typographical and in many cases the correct data could be deduced. In some cases we determined that an error was present because the allele frequencies did not add to sufficiently near to 1. In approximately half of the cases of error we received a helpful answer from the corresponding author, but in the remainder there was either no answer or an unhelpful answer. In these cases we have either omitted the data or used our own deduction. We also struggled with different nomenclatures for rare alleles; however this should have only a minor effect on the analysis. Because of the extensive nature of the reference list associated with the data, we have only given selected references.

$\hat{\beta}$ values were estimated using methods from Weir (pers comm) extended from Bhatia et al.[539] We would suggest that $\hat{\beta}$ be used in the Balding and Nichols equations in place of $\hat{\theta}$ when the allele probabilities are from a general population.

The average $\hat{\beta}$ values differed between loci (see Table 5.7). This would suggest that different values should be used for every locus. This is a level of complexity that we think is unlikely to pay any dividend.

The average $\hat{\beta}$ values for some commonly used multiplexes appears in Table 5.8. Average across the common multiplexes, the locus effect tends to average out. There is really quite a small difference in $\hat{\beta}$ expected for different multiplexes and we suggest this effect can be ignored.

Table 5.7	The Average Across All Populations by Locus		
D1S1656	0.014	D18S51	0.018
D2S1338	0.031	D19S433	0.025
D2S441	0.032	D21S11	0.020
D3S1358	0.026	D22S1045	0.020
D5S818	0.033	CSF1PO	0.011
D6S1043	0.021	FGA	0.014
D7S820	0.026	Penta D	0.022
D8S1179	0.018	Penta E	0.019
D10S1248	0.010	SE33	0.021
D12S391	0.011	TH01	0.074
D13S317	0.038	TPOX	0.033
D16S539	0.024	vWA	0.019

Table 5.8	The Multiplex Effects per Locus for Some Commonly Used Multiplexes						
Multiplex	SGMPlus	CODIS	Identifiler™	Powerplex 16	PP21	Fusion	GlobalFiler
Average $\hat{\beta}$ across loci	0.027	0.027	0.028	0.027	0.025	0.024	0.025

We present in Table 5.9 a summary of our findings for each of eight clusters. Each cluster is summarized by its mean, median and 95th percentile. We also provide, for each cluster, the populations which have an estimated $\hat{\beta}$ value which is greater than the 95th percentile. We might regard these populations as being outlying in some sense. In Figure 5.7 we give the distributions for those clusters with reasonable sample number. In Figure 5.8 we give a neighbour joining tree for the different populations.

Given the data in Table 5.9 there is still a question of what value should be selected for use in forensic work.

A rational approach might be to routinely use the 50th percentile figures, but if the suspect is from one of those populations given in Table 5.9 that had a $\hat{\beta}$ high value, then use the actual value for that population. We emphasize that this makes the assumption that the offender is from the same subpopulation as the suspect. This approach adds a conservatism in the assignment of $\hat{\beta}$ to a model already believed to be conservative.

There is a coherent argument that any additional level of conservatism in the assignment of $\hat{\beta}$ is unnecessary since there is reason to believe that equations 3.5 are inherently conservative.[365,366,370,371]

Dealing with Diverse Populations

What should we do if a part of our population includes individuals from a race that we have not sampled extensively or if the suspect belongs to a race we have not sampled? NRC II[176] Recommendation 4.3 addresses this issue. 'If the person who contributed the evidence sample is from a group or tribe for which no adequate database exists, data from several other groups or tribes thought to be closely related to it should be used. The profile frequency

Table 5.9 Summary Statistics and Populations Outside the 95th Percentile for the Clusters

Cluster	Percentile 50th	95th	N	Populations above the 95th Percentile and $\hat{\beta}$ Value	
European ancestry, Middle Eastern and North African	0.019	0.041	172	Vojvodina, Slovakia[540]	0.042
				El Minya, Egypt	0.044
				Basque[541]	0.044
				Belarus[542]	0.059
				Italy[543]	0.061
				Romani Croatia – north-west[544]	0.070
				Innsbruck, Austria[545]	0.080
				Zagreb, Croatia[545]	0.080
Australian Aboriginal	0.000	0.025	17	Tiwi[546]	0.070
Hispanic or mixed Native American	0.014	0.057	41	Metztitlan, Mexico[547]	0.057
				Argentina[548]	0.068
Indian subcontinent and Afghanistan	0.035	0.062	30	Indians – United Arab Emirates[549]	0.071
				Pakistani – United Arab Emirates[549]	0.072
Inuit	0.026	0.036	3		
Native American	0.054	0.106	34	Tojolabal[550]	0.111
				Lacandon[550]	0.169
Polynesian	0.000	0.011	4		
Sub-Saharan Africa, African American, Bahamas and Afro-Caribbean	0.032	0.047	37	Andean, Amazonian and Orinoquian – Columbia[551]	0.052
				South African, South-West African[552]	0.063
Asian	0.033	0.070	85	Bao'an, China[553]	0.070
				Lisu of China[554]	0.075
				Southern Han of China[555]	0.092
				Tibeto-Burman Nu of China [556]	0.116
				Tibeto-Burman Derung of China[556]	0.131
Andaman Islanders	0.068	0.152	3		

should be calculated as described in Recommendation 4.1 for each group or tribe.' Of course the population to be modelled is not necessarily dictated by the group or tribe of the defendant but that aside this is a sensible approach to the problem. However it should be accepted that, on average, a person's genotype tends to be more common in their own group than others. Hence we should expect a person's genotype estimate to be more common on average in their own group than even in several closely related groups. This effect is likely to be very minor. However an effective mechanism for making estimates of groups that have not been sampled is provided by the Balding and Nichols[358] equations with a suitable value of θ. Using this approach we would sample the closely related groups *and* then use the Balding and Nichols formulae with an appropriate estimate of θ. This approach is a preferable refinement of Recommendation 4.3.

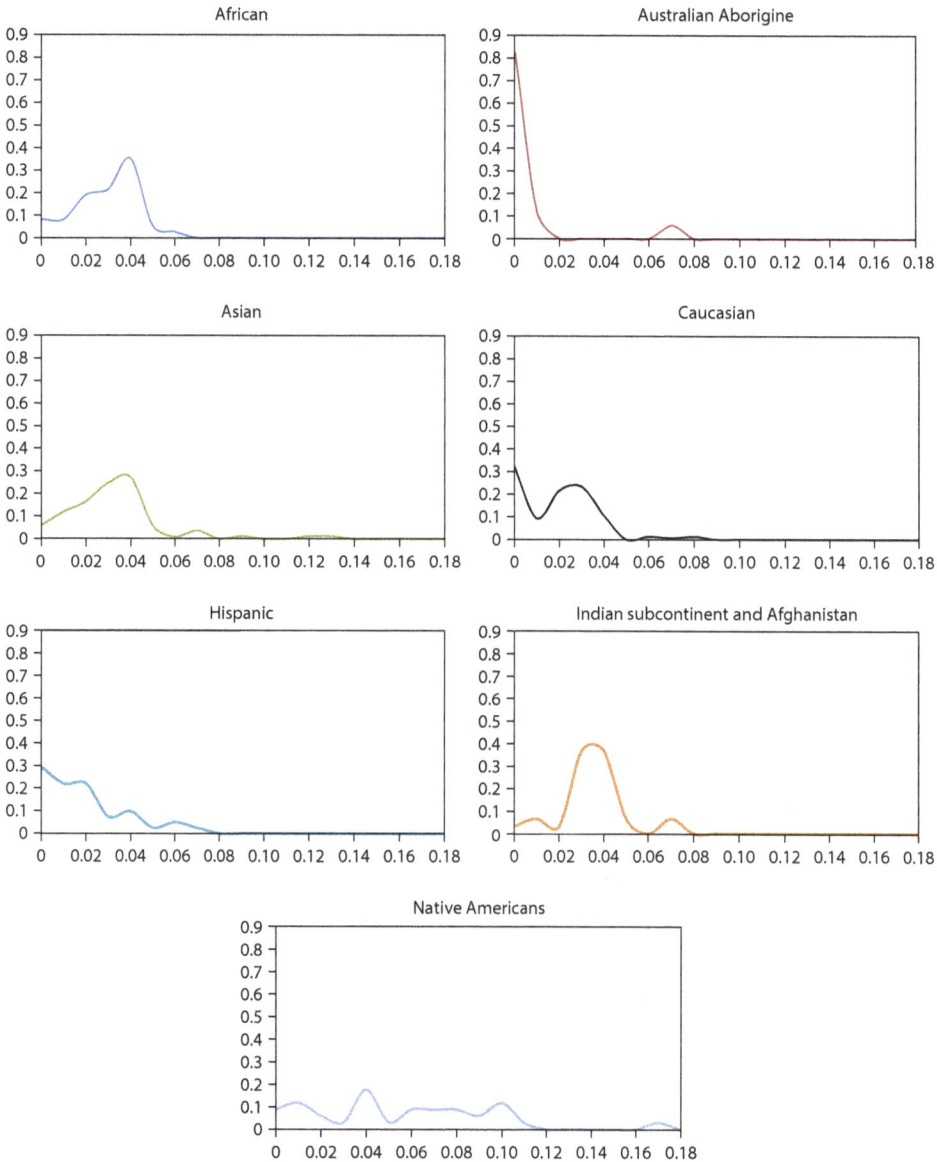

Figure 5.7   Distributions of $\hat{\beta}$ for the clusters with good sample numbers.

Descriptive Statistics for Databases

Most laboratories that are validating their databases publish the data. This is a very desirable activity. This policy is supported by the editors of many journals who have developed sections specifically for this purpose.

These publications typically give a summary of the allele probabilities. This is useful for other scientists who may wish to use these data or to compare them with their own or other populations.

Many publications also include some summary statistics used to describe the data. This move has been facilitated by the provision of software such as PowerStats.[557] The purpose of this section is to give the mathematical definitions of some of these statistics and to make recommendations for their use.

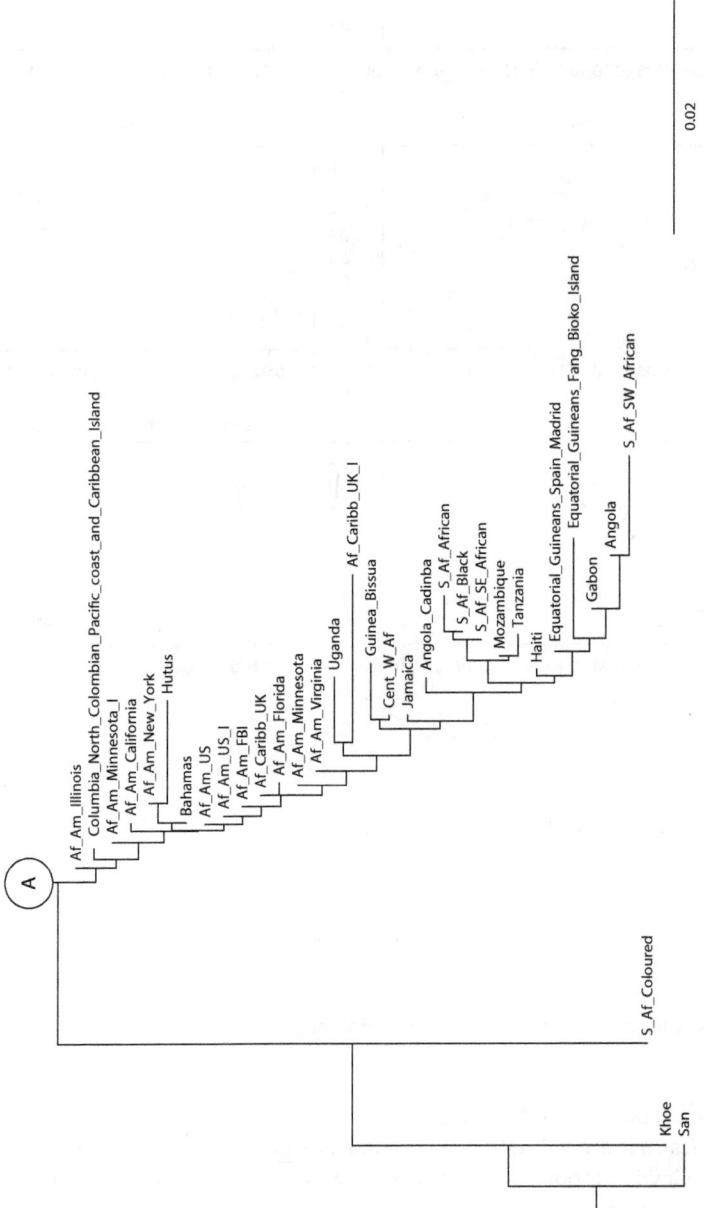

Figure 5.8   A Neighbour Joining tree for human population samples.

(Continued)

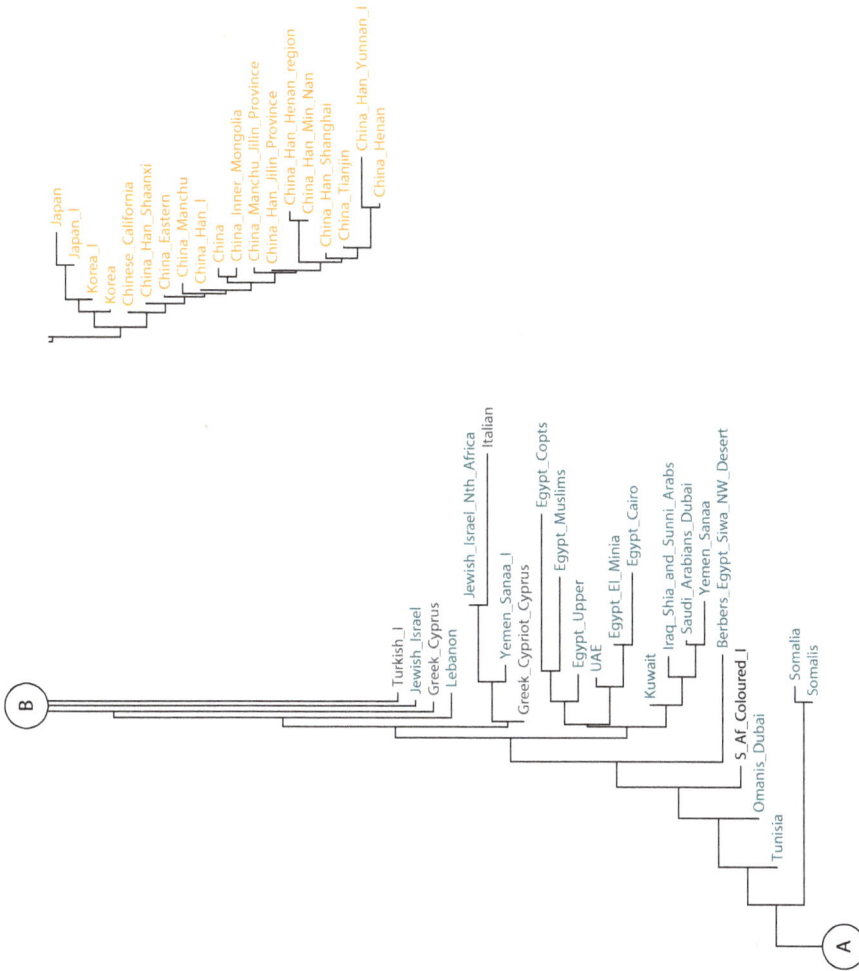

Figure 5.8 (Continued)   A Neighbour Joining tree for human population samples.

(Continued)

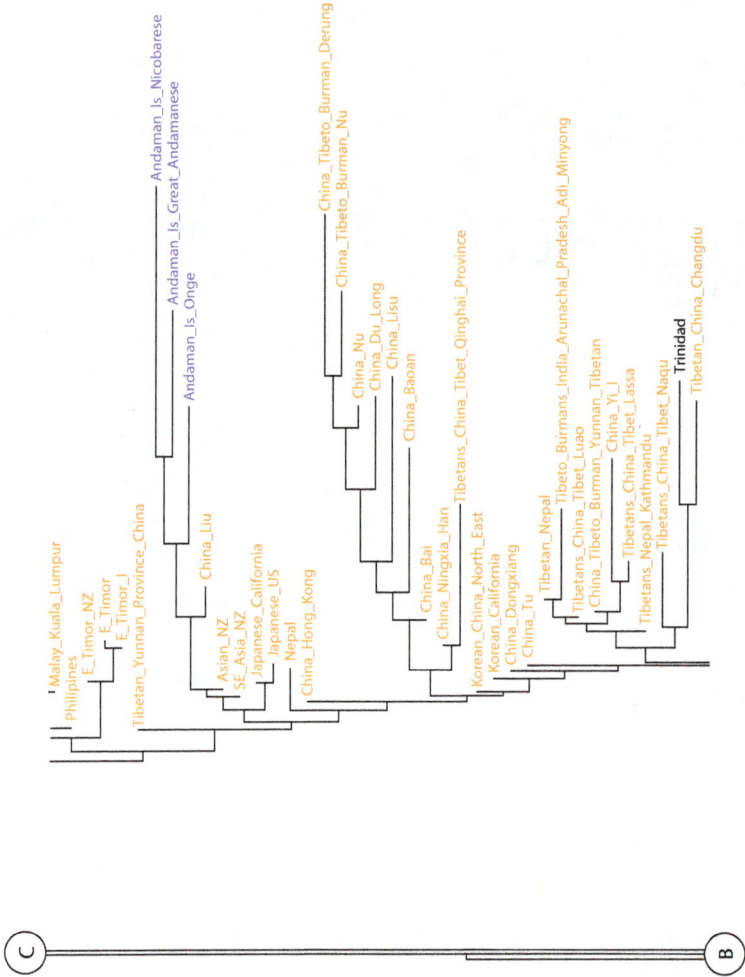

Figure 5.8 (Continued) A Neighbour Joining tree for human population samples.

(Continued)

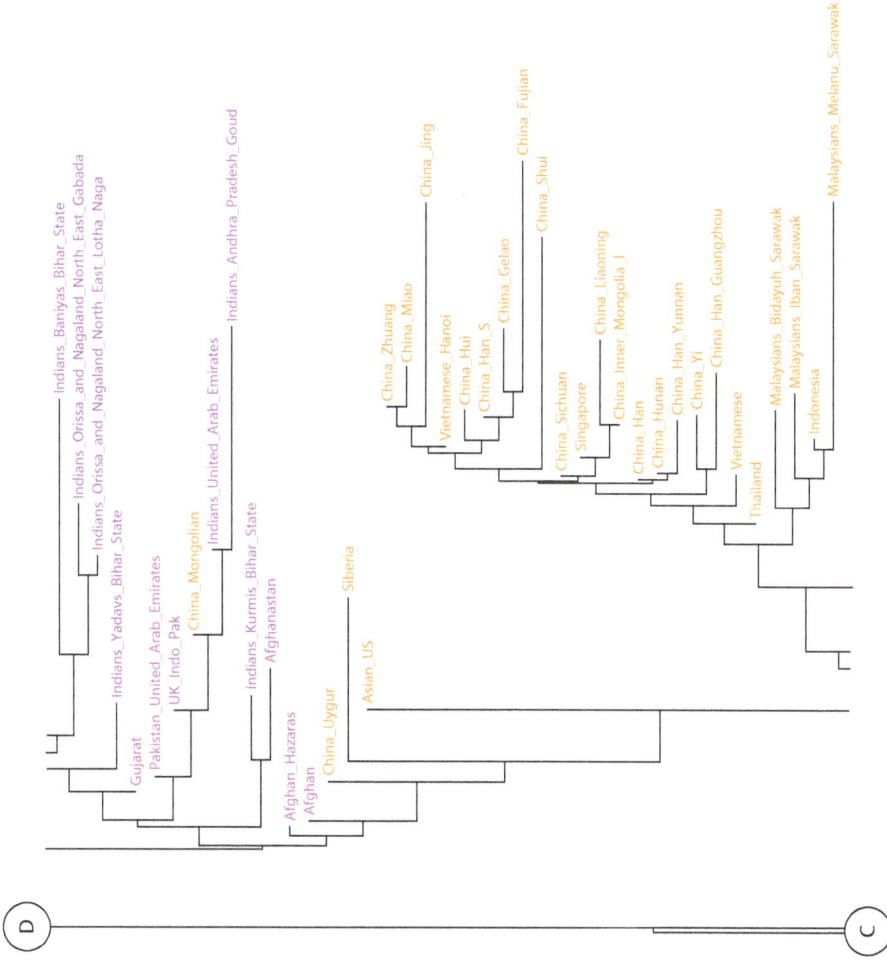

Figure 5.8 (Continued)   A Neighbour Joining tree for human population samples.

(Continued)

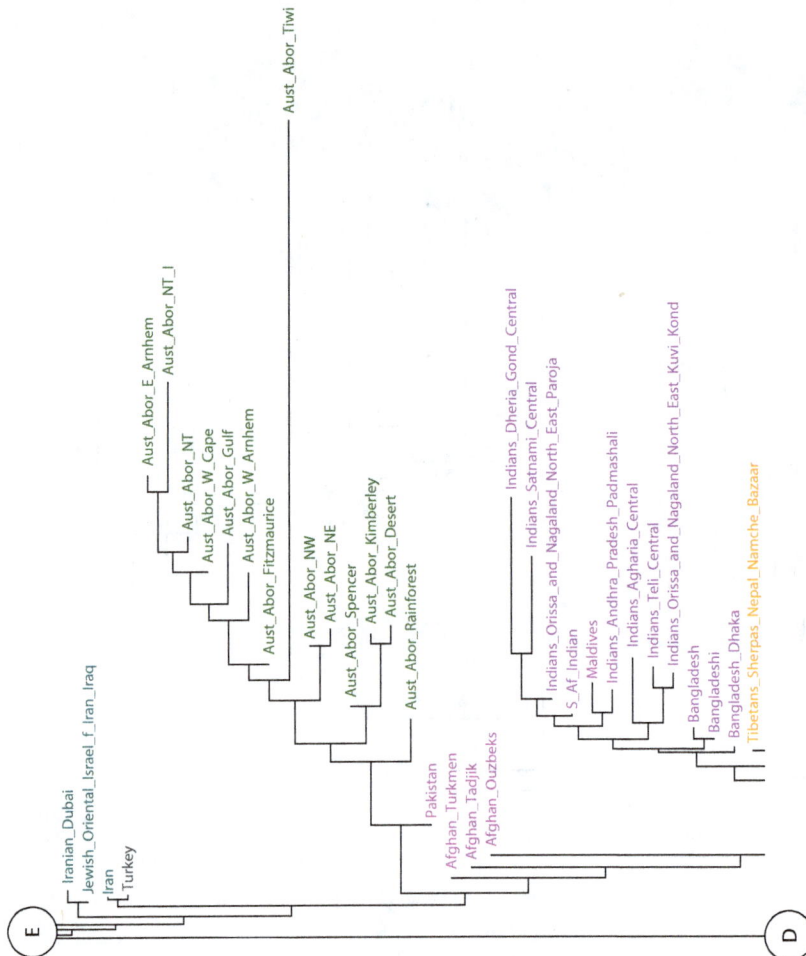

Figure 5.8 (Continued) A Neighbour Joining tree for human population samples.

(Continued)

(Continued)

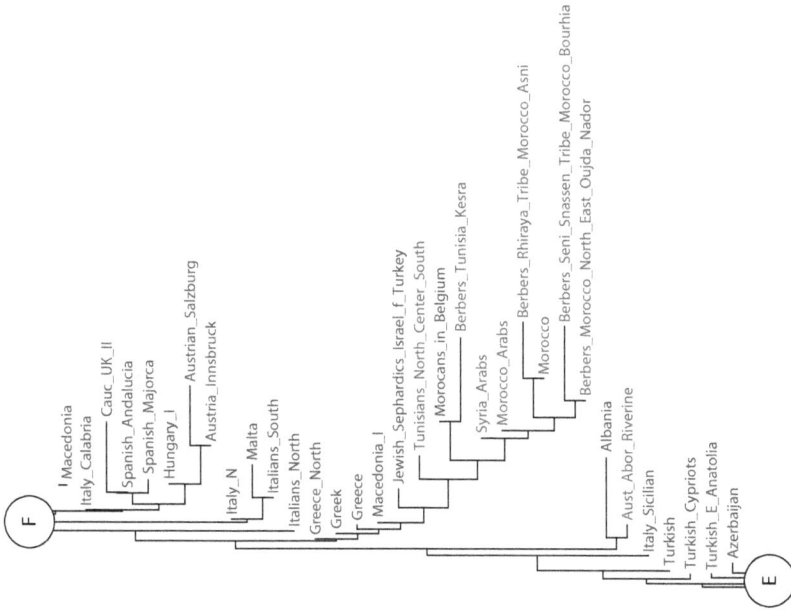

Figure 5.8 (Continued)   A Neighbour Joining tree for human population samples.

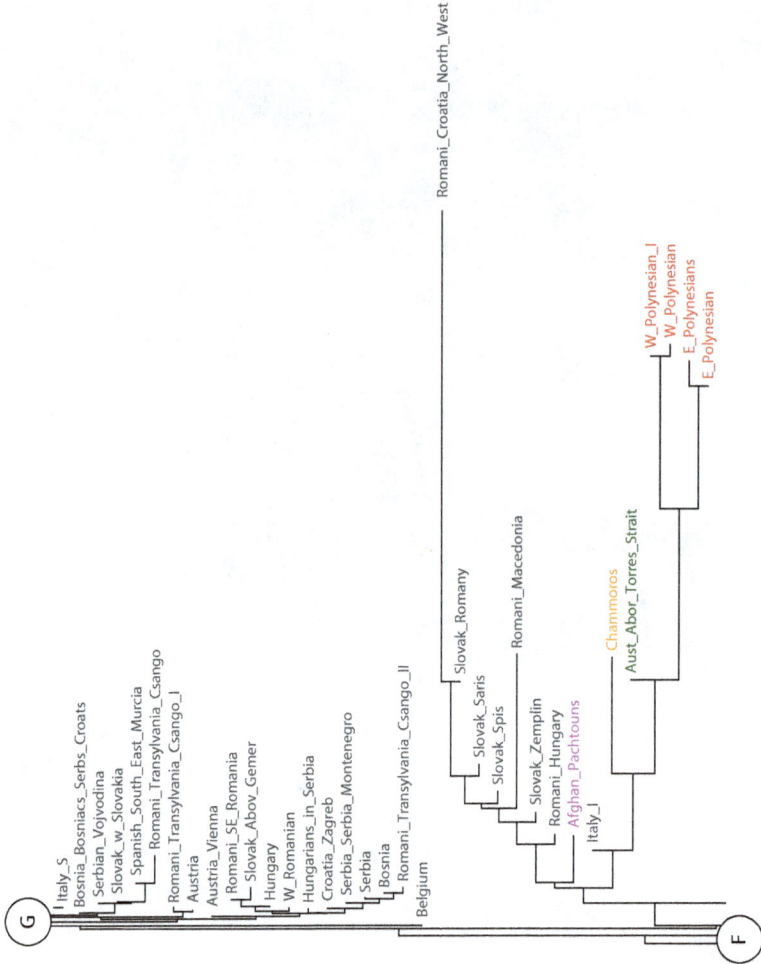

Figure 5.8 (Continued)   A Neighbour Joining tree for human population samples.

(Continued)

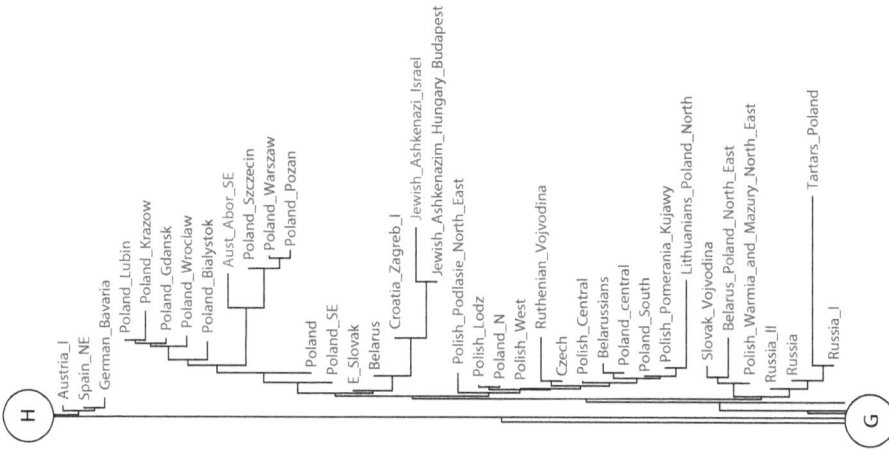

Figure 5.8 (Continued)   A Neighbour Joining tree for human population samples.

(Continued)

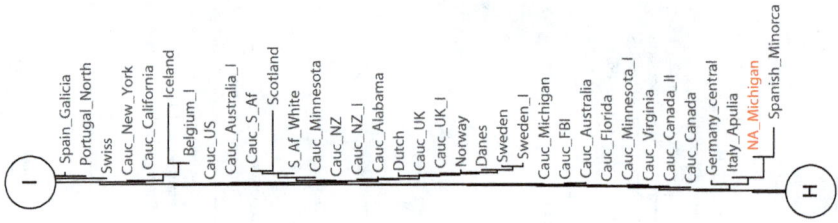

Figure 5.8 (Continued)   A Neighbour Joining tree for human population samples.

(Continued)

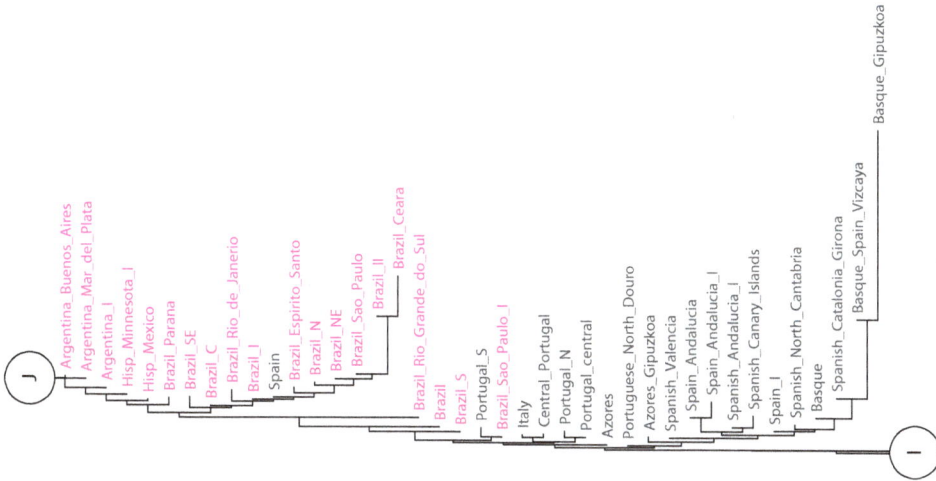

Figure 5.8 (Continued)   A Neighbour Joining tree for human population samples.

(Continued)

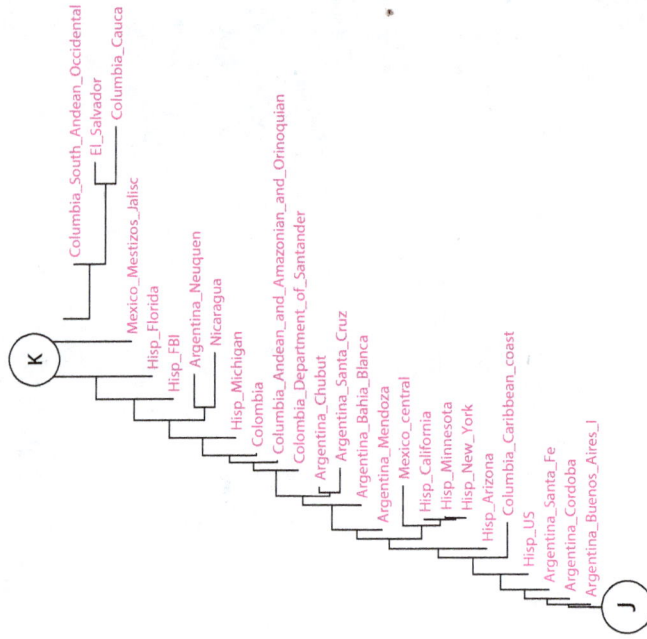

Figure 5.8 (Continued)   A Neighbour Joining tree for human population samples.

(Continued)

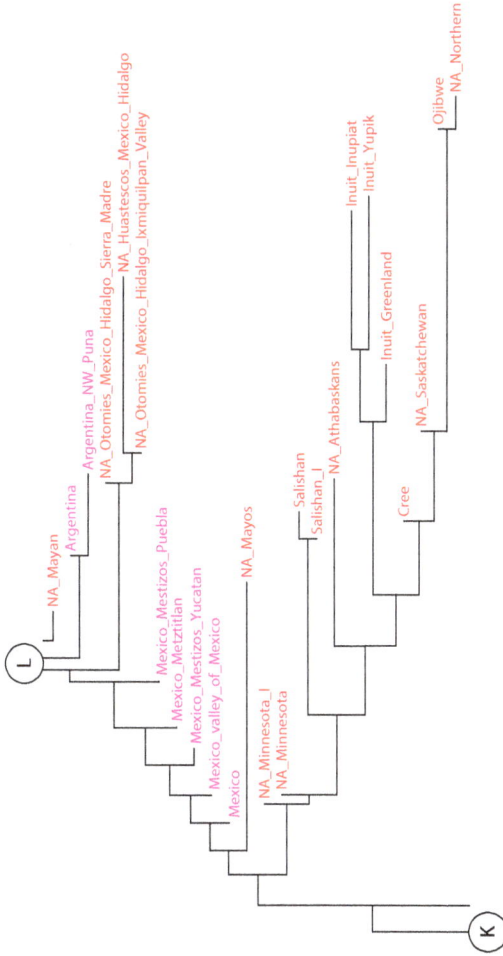

Figure 5.8 (Continued)   A Neighbour Joining tree for human population samples.

(Continued)

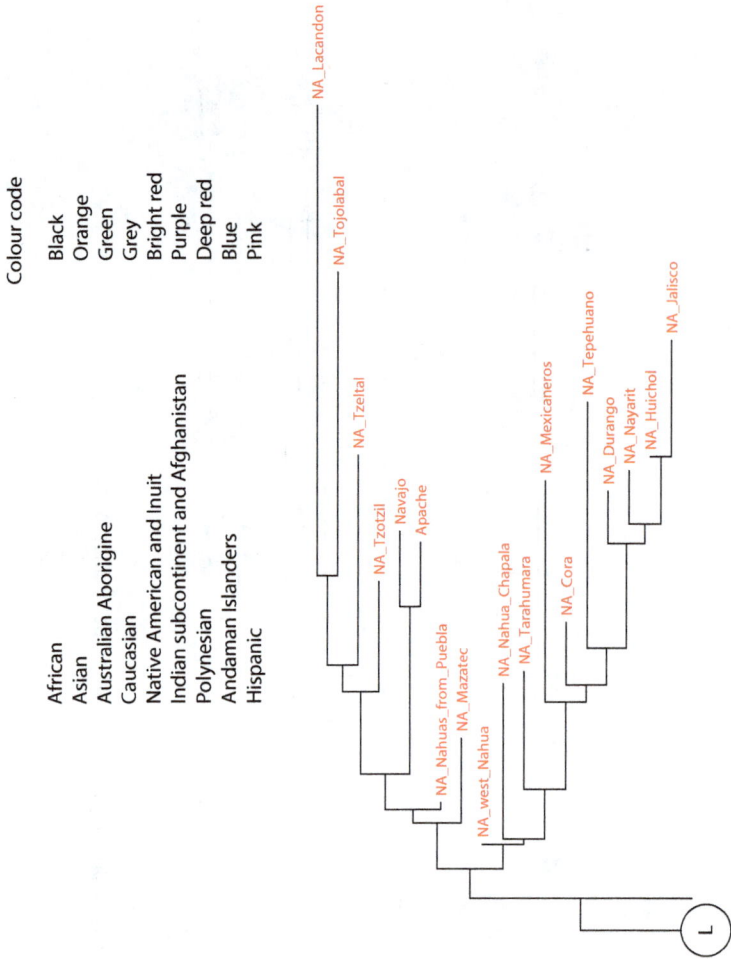

Colour code

African	Black
Asian	Orange
Australian Aborigine	Green
Caucasian	Grey
Native American and Inuit	Bright red
Indian subcontinent and Afghanistan	Purple
Polynesian	Deep red
Andaman Islanders	Blue
Hispanic	Pink

Figure 5.8 (Continued)   A Neighbour Joining tree for human population samples.

When describing descriptive statistics it is vital to draw a careful distinction between the value of the population parameter and the estimate of that parameter calculated from the sample actually observed.

Heterozygosity

This term is applied to a measure of the fraction of heterozygotes[424] in the population. Let us term the population heterozygosity at locus l in population q, h_l^q. To avoid the proliferation of superscripts and subscripts we will use h as shorthand, but it must be recalled that this is at a certain locus and in a certain population.

The simplest estimate of this parameter is the fraction in the sample, $\tilde{h}_l^q$, where the tilde (~) is used to signify the sample value. Again we will occasionally shorten this to $\tilde{h}$. This is assessed by taking the count of heterozygotes in the database at this locus, n_l, and dividing by the total samples, N_l:

$$\tilde{h}_l^q = \frac{n_l}{N_l} \text{ (heterozygosity at locus } l \text{ in population } q)$$

The observed sample proportion, $\tilde{h}_l^q$, is expected to be an unbiased estimator of the true parameter, h_l^q; $\sum \tilde{h}_l^q = h_l^q$ with variance

$$\mathrm{Var}\,\tilde{h}_l^q = \frac{h_l^q(1 - h_l^q)}{n_l}$$

if the sampling of individuals is independent.

Weir[424] gives the average over m loci as the simple arithmetic average.

$$\tilde{h}^q = \frac{1}{m}\sum_{l=1}^{m} \tilde{h}_l^q = \frac{1}{m}\sum_{l=1}^{m} \frac{n_l}{N_l} \text{ (average heterozygosity across } m \text{ loci in population } q)$$

This overall average will rarely be required in forensic work as it is customary to report locus-specific heterozygosities. Weir states that this remains an unbiased estimator but that the variance requires cognizance to be taken of the covariance between the estimates at each locus.

Homozygosity

Homozygosity, H, can be similarly defined as the fraction of homozygotes in the sample:

$$\tilde{H}_l^q = \frac{p_l}{N_l}$$

where p_l is the count of homozygotes in population q at locus l. We see directly that

$$\tilde{H}_l^q = 1 - \tilde{h}_l^q$$

Gene Diversity (Often Termed H_{ex})

Heterozygosity is estimated as the fraction of heterozygote genotypes at a locus in a sample. An alternative strategy would be to proceed from allele frequencies. Let $\tilde{p}_{lu}^q$ be the frequency of the uth allele at locus l in a sample from population q of size n individuals. For simplicity we drop the subscript for the locus and the superscript for populations. The maximum likelihood estimator for gene diversity is given by

$$\hat{D} = 1 - \sum_u \tilde{p}_u^2$$

where the summation is over all alleles at this locus. Weir notes that

$$\varepsilon \hat{D}_l = \left(1 - \frac{1+f}{2n}\right)D_l$$

hence there is a small downward bias, $\frac{2n-1}{2n}$, for non-inbred populations ($f = 0$) and a slightly larger one for inbred populations. He also gives expressions for the variance and covariance of $\hat{D}_l$.

This suggests the use of

$$\hat{D} = \frac{2n}{2n-1}\left(1 - \sum_u \tilde{p}_u^2\right)$$

to compensate for this bias,[558,559] where n is the number of individuals sampled.

Gene diversity is expected to be similar to, but not exactly the same as, heterozygosity. The difference will be larger for samples that differ from Hardy–Weinberg proportions markedly. Gene diversity should have smaller sampling variance than heterozygosity.

Nei[559] also suggests that the quantity $1 - \hat{D}$ that he terms *gene identity* may be useful.

Match Probability

The probability of a match at locus l, PM_l, was first described from genotype data. Fisher[560] gave

$$PM_l = \sum_i \tilde{G}_{il}^2,$$

where $\tilde{G}_i$ is the sample frequency of the ith genotype at locus l. Jones[561] suggests setting

$$PM_l = \frac{\sum_{i=1}^{n} \tilde{G}_{il}^2 - \frac{1}{N_l}}{1 - \frac{1}{N_l}} \approx \sum_{i=1}^{n} \tilde{G}_{il}^2$$

where the first part of this equation is for a sample of size N_l at locus l. An alternative does exist, which would proceed from allele probabilities.

$$PM_l = \sum_i \tilde{p}_{il}^4 + 2\sum_{i\neq j} \tilde{p}_{il}^2 \tilde{p}_{jl}^2$$

$$= \left(\sum_i \tilde{p}_{il}^2\right)^2 + \sum_{i\neq j} \tilde{p}_{il}^2 \tilde{p}_{jl}^2$$

$$= \left(1 - \hat{D}\right)^2 + \sum_{i\neq j} \tilde{p}_{il}^2 \tilde{p}_{jl}^2$$

Across k loci Jones gives

$$PM = 1 - \prod_{j=1}^{k} PM_j$$

Power of Discrimination
The power of discrimination is often given as

$$1 - PM = 1 - \left(1 - \prod_{j=1}^{k} PM_j\right) = \prod_{j=1}^{k} PM_j$$

Polymorphism Information Content
Botstein et al.[562] give

$$\text{Polymorphism information content (PIC)} = 1 - \sum_{i=1}^{n} p_i^2 - \sum_{i=1}^{n-1}\sum_{j=i+1}^{n} 2p_i^2 p_j^2$$

where
   n is the number of alleles
   p_i is the allele probability of the ith allele

Probability of Excluding Paternity
Ohno et al.[563] give the probability of excluding paternity

$$Q_n = \sum_{i=1}^{n} p_i(1 - p_i)^2(1 - p_i + p_i^2) + \sum_{i=1}^{n-1}\sum_{j=i+1}^{n} p_i p_j (p_i + p_j)(1 - p_i + p_j^2)$$

where
   n is the number of alleles
   p_i is the allele probability of the ith allele

Average Paternity Index
Brenner and Morris[564] give

$$\overline{PI} = \frac{1}{1 - \overline{A}}$$

for fathers and non-excluded non-fathers, where $\overline{PI}$ is the average paternity index and $\overline{A}$ is the mean exclusion probability. They further give the approximation $\overline{A} \approx h^2$ or more accurately $\overline{A} \approx h^2(1 - 2hH^2)$ and reference Nijenhuis.[565] The posterior probability of paternity, W, would be

$$W = \frac{1}{2 - \overline{A}}$$

(referenced in Brenner and Morris to Morris JW pp. 267–276 of the same volume).[565] As usual prior odds of 1:1 are assumed.

Haplotype Diversity

$$H = \frac{n}{n-1}\left(1 - \sum_{i=1}^{k} p_i^2\right)$$

where H is the *haplotype diversity* and k is the number of allele classes.[559,566]

Summary

The purpose of a descriptive statistic is to give an overall impression of the usefulness of a locus for forensic, paternity or other purposes. Most of the measures differ very little in their utility. Since the allele frequencies have a value in themselves, we assume that they will be presented in such publications. Many of the statistics may be derived directly from these allele probabilities. The presentation of multiple summary statistics seems excessive.

The most informative statistics are the two simple measures: heterozygosity and gene diversity. The first cannot be checked against the data, the second can. It would be better for the forensic community to agree on one of these as the summary statistic of choice.

The p-value from the exact test for Hardy–Weinberg proportions is also valuable and should be presented without comment as to whether or not the value is significant. The p-values from linkage equilibrium tests are also valuable. They would not fit into the type of table currently published but could be deposited as supplementary data or placed in a separate table.

6

Sampling Effects

John S. Buckleton, Duncan Taylor, Jo-Anne Bright and James M. Curran

Contents

Introduction

It is usual to attach a numerical weight to a match between DNA obtained from a crime sample and DNA taken from a sample given by a suspect. In Chapter 2, we discussed the possibilities of using a frequency, an exclusion probability or a likelihood ratio (*LR*) for this purpose. A frequency or an exclusion probability is based on data and the result is termed an *estimate*. The fact that what is given is an estimate leads to the following question: Should this numerical estimate be a best estimate or should some consideration be given to the uncertainty in this estimate? This is a matter where opinions in the forensic community differ.

With an *LR* when applied in the purest form, an estimate is not produced. Rather the resultant *LR* is termed an *assigned LR* to embrace the subjective probabilities that may have been used in its formation.

Part, and maybe the smaller part, of the uncertainty in the estimate is often referred to as *sampling error*. The word *error* does not refer to an analytical error but rather the variation that would occur if a different sample of individuals were taken to create the population database. Nor does the word *sampling* have anything to do with the physical act of taking a DNA sample, but rather the selection process whereby someone's DNA profile ends up in the database used for statistical calculations. This selection process induces sampling error in the resulting estimate regardless of the population genetic model used to construct it or the size of the reference database.

The argument for the assessment of sampling error is best made with an example. Take a situation involving a single suspect and a single stain from a scene. The questioned item (the stain from the scene) and the known sample (from the suspect) are sent to the laboratory. After DNA testing, on the basis of whatever typing system is in use, it is decided that there is a match between the suspect and the scene. It remains for us to assess the statistical weight of the evidence. Based on a database of genotypes and a population genetic model, the estimate for the frequency of this genotype* is one in a billion (10^{-9}). This is obviously compelling evidence. Now let us add, unrealistically, an additional fact: we are somewhat uncertain about this estimate. In fact, rather than being exactly one in a billion it may be anything from one in ten (10^{-1}) to one in a billion billion (10^{-18}). We believe that most people would now regard the original estimate of one in a billion somewhat differently.

Brenner[567] offers the following allegory for our consideration:

> Suppose you plan to drive to some point in the desert and must carry enough fuel for the round trip. Your best estimate is that ten gallons will be enough, but you know that this estimate carries some uncertainty, and there is, let us say, a 1% chance that you really will need 15 gallons. So 15 gallons is the '98% (or maybe 99%) upper confidence estimate', and you may well judge it prudent to carry this amount of gas, rather than the 'point estimate' of 10 gallons. (Reproduced with the kind permission of Dr Brenner.)

In our DNA example the uncertainty about the statistical evidence varies from moderate (10^{-1}) to extremely strong (10^{-18}). Sampling error has been investigated by a number of authors[176,258,473,568–571] and in reality the variability in a DNA estimate is not as large as this (at least for a database of moderate size ≈ 200 individuals). One may ask whether it is sufficient to rely on these published results. While we believe that the results generalize to any DNA database, we encourage forensic scientists to think about what should be accepted practice in their own laboratories and institutions and consider the following questions:

Should sampling error be assessed in every case?

Should it be done once for a sample of profiles from a database and published?

Should it be never done at all?

We attempt to address these questions here.

Not all commentators believe that an assessment of sampling error is necessary. Brenner[567] makes explicit his doubts of the usefulness of assessing sampling uncertainty with the following challenge:

> Will someone tell me, please, what rational difference it ever can make to know the confidence limits in addition to knowing the best point estimate? Specifically, can you give premises under which,

---

* In fact this is an estimate of the probability that someone who is unrelated to the suspect has this same genotype, which happens to be numerically identical to the frequency of the genotype in the population when substructure is not an issue.

for a fixed point estimate, the decision to convict or not to convict would depend on the size of the confidence interval? (Reproduced with the kind permission of Charles Brenner.)

There is a lot of substance to Brenner's challenge. However these comments may not have taken full account of the cross-examination process, in which any uncertainty or doubt should be, and often is, explored at length. An analyst who has prepared for such a cross-examination will definitely present better evidence to the court than one who chooses to answer 'would it make any difference?' Furthermore, and perhaps more importantly, it is accepted in adversarial systems that all reasonable uncertainty should be conceded to the defendant.

For example, consider the testimony of Professor Angela van Daal in *R v Cannell*. In that case a statistic with a probability interval had been reported for the *LR* for H_{d1} (the donor of the DNA is unrelated to Mr Cannell). An *LR* was reported without a probability interval for H_{d2} (the donor of the DNA is a brother of Mr Cannell).

van Daal was particularly troubled that a 'confidence interval' [sic] was not applied to the *LR* obtained for a sibling match.

> ... given that an estimate was being made of something where we don't know the true answer it's important to determine with what confidence we have in that estimate and that is done by obtaining a range of values by which we are confident that the true value falls within, and in the case of a forensic database the one end of that range is given, the conservative end of that range is given.

The newspapers emphasized the dramatic in their reporting:

> 'The confidence interval takes into account the number of people in the database ... one with 100 or 200 people isn't going to give the same confidence as one with 1000 or one million people,' van Daal said.
>
> That is a very fundamental concept of statistics, something that any student would have done ... it's very elementary.
>
> Any estimate can, obviously, be incorrect ... given you do not know the true answer, it's important to determine the confidence had in the estimate.

van Daal did not furnish the confidence interval and has not done so subsequently.

Commenting on statistical evidence in general, rather than DNA in particular, Good stated: 'The court expects us to provide both an average based on our sample and some measure of the accuracy of our average'.[174]

Almost any measurement in science has an associated measure of uncertainty.

During a meeting of the New York State Subcommittee on DNA Evidence, Ken Kidd asked about the verbal scale associating words with *LR* ranges: Should 1–10 be described as *slight support* when it might not be significantly different from 1? This gives voice to the observation that uncertainty in the *LR* is part of the likely thinking process of a judge or jury.

Well-prepared lawyers correctly investigate this avenue of questioning. In our experience this is most commonly done by asking a question along the lines, 'Is your database of 180 individuals big enough?'

Is there any reason why DNA evidence should be exempt from this line of questioning? The position advocating a consideration of sampling uncertainty is also taken by many authors.[176,258,568,570–573] In most cases, even with the inclusion of an estimate of sampling uncertainty, the final answer is not vastly different to the point or 'best' estimate.

In the first edition of this book the position was adopted that, on balance, it was better to make the assessment of sampling uncertainty than not to. At the time this was a guarded conclusion really based on the balance of comment in the literature. In the intervening decade we have developed even more significant doubt that this assessment achieves any worthwhile aim.

At the end of this chapter we will debate this subject with ourselves in a section entitled 'Discussion of the Appropriateness of Sampling Uncertainty Estimates'. However in the interim, and for the interested reader, we will review the existing methodology and other considerations if an assessment of sampling uncertainty is desired.

Bounds and α-Level

We assume that the sampling uncertainty will be described simply by its confidence or probability bounds. Weir at al.[574] and Curran et al.[571] discuss one- and two-sided intervals and α-levels in the DNA context. This is a simple extension of classical theory. A two-sided, say 95%, confidence interval would allow the following type of statement to be made: '95% of intervals constructed in this way will contain the true frequency'.

The one-sided equivalent is: 'In 95% of intervals constructed in this way, the true frequency will be higher than this value'.

The practical differences between a one-sided and two-sided interval are that the upper limit changes slightly and that the one-sided confidence limit has an upper bound rather than both a lower and an upper bound. The philosophical differences are larger. The two-sided bound attempts to bracket the 'true value' above and below. The one-sided bound attempts to give a value above the true value for frequencies or below it for *LRs*. The argument for a two-sided interval is that it is more scientific and balanced to bound above and below. The one-sided advocates, including us, argue that there is one fewer number to give in court. The court may be more interested in the weakest that the evidence could reasonably be, and the one-sided limit corresponds more with this.

It is not acceptable to substitute the word *probability* for *confidence* in statements regarding confidence intervals. '...A report issued by the NRC[473] that contains (p. 76) "the traditional 95% confidence limit, whose use implies the true value has only a 5% chance of exceeding the upper bound" must lose credibility with statisticians'.[345] The report in question wrongly confuses a confidence interval with a probability interval. Strictly speaking any particular confidence interval either contains the true value or it does not, but 95% of intervals should contain the true value. We cannot say, 'It is 95% probable that *this* confidence interval contains the true value'. The difference appears academic but could easily lead to difficulty in court.

The Bayesian posterior method given by Curran et al.[571] would allow the statement: 'It is 95% probable that the true frequency is not more than one in 1.1 billion'.

This latter statement seems easier to understand but can only be made using Bayesian methods.

Methods for Assessing Sampling Uncertainty

We briefly review the suggested methods below to allow comparison of their accuracy and the relative ease of their implementation and use. For the more widely used mathematical methods we include discussion of their derivations.

Method: NRC I

Requirements: Pen and paper.[473]

Applicability: Cases where a suspect matches a simple unmixed stain from the scene.

Comments: There is no need to discuss further the first NRC suggestion of replacing $\tilde{p}_{ij}$ by its binomial-based confidence limit $\tilde{p}_{ij} + 1.96\sqrt{\tilde{p}_{ij}(1-\tilde{p}_{ij})/2n_i}$ as that is clearly invalid. Confidence limits for products are not obtained as products of confidence limits.[574] (See also Weir.[575])

Implementation: This approach has no statistical credibility and its implementation is not discussed here.

Method: Factor of 10
Requirements: Pen and paper.[176]

Applicability: This method applies to cases where a suspect matches a simple unmixed stain from the scene. This method was not developed for mixtures, relatives, paternity or missing person cases and its performance in these instances is unknown.

Comments: Similarly, the second NRC suggestion of constructing the interval $(\hat{P}/10, 10\hat{P})$ has limited theoretical validity. There must at least be an effect of sample size.[574]
  The 'Factor of 10' approach has little to recommend it from a theoretical standpoint, and we must prefer the other methods which have a more firm statistical backing. As mentioned previously there must be an effect of sample size and number of loci.… However our own simulation may be viewed as further empirical support for the 'Factor of 10' approach. In general the 'Factor of 10' approach performed in a broadly similar way to the other methods or was excessively conservative.[571]

Implementation: Suppose that the match probability is estimated as, say, one in a billion. This approach would suggest that the bounds for uncertainty (sampling and population model) are 1 in 100 million to 1 in 10 billion.

Method: Asymptotic Normality of the Logarithm Extended by the NRC to Allow for Population Structure
Requirements: May be easily applied by an MS Excel spreadsheet for unmixed stains.[176,568]

Applicability: This method can be applied to unmixed or mixed stains. In the case of unmixed stains the mathematics is simple enough that it can be easily entered into a spreadsheet. Weir and Beecham[576] extended this method to deal with mixed stains; however the complexity requires a custom written program.

Comments: Curran et al.[571] scored the performance of this method as adequate in most situations except for small database sizes, reporting that 'for single-contributor stains, such as those considered here, it does appear that these normal methods are completely suitable'. However this method does not easily extend to mixed stains, nor does it generalize for such situations. This shortcoming limits its overall usefulness.

Implementation: An excellent explanation is given in NRC II.[176] Here we present a spreadsheet layout to apply this approach with the subpopulation correction, θ (Figure 6.1). If the product rule is desired, the more simple formulae in NRC II used or this spreadsheet may be utilized with θ set to zero.

Theoretical Basis:[*] Methods based on asymptotic normality have the advantage of leading to relatively simple analytical expressions. Let P be the match probability and $\hat{P}$ the estimate.

---

[*] Following Weir et al.[574]

		Locus	D3	vWA
			17	14
	Observed genotype			16
Heterozygote allele frequencies		p	0.2005	0.0932
		q		0.2082
	N total alleles in database at this locus		818	826
Theta, called F hereafter		0.03		
Confidence interval (95, 99, 99.9) called X		99%	Recommended 99%	
One- or two-tailed (enter 1 or 2) called Y		1	Recommended one tail	
Z value		2.576	←ABS(NORMSINV $((1 - X)/Y))$	

Genotype frequency (heterozygote, Balding formula)

$$\frac{2(F+(1-F)p)(F+(1-F)q)}{(1+F)(1+2F)} \rightarrow \qquad 0.0512$$

Genotype frequency (homozygote, Balding formula)

$$\frac{2(F+(1-F)p)(3F+(1-F)p)}{(1+F)(1+2F)} \rightarrow \qquad 0.0663$$

Variance component (heterozygote, $NRC\ II$ with theta)

$$\left(\frac{p(1-p)}{(F+(1-F)p)^2} + \frac{q(1-q)}{(F+(1-F)q^2)} - \frac{2pq}{(F+(1-F)p)(F+(1-F)q)} \right) \frac{(1-F)^2(1+F)}{N} \rightarrow \qquad 0.0088$$

Variance component (homozygote, $NRC\ II$ with theta)

$$\left(\frac{1}{(2F+(1-F)p)} + \frac{1}{(3F+(1-F)p)} \right)^2 \frac{(1-F)^2(1+F)p(1-P)}{N} \rightarrow \qquad 0.0105$$

Point estimate (includes theta): 1 in 295

$$\leftarrow \frac{1}{\prod_{loci} \text{genotype frequencies}} = \frac{1}{P_M}$$

Upper confidence limit: 1 in 206

$$\leftarrow e^{\left(ln(P_M)+Z \sqrt{\sum_{loci} \text{variance components}} \right)}$$

Lower confidence limit: 1 in 422

$$\leftarrow e^{\left(ln(P_M)-Z \sqrt{\sum_{loci} \text{variance components}} \right)}$$

Figure 6.1   A spreadsheet layout to implement the asymptotic normality of the logarithm method.

The procedure assumes that $\ln(\hat{P})$ is normally distributed, so that a 99% confidence interval for P is $\hat{P}/C, C\hat{P}$, where $\ln(C) = 2.57\sqrt{\mathrm{Var}[\ln(\hat{P})]}$. The task is to compute the variance of $\ln(\hat{P})$. Assuming independence between loci this is approximated by

$$\mathrm{Var}\left[\ln(\hat{P})\right] = \mathrm{Var}\left[\sum_i \ln(\hat{P}_i)\right] \approx \sum_i \mathrm{Var}\left(\hat{P}_i\right)\big/\hat{P}_i^2$$

As θ is generally assigned a numerical value[577] such as 0.03 in this context, rather than being estimated from sample data, it will be assumed constant.

For a homozygous profile at locus i:

$$\mathrm{Var}\left(\hat{P}_i\right) \approx \left(\frac{\partial \hat{P}_i}{\partial \tilde{p}_{i1}}\right)^2 \mathrm{Var}\left(\tilde{p}_{i1}\right)$$

and for a heterozygous profile

$$\mathrm{Var}\left(\hat{P}_i\right) \approx \left(\frac{\partial \hat{P}_i}{\partial \tilde{p}_{i1}}\right)^2 \mathrm{Var}\left(\tilde{p}_{i1}\right) + \left(\frac{\partial \hat{P}_i}{\partial \tilde{p}_{i2}}\right)^2 \mathrm{Var}\left(\tilde{p}_{i2}\right)$$

$$+2\left(\frac{\partial \hat{P}_i}{\partial \tilde{p}_{i1}}\right)\left(\frac{\partial \hat{P}_i}{\partial \tilde{p}_{i2}}\right)\mathrm{Cov}\left(\tilde{p}_{i1}, \tilde{p}_{i2}\right)$$

When $\theta = 0$, these expressions become

$$\mathrm{Var}\left[\ln(\hat{P}_i)\right] = \begin{cases} \dfrac{2(1-p_{i1})}{n_i\, p_{i1}}, & A_{i1} = A_{i2} \\[2ex] \dfrac{p_{i1}+p_{i2}-4p_{i1}p_{i2}}{2n_i\, p_{i1}p_{i2}}, & A_{i1} \neq A_{i2} \end{cases}$$

as given previously.[568,577] Use was made of the binomial variances and covariances of allele proportions:

$$\mathrm{Var}\left(\tilde{p}_{ij}\right) = \frac{p_{ij}(1-p_{ij})}{2n_i}$$

$$\mathrm{Cov}\left(\tilde{p}_{ij}, \tilde{p}_{ij'}\right) = -\frac{p_{ij}p_{ij'}}{2n_i}$$

in the derivation of $\mathrm{Var}\left[\ln(\hat{P}_i)\right]$.

When $\theta \neq 0$, the conditional probabilities shown above take into account the variation among populations. It is not appropriate, therefore, to use variance formulae that consider only variation within populations as did the NRC.[176]

The total variances and covariances for allele proportions[424] in this case can be calculated with two common methods in regular use. Method 1[176,571] accounts for sampling variation and Method 2[576] accounts for sampling variation and genetic variation. Method 2 can account for genetic differences between the subpopulation of the individual(s) involved in the calculation and the population as a whole. It is able to be used with a sampling scheme where the alleles in the database are drawn from a population-wide sample (sometimes referred to as a *general database*).

Method 1:

$$\text{Var}(p_A) = p_A(1-p_A) \times \frac{(1+\theta)}{2n}$$

$$\text{Cov}(p_A, p_B) = -p_A \times p_B \times \frac{(1+\theta)}{2n}$$

Method 2:

$$\text{Var}(p_A) = p_A(1-p_A) \times \left[\theta + \frac{(1-\theta)}{2n}\right]$$

$$\text{Cov}(p_A, p_B) = -p_A \times p_B \times \left[\theta + \frac{(1-\theta)}{2n}\right]$$

where n is the number of individuals in the database.

If the number of individuals in the database was one, then the two forms of calculating variance and covariance would be equal. As the population database becomes large, the variance and covariance using Method 1 become effectively zero, and the upper and lower bound confidence intervals equal the LR point estimate. Looking at Method 2, as the number of individuals in the database increases, θ quickly becomes the term that will dominate the equations, as $\frac{(1-\theta)}{2n} \to 0$. Using Method 2 as n approaches infinity:

$$\text{Var}(p_A) \to p_A(1-p_A) \times \theta$$

$$\text{Cov}(p_A, p_B) \to -p_A \times p_B \times \theta$$

(and using either method these covariance and variance terms reduce to the binomial terms when $\theta = 0$). Using Method 1 the required expressions are as follows:

$$\text{Var}\left[\ln\left(\hat{P_i}\right)\right] =$$

$$
\begin{bmatrix}
p_{i1}(1-p_{i1})(1-\theta)^2 \left(\theta + \dfrac{1-\theta}{2n_i}\right) \left(\dfrac{5\theta + 2(1-\theta)p_{i1}}{[3\theta + (1-\theta)p_{i1}][2\theta + (1-\theta)p_{i1}]}\right)^2, \quad A_{i1} = A_{i2} \\[3ex]
\left\{(1-\theta)^2\left(\theta + \dfrac{1-\theta}{2n_i}\right)\left(\dfrac{p_{i1}(1-p_{i1})}{[\theta+(1-\theta)p_{i1}]^2}\right)\right. \\[3ex]
\left. -\dfrac{2p_{i1}p_{i2}}{[\theta+(1-\theta)p_{i1}][\theta+(1-\theta)p_{i2}]} + \dfrac{p_{i2}(1-p_{i2})}{[\theta+(1-\theta)p_{i2}]^2}\right), \quad A_{i1} \ne A_{i2}
\end{bmatrix}
$$

Balding[570] discussed a four-locus profile given by Chakraborty et al.[568] We show component sample allele counts in Table 6.1 and 99% confidence intervals for the match probability based on asymptotic normality in Table 6.2. Setting $\theta \ne 0$, with an implicit requirement that between-population variation be taken into account, clearly increases the estimated match probability and widens the confidence intervals. For $\theta = 0.03$, the 99% confidence interval in this example is not very different from the NRC factor of 10 rule.

Table 6.1	Sample Allele Counts for Four-Locus Profile of Chakraborty et al.		
Locus (i)	Sample Counts		Sample Size (n)
	Allele 1 (x_{i1})	Allele 2 (x_{i1})	
1	74	35	595
2	131	169	729
3	156	128	594
4	309	408	776

Table 6.2	99% and 95% Confidence Intervals for Profile in Table 6.1				
	$10^7 \hat{P}/C$			$10^7 C\hat{P}$	
θ	99%	95%	$10^7 \hat{P}$	95%	99%
0.000	1.0	1.2	1.9	3.1	3.7
0.001	0.79	0.99	2.1	4.3	5.4
0.010	0.51	0.82	3.9	18	29
0.030	0.80	1.5	12	91	170

Method: Bootstrap

Requirements: This method requires a purpose written programme.[574] A very adaptable one that can handle any forensic situation has been developed by Curran.[578]

Applicability: Simple stains, mixtures, paternity cases, missing persons, all forensic casework.

Comments: Curran et al.[571] scored the performance of this method as adequate in most situations except for small database sizes. As they explained, '...the relatively poor performance of normal-based limits or bootstrap limits for small sample sizes [small databases] is a consequence of specific alleles not appearing in these samples. The problem disappears when θ is assigned a non-zero value'.

Implementation: Consider a database of individuals indexed 1 ... N. We wish to assess, say, the genotype probability across 13 loci. The steps are as follows:

- Assess the multilocus genotype using whatever formula is preferred. This formula could be the product rule, a theta correction, the brother's formula, a paternity calculation or another.

- Select an individual at random between 1 and N and put a copy of this genotype into the 'new database' but do not remove this individual from the original database (that is, we sample genotypes – or individuals – from the database with replacement).

- Repeat these processes N times. We now have a new database of N individuals. Some of the initial individuals may be represented twice or three times, some once or some not at all.

- Recalculate the allele frequencies using our new database.

189

- Recalculate the formula of interest using these allele frequencies.

- Repeat this 1000 times.

- Sort the 1000 results of the formula in ascending order. The 25th and 976th results represent the bounds of the 95% two-sided confidence interval. The 951st represents the 95% one-sided confidence interval.

Method: Balding's Size Bias Correction Amended in Evett and Weir

Requirements: Pen and paper.[258,570]

Applicability: This method was developed for simple unmixed stains; 'there appears to be no simple general extension to mixed stains and paternities'.[571]

Comments: Curran et al.[571] score the performance of this method as poor if the intent is to assess sampling error. 'An unfortunate consequence of Balding's discussion of "conservative Bayesian estimates" is that some forensic agencies have taken to presenting only point estimates based on sample allele proportions calculated by adding crime and suspect profiles to a database. These modified point estimates do not address sampling error. As sample size increases they are more likely to provide intervals (bounded above by these values) that do not contain the true values. It would be misleading to regard them as acting like confidence limits … we are disappointed in the lack of scientific rigor both in its derivation and application. However for small databases or rare profiles it is probably acceptable as a coarse correction for sampling error. For larger databases and common profiles it performs more as a mean estimate'.[574] The performance of this method may be adequate when applied to very small databases and rare profiles. It is difficult to predict this method's performance in any given case.

The theoretical support for this method is given under the headings 'Support Intervals' and 'Uniform Allele Prior Distribution'. A discussion of the possible use of non-uniform priors is also included.

Implementation: Suppose that we have a database of size $2N$ alleles. To calculate the probability of observing an aa homozygote take the count, x, of the a allele in the database and use

$$\hat{P}_{aa} = \left(\frac{x+4}{2N+4} \right)^2$$

To calculate the probability of observing an ab heterozygous profile, count the number of α and β alleles in the database, x_a and x_b, and use

$$\hat{P}_{ab} = 2\left(\frac{x_a+2}{2N+4} \right)\left(\frac{x_b+2}{2N+4} \right)$$

Theoretical Support:[*] *Support Intervals*
Suppose that the population probability of allele j at locus i is p_{ij}, and a sample from the population contains x_{ij} copies of that allele. For locus i, the likelihood function for the alleles in the profile is

$$L\left(\{p_{ij}\}\right) \propto \begin{cases} p_{i1}^{x_{i1}}(1-p_{i1})^{2n_i-x_{i1}}, & A_{i1} = A_{i2} \\ p_{i1}^{x_{i1}} p_{i2}^{x_{i2}}(1-p_{i1}-p_{i2})^{2n_i-x_{i1}-x_{i2}}, & A_{i1} \neq A_{i2} \end{cases}$$

---

[*] Following Weir et al.[574]

where the sample has n_i individuals scored at locus i. The likelihood has a maximum value of

$$L\left(\left\{\tilde{p}_{ij}\right\}\right) \propto \begin{cases} \left[\left(\dfrac{x_{i1}}{2n_i}\right)^{x_{i1}}\left(\dfrac{2n_i-x_{i1}}{2n_i}\right)^{2n_i-x_{i1}}, & A_{i1}=A_{i2} \\[3ex] \left[\left(\dfrac{x_{i1}}{2n_i}\right)^{x_{i1}}\left(\dfrac{x_{i2}}{2n_i}\right)^{x_{i2}}\left(\dfrac{2n_i-x_{i1}-x_{i2}}{2n_i}\right)^{2n_i-x_{i1}-x_{i2}}, & A_{i1}\neq A_{i2} \end{cases}$$

Balding[570] considered support intervals obtained by constraining the multinomial proportions to give a fixed profile probability, P_0, introducing a Lagrange multiplier λ to maximize the expression $\sum_i\left[\ln L\left(\left\{p_{ij}\right\}\right)\right] + \lambda\left[\sum_i \ln\left(P_i\right) - \ln P_0\right]$. The constrained solutions are

$$P_{0i} = \begin{cases} \dfrac{(x_{i1}+2\lambda)^2}{(2n_i+2\lambda)^2}, & A_{i1}=A_{i2} \\[3ex] \dfrac{2(x_{i1}+\lambda)(x_{i2}+\lambda)}{(2n_i+2\lambda)^2}, & A_{i1}\neq A_{i2} \end{cases} \tag{6.1}$$

that correspond to the addition of λ copies of the profile to the sample. The ratio of the constrained to the unconstrained maximum likelihoods is

$$R_i(\lambda) = \begin{cases} \dfrac{(1+2\lambda/x_{i1})^{x_{i1}}}{(1+2\lambda/2n_i)^{2n_i}}, & A_{i1}=A_{i2} \\[3ex] \dfrac{(1+\lambda/x_{i1})^{x_{i1}}(1+\lambda/x_{i2})^{x_{i2}}}{(1+2\lambda/2n_i)^{2n_i}}, & A_{i1}\neq A_{i2} \end{cases}$$

which differ from Balding's equation 15 in detail. Over the whole profile, the LR is

$$R(\lambda) = \prod_i R_i(\lambda)$$

A 99% profile likelihood interval is found by choosing those two values of λ such that $\ln R(\lambda) = -(1/2)\chi^2_{1;0.99} = 3.317$. For the profile in Table 6.1 the values are $\lambda = -9.54$, 10.85 and the corresponding profile probabilities are 0.98×10^{-7} and 3.59×10^{-7}, which are similar to the confidence limits from the normal-based values in Table 6.2 for $\theta = 0$. The corresponding limits for a 95% profile likelihood interval are $\lambda = -7.38$ and 8.14. Use of $\lambda = 2$, as suggested by Balding,[570] corresponds to using a one-sided interval with a coverage probability of 0.51 in this case.

The example does not support Balding's claim that the λ value for the upper support limit should be 2, corresponding to the addition of the crime stain profile and the suspect's profile to the sample. Without this appealing way to choose λ there seems little numerical advantage to the use of profile likelihood support intervals over conventional confidence intervals. The bounds of λ will depend on the number of loci in the profile, the population probabilities of the profile alleles and the size of the sample as well as on the probability ordinate used to construct the interval. Adding the crime stain profile and the suspect's profile to the sample before constructing allele sample frequencies neither accounts for the sampling variation induced by finite samples nor corrects for the presence of population substructure.

Uniform Allele Prior Distribution

Balding[570] also considered a Bayesian approach by assuming a Dirichlet prior distribution for allele probabilities. The probability density for values p_{ij} in a particular population was taken to be

$$\pi\left(p_{i1}^{*}\right) \propto \left(p_{i1}^{*}\right)^{\gamma_{i1}-1}\left(1-p_{i1}^{*}\right)^{\gamma_{i\bar{1}}-1}, \qquad A_{i1}=A_{i2}$$

$$\pi\left(p_{i1}^{*}, p_{i2}^{*}\right) \propto \left(p_{i1}^{*}\right)^{\gamma_{i1}-1}\left(p_{i2}^{*}\right)^{\gamma_{i2}-1}\left(1-p_{i1}^{*}-p_{i2}^{*}\right)^{\gamma_{i\overline{12}}-1}, \qquad A_{i1} \neq A_{i2}$$

The quantities $\gamma_{i\bar{1}}$ and $\gamma_{i\overline{12}}$ are the Dirichlet parameters for the allelic classes 'not 1' and 'not 1 or 2' at locus i. Combined with multinomial sampling of alleles from the population, the posterior profile probability (i.e. the expectation over populations of $\left(p_{i1}^{*}\right)^{2}$ for $A_{i1}A_{i2}$ profiles and of $2p_{i1}^{*}p_{i2}^{*}$ for $A_{i1}A_{i2}$ profiles) is

$$E(P_{0i})=\begin{cases} \dfrac{\Gamma\left(\gamma_{i1}+\gamma_{i\bar{1}}+2n_{i}\right)}{\Gamma\left(\gamma_{i1}+\gamma_{i\bar{1}}+2n_{i1}+2\right)}\dfrac{\Gamma\left(\gamma_{i1}+x_{i1}+2\right)}{\Gamma\left(\gamma_{i1}+x_{i1}\right)}, & A_{i1}=A_{i2} \\[3mm] \dfrac{2\Gamma\left(\gamma_{i1}+\gamma_{i2}+\gamma_{i\overline{12}}+2n_{i}\right)}{\Gamma\left(\gamma_{i1}+\gamma_{i2}+\gamma_{i\overline{12}}+2n_{i}+2\right)}\dfrac{\Gamma\left(\gamma_{i1}+x_{i1}+1\right)}{\Gamma\left(\gamma_{i1}+x_{i1}\right)}\dfrac{\Gamma\left(\gamma_{i2}+x_{i2}+1\right)}{\Gamma\left(\gamma_{i2}+x_{i2}\right)}, & A_{i1} \neq A_{i2} \end{cases}$$

(6.2)

Balding then simplified this to allow for uniform priors, $\gamma_{i1}=\gamma_{i\bar{1}}=1$ for homozygotes and $\gamma_{i1}=\gamma_{i2}=\gamma_{i\overline{12}}=1$ for heterozygotes. Then the expected profile posterior probabilities are

$$E(P_{0i})=\begin{cases} \dfrac{(x_{i1}+2)(x_{i1}+1)}{(2n_{i}+3)(2n_{i}+2)}, & A_{i1}=A_{i2} \\[3mm] \dfrac{2(x_{i1}+1)(x_{i2}+1)}{(2n_{i}+4)(2n_{i}+3)}, & A_{i1} \neq A_{i2} \end{cases}$$

(6.3)

which again differ slightly from the expressions given by Balding. An advantage of the Dirichlet distribution is that all moments have simple expressions, so that with a uniform prior the expectations of $\left(p_{i}^{*}\right)^{4}$ and of $\left(2p_{i1}^{*}p_{i2}^{*}\right)^{2}$ give

$$E\left(P_{0i}^{2}\right)=\begin{cases} \dfrac{(x_{i1}+4)(x_{i1}+3)(x_{i1}+2)(x_{i1}+1)}{(2n_{i}+5)(2n_{i}+4)(2n_{i}+3)(2n_{i}+2)}, & A_{i1}=A_{i2} \\[3mm] \dfrac{4(x_{i1}+2)(x_{i2}+1)(x_{i1}+2)(x_{i2}+1)}{(2n_{i}+6)(2n_{i}+5)(2n_{i}+4)(2n_{i}+3)}, & A_{i1} \neq A_{i2} \end{cases}$$

(which also differ slightly from the expressions given by Balding). The ratio of these two expectations can be regarded as the probability of the profile occurring twice given that it has occurred once (i.e. the match probability):

$$\frac{E(P_{0i})}{E\left(P_{0i}^{2}\right)}=\begin{cases} \dfrac{(x_{i1}+4)(x_{i1}+3)}{(2n_{i}+5)(2n_{i}+4)}, & A_{i1}=A_{i2} \\[3mm] \dfrac{2(x_{i1}+2)(x_{i2}+2)}{(2n_{i}+6)(2n_{i}+5)}, & A_{i1} \neq A_{i2} \end{cases}$$

(6.4)

This is almost the expression that would result for the simple product rule if the profile in question were added twice to the database.

Balding suggested this method as a way to incorporate sampling effects into estimated match probabilities, in the sense that the sample database was allowed to modify the assumed uniform prior for allele probabilities. Weir et al.[574] believe, however, that these estimates are posterior means for match probabilities when the prior means for the probabilities are 1/3 for homozygotes and 1/6 for heterozygotes, as can be seen by setting $x_{i1} = x_{i2} = n_i = 0$ in Equations 6.3.

There are several unfortunate consequences of this work:

1. It has become a prevalent but false view that the foundation of the method is adding the person of interest (POI) and offender to the database. For example 'Alternatively, point estimates for probabilistic approaches are often given by $(X + 1)/(N + 1)$ or $(X + 2)/(N + 2)$ ... which takes the conceptual approach of adding the case profiles to the database, under the hypothesis that the profiles observed in the case may have come from two different individuals'.[579]

2. There is a view that this accounts for sampling uncertainty in some way.

Non-Uniform Allele Prior Distribution

As Balding remarks, it is illogical to assign uniform priors for allele probabilities that differ with the number of alleles (1 or 2) that occur in the evidentiary profile. There is population-genetic logic in the non-uniform Dirichlet, which invokes the parameter θ via

$$\gamma_{ij} = \frac{(1-\theta) p_{ij}}{\theta}$$

as discussed by Balding and Nichols[453] and Evett and Weir.[257] The posterior match probabilities are then

$$\frac{E(P_{0i})}{E(P_{0i}^2)} = \begin{cases} \dfrac{\left[(3+x_{i1})\theta+(1-\theta)p_{i1}\right]\left[(2+x_{i1})\theta+(1-\theta)p_{i1}\right]}{\left[1+(1+2n_i)\theta\right]\left[1+(2+2n_i)\theta\right]}, & A_{i1} = A_{i2} \\ \dfrac{2\left[(1+x_{i1})\theta+(1-\theta)p_{i1}\right]\left[(1+x_{i2})\theta+(1-\theta)p_{i2}\right]}{\left[1+(1+2n_i)\theta\right]\left[1+(2+2n_i)\theta\right]}, & A_{i1} \neq A_{i2} \end{cases} \tag{6.5}$$

There is a problem in knowing what values to use for the unknown allele probabilities p_{ij}. Simply using sample proportions from current populations appears to ignore the variation that the Dirichlet distribution is designed to incorporate, although the problem is lessened when the x_{ij} values are large. Balding does not comment on the fact that the sample of size n_i individuals in Equations 6.5 is from the specific subpopulation relevant to the crime. It is not a sample that would furnish an estimate of the population-wide frequencies p_{ij}, further explaining why there is no simple interpretation of these results in terms of adding copies of the matching profile to the database.

Note that, as the sample size n_i increases, Equations 6.5 reduce to

$$\frac{E(P_{0i})}{E(P_{0i}^2)} = \begin{cases} p_{i1}^2, & A_{i1} = A_{i2} \\ 2 p_{i1} p_{i2}, & A_{i1} \neq A_{i2} \end{cases} \tag{6.6}$$

which are just the product rule expressions for the relevant subpopulation. The product rule expressions are also obtained when $\theta = 0$ because there is then no distinction between subpopulations and the whole population. When there are no data from the relevant subpopulation, $x_{i1} = x_{i2} = n_i = 0$, and Equations 6.6 are recovered.

If only the two samples from the crime stain and the suspect are available from the relevant subpopulation, $n_i = 2$ and $x_{i1} = 4$ for homozygous profiles $A_{i1}A_{i1}$ or $x_{i1} = x_{i2} = 2$ for heterozygous profiles $A_{i1}A_{i2}$:

$$\frac{E(P_{0i})}{E(P_{0i}^2)} = \begin{cases} \dfrac{\left[7\theta+(1-\theta)p_{i1}\right]\left[6\theta+(1-\theta)p_{i1}\right]}{[1+5\theta][1+6\theta]}, & A_{i1} = A_{i2} \\[4mm] \dfrac{2\left[3\theta+(1-\theta)p_{i1}\right]\left[3\theta+(1-\theta)p_{i2}\right]}{[1+5\theta][1+6\theta]}, & A_{i1} \neq A_{i2} \end{cases} \tag{6.7}$$

In Australasia we initially implemented a Dir $(1,1,\ldots 1)$ prior, assuming this to be 'uninformative' and not biasing the process with unsubstantiated prior opinion. In operational practice it was observed that if the number of allele types at a locus, K, was large, then the posterior mean was $\dfrac{x_i + 1}{2N + K}$ and could be well below the sample estimate. Implementation of the previously advocated[580] $Dir\left(\dfrac{1}{K}, \dfrac{1}{K}, \ldots, \dfrac{1}{K}\right)$ leads to a posterior mean $\dfrac{x_i + \dfrac{1}{K}}{2N+1}$ and the prior has a negligible effect on the posterior. This prior also appeared to have superior sampling properties.[581] This is the approach (and prior) that is currently implemented in Australasia.

Method: Posterior Density[*]

Requirements: This method requires a purpose written program. A very adaptable one that can handle any forensic situation has been developed by Curran.[578]

Applicability: All forensic casework.

Comments: Curran et al.[571] scored the performance of this method as adequate in most situations.

Implementation: This is the most mathematically intimidating of the various approaches, but in concept it is the most familiar and most intuitive. It helps to start by thinking about the problem without the hindrance of the mathematics.

One way 'into' the problem is to think about a situation where we have no alleles of type a in our database but have just done a case where the suspect and crime stain have this allele. Our allele probability estimate from our database is 0 (please ignore minimum allele probabilities at this point). However we have just seen one copy of allele a (in the suspect). So we certainly no longer believe that the frequency is zero.

Next we ask ourselves why we are calculating a frequency at all. It is to assess the chance of this evidence *if* the suspect did not leave the stain. Hence the whole calculation of a frequency is based on the assumption that the suspect did not leave the stain. Now if the suspect did not leave the stain, someone else did. Hence we have two, not one, observations of allele a. Thinking of this type led Scranage and Pinchin[582] to add the 'suspect and offender' to the database when they wrote the ground breaking programme DNASYS.

This is what the Bayesian approach does. It starts from a position, observes the database *and* the suspect *and* the offender. This results in an estimate *and* the variability in that estimate. We feel that the court would also respond well to an explanation that we had 'updated' our view of allele probabilities based on the suspect and offender profiles. A programme is required to implement this approach but one is available.

---

[*] We attribute this method to the suggestion of Dr Ian Painter. It is an extension of the method of Professor David Balding.

An Explanation of the Bayesian Highest Posterior Density

This approach is not explained in simple terms elsewhere in the literature. We attempt this here.

Bayes' Theorem and Bayesian Estimation

In forensic applications the odds form of Bayes' theorem is used to show how the *LR* can be combined with the prior odds on guilt to give us the posterior odds on guilt. In Bayesian estimation we are interested in the value of an unknown population parameter such as an allele probability. To estimate this parameter we combine our prior probability about the possible values for this parameter with the data that have been observed to get the posterior probability on the possible values the parameter may take.

Bayes' theorem tells us how to do this. We write

$$Pr(\lambda \mid data) = \frac{Pr(data \mid \lambda)Pr(\lambda)}{\int Pr(data \mid \lambda)Pr(\lambda).d\lambda}$$

or

$$Pr(\lambda \mid data) \propto Pr(data \mid \lambda)Pr(\lambda) \tag{6.8}$$

where λ represents the parameter(s) of interest. In forensic casework λ is likely to be an allele probability. In words, Equation 6.8 states, 'the probability of the parameter given the data is proportional to the probability of the data given the parameter times the probability of the parameter'. The first equation shows the 'scaling' factor that we need to calculate the probability.

We start with some belief about a parameter. Possibly we have no knowledge at all. This can be modelled by various functions. For instance, 'no knowledge at all' is often modelled by a function that assigns all values between 0 and 1 the same probability. An experiment is performed to collect some information about the parameter. In our case this is the database *and* the suspect and offender profiles. Then the prior belief and the data are combined to give an updated idea about the parameter. The equation can be broken down into the posterior, $Pr(\lambda \mid data)$, the likelihood, $Pr(data \mid \lambda)$, and the prior $Pr(\lambda)$. The likelihood is usually straightforward to compute and is suggested by the problem. Choice of the prior can be very problematic.

Prior Probabilities

Assume that we wish to assess the frequency (probability) of various alleles at a locus. Furthermore let us assume that this particular locus has only alleles a and b. Since people can only have A or B alleles, then $Pr(A) + Pr(B) = 1$, or $Pr(B) = 1 - Pr(A)$. Therefore it suffices to estimate the probability of allele A denoted by π_A.

A sample of people is taken and typed. Our maximum likelihood estimate for the probability of the A allele is

$$f_A = \hat{\pi}_A = \frac{\# \text{ of } A's}{2N}$$

where N is the number of individuals in our database. The hat character ($\wedge$) is used to indicate that this is an estimate. Imagine that in a sample of, say, 10 people, there were seven type A alleles, then our estimate is 7/20 = 0.35. However before this sample was taken what did we know about π_A? Regardless of what we assume, we need a way of representing our knowledge. We do this by saying how probable we think certain values of π_A are. For example, we might say that there is a 10% chance that π_A is less than 0.2, $Pr(\pi_A < 0.2) = 0.1$, a 10% chance that π_A is greater than 0.9, $Pr(\pi_A > 0.9) = 0.1$, and an 80% chance that π_A is between 0.2 and 0.9, $Pr(0.2 < \pi_A < 0.9) = 0.8$. Together these probabilities add up to 1, and what we've described is called a *cumulative density function*. They describe the area under a curve called a *probability density function*. The key fact is that the area, not the height of the curve, measures probability.

The proportion may have been estimated as 0.53 using a database in Scotland so it might be similar in Ireland. Or we may choose to say that we know nothing – all values of π_A are equally likely. We can choose prior densities that have these probabilities. Typically these are chosen (to simplify the mathematics) from a family of probability density functions with well-known properties. In the case of a single proportion this family of curves is called the *beta family*. The shape of distributions in the beta family is defined by two parameters, α and β. Any choice of α and β that differs from 1, gives substantial shape to the curve. The shape of the curve of course will affect the posterior distribution, so some people would say that if α and β are not 1, then we have chosen an *informative* prior. If we set α and β to 1, we have an *uninformative* prior and are assuming that all values of π_A are equally likely.

A convenient property of the beta distribution is that if our prior is beta (α, β), and we observe x A alleles in a sample of $2N$ then the posterior distribution is beta$(x + \alpha, 2N - x + \beta)$. The mean of this posterior distribution is $\dfrac{x+\alpha}{2N+\alpha+\beta}$. This is known as the *beta binomial*.

In many cases, especially mixtures, we need to consider the allele probabilities of two or more alleles. The multidimensional equivalent of the beta binomial is the Dirichlet multinomial. If the prior is $Dir(\alpha_1, \alpha_2, ..., \alpha_k)$ and the sampling is multinomial with counts $x_1, x_2, ..., x_k$ for alleles $a_1, a_2, ..., a_k$, then the posterior distribution is $Dir(\alpha_1 + x_1, \alpha_2 + x_2, ..., \alpha_k + x_k)$ and the posterior mean of each allele probability is

$$\frac{\alpha_1 + x_1}{\sum_i \alpha_i + 2N} \text{ where } \sum_i x_i = 2N.$$

Highest Posterior Density Intervals

The highest posterior density (HPD) method[570,571,581] (sometimes referred to as *Bayesian credible intervals*) uses a Dirichlet distribution to describe the frequencies of alleles in a database. The general form of a Dirichlet distribution is

$$f(\alpha_1 ... \alpha_n) = \frac{\Gamma\left(\sum_{i=1}^{k} \alpha_i\right)}{\prod_{i=1}^{k} \Gamma(\alpha_i)} \prod_{i=1}^{k} x_i^{\alpha_i - 1}$$

referred to as a Dirichlet $(\alpha_1, ... \alpha_n)$ distribution, where α_i is the frequency of allele i, x_i is the count of allele i from the database and k is the number of alleles at the locus with non-zero count. For a two-allele system this function simplifies to a beta distribution.

We utilize a $\dfrac{1}{k}$ prior distribution, i.e. a Dirichlet $\left(\dfrac{1}{k}, \dfrac{1}{k}, ..., \dfrac{1}{k}\right)$, distribution to produce a Dirichlet $\left(x_1 + \dfrac{1}{k}, x_2 + \dfrac{1}{k}, ..., x_k + \dfrac{1}{k}\right)$ posterior density. To calculate an exact credible interval would require the derivation of a probability density function for each LR formula based on the Dirichlet distributions. This is difficult even for simple equations and so a Monte Carlo simulation method can be used that generates sets of allele frequencies (or vectors of allele frequencies) from a Dirichlet probability density function and then use these allele frequencies to generate LRs.

A fast method to sample a random vector $f_1 ... f_k$ from the k-dimensional Dirichlet distribution with parameters $(\alpha_1 ... \alpha_k)$ is to draw k independent random samples $g_1 ... g_k$ from gamma distributions each with density $Gamma(\alpha_i, 1) = \dfrac{g_i^{\alpha_i - 1} e^{-g_i}}{\Gamma(\alpha_i)}$ and then set

$$f_i = \frac{g_i}{\sum_{j=1}^{k} g_j}$$

(so that the sum of all f_i frequencies is 1).

Gamma number generation may be carried out using the GS and GD algorithms of Ahrens and Dieter.[583,584]

If, say, the lower bound is taken, then it should be borne in mind that a statement that the *LR* is greater than the bound 0.99 of the time is only true if the only source of uncertainty is the sampling uncertainty. It may be better to accept that there are a great many sources of uncertainty and to assign the *LR* at this (or some other) bound as a subjective judgment of a fair and reasonable approach.

Minimum Allele Probabilities

The concept of a minimum allele probability replaces zero or very small allele probabilities derived by counting from some database with some minimum probability. This avoids the genotype probability estimate being zero and stems largely from the concern that these small allele probabilities are very poorly estimated. Minimum allele probabilities are unnecessary when either the Bayesian support interval (Balding's size bias correction) or the highest posterior density interval is used as these methods can 'handle' a zero estimate. Consider Balding's size bias estimator for a homozygote, $\hat{P}_{aa} = \left(\dfrac{x+4}{2N+4} \right)^2$. This returns a non-zero value for $\hat{P}_{aa}$ even when the count in the database, x, is zero.

When a non-zero value is assigned to θ, the genotype estimate will be non-zero even when the count of the allele or alleles is zero in the database. However the bootstrap, the factor of 10 and the assumption of asymptotic normality of the logarithm will not correctly estimate sampling variation in these circumstances. The typical solution has been to apply a minimum allele probability.

Budowle et al.[573] discuss two options for the $1 - \alpha$ upper confidence interval:

Following Chakraborty,[572] $p_{\min} = 1 - [1 - (1 - \alpha)^{\frac{1}{c}}]^{\frac{1}{2n}}$, where $p_{\min}$ is the minimum allele probability, c is the number of common alleles and n is the number of individuals in the database.

Following Weir,[585] $p_{\min} = 1 - \alpha^{\frac{1}{2n}}$. Chakraborty's approach typically gives a higher minimum allele probability and behaves in an unusual manner. We wonder if it has any merit.

The United States has an established precedent of using $5/2N$ as a minimum allele probability. This may have arisen from the NRC II paragraph below:

> A similar expedient for rare alleles is to use the maximum of 5 and k, where k is the actual number of alleles from the database that fall within the match window.[176, p. 148]

It is difficult to see this comment by NRC II as a recommendation. The word *recommended* does appear earlier in the paragraph in relation to rebinning for fixed bin VNTR analysis. The part referring to $5/2N$ describes this as an expedient. No numbered recommendation to this effect appears at the end of the chapter in the NRC II report. The value $5/2N$ is about the upper 99.3% bound of the confidence interval for 0 out of $2N$ trials. However recall that the confidence interval of the full multilocus probability estimate is not obtained by confidence intervals on each allele.

NRC II did state,[176, p. 146] 'To account for the fact that match probabilities are based on different databases and might change if another dataset were used, it is helpful to give confidence intervals for those probabilities'.

SWGDAM[106] states: '4.6. The formulae used in any statistical analysis must be documented and must address both homozygous and heterozygous typing results, multiple locus profiles, mixtures, minimum allele frequencies, and, where appropriate, biological relationships'.

Taking this together we would suggest that neither NRC II nor SWGDAM have recommended $5/2N$ as a minimum allele probability. NRC II do mention $5/2N$ but realistically come closest to recommending a confidence interval, describing it as helpful.

Coverage

The performance of each of these methods was examined through simulation. The results of these simulations are shown in Table 6.3. Use was made of the 210 African-American profiles published by Budowle et al.[502] and an unpublished New Zealand Caucasian database of 12,163 profiles which were typed using the Second Generation Multiplex Plus (SGM Plus) system. We used the CODIS (Combined DNA Index System) core loci from the Budowle et al. publication profiles. The performance of each method was tested using a 'common' profile and a 'rare' profile. More common (or rarer) profiles could have been artificially generated.

The sample allele proportions from each database were used to generate 1000 'databases' of N profiles for $N = 100, 400, 1000, 5000$ and $10,000$. This simulates the act of sampling from the population. As the databases were generated without any population substructure, the appropriate estimator of the match probability is given by the product rule.

An estimate of sampling error was calculated for the match probabilities estimated from each database. Balding's Bayesian method used the corrected equations 5 (from Evett and Weir[257]). After some reflection we have changed from our previous work and added the POI profile to the database prior to applying the bootstrap, the factor of 10, the lognormal and the HPD with the $1/k$ prior. However doing this is not appropriate for the size bias correction. The upper 99% bound was calculated.

The proportion of times that the upper bound is higher than the true match probability is called the *estimated coverage*. Recall that we know the true match probability since we know the true probabilities from which we have drawn the samples.

Our first requirement for an ideal method is high coverage. It is simple to maximize coverage, by making the upper bound absurdly high. Such an action is excessively conservative and may rob the court of useful information. Therefore our second property of an ideal method is that the coverage should be close to the expected 99% value.

Discussion of Appropriateness of Sampling Uncertainty Estimates

To conclude we review some published and unpublished opinions as to the appropriateness of various sampling uncertainty corrections. No uniform consensus exists and there are some quite polarized views. Our own opinions are directly ascribed.

It is worthwhile to begin this discussion by considering the potential sources of uncertainty in determining a match probability. The larger ones relate to errors in laboratory work or in assigning genotypes. We begin the mathematical consideration by assuming that these functions have been correctly carried out. However it must always be remembered that everything from here onwards is conditional on the profiles being correctly assigned.

Probably the next largest source of uncertainty would be the existence of a monozygotic twin or other close relatives in the population of potential suspects. This possibility is becoming more important as more loci are added. The addition of further loci focuses attention away from unrelated persons and onto close relatives and members of the same subpopulation. This was discussed in Chapter 4.

Next we come to uncertainties in the appropriateness of the population genetic model, sampling uncertainty and minimum allele probabilities. These last two are manifestations of the same thing.

Table 6.3   Coverage of Different Sampling Methods

Method	2N	Coverage after the Addition of the POI Profile			
		African-American Database (CODIS Loci)	New Zealand Caucasian Database (SGM Plus Loci)	African-American Database (CODIS Loci)	New Zealand Caucasian Database (SGM Plus Loci)
		Common Profile		Rare Profile	
Bootstrap	100	0.994	0.986	1.000	1.000
	400	0.994	0.984	0.999	0.998
	1000	0.991	0.988	0.994	0.985
	5000	0.998	0.992	0.992	0.992
	10,000	0.995	0.986	0.991	0.991
Factor of 10	100	0.999	1.000	1.000	1.000
	400	1.000	1.000	0.999	1.000
	1000	1.000	1.000	0.999	1.000
	5000	1.000	1.000	1.000	1.000
	10,000	1.000	1.000	1.000	1.000
HPD, $1/k$ prior	100	0.993	0.983	1.000	1.000
	400	0.992	0.981	1.000	1.000
	1000	0.991	0.987	1.000	1.000
	5000	0.998	0.992	0.996	0.994
	10,000	0.993	0.987	0.993	0.993
Log normal	100	1.000	0.996	1.000	1.000
	400	0.997	0.992	1.000	1.000
	1000	0.996	0.990	1.000	1.000
	5000	0.999	0.996	0.998	1.000
	10,000	0.994	0.989	0.996	0.996
Size bias (no addition of POI prior to applying)	100	0.902	0.701	1.000	1.000
	400	0.764	0.616	0.999	0.999
	1000	0.651	0.581	0.952	0.958
	5000	0.583	0.519	0.762	0.772
	10,000	0.540	0.534	0.723	0.694

Note: POI, person of interest; CODIS, Combined DNA Index System; HPD, highest posterior density.

We are aware of opinion that supports the use of the following:
* Minimum allele probabilities and the product rule
* Minimum allele probabilities, the product rule and sampling uncertainty assessment
* Minimum allele probabilities, a conservative θ correction and Balding's size bias correction
* A conservative θ correction and sampling uncertainty assessment

A key question is, are we seeking the best assignment or a conservative one with known properties? The best assignment may be the product rule and Balding's size bias correction. We have formed this opinion from simulation studies. This is the only way that has been developed, since we do not *know* the true answer. This approach would be highly appropriate in civil cases where the least biased answer is required.

A problem in criminal cases when giving only the 'best assignment' is that it immediately leads to legitimate debate in court about the uncertainty inherent in that assignment. We had previously suggested that if the analyst is unprepared for this debate, then she may be in for a rough time and may appear unscientific and underprepared. The discussion in *R v Cannell* involving Angela van Daal and Duncan Taylor confirms this fear. A similar disappointing discussion occurred in a footwear impression case, *R v T*.[198,586] In that case the court commented unfavourably on a footwear database of size 8122. It is probably wise for us to accept that the size of our databases is likely to be a subject of some interest and perhaps adverse comment in court.

The next fact that needs consideration is that robust methodology exists that can handle both sampling uncertainty and minimum allele probabilities. These methods have been summarized in this chapter. The behaviour of these methods is known, and there is a large body of support for their use.

However since the first edition we have become aware of a serious negative aspect to giving confidence or probability intervals. Our awareness was brought into focus during an interchange about the wording of a probability interval. The suggestion was that the written statement should read, 'With 99% probability the true likelihood ratio is greater than *x*'. We took objection to this suggestion for two reasons, one philosophical and one practical. We suspect the practical one will carry greater weight so we will concentrate on that, but the philosophical one has great merit as well.

Our practical problem is that the statement is wrong. The statement is approximately correct if the only source of uncertainty is sampling. However there are a great many sources of uncertainty and some of these may yield much larger uncertainty than that associated with sampling. For example, we believe we use a value for θ at the upper end of the plausible distribution. If this is so, then the effect on the 99% could be considerable (in the direction of 100%). However there are a great many other possible effects such as the effect of threshold and allele calling.

Why is anyone so interested in coming up with such a wording? Is this some search for certainty in a world that offers little? We believe it is. We believe the understandable and valid motivation is to find some solid lower bound below which the true value of the evidence would never fall. This lower bound is not possible to find with our current knowledge, and if found it would be such a pale underestimation of the evidence that it would do a significant disservice to justice.

We suggest that all practical forensic scientists stop reading at this point. Further we suggest that all advocates of subjectivist probability also stop reading. We therefore recommend that almost no one should read further.

If we could develop a strong prior belief about the prior probability of all inputs, we could 'absorb' this uncertainty (strictly speaking integrate it out) into the assignment process and hence produce one assignment that correctly reflects the uncertainties in the process. This method is beyond current scientific understanding. Many of our respected colleagues suggest *sensitivity analysis*. This involves varying the inputs in some sensible range and observing the outputs. We still need some help in how to decide what to do with the varying outputs and for us, personally, we could use the HPD method to inform sensible ranges. In some sense DNA is 'too easy'. The immense power of the technique allows us the luxury of 'wasting' evidence. We can vary the inputs in the sensible ranges and take some fair and reasonable value from the lower tail of the *LR*s produced. For us, this is a dangerous process to begin. Once we accept the principle of varying inputs and accepting underestimates, we empower a process that seeks to push the limits of sensible ranges and force lower values. This is a reality we recognize.

The philosophical argument is much harder for us to form, largely because we are unsure whether we have understood the point that such distinguished commentators as Ian Evett have tried to teach us. Consider the question, what is the chance it will rain tomorrow? First let us reopen the question we parked in Chapter 3 relating to the true answer. What is the 'true' probability that it will rain tomorrow? How could we answer such a question? Let us imagine that tomorrow comes and it either rains or not. Does this help us with the true probability that it would rain? Not at all. It either rained or it did not. This information would not inform us whether a probability of, say, 70% rain was correct or not. Could we envisage a great many tomorrows all equivalent to the one tomorrow we are considering? Not really. They are all different in some sense. The time of year may differ; the state of La Niña or El Niño may differ. The extent of global warming and the Earth's orbit and inclination may differ year to year. Can we score our predictor? Yes to some extent. If our predictor says 70% *rain* and it does rain, we could score +0.70 and if it does not rain we could score –0.70. Over the long run we could score people or systems. Strangely our predictor who *says* 0.70 is likely to be outscored by someone who uses only 100% and 0% with some accuracy. However none of this helps us with the true probability that it will rain tomorrow.

Now consider the statement that there is a 95% probability that the chance of rain is between 50% and 90%. Is there any situation where one of the extremes of this range or the whole range would be of more use than the point estimate?

Of no forensic interest, I (JSB) worked in Australia for a while. I asked some Australians why Australia is so dry. They answered that it does not rain much. I was hoping for more.

Provided by David Balding, 2012

What I would regard as the most satisfactory analysis is one that doesn't use any point estimates for population allele fractions or F_{ST} or anything else. Instead you put all the relevant data that you have into one big computation and turn the handle and get a single number out as the likelihood under H_p, and then again under H_d. You then take the ratio. If you don't have much or good data (small database or poor match with suspect's ethnicity or no relevant studies on F_{ST}), your perfect probability model will account for the resulting uncertainty and you automatically get a smaller LR. Instead of confidence intervals you do a sensitivity analysis and show that the LR does not change very much under a range of reasonable assumptions. There are some reasons, good and less good, that we do not do this in practice, the main one being that it's too hard. Nobody currently has a working theory for everything.

In the real world we simplify by using plug-in estimates for allele fractions and F_{ST}, instead of integrating them out in an ideal analysis. Smaller values of these tend to be bad for the suspect (Q); errors are not necessarily symmetric and so do not average out. The ideal analysis of integration over distributions for these parameters usually gives a larger result than does plugging in, say, the means of those distributions as fixed values. Thus this 'plug-in estimates' approach often tends to go against Q. To avoid this we can bias our estimates upwards: for the allele fractions we often throw into the database some imaginary extra copies of the alleles of Q (pseudocounts). For F_{ST} I would always advocate using a larger value than is typically reported in population genetic studies (for a number of reasons). These are both *ad hoc* ways to try to crudely approximate what we have in mind as the ideal but not really feasible analysis.

It is not surprising that whenever point estimates are used, a statistician will want to calculate confidence intervals. It is not entirely illogical but I think it's taking the wrong direction; instead of a crude (but conservative) approximation to something sensible, we end up with something not very helpful because it is a confused hybrid of different ideas. The allele fraction sampling error that is addressed by a confidence interval is less important than the effect of F_{ST}, which is not amenable to being included in a confidence interval (CI) calculation, and so reporting a CI may give the impression that uncertainty has been dealt with when it has not. Moreover it does not recognize that uncertainty has been dealt with by using upwardly biased point estimates. F_{ST} is usually (but not always) much less than 1% for European-origin populations. It may be argued that 1% is sufficiently conservative but I would suggest using at least 2%: the magnitude of that effect in favour of defendants puts all concerns about sampling error into the shade.

More recently Taylor et al.[587] investigated the relative magnitude of the uncertainty associated with database size, uncertainty in the value for θ and unexcluded relatives in the population. Their work showed that any of the sources of variation could dominate the total variation in the LR distribution under certain circumstances.

Given that it is possible to evaluate all these uncertainties within the LR calculations, what value should be reported to a courtroom? It has been argued that the most relevant figure to provide is the point estimate.[567] Our own experience is that the court often concerns itself with exploring potential sources of uncertainty. If a decision is made to report a CI, then this should attempt to consider total variation.

7

Single Source Samples

John S. Buckleton, Duncan Taylor, Peter Gill and Jo-Anne Bright[*]

Contents

Introduction

In this chapter we consider the interpretation of single source samples. A distinction is drawn in the minds of forensic practitioners between single source and mixed samples. This distinction is unnecessary and possibly unhelpful; however it is so prevalent that we fall into line. The chapters treating single source and mixed samples are back to back to make our point.

---

[*] We sincerely acknowledge valuable comments from Ian Evett and David Balding.

BOX 7.1   SCIENTIFIC WORKING GROUP ON DNA ANALYSIS METHODS

The Scientific Working Group on DNA Analysis Methods maintains a page of frequently asked questions at http://swgdam.org/faq.html. There are two questions on this page that might be good points for discussion.

Q: The document contains a fallacy that low copy DNA is a method not an amount. Low copy or low template refers to an amount of DNA. That amount should be stated in this document and it is 100–200 pg, based on numerous scientific and internal validation studies.

Our answer: We are not sure we agree with the questioner that this is a fallacy. There was a need at one point to have two terms, one that described a method and one that described template amount. At that time the low copy number (LCN) label was attached to a method, specifically 34 cycle amplification with duplication and a consensus interpretation strategy. The term *low template DNA*[36] was coined, we think usefully, to describe any low template sample whether at 34 cycles or any other number. However we do not want to quibble terms here. We do want to argue that *low template* cannot be defined by a quantification value, which is what we assume the 100–200 pg refers to. Such a definition would miss the low template of component of mixtures and of degraded samples.

Q: The document [ignores] the issue of replicates. The scientific literature is very clear. Replicate analysis must be used when performing enhanced detection methods.

Our answer: We feel that the questioner overstates the case. Replication is advantageous in many but not all cases. However this does not render a single analysis worthless.

There is a level of debate about uncertainty in the number of contributors. This debate exists in the mixture area. However in truth the number of contributors to a stain is never known with certainty, and it is at least theoretically possible that an apparently single sourced stain is in fact from two contributors. For modern multiplexes with many, say 24 loci, it is really quite hard to imagine how this could happen and for all practical purposes practitioners can reliably detect a single sourced stain. However in other fields, such as Y chromosome STR, particularly at low level, the risk is more realistic.

Single sourced DNA samples may have any number of template molecules. This affects the interpretation. Low template is not readily defined, and clearly there is a gradual change from low to 'normal' template as the number of template molecules increases. We emphasize that low template cannot be defined on cycle number or on quantification result and the prevalent attempts to do so are misguided. There is, in theory, no distinction, between the treatment of low and normal template samples of one or many contributors. In a perfect world one system could interpret all variants using the same principles see Box 7.1 for some discussion.

Single Source Samples Small Probability of Dropout

If template levels are good and the polymerase chain reaction (PCR) process has proceeded normally, peak heights will be such that the probability of dropout will be very small. If the sample is assigned as coming from a single source, this is the simplest type of evidence with which the forensic biologist may be presented. The issues in this subject area relate to the choice of proposition and the possibility of relatives, the process of interpretation and choice of database and the phrasing of the result.

The default situation in most forensic laboratories is to quote either a match probability or a likelihood ratio (Equation 2.3) for the following propositions:

H_p: The person of interest (POI) is the donor of the DNA.

H_d: The true donor is unrelated to the POI.

These are termed the *unrelated propositions*. These propositions may be supplemented, but rarely are with a match probability or likelihood ratio (LR) for a number of possible relationships between the accused and the true donor. It is worthwhile calibrating current practice against the optimal solution, which is the full Bayesian approach (Equation 2.4), currently implemented to our knowledge only in New Zealand and Adelaide, Australia. Examination of the behaviour of the posterior probability for feasible priors suggests that for modern multiplexes the bulk of the probability if the accused is not the donor resides on an unexcluded sibling. We cannot, as yet, conceive of a reporting policy that dispenses with reporting the statistic for the unrelated proposition and substituting the statistic for a sibling. Yet this is the scientifically correct conclusion. We are aware of court work where the court has examined the possibility that a sibling is the donor in a way consistent with attempting to assign a prior to this proposition.

The Race of the Accused

The question has arisen as to whether the race of the accused has any bearing at all on the interpretation. If we look at the form of the match probability or the denominator of the LR, it is $\Pr(G_c| G_s, H_d)$. Recall that H_d represents the hypothesis that an unknown person is the donor of the stain. The very reasonable line of logic is that if the accused is not the donor of the stain, then 'he has nothing to do with it' and it is from someone else. How then could his genotype or his race have any effect on the interpretation? The mathematical way into this discussion is via Equation 2.4, but we thought we might try a more verbal line of argument here.

We ask you to dispense with the thought of the crime stain entirely for the time being. We inform you that the accused has genotype G_S and we ask you to place your best bet on where you might find a second copy of this genotype. We assume you would choose a sibling. Hence we accept that the chance that a sibling has G_S is elevated by the knowledge that the accused has it. We assume you would also elevate the chance that a parent or child has this genotype, albeit you would elevate it less. You would elevate cousins a bit, second cousins a small bit and people in the general gene pool a very small amount. We assume that this argument would allow us to sustain the concept that the match probability in the race of the accused is elevated a small amount by knowledge of the accused's genotype.

We hasten to add that this effect is small and we are not advocating that the match probability for the race of the accused should take predominance in the interpretation unless other evidence such as a reliable eyewitness suggests that the offender is of a certain race. For the record we state that the offender is the person who committed the crime. The person of interest may or may not be this person and his ethnicity does not inform the ethnicity of the offender directly.

Choice of Database

In the United Kingdom the policy is to quote the match probability for the race of the POI and make an appeal to simplicity and pragmatism.[60,264] This policy is typically conservative, but we would have been warmer to a more rigorous approach.

The default situation in most other laboratories of which we are aware is to quote either a range of match probabilities for various racial groups that predominate in the area of the crime or the most common match probability from among these groups. This set is typically supplemented by another probability assignment often made from literature sources if the accused is of some race not represented in the default set. This approach is perfectly supportable scientifically and has the beneficial potential to give a feel for the behaviour of the estimates across racial groups.

If there is some reason to focus on one racial group such as eyewitness evidence or because the alternative suspects are largely from one racial group, then that match probability may be used.

The match probability is usually, but not always, highest for the racial database to which the accused belongs. This is true whenever there is heterogeneity in allele probabilities across ethnic groups; it is the basis of ethnic inference.[264]

There is a seldom applied method that is likely to be superior and in our view to reduce the chance of confused lines of thinking in court. That is modelling the general population as the sum of the component races. Each racial estimate is weighted in some sensible way such as the census frequency or from assignments made with regard to the circumstances of the crime. This method can remove any mention of the race of the accused at all and may ameliorate the risk of the line, 'my client is half Abernaki, half French Canadian, what is the match probability in that group'.[503,507]

Choice of Population Genetic Model

In Chapter 3 we described three population genetic models in common use. These are the product rule and NRC II Recommendations 4.1 and 4.2. It is a great pity that we do not have a better set of names for NRC II Recommendations 4.1 and 4.2. This situation has allowed the very false impression to grow that these recommendations are both a subpopulation correction. NRC II Recommendation 4.1 corrects for within-person correlations, and since we are interested only in the chance of a second person having a certain profile, it is only the between-person correction behind Recommendation 4.2 that has any logical basis. This is unfortunate because Recommendation 4.1 is incumbent in the United States.

The two approaches with a logical basis are the product rule and Recommendation 4.2. Since the product rule is Recommendation 4.2 with $\theta = 0$, they may be viewed as variants of each other.

Simulation testing[365,366] suggests that the product rule has a mild bias in favour of the prosecution relative to the known truth of the simulation. Please note the words *the known truth of the simulation* and differentiate this wording from a statement that we cannot make about a truth in a population. Recommendation 4.2 has a large bias in favour of the defence relative to this known truth in the simulation. This suggests that Recommendation 4.2 is suitable for criminal work but unsuitable for civil work. In civil work the product rule is preferred.

Tippett testing (see Chapter 3) of Recommendation 4.2[367-371] has been undertaken out to about 1 in 10^{10}. The relatively low values for θ needed to get acceptable fits of observed and expected suggest that all three models, the product rule and Recommendations 4.1 and 4.2, will have acceptable performance as long as close relatives are considered and we are prepared to overlook the claims of logic.

We are prepared to subjectively accept that, however probable an x locus match may be, an $x + 1$ locus match will be less probable. We believe this to be true until such a time as the only matches are monozygotic twins. Therefore if we can empirically support Recommendation 4.2 out to 1 in 10^{10}, we are prepared to assert that the probability continues downwards as more loci are added. We cannot see any other conclusion as supportable from theory and experiment. Whether the extrapolation of Recommendation 4.2 is exact when the match probability is 1 in 10^{20} is unknown, but although the relative uncertainty may be large the absolute uncertainty, we believe, is minimal. We therefore assert that, from our own understanding, we are prepared to work with the assignment of Recommendation 4.2 to any level of extrapolation.

General Match Probability Values

In their work to validate Second Generation Multiplex Plus (SGM Plus) for its first use in the United Kingdom, Foreman and Evett[458] have suggested that 'case specific match probabilities should not be calculated as a matter of principle'. Instead they suggest the use of 'general figures'. Below we give the calculated figures for the most common profiles for an SGM Plus 10 locus match and the suggested reported value:

- One in 8300 for siblings, which they suggest reporting as 1 in 10,000

- One in 1.3 million for parent/child reported as one in a million

- One in 27 million for half-siblings or uncle/nephew reported as one in 10 million

- One in 190 million for first cousins reported as one in 100 million

- One in 2.4 billion for members of the same subpopulation reported as one in a billion

- One in 5 billion for unrelated persons, also reported as one in a billion, irrespective of the ethnicity of the individuals concerned

Ian Evett has consistently stated that this position was provisional and that it would be modified when new data enabled the investigation of the robustness of the independence assumptions necessary to assign smaller match probabilities. His view has always been that a rational basis for assigning a match probability of the order of one in a trillion can only follow from an experiment that has enabled around one in a trillion comparisons between unrelated people.

This approach has been accepted practice in the United Kingdom. Foreman and Evett motivate their approach by stating that 'the independence assumptions are sufficiently reliable to infer probabilities that are of the order of 1 in tens of millions' but that SGM Plus case-specific match probabilities would 'invoke independence assumptions to a scale of robustness which we could not begin to investigate by statistical experiment....'

Hopwood et al.[468] continue the UK line when considering a new set of 15 loci, the European standard set (ESS), reprising the 'independence assumption' argument of Foreman and Evett. They argue that Tippett tests have been undertaken up to about a billion trials[368] and hence one in a billion may be substantiated but no further.

In Chapter 3 we discussed the Tippett test undertaken by Tvedebrink.[368] There are six matches at ten out of ten loci. We accept that these are most likely to be the same person sampled twice and hence are comfortable with their removal from the analysis. Others differ. Recall that there are 1.3×10^{10} pairs of nine locus comparisons. If we assign the probability of a 10 locus match as one in a billion (1×10^{-9}), we would suggest that the match probability for a nine locus match would be greater. Since we would expect more than 13 such matches and we see none we would interpret this as evidence that one in a billion is too large a probability for a nine out of ten locus match and hence too large for a 10 locus match.

The approach of Foreman and Evett appeared to follow the logical line of calculating a match probability for unrelated, same subpopulation and different classes of related using the most common SGM Plus genotype. The calculation method used was their 'current practice', which included most importantly the use of a subpopulation correction assigned at 0.02. Subsequent to this calculation a probability was assigned higher (in most cases) than this number. There is an inevitable subjective element to probability. In the above we have avoided the word *estimate* and used *calculate*. However we have some level of belief in the performance of the Recommendation 4.2 model and that the θ used is at the upper end of the plausible distribution. Is the output of this calculation a fair and plausibly conservative assignment of probability?

The assigned *LRs* for the most common genotypes assuming various relationships for the ESS accounting for subpopulations and linkage are given in Table 7.1.

We again have a transatlantic split in procedure with North America typically quoting the estimate however small it may be. The Foreman and Evett and Hopwood et al. papers make the statement that numbers lower than one in a billion 'invoke independence assumptions to a scale of robustness which we could not begin to investigate by statistical experiment'. We are unaware of this statement being used in court in challenge to smaller match probability assignments. In fact the general probability selected in Australia is 1 in 100 billion. Hence we would conclude that the between-locus assumptions must be more robust in Australia than in the United Kingdom.

Christophe Champod of the Université de Lausanne stated, 'I still favor an order of magnitude (10^9 or 10^{10}) is adequate to convey the extreme strength of the information with the great benefit of not falling into the "uniqueness" pitfall'.

Table 7.1 The Assigned Likelihood Ratios for the Most Common Genotypes for Various Relationships for the European Standard Set Accounting for Subpopulations and Linkage Following Bright et al.[56,588]			
Relationship	Caucasian	Indo-Pakistani	Afro-Caribbean
Unrelated	6.01×10^{13}	1.06×10^{14}	1.24×10^{14}
Full siblings	2.20×10^{5}	3.43×10^{5}	2.88×10^{5}
Parent/child	6.40×10^{7}	1.56×10^{8}	9.49×10^{7}
Half-siblings or grandparent/ grandchild	2.02×10^{10}	6.46×10^{10}	3.93×10^{10}
Uncle/nephew	2.05×10^{10}	6.58×10^{10}	4.00×10^{10}
First cousins	7.97×10^{11}	2.14×10^{12}	1.93×10^{12}

Franco Taroni of the Université de Lausanne stated, 'I favour an order of magnitude of, for example, 10^{9}, because I believe that a scientist should be able to defend the "reality" of the number he/she presents in front of a Court of Justice. Could we be able to justify orders of magnitude greater than 10^{10}?'

More recently during discussions about the Australasian standard for DNA interpretation, the argument has been advanced that avoiding the case-specific calculation saves time or training.

We admit the pragmatism and intuitive appeal of this approach. Objections would range from the practical to the philosophical and will be mentioned briefly here.

- The relative reliance upon independence assumptions and Mendel's laws differs markedly between the calculations for siblings to the use of the product rule. For siblings most of the procedure leading to a probability assignment is based on the assumption that alleles assort in a Mendelian fashion and only to a very small extent on independence assumptions within a population. Hence these calculations are much less affected by uncertainties about independence.

- The probability assignments that are advocated in this chapter are really based on belief in a model.

In the first edition of this book the following was written:

- A general match probability of one in a billion is not likely to induce further refinements of the model or simulate further sampling and study.

- What would we do if we added more loci?

If we come to the subject of saving, training one must really despair. Is this really to be the future of our science?

This is a subject that appears to evoke strong opinions although Evett has regularly expressed his flexibility if new data become available. However this is a case where there is a balance of rational argument on either side and a strong position appears, to us, unwarranted.

In general we would on slim balance prefer to assign a probability, whatever it may be, but to accept and make explicit that very low probabilities cannot yet be verified experimentally. We would greatly prefer to press for research, experimentation and higher standards of training and reporting. If general values are used, we would prefer that they be based on the reasonable line of Champod or Taroni, which suffices to give the impression of rarity; smaller numbers run the risk of ridicule.

In any case, for 24 loci, it is all about relatives.

Same Source?

The following apparently reasonable question has arisen: when can a DNA profile match be considered proof that two DNA samples have come from the same source? In 1997 a policy of source attribution[589,590] was suggested when the assigned match probability was below a certain value, set at 2.6×10^{10}. This approach harked back to a statement by the National Research Council report.[176] The approach has been implemented in some, but not all, jurisdictions in the United States.[591] The source attribution paper was followed by a critique of the mathematics by Weir.[475] Weir, a highly respected population geneticist, stated

> A forensic scientist may well decide not to present any numerical testimony in a DNA case and simply state that the failure to exclude a defendant from an evidentiary profile based on many loci provides very powerful evidence. However, if that statement rests on false numerical calculations then the cause of forensic science is not advanced. It may be that the false calculations are conservative, but this is not a scientific basis. There is also the danger that they are not conservative. In an age when profile probability calculations are performed by computer, there is no justification for violating population genetic theory simply to invoke simple equations.

The reply from the authors of the original paper appealed to pragmatism.

The term *same source* is used in this discussion to describe this situation as it best approximates the underlying forensic question. Other terms such as *uniqueness*, *source attribution* and *individualization* have been used elsewhere. This situation has led to considerable discussion of the use of these terms, which has also produced useful philosophical debates about their meaning. We cannot do justice to these arguments and simply direct the reader to the well-written work by Champod and Evett[235] on the equivalent subject in the area of fingerprints (see also the response by McKasson[592] and the more balanced commentary by Crispino[593] or the excellent writing of Inman and Rudin[175]).

The question of whether we can ever base a conclusion of common source on a probabilistic argument has also been examined, most notably by Stoney,[594,595] Champod[596] and Evett et al.[457] In the DNA context we can see that, using the current population genetic models, the more loci we add, the smaller are the match probabilities produced by our model. There are three important points with regard to this. First, the match probability derived from the model can approach zero but never actually equal zero. Second, very small match probabilities arising from models cannot be directly tested. They are as reliable or unreliable as the models themselves. Third, we recognize that we are considering an extreme extrapolation using these models. We are not operating near the centre of their prediction range where they are more testable and tested. The models have been extensively tested in this central range and there is some considerable reason to believe that they are robust there, but they are still models and the probabilities produced by them are still untestable.*

To conclude same source from a probabilistic model someone has to decide that the match probability produced by that model at this extreme end of extrapolation is sufficiently reliable that it can be trusted and the probability sufficiently small that it can be ignored. Stoney terms this the 'leap of faith'.

Inman and Rudin[175] in describing this situation state, 'at some subjective point, most qualified authorities would agree that, for practical applications, the likelihood … is so small that it can be ignored'. In the text following this quote they very clearly set out the subjective nature of this decision.

There has been considerable argument about whether a scientist should do this or leave the matter to the court. Certainly in England and Wales the court direction appears to be that the scientist should abstain from deciding whether the probability is small enough to ignore.[172]

---

* To quote Ian Evett, 'Is it rational for me to assign such a small match probability?'.

Inman and Rudin[175] agree: 'It is the purview of the fact finder to draw inferences from circumstantial evidence, and, of course, potentially individualising physical evidence is circumstantial evidence. However, there are pieces of information that only science can legitimately provide to the fact finder, such as population frequencies, transfer and persistence data, and limitations of the evidence and the test'.

It is unclear whether the scientists should even be the persons who decide on the reliability of the model. It is regrettable to us that, as we add more loci, we extrapolate the model further and further, but we have added some, but we wish much more experimental data on the reliability of the model at this extreme extrapolation. Robertson and Vignaux[163] complained about a similar lack of fundamental research in the area of fingerprints:

> ... the expert is giving evidence of identity ... This may have had the unfortunate effect of removing the incentive to carry out the basic research to build appropriate models.

Source attribution is the norm in many disciplines of forensic science. These are largely areas where numerical evaluation is not currently possible. Examples include firearms, toolmarks and shoeprints. The area of fingerprints has also been treated this way, but its history appears different. In its early development, numerical treatments were attempted[597-602] and there have been many efforts over the duration of fingerprint evidence to refine the models.[235,603-613] Source attribution in fingerprints, therefore, may not have been a response to perceived impossibility of numerical presentation.

In DNA work early presentation of evidence inherited its conceptual framework from serology. Serology had been quoting a match probability for a certain blood type and this approach was adopted into DNA presentation. As systems became more discriminating, the assigned match probability became smaller. There had always been a suggestion that DNA profiles might be individual specific. In fact Sir Alec Jeffreys published a paper in 1985 that was entitled 'Individual specific fingerprints on human DNA'.[9] Certainly by the 1990s the question 'what do such numbers mean?' was often asked. In an apparent desire to spare the jury from contemplations with probabilities of an unfamiliar magnitude, there was a desire to give a plain English expression of the evidence.

> Academic quibbling does not justify exposing the jury to mind-numbing numbers that, as many defense attorneys will tell you, may well actually be prejudicial to the defendant (since they invite the jury to conflate them with probability of innocence.)[614]

A reasonable distinction has been made between the judgment in one particular case and the judgement in all potential cases.[591] We could imagine a criterion that was considered reasonable in an individual case, and Budowle et al.[591] suggest '99% confidence'.* They go on to suggest that this may correspond with the expression *a reasonable degree of scientific certainty*. This phrase has been selected because of its legal implications.

> From the medical model has come the phrase "to a reasonable scientific certainty." Both the judicial system and some experts have latched onto this phrase as a convenient way to render an opinion as fact. As convenient as it might be, it is a non sequitur. As we have repeatedly discussed throughout this book, the notion of scientific certainty does not exist. In our opinion, scientific experts should refrain from resorting to that phraseology in expressing their opinions.[175]

This raises the interesting but unimportant matter of the various colours of certainty. In the literature we have met absolute certainty, moral certainty and practical certainty, as well as scientific certainty. Dr Tacha Hicks-Champod has even brought the notion of ballistic certainty to our attention.[615,616]

---

* This term needs thought. There is a distinction between the use of the words *confidence* and *probability*.

Kaye[616] is critical of certainty statements that actually obscure uncertainties: '...experts should not be permitted to avoid the limitations in their knowledge simply by qualifying assertions of uniqueness with a fig leaf such as "to a reasonable degree of ballistic certainty"'.

More recently the US National Commission on Forensic Science stated: 'Forensics experts are often required to testify that the opinions or facts stated are offered "to a reasonable scientific certainty" or to a "reasonable degree of [discipline] certainty"…. It is the view of the National Commission on Forensic Science (NCFS) that the scientific community should not promote or promulgate the use of this terminology'.[617]

The method used by Budowle et al. stems from a suggestion by NRC II, who discussed the use of the formula $p_x \leq 1-(1-\alpha)^{1/N}$, where p_x is the match probability, N is the size of the suspect population and $1 - \alpha$ is the confidence interval. They give an example using a 99% confidence interval $(1 - \alpha) = 0.99$, implying $\alpha = 0.01$ and $N = 260,000,000$, the approximate population of the United States at that time. This logic suggests a match probability of $p_x = 3.9 \times 10^{-11}$. It is suggested that the estimated p_x be decreased by a factor of 10 to provide additional conservativeness. Weir[475] correctly points out the flaws in this approach, which unreasonably assumes independence of trials.

Also included in the original publication is a brief mention of relatedness. In particular they recommend typing of relatives. The typing approach to dealing with relatedness is admirable but is applied only rarely in the United States, Australia, United Kingdom and New Zealand. In the absence of typing they suggest that the match probability for brothers be calculated or that calculations should be performed (when required) for three classes of people: unrelated, subpopulation members and relatives. They do not give a specific formulation of how to amalgamate the contribution from relatives and unrelated people, directing the reader, correctly, to Balding.[618]

This division of the population into unrelated, subpopulation and related persons is akin to the coarse division undertaken by Balding. The unifying formula suggests that it is the weighted sum of all three contributions that should be considered, not simply one of these probabilities.

The unifying formula will assign a posterior probability to the proposition that the suspect is the donor of the stain material. This appears to be the probability that is desired in 'source attribution'. However, the unifying formula will require an assignment of prior probabilities, which cannot be avoided. It is central to the concerns about the concepts of source attribution and a reasonable degree of scientific certainty. We see therefore that any approach to assigning a posterior probability involves a prior. This idea is, of course, not an original insight and was reported as long ago as 1983[226] in forensic science and much earlier in other sciences.

There is an interesting interplay between the prior for the suspect and the probability that someone else possesses this profile. Balding and Donnelly explained this[275]:

> Finally, we remark that the magnitude of the size biasing effect … is related to the prior distribution. Intuitively, the effect occurs because, under the hypothesis of innocence, two distinct τ-bearers* have been observed. Such an observation stochastically increases the number of τ-bearers, thus decreasing the strength of the evidence against the suspect and decreasing the probability of guilt. Decreasing the prior probability of guilt increases the chance that the suspect and criminal are distinct, hence increasing the effect of size biasing. (David Balding and Peter Donnelly quoted with the kind permission of CRC Press.)

This effect can easily be illustrated. Suppose that we have a certain profile at a crime scene and that it matches a suspect. However the suspect, for whatever reason, cannot have been the

---

* This is the term used to describe the people carrying the matching profiles. In this case the defendant and the true perpetrator.

donor (his prior is 0). Then the probability that someone else possesses this profile goes from whatever value it was before to 1.

> Consider a crime scene DNA profile which is thought to be so rare that an expert might be prepared to assert that it is unique. Suppose that, for reasons unrelated to the crime, it is subsequently noticed that the crime scene profile matches that of the Archbishop of Canterbury. On further investigation, it is found to be a matter of public record that the Archbishop was taking tea with the Queen of England at the time of the offence in another part of the country. (You may consider your preferred religious leader, beverage, and head of state in place of those named here.) A reasonable expert would, in light of these facts, revise downwards any previous assessment of the probability that the crime scene profile was unique. However, this is just an extreme case of the more general phenomenon that any evidence in favour of a defendant's claim that he is not the source of the crime stain is evidence against the uniqueness of his DNA profile.[618] (David Balding, quoted with the kind permission of *Science & Justice*.)

David Balding warns

> Although attractive in some respects, a practice of declaring uniqueness in court would lead to substantial difficulties. [Later in the same article] Perhaps the most problematic assumption underlying the calculation of a probability of uniqueness is the assumption that there is no evidence in favour of [the defendants]. In some cases there is evidence favouring the defendant. More generally, it is usually not appropriate for the forensic scientist to pre-empt the jurors' assessment of the non-scientific evidence.[618]

We could also envisage a great many other types of non-DNA evidence that could affect our view that a certain profile was unique or not. However the key point to note is that the question of the probability of a second copy of a profile cannot be answered fully from the knowledge of the match probability and the population size alone.

To quote Evett and Weir, 'we have difficulty with a statement of the form, "In my opinion, the crime sample was left by the suspect" ... such a statement cannot be made without invoking a prior of some kind – unless, like the fingerprint expert, we believe the *LR* to be so large that it does not matter how small the prior is'.

Balding[618] also makes the valid point that one brother in a population may have a more significant effect on the probability of a second copy than all the other unrelated people. This point was picked up by Buckleton and Triggs.[373] The original authors of the source attribution paper[589] did produce a criterion for related and unrelated individuals separately. However the key point in the work of Balding and Buckleton et al. is that there is no need for evidence specifically pointing to a relative; all that is required is for the relative to be among the non-excluded alternative donors.

The supposition that the Budowle et al. approach is necessarily conservative is of concern. An appeal is often made at this point to the increase in the frequency assignment by a factor of 10 and the relatively large value chosen for N (260 million). The factor of 10 was intended to compensate for potential sampling error or subpopulation effects or both. Examination of the unifying formula suggests that it may be inadequate especially when many loci are considered. It is also likely to be inadequate to compensate for both subpopulation effects and sampling error, and it certainly cannot compensate for the effect of uneliminated brothers.

Budowle et al. make it clear that this approach is designed for a case by case application. If we misapply this method to the question of 'are such profiles unique in the United States', we will soon be embarrassed. There are 3.38×10^{16} pairs of people in the United States. If we use the match probability suggested for the 99% probability interval $p_x = 3.9 \times 10^{-11}$ and assume that the factor of 10 recommended as additional conservativeness was included, then $p_x = 3.9 \times 10^{-12}$. This match probability suggests that there will be an expectation of about 132,000 matching pairs of unrelated people in the United States. In fact a database of about 716,000 profiles all with a match probability of $p_x = 3.9 \times 10^{-12}$ would have an expectation of about one match. In reality full CODIS (Combined DNA Index System) profiles produce match probabilities less than this.

Table 7.2 The Size of Databases That Give the Expectation of One Match		
	$\theta = 0.00$	$\theta = 0.03$
US African Americans	43,000,000	11,000,000
US Caucasians	34,000,000	9,300,000
US South-Western Hispanics	21,000,000	5,900,000

Bruce Weir[497] estimates that we would expect a full CODIS match among unrelated people if the databases were of the size shown in Table 7.2.

Despite the careful wording in the paper of Budowle et al., our suspicion is that it will be read as providing a declaration of uniqueness among all people and hence such an adventitious match will cause a public embarrassment. Certainly the view is developing among the public that DNA profiles are unique.

The situation is probably slightly worse when we consider relatives. The expected number of matches when relatives are included in the population or database will be larger. It is likely that there are a number of pairs of persons matching at the 13 CODIS loci in the whole US population. Many of these matching sets will be brothers. The chance that two of these would be involved in the same crime is small, but the matches will eventually be revealed as the size of databases increases and will embarrass forensic science if we have declared such profiles unique.

Findlay and Grix[197] have studied juries and report a strong pre-existing prejudice that is pro-DNA. It is likely that many jury members wrongly believe that all DNA findings represent certain identification. It would be worrying to foster this belief.

There is a considerable body of publication by science and law commentators almost ubiquitously opposed to forensic scientists making statements of source attribution. Largely these criticisms may be divided into those that state that such a proposition is unproven or unprovable, that it is not the province of a scientist to make such a statement or that it inappropriately makes assumptions about the non-DNA evidence.

Many of the articles arguing against the policy of source attribution argue that it is not proved or impossible to prove (see for example Ref. 619). The approach used in the DNA context proceeds via statistics although other means of proof could be envisaged. However in the DNA context we proceed by assigning a match probability and then asserting that the chance of a second copy of this profile in a population of size N is sufficiently low that it may be ignored. As previously discussed this ignores information of relevance to the problem, but for the purposes of this argument all we need to note is that the probability of a second copy, however calculated, is never zero. Therefore a statement of source attribution based on statistics is in itself probabilistic. It is a match probability reprocessed with a set of further assumptions. Although this method may sound simple, it is more complex mathematically and conceptually and makes more assumptions than the underlying match probability. For the interested reader the extra assumptions include the following:

1. The size of the relevant population

2. That there is no non-DNA evidence in favour of the suspect

3. That the profiles in the population are independent

4. That there are no relatives in the population of interest

The New Zealand code of conduct for expert witnesses[620] states that a witness should 'state the facts and assumptions on which the opinions of the expert witness are based'. It could easily be argued that a bald statement of source attribution fails in this regard, or at best that all the assumptions are rolled in to the clause 'a reasonable degree of scientific certainty'. In a recent court ruling in the area of shoeprint comparison[586] their Lordships were critical of the lack of disclosure of a formula lying behind a verbal opinion. Again this criticism would appear to apply to a statement of source attribution.

If we accept that a statement of source attribution is to be made via a statistical approach, then there are two elements. First, we need to accept that the match probability statistic is sufficiently reliable, and the other assumptions such as the size of the population and the relevance of relatives are met or approximately met. Second, we need to accept that the assigned probability of a second copy of the profile is sufficiently low that it may be ignored. The argument, which is ubiquitously supported in our search by legal writers, is that the decisions as to the reliability of the statistic and the acceptability of the other assumptions are for the judge and jury, not the scientist (see for example Refs. 621–623). It would be very difficult to assert that a scientist is better prepared to make these decisions especially as they may not have heard all the admissible evidence and further may have heard some inadmissible evidence.

Stoney[595] argues that there is no route to source attribution via statistics. He argues that, however small the statistic may be, the move to an assertion of source attribution is a 'leap of faith'. He adds the telling comment that such approaches are only superficially objective. He defines probabilities as objective when they can be tested and reproduced. Microprobabilities fail in the testability criterion, at least at this time, because we can only test the models behind them to a certain extent. Probabilities of the order of 10^{-12} are at this time untestable, although good efforts have been made out to 10^{-10}.[367,369-372]

Kaye[616] argues '... the problem with using probability theory to demonstrate uniqueness is not that the probability of duplication always exceeds zero. The difference might be too small to matter. Such demonstrations are generally unconvincing because it is so hard to establish that the models are sufficiently realistic and accurate to trust the computed probabilities'.

Kaye's statement would appear to indicate the pragmatic stance that such small probabilities may be disregarded but that the weak point is that some models cannot be trusted at this level of extrapolation. Kaye is referring to identification sciences in general, which include DNA, fingerprints, shoeprints and toolmarks at least. It is plausible that the models in DNA are the strongest of these and hence the objection in DNA may be lessened but not completely removed.

Later in the same article Kaye[616] concludes,

> In sum, a well founded and extremely tiny random-match probability indicates that, ... the match at issue is not merely a coincidence; rather, it is a true association to a single source. It is therefore ethical and scientifically sound for an expert witness to offer an opinion as to the source of the trace evidence. Of course, it would be more precise to present the random-match probability instead of the qualitative statement, but scientists speak of many propositions that are merely highly likely as if they have been proved. They are practicing rather than evading science when they round off in this fashion.

We would read this as stating that source attribution is acceptable if the models are judged to be sufficiently reliable and the match probability sufficiently small but that he would still prefer the actual number to be given.

In an in-depth review on the subject, Roth[624] appears to argue for a threshold based on the match probability alone in the context of whether a judge should let a DNA case that only has DNA evidence go to a jury. This situation is obviously different from a scientist asserting source attribution.

Dr Hicks-Champod brings to our attention the realistic risk that a threshold on certainty might mean that all evidence below this threshold is discarded or severely discounted even though it has considerable value.

There is significant pressure, for example from the National Academy of Sciences report,[323] to rethink the policy of source attribution for areas such as fingerprints or firearms. It would seem a great pity for DNA to proceed in the opposite direction. Forensic DNA consultant Norah Rudin has provided us with the telling quote,

> Forensic DNA evidence should not stand apart from other forensic disciplines. The presentation and communication of the strength of forensic DNA data must be considered in the context of forensic science as a whole. Ideally, a comprehensive model would support the determination and expression of the weight of evidence across the breadth of forensic disciplines.

Policy in science is usually made via the international peer-reviewed literature. In forensic science there is also the effect of court rulings. Given the lack of published support for a policy of source attribution and criticism by some very respected commentators, we must ask why the policy persists. Butler[258, p. 297] gives a very balanced review. Butler also reprises the example of two Israeli brothers from an endogamous community that share 31 of 32 alleles[625] and more recently an example of brothers sharing 27 of 30 alleles was reported.[626]

If we do not take a source attribution approach, we are assigned the task of stating that the evidence is extremely powerful and remains so regardless of almost any factor of which we can realistically conceive without actually stating that it is conclusive.

Our feeling is that we would be unwise to conclude that two samples come from the same source because it is not our place to do so. If we do so, we would prefer the standard to be much higher than previously suggested *and* we would like to make it transparent that we have subjectively decided to round a probability *estimate* off to zero. On balance we cannot see much positive coming from a policy of declaring that two samples have a common source.

Single Source Samples: Significant Possibility of Dropout

This section deals with the forensic analysis of low levels of DNA. Previously terms such as *low copy number* (LCN) or *touch DNA* have been used to describe this or related fields, and nomenclature has become confused. This topic will be discussed in this chapter.

Many strategies to increase sensitivity have been employed. Increasing the number of cycles,[29] whole genome analysis nested PCR,[627–629] post-PCR clean-up,[144] reduced reaction volumes[630,631] and increased injection volume.[632] Useful comparisons of the methods exist, one favouring increased cycle number over whole genome amplification or nested PCR[633] and others favouring post-PCR clean-up over increased cycle number.[145] Reducing reaction volumes can also be useful to save on reagents or to preserve sample for subsequent reanalysis. However for the purpose of this section the significant finding is that reducing the reaction volume but maintaining the template DNA quantity leads to increased signal to noise ratio and hence enhanced sensitivity.

Modern multiplexes appear to have much improved sensitivity even at 28, 29 or 30 cycles. It has become recognized that the effects of low template levels may occur independently from the technology. We will discuss changes in profile morphology that occur when there are very few starting templates and the issue of contamination. In addition we will consider the ideas that have been offered on interpretation of profiles that have been or may have been affected by the morphological changes and contamination risks associated with ultra-trace work.

The analysis of trace evidence was anticipated in 1988 by Jeffreys et al.[634] Subsequently, the successful typing of single cells was first reported in the mid-1990s.[29,127,635–640] The typing of DNA from fingerprints,[640–643] touched paper,[644] latex gloves,[645] debris from fingernails,[646,647] epithelial cells,[648,649] single hairs[650,651] clothing,[652,653] cigarettes,[654] formalin-fixed, paraffin-embedded tissues[655] and biological material on strangulation tools[656] has been reported. Full or partial profiles of transferred DNA were obtained up to 10 days after simulated strangulation.[332]

The author of the simulated strangulation work also noted the presence of DNA from a third party in some experiments. Sutherland et al. report the typing of fingerprints after development with fingerprint powder but warn, wisely, that the brush and powder may be a source of carry-over from previous brushings since the brush is usually placed back into the powder multiple times when brushing previous prints.[657]

The approach to using enhanced sensitivity in DNA analysis originated largely in Australia and has led to a field of forensic work that was subsequently termed *LCN* in the United Kingdom. This term has become problematic. For historic reasons and so that this discussion may be placed in the larger context, we will retain the term but will restrict its use to describe a 34-cycle method. This approach was launched into casework in January 1999 in the United Kingdom and subsequently in New Zealand and the Netherlands. However closely related approaches are in use in many European countries and New York in the United States (albeit 31 cycles). Aside from the variation in the number of PCR cycles used to increase sensitivity, there is also variation in interpretation strategy. The variation among European Network of Forensic Science Institutes members was demonstrated in a reported summary. Of note, 11 laboratories report using elevated cycle number (greater than 28 cycles but not necessarily 34 cycles) in some cases for low template DNA (LTDNA).[658]

These methods broaden the potential impact of forensic science but may also bring with them additional challenges with regard to interpretation issues.[659] More recently we have realized that there was nothing new in these challenges. They had existed in traditional 28 cycle work whenever the profile was low level. Modern multiplexes often are run at 29 or 30 cycles. This further emphasizes that a 28 versus 34 cycle divide is unhelpful.

LTDNA and LCN

One approach to analyzing samples suspected of having low levels of DNA is to raise the number of PCR amplification cycles from 28 to 34. This technique has become known commonly as *LCN analysis*. This label has not proved helpful as it confuses the issues of a technique (34 cycles) with the sample on which the technique is used.[660] The very name, *LCN*, encourages this confusion. As noted, there are other methods available for increasing the sensitivity.

To begin to clarify this situation Caddy et al.[36] introduced the term *LTDNA* for DNA with low levels of DNA. This has proved to be a marked step forward. Clearly the quality of the result from a technique may depend on the quality of the sample. Even the result from a very low quality sample is not invalid as long as it is correctly interpreted.

We will refer to the particular variant of 34 cycle work used in the Netherlands and in New Zealand as *LCN* to clearly differentiate a technique (LCN) from a type of sample (LTDNA). However we support the suggestion of Gill et al.[660,661] for a complete abandonment of the term *LCN*.

Template levels are strictly integral in that there can be 1, 2, 3, ... copies of any particular template. However amplification is a stochastic process such that the final signal is essentially continuous. If we persist with the use of the term *LTDNA*, we need to recognize that we are referring to one end of an essentially continuous scale. Gill et al.[662] suggest dealing with the continuous nature of the scale by assessing a probability of dropout based on the height of the survivor allele (the allele that is above-threshold).

If we are to have LTDNA, we need a label for DNA that is not *low template* and the term *conventional* has been used. However, perhaps there is a deeper issue: arbitrary thresholds on continuous scales have not been particularly successful in the past. The impression is given that above the threshold all is good and below it all is bad. This impression is false and laced with traps into which the adversarial process could happily lead discussion. Using the terms *LTDNA* and *conventional* may enhance the misconception of a clear divide rather than emphasizing continuous variation. The Forensic Science Service in England and Wales had, for some time prior to its demise, used a three level scale using the terms *red*, *amber* and *green*. Three levels more nearly express the underlying continuous variation. The red, green and amber zones are defined almost exclusively on peak height.

The amount of DNA in a sample is not known *a priori*. Methods are available to assess the starting DNA, and many laboratories include this step, known as *quantification*. Quantification is now recommended for all DNA samples. However quantification results tend to be unreliable especially at low levels. There are very clear examples of low or nil quantification results giving full profiles and considerable quantification results giving nil profiles. In addition the quantification result refers to the total human DNA present and hence does not directly inform the template levels of the minor component of a mixture. This subject is reviewed well in Butler.[258, p. 159]

Gill et al.[660] have suggested diagnosing the existence of low template levels *post hoc* by effects observed in the profiles themselves. These effects include locus dropout, allele dropout, extreme heterozygote imbalance, extreme stuttering, allele drop-in and differences between duplicates from the same sample. Such results are the normal result of low template levels and are collectively termed *stochastic effects*.

- *Locus dropout* describes the event when no alleles are observed at a locus.

- *Heterozygote balance* refers to the relative heights of the two peaks of a heterozygote. All things being perfect these two peaks are expected to have the same height.

- *Allelic dropout* describes the event when one of the two alleles of a heterozygote cannot be observed. Allelic dropout is the extreme expression of heterozygote imbalance. We note that allelic dropout should not be diagnosed from a profile by assuming the POI is a contributor but could reasonably be inferred from sub-threshold peaks.

- *Stutters* arise during the PCR and produce small peaks usually one repeat unit smaller than the parent allele peak.[135] Stutters can be assessed by a ratio (stutter ratio) of the height of the stutter peak height to the parent allele peak height.[661,663]

- *Allelic drop-in*[117] is the observation of single alleles detected in a profile that are not from the sample. They are most often from traces of randomly fragmented DNA found either in the laboratory environment or from reagents and plasticware used in the DNA profiling process.

The concept of defining *LTDNA* from a diagnosis of the likely presence of significant stochastic effects appears a sensible approach. The availability of duplicate profiles that differ in allele presence and significantly in peak imbalances is proof of the existence of stochastic effects.

Experienced examiners appear to be able to infer that stochastic effects should be expected even from a non-replicated profile. They do this largely from the peak heights but may also make some holistic assessment of the profile describing profiles as 'clean' or 'balanced'. When questioned about the process, these examiners mention a number of factors:

- Are the peak heights above a preset threshold?

- Are the peaks balanced across the loci in the lane? This compares the heights of the peaks in the low molecular weight and high molecular weight loci.

- Is the baseline noisy?

- Is there evidence of a mixture? If not, are the peaks at a locus balanced?

Other suggestions exist. For example, Budowle et al.[31] suggest that all profiles that give a quantification value of 200 pg or less should be both defined and treated as LTDNA. Defining LTDNA on a quantification result appears unsound to us not only because of the uncertainty in the actual template level, but also because it is one further step removed from the nub of the matter: the magnitude of expected stochastic effects. We have been approached by lawyers soliciting comment for the defence who want an answer to the question, 'What level in pg do you consider to be the threshold between LTDNA and normal template?' This is silly. We are probably guilty of fostering this with the title of one of our early papers 'An investigation of the rigor of interpretation rules for STRs derived from less than 100 pg of DNA'.[117]

This then is a key point of differentiation among commentators and is also one where the wording of terms is not always helpful. For the purposes of interpreting DNA it is not the template level that we require, per se, but an assessment of the likely extent of stochastic effects. The differentiation between commentators then is whether we are to infer the likely presence of stochastic effects from either a quantification result, failure at 28 cycles, observed stochastic effects in replicates or inferred from peak heights in the resulting profile.

In the first edition of this book we had a separate chapter for mixtures and for LCN. In this edition we have retained a chapter for mixtures and rewritten the LCN chapter as a LTDNA section. In the intervening years it has become apparent that LTDNA issues pervade other work and especially mixtures with minor or trace components. The distinction between normal and LTDNA work has become unhelpful, and it has become apparent that LTDNA is simply one end of a continuum that affects all our work.

There is another term often associated with this field. This is *touch DNA*.[35] We must advocate strongly against its use. *Touch DNA* gives the impression that we know how a latent DNA stain was deposited. This may be true in research but will seldom if ever be true in casework. Equally, in research trials, touch DNA is not necessarily LTDNA and LTDNA not necessarily touch.

Non-Concordance

Concordant allele: This term was introduced by Balding and Buckleton[113] to replace the previously commonly used term, *surviving allele*. Consider an *ab* suspect and a crime profile that shows an *a* peak only. This peak is termed the *concordant allele*. The term *surviving allele* has an unfortunate implication that the true donor is *ab*.

Non-concordant allele: This is an allele in the suspect profile, the *b* in the example, that is not present in the crime profile. These have also been termed *voids*, which has the same poor implications as the term *surviving allele*.

Transfer and Persistence

Increased sensitivity methods readily allow the examination of less than 100 pg of total genomic DNA.[29,104] It is expected that 3.5 pg contains one haploid DNA template, therefore 100 pg should equate to approximately 30 templates. This increase in sensitivity facilitates the examination of a whole new range of evidence types that previously could not be analyzed because of the very low amounts of DNA recoverable from the sample. Variables affecting recovery of DNA have been discussed.[664]

The amount of DNA deposited by contact between a donor and an object appears to depend on the donor. Some people are observed to be 'good shedders', which means that their DNA is easily transferred to objects simply by touching them. There appears to be day-to-day variability in this property. Others people are 'poor shedders' who deposit little DNA, with a range of propensities in between[640,643,648,665-667] (for a different result see Balogh et al.,[644] who found no difference for their four subjects). The reason for these differences between people are as yet unknown but are not thought to be sex dependant. Quinones and Daniel[668] have also challenged the conclusion that individuals can be classified as *good* or *poor shedders*. They suggest that DNA deposition is a *multifactorial trait* related to the amount of cell-free nucleic acids present in an individual's sweat and also to an individual's habits such as how often a person might rub his or her eyes. Kamphausen et al.[669] demonstrated that individuals with active skin diseases (atopic dermatitis and psoriasis) are more likely to transfer epithelial cells suitable for DNA analysis prior to treatment for their skin condition. Both sets of authors agree that extrinsic factors such as temperature or air moisture are likely to influence profiling success and more research is warranted.

Secondary transfer has also been observed. In such a case DNA has been seen to transfer from a good shedder to the hand of a poor shedder and then subsequently onto a touched object, usually as part of a mixed profile including both the good and poor shedder (see Lowe et al.[670] for an excellent review). This finding was not replicated when Ladd et al.[666] repeated the work.

Transfer probabilities have been used to predict expected transfer in multistep transfers. It was found that unrealistically large initial amounts of DNA may be needed to explain detectable levels after multiple transfer steps.[671]

The time of day that a person touched paper or whether or not they had recently exercised did not affect the amount of DNA detected.[644] The strongest signal in a mixture is not necessarily from the last person to touch the paper.[640,644]

Along with the increased sensitivity has come a greater need for strict efforts to reduce contamination at the scene, in the consumables[328,672] and in the mortuary[673,674] and laboratory[675] (again Balogh et al.[644] have dissenting results finding no contamination issue in their study). The use of protective clothing[330] and masks at scenes reduced, but did not eliminate, the possibility of transfer from the scene officers. Talking and coughing increased transfer, hence it is advisable to wear face masks and full protective clothing in the laboratory. A 'no talk' policy in the laboratory has been mooted. Negative controls may have to be introduced from the scene onwards.[141] Decontamination procedures such as UV irradiation may not be adequate.[676]

The presentation of this, and indeed all, evidence requires care. For example, it should be made explicit to the court that issues of transfer and relevance, which are always pertinent, come into even greater prominence for LTDNA.[665,677]

The Interpretation of Profiles Where Dropout Is Possible

In this section profiles will be described as having spurious alleles or having undergone dropout. These statements would be accurate only if we knew the true genotype that should appear in the profile. In real casework this genotype will never be known. The correct phrasing would be to describe bands as spurious or as having dropped out *if* the prosecution proposition, H_p, were true. This phraseology is cumbersome and will be dropped in the remainder of this discussion. However we emphasize that bands are not known to be spurious or to have dropped out. We are simply naming them as such.

Most laboratories define a threshold, T or *Mixture interpretation threshold (MIT)*, below which dropout is deemed possible. This threshold is typically assigned from validation data either as the largest surviving peak of a heterozygote where one peak has dropped out or somewhere near the maximum ever observed.

Loci with this situation have historically been omitted or interpreted with the $2p$ rule. We discuss this strategy below.

The Selection Model

Most laboratories replicate on an as-needed basis at 28 or 29 cycles, although at higher cycle numbers the policy is often to replicate routinely. When replication is undertaken at 28 or 29 cycles, it is usually because the first attempt has not produced a satisfactory outcome. In such cases the conditions are usually changed. More or less DNA may be injected depending on what was thought to be the problem, the sample may be diluted or other conditions changed. As such the repeat sample is not a true replicate.

If one profile is close to valueless the scientist may disregard it and base the interpretation entirely on the other. This is perfectly fair.

By selecting the most informative or reliable profile, forensic biologists can be accused of bias (choosing a profile that 'fits' the prosecution proposition) or 'replicate shopping'. Having preset rules for the selection of the most informative profile typically ameliorates this bias as would ignorance of the reference profiles at the time of the decision. Conversely, selecting the least informative profile wastes information.

If the two profiles are both informative in some sense, selecting one must waste some information.

The Composite Model

In its most pure form a composite profile relates to replicate amplifications from one extract. Any allele that is confirmed in any replicate is assembled into a composite profile. Hence if an *a* allele is observed in replicate 1 and a *b* allele in replicate 2, then the composite profile is *ab*. Variants on this process occur, in that there may be a composite of injections from different amplifications of either the same or a closely related sample. We are, for example, aware of composites being developed from swabs of items taken from close but different areas.[678]

A composite DNA profile is described as a 'virtual profile' because it is an artificial construct. This approach seeks to generate a more complete (virtual) profile by including all alleles observed in all of the replicates in a combined profile.

Composite profiles are the least conservative option resulting in the highest number of loci incorrectly called heterozygotes and mixtures, due predominantly to drop-in or stutters incorrectly identified as alleles.[679]

A comparison of the composite method versus a semi-continuous model (described below)[680] for the analysis of replicate DNA profiles has shown that the composite method is conservative with respect to, or approximates, the semi-continuous model, when certain conditions are met. These include where the rate of drop-in, C, is low or preferably zero and due care is taken regarding non-concordant alleles and the number of contributors. These warnings were also described by Benschop et al.[679] Where the composite profile contains non-concordances with the person of interest, a consideration of the probability of dropout is required.

The composite approach should never be preferred to the semi-continuous model and should not be used at all unless these conditions are met. The traditional complexities around uncertainty in the number of contributors[681,682] and around non-concordant alleles[114,115] still exist but, as far as we can see, no new complexities have been introduced, provided that all of the suspect's alleles have been observed in the composite result under H_p.

The ability to sustain the composite approach was a surprising outcome to us. The composite profile approach has developed without any formalization or application of caveats. Consequently we had, and retain, intuitive reservations about the approach. However we can only support a composite approach as an interim, 'low tech' solution. Better solutions exist that utilize the full information present in the replicates. These include the semi-continuous model[114,117] and the continuous model (such as TrueAllele and STRmix).[110,111]

The Consensus Model

A consensus profile is one where an allele is only reported provided that it appears in at least two replicate analyses – where replicates are typically carried out in duplicate or in triplicate. There are variants of this generalized approach which are discussed and summarized at length by Benschop et al.[679] Benschop et al. introduced a useful nomenclature where the number of replicates is n and the number of instances of an allele that is required for reporting is x. Hence the consensus method could be $n = 2^+$, $x = 2$, whereas the composite method could be $n = 2^+$, $x = 1$.

Sometimes the terms are confused. For example, the recommended checklist of questions pertaining to LCN evidence provided by the UK crown prosecution service[683] specifically asks the following: 'Does the evidence include composite results obtained by taking DNA information from different stains or sources (on a garment for example)?' The word *composite* is substituted for *consensus* and further confused with results that have not been obtained from the same DNA extract. Clear definition is important.

Guidelines for reporting LCN (recall we mean a certain 34-cycle technology) profiles have been developed and published.[104] These guidelines are based on concept that all LCN samples will be analyzed in duplicate, at least.

The first step in this process is to compare duplicate profiles and note which alleles are present in both profiles. These alleles are scored in the consensus profile. After this process there may be zero, one, two or more alleles at each locus. It can be very difficult to determine whether the resulting consensus profile represents one or more individuals. In normal 28-cycle casework we conclude that if there are more than two alleles scored at a locus, then there is more than one individual present. In LCN casework these rules break down. Three alleles may be the result of a reproduced contaminant and zero, one or two alleles at each locus or may still represent two individuals with allelic overlap or dropout. Hence the decision as to how many individuals are present in the consensus profile is one of the more problematic decisions in LCN casework. Currently this decision[*] is based on a subjective assessment of the quality of the profile and peak areas, but this decision is always tentative.

Let us assume that the consensus profile is thought to be from a single individual. Any loci that have zero alleles in the consensus profile are typically treated as inconclusive and assumed not to affect the *LR*. Under this model the loci with two alleles, both of which match, are interpreted as normal, although it is important to remember that LCN work cannot be reported with the same confidence as normal work and important caveats should be made. The loci with one allele will have been denoted by, say, 16F, indicating the presence of the 16 allele and 'anything else'. These are typically reported using the $2p$ rule or an equivalent.

These intuitive guidelines are based on biological principles. We have compared them against a statistical model and have identified some areas of concern. Of note is that we can no longer state that the $2p$ rule is always conservative. The model and the insights we have developed from it are the subject of the next section.

The Semi-Continuous Model

Since we accept that LTDNA profiles can be affected by dropout, the appearance of spurious alleles (termed *drop-in*), high levels of heterozygote imbalance and variable stuttering, we believe that they suit a different method of interpretation. Consider the procedure for interpreting 'normal' single contributor DNA profiles, which proceeds via a series of steps including the following:

- Consider which propositions are relevant in this case.

- Assign the alleles present in the profile. This step will involve assigning peaks as allelic, artefactual or ambiguous.

- Determine whether the comparison is a match or a non-match.

- Estimate a match probability or preferably an *LR* for this evidence.

When we discuss mixture cases (Chapter 8) we will introduce the well-accepted concept that there may be ambiguity in the genotypes present. For instance, a locus showing four alleles a, b, c and d of approximately the same peak heights may be a mix of ab and cd, or ac and bd, or any other combination of alleles. The inability to explicitly nominate which genotypes are present in a mixture is not an impediment to interpreting the mixture as long as reasonable safeguards are followed. This interpretation is especially facilitated by the semi-continuous model approach. At least with many mixtures we can nominate which peaks are allelic and which are not. However with mixtures where one component is present in low proportions it may be impossible to decide, say, whether a peak is allelic or is due to stuttering from a larger adjacent peak. Again this inability to nominate peaks as allelic or not is not a fatal impediment to interpretation, and methods exist to handle this ambiguity. These methods are explicitly incorporated into David Balding's software LikeLTD.[684] When we consider LTDNA, we must accept that we have even further levels of ambiguity, specifically:

- Peaks that are present may be allelic, stuttering or spurious.

- Alleles that should be present may have dropped out.

---

[*] Again this issue is markedly ameliorated by the semi-continuous model approach. A 'decision' as to how many individuals are present is not needed. In fact the consensus approach is not required at all. Rather the probability of the replicates is calculated conditional on each of all the realistic possibilities.

Under these circumstances it may be unrealistic to unambiguously assign a genotype to a sample. It may, in fact, be very difficult to determine whether the evidence supports the presence of one or more contributors. These factors suggested that a completely different approach to interpreting profiles was warranted. Rather than try to assign genotypes from the sample, we are better served to consider the probability of the electropherogram (epg) *given* various genotypes. In the following section we will outline an approach to this. However the reporting officer must be warned that not only will the evidence take greater skill to interpret and explain, but also the very concept that the scene profile and the genotype of the suspect may differ will undoubtedly be a source of questioning in court. The key to interpreting and understanding this type of evidence is to think of the probability of the evidence *given* a genotype, not the other way around. The semi-continuous model has been extended and programmed by James M. Curran for the UK Forensic Science Service into a software called LoComatioN that was never released publicly and into LRmix by Gill et al.,[685] LikeLTD by Balding,[684] FST by Mitchell et al.[686] and Lab Retriever by Rudin and Lohmueller.[107]

The semi-continuous model that we are about to present contains a number of assumptions. It treats bands as present or absent and takes no account of peak height. In the LTDNA context it is likely that this loss of information is not too extreme as peak height is less informative than at higher template levels.[687] The model has allowed us to examine the behaviour of the binary and consensus models in a useful way. The *LRs* produced by this statistical model suffer from all the uncertainties associated with the assignment process for any DNA profile plus a few new and larger uncertainties. Hence *LRs* calculated for LTDNA will be more reliant on modelling assumptions than those calculated for ordinary template levels.

The Gill et al.[103] model was adapted by Balding and Buckleton[113] and it is this latter adaption that we follow here:

Term	
D	The probability that an allele of a heterozygote drops out (averaged across alleles and loci).
D_2	The probability that both alleles of a homozygote drop out (averaged across alleles and loci).
C	The probability that a contaminant allele appears at a locus.
St	The probability that an allele makes a stutter peak above threshold.
Q	Stands for any allele other than those already named in the equations.
$P_{i\|j}$	The probability of alleles i (ordered if more than one) given alleles j. Because of the way we are writing this the heterozygote *ab* is written $2P_{ab\|j}$.
α	Is defined by the equation $D_2 = \alpha D^2$.

To keep the nomenclature under control we write $\bar{D} = 1 - D$, $\bar{D}_2 = 1 - D_2$ and $\bar{C} = 1 - C$.

For simplicity we model the continuous events of contamination or dropout as discrete. Under this simplified model an allele either drops out or it doesn't; contamination either happens or it doesn't. Ignoring peak area in this way leads to a loss of information. We suggest that the probabilities C, D and D_2 should be estimated from experimental data.

A Binary Statistical Treatment*

Suppose that n replicates have been analyzed. We term these $R_1, R_2, ..., R_n$.

---

* Hereinafter referred to as the *semi-continuous model*. The term *drop model* is also in use internationally and we may lapse into that usage sometimes.

Propositions are defined as follows:

H_p: The DNA in the crime stain is from the suspect.

H_d: The DNA in the crime stain is from someone else.

We can write

$$LR = \frac{\Pr(R_1 R_2 ... | H_p)}{\Pr(R_1 R_2 ... | H_d)} \qquad (7.1)$$

We assume that the events of dropout, drop-in and stutter in one replicate are independent of those in the others. We accept that this assumption is unlikely to be true if fixed values are used for their probabilities.

> But there will be values of C and D for which independence holds – this is an argument for estimating C and D or integrating them out rather than assigning them.
>
> **David Balding**

Using this assumption we obtain

$$\Pr\left(R_1 ... | M_j\right) = \prod_i \Pr\left(R_i | M_j\right) \qquad (7.2)$$

It is necessary to specify the 'components' of H_d. By this we mean that the 'expert' determines a set of possible 'random man' genotypes worth considering, M_1, M_2, ..., M_n. These genotypes will be exclusive but not necessarily exhaustive. This step is actually unnecessary as it is possible to postulate all possible random man genotypes and sum over all possibilities. It does however markedly simplify manual implementation if the list can be shortened by judgement.

$$LR = \frac{\Pr\left(R_1 R_2 ... | H_p\right)}{\sum_i \Pr\left(R_1 R_2 ... | M_j\right)\Pr\left(M_j\right)} \qquad (7.3)$$

Hence:

$$LR = \frac{\prod_i \Pr\left(R_i | H_p\right)}{\sum_j \prod_i \Pr\left(R_i | M_j\right)\Pr\left(M_j\right)} \qquad (7.4)$$

We evaluate the LR using Equation 7.4. To calculate $\Pr(R_i|M_j)$ we assume that the events of drop-in and dropout are independent both of each other and of M_j. We assume that the M_j profiles are from the same subpopulation as the suspect. Drop-in alleles are modelled without a subpopulation correction. It is convenient to analyze the components separately in tabular format. This will be demonstrated by example.

Example 7.1: A Heterozygotic Suspect and Replicates Showing Apparent Dropout

We begin by considering profiles which potentially include spurious peaks and dropout. Later we will consider stuttering. Suppose a crime stain was analyzed in two separate replicates (R_1 and R_2) and two different results were observed at the D18S511 locus: R_1 = 12; R_2 = 12,16. The suspect (S) was 12,16.

Consider the following propositions:

H_p: The DNA in the crime stain is from the suspect.

H_d: The DNA in the crime stain is from someone else.

For these propositions, we calculate the LR, using the format in Table 7.3, and proceed as follows.

Step 1: Assess the reasonable random man genotypes from the information in the replicates. List these in column M_j.

Step 2: Calculate $Pr(M_j)$ in the second column.

Step 3: Calculate $Pr(R_i|M_j)$ in the rows R_1, R_2 and R_3.

Step 4: Calculate the products of each row.

Step 5: Sum the products $= \bar{D}\bar{D}_2 C\bar{C} P_{12,12|12,16} P_{16} + 2\bar{D}^3 D\bar{C}^2 P_{12,16|12,16} + \bar{D}_2 DC^2 P_{12} P_{12} P_{16,16|12,16}$.

Step 6: The numerator is the product $Pr(R_i|M_j)$ corresponding to the genotype of the suspect. In the example (Table 7.3) this appears as part of the term at the right-hand side of the second row corresponding to the genotype 12,16 but without the frequency term for $Pr(M_j)$ $\bar{D}^3 D\bar{C}^2$.

Step 7: Assemble the LR by taking the appropriate terms in the numerator and the appropriate sum in the denominator.

$$LR = \cfrac{1}{\cfrac{\bar{D}_2 C}{\bar{D}^2 DC} P_{12,12|12,16} P_{16} + 2P_{12,16|12,16} + \cfrac{\bar{D}_2 C^2}{\bar{D}^3 \bar{C}^2} P_{12} P_{12} P_{16,16|12,16}} \quad (7.5)$$

Provided that C is small (<0.3) the expression is approximately

$$LR \approx \frac{1}{2P_{12,16|12,16}} \quad (7.6)$$

Table 7.3	A Layout for Example 7.1			
Possible Random Men, M_j	$Pr(M_j)$	$Pr(R_1 = 12\,|M_j)$	$Pr(R_2 = 12,16\,|M_j)$	Product
12,12	$P_{12,12|12,16}$	Allele 12 not dropped No drop-in $\bar{D}_2 \bar{C}$	$\bar{D}C P_{16}$	$\bar{D}\bar{D}_2 C\bar{C} P_{12,12|12,16} P_{16}$
12,16	$2P_{12,16|12,16}$	Allele 12 not dropped Allele 16 dropped No drop-in $\bar{D}D\bar{C}$	$\bar{D}^2 \bar{C}$	$2\bar{D}^3 D\bar{C}^2 P_{12,16|12,16}$
16,16	$P_{16,16|12,16}$	Allele 16 dropped drop-in by allele 12 $D_2 C P_{12}$	$\bar{D}_2 C P_{12}$	$\bar{D}_2 DC^2 P_{12} P_{12} P_{16,16|12,16}$

The biological model would have given a consensus profile of 12 and would have reported a LR of $LR \approx \dfrac{1}{2\, p_{12|12,16}}$. Hence we see that the biological model is conservative relative to the semi-continuous model in this case.

Applying the Semi-Continuous Model

We have applied this approach to a number of common situations. The results are given in Table 7.4.

A large simplification is possible if we can express D_2 in terms of D. The simplest suggestion is to write $D_2 = D^2$, which is equivalent to assuming that an allele drops out independently with known probability D.[99,688] This is likely to overstate D_2 if both alleles can generate partial signals that combine to reach the reporting standard, whereas each individual signal would fail to reach this standard.[114] Some limited empirical data exists in support of this suggestion. At 34 cycles it may be that a single template can produce an above-threshold peak. If true, then the independence assumption may be reasonable.

Another plausible assumption is that $C = 0$ at 28 cycles. Certainly experienced biologists have asserted that they have not observed drop-in at 28 cycles. These two assumptions, while each strictly false, lead to such a simplification of the equations in Table 7.4 that a comparison with current practice is much facilitated.

Is the 2p Rule Conservative?

We consider the situation where a locus shows one peak, say a, below the stochastic threshold (termed *MIT* by Budowle et al.[102]). It is customary, and correct, to allow that this may be either a homozygote aa or a heterozygote aQ, where Q stands for any other allele, this other allele, Q, having dropped out. A rather simplistic approach, and one to which we all subscribed until a few years ago, is that a conservative approach was to assess the frequency of such a profile as $2p$, where p is the frequency of the a allele. This is the origin of the term $2p$ *rule*.

Table 7.4		The Formulae for the Semi-Continuous Model for Apparently Single Source Stains		
		Numerator of the *LR*		
R_1	R_2	$S = aa$	$S = ab$	**Approximate Denominator of the *LR*[a]**
aa	–	$\bar{D}_2\bar{C}$	$DD\bar{C}$	$\bar{D}_2\bar{C}P_{aalj} + 2DD\bar{C}P_{aQlj}$
	aa	$\bar{D}_2^2\bar{C}^2$	$D^2\bar{D}^2\bar{C}^2$	$\bar{D}_2^2\bar{C}^2 P_{aalj} + 2D^2\bar{D}^2\bar{C}^2 P_{aQlj}$
	ab	$\bar{D}_2^2\bar{C}CP_b$	$DD^3\bar{C}^2$	$\bar{D}_2^2\bar{C}CP_b P_{aalj} + 2D^2\bar{D}^2\bar{C}CP_b P_{aQlj} + 2DD\bar{D}^3\bar{C}^2 P_{ablj}$
ab	–	$\bar{D}_2CP_b$	$\bar{D}^2\bar{C}$	$\bar{D}_2C\left(P_bP_{aalj} + P_aP_{bblj}\right) + 2\bar{D}^2\bar{C}P_{ablj}$
	ab	$\bar{D}_2^2C^2P_b^2$	$\bar{D}^4\bar{C}^4$	$\bar{D}_2^2C^2\left(P_b^2 P_{aalj} + P_a^2 P_{bblj}\right) + 2\bar{D}^4\bar{C}^4 P_{ablj}$
abc	–	$2\bar{D}_2C^2P_bP_c$	$\bar{D}^2CP_c$	$2\bar{D}^2C\left(P_cP_{ablj} + P_bP_{aclj} + P_aP_{bclj}\right)$
	ab	$2\bar{D}_2^2C^3P_b^2P_c$	$\bar{D}^4CP_c\bar{C}$	$2\bar{D}^3C\left(\bar{D}CP_cP_{ablj} + DC\left[P_b^2 P_{aclj} + P_a^2 P_{bclj}\right]\right)$

Note: The – symbol means that no second test was done. Since the order of the replicates does not matter some combinations are not entered.

LR, likelihood ratio.

[a] The conditioning alleles are termed j.

Table 7.5 A Layout for the 2p Rule Example

Possible Random Men, M_j	$Pr(M_j)$	$Pr(R_1 = a \mid M_j)$	Product
aa	$P_{aa\mid ab}$	$\bar{D}_2\bar{C}$	$\bar{D}_2\bar{C}P_{aa\mid ab}$
aQ	$P_{aQ\mid ab}$	$\bar{D}D\bar{C}$	$\bar{D}D\bar{C}P_{aQ\mid ab}$

To progress further it is helpful to call the probability of the ith allele p_i and hence the frequency of the a allele is p_a. Since the genotype of the true contributor is either aa or aQ, we assess the probability of this, using the product rule, as $p_a^2 + 2p_a(1-p_a) = 2p_a - p_a^2 < 2p_a$. This was the (false) rationale that led to the (false) belief that the $2p$ rule was always conservative.

There was a clue that this thinking was false and we all should have noticed earlier. Let us imagine that the stochastic threshold is 200 rfu. Imagine that we have an ab suspect. If we have a single a peak at 201 rfu this is an exclusion; however if this peak is 199 rfu, then it is an inclusion assigned a frequency $2p_a$. We should have noticed that this sharp transition from exclusion to inclusion was an indication that something was awry in our thinking.

Our own way into the problem came from application of the semi-continuous model described above. Since we only consider one replicate, the algebra is much easier. Above (Table 7.5) we give our standard layout for this problem.

Let us consider two propositions:

H_p: The suspect (ab) is the donor of this stain.

H_d: A random man is the donor of this stain.

For these propositions, we obtain

$$LR = \frac{1}{2P_{aQ\mid ab} + \frac{\bar{D}_2}{\bar{D}D}P_{aa\mid ab}} = \frac{1}{2P_{a\mid ab}\left(P_{x\mid aab} + \frac{\bar{D}_2}{2\bar{D}D}P_{a\mid aab}\right)}$$

Clearly the term $\frac{\bar{D}_2}{2\bar{D}D}P_{a\mid aab}$ can be larger than 1 depending to a considerable extent on the magnitude of D. Hence the LR can be much less than $LR = \frac{1}{2P_{a\mid ab}}$, which is the equivalent of the $2p$ rule. In fact it can be less than 1. Accordingly we conclude that the $2p$ rule is not always conservative and, since the LR may be less than 1, we cannot even advocate omitting this locus as conservative.

Non-conservativeness arises if there is other evidence to suggest that dropout is unlikely, such as a high height for the observed allele or no indication of stochastic features in the rest of the profile.

David Balding

This aligns with those of the DNA commission of the International Society of Forensic Geneticists,[689] the UK Technical Working Group,[660] the European Network of Forensic Science Institutes[690] and the Biological Scientific Advisory Group.[691]

If the $2p$ rule or omitting the locus is not reliably conservative, what can we do? At this stage we can envisage three options:

1. Change to the semi-continuous or continuous model and report an LR based on that. This method will require numerical assessment of the probability of dropout and drop-in.

2. Use the semi-continuous or continuous model to assess an *LR* and use that to check that the 2*p* rule, omitting the locus or other action is reasonable. Then proceed with the 2*p* rule, omitting the locus or other action.

3. Develop a set of heuristics that suggest when the 2*p* rule, omitting the locus or other action is reasonable. These heuristics could include the height of the concordant allelic peak and the presence of a sub-threshold (alternatively referred to as *PAT*) peak in the non-concordant allelic position. Presumably we would do experiments modelling the risk of falsely reporting the weight of evidence to assess what heuristics were viable.

We now consider the same crime profile but with an *aa* suspect:

$$LR = \frac{1}{2P_{a|ab}\left(\dfrac{P_{a|aab}}{2} + \dfrac{\bar{D}\bar{D}}{\bar{D}_2}P_{Q|aab}\right)}$$

Since $\bar{D} < \bar{D}_2$ and $D < 1$ the term $\dfrac{\bar{D}\bar{D}}{\bar{D}_2} < 1$ and hence $\dfrac{P_{a|aab}}{2} + \dfrac{\bar{D}\bar{D}}{\bar{D}_2}P_{Q|aab} > 1$. This suggests that the 2*p* rule is always conservative for an *aa* suspect.

This analysis and examination of the tables suggests a general principle that is as yet unproved but highly intuitive. This principle would be that the biological model is likely to be unsafe whenever the suspect possesses alleles that cannot be seen in the profile.

We draw one further conclusion from this examination: it is not possible to decide whether the biological model, the 2*p* rule or any other interpretation method, such as RMNE, is likely to be conservative without knowing the genotype of the suspect.

Dropping Loci

The argument given above extends straightforwardly to the concept of dropping loci in either single source or mixed profiles. In a single source profile, a locus with no peaks at all above threshold (a blank locus) would often be omitted from the calculation. This has a very minor, and we suggest inconsequential, risk. It is slightly easier to drop out both peaks of a heterozygote than the single peak of a homozygote of the same total template. Hence there is very mild evidence that a blank locus is a heterozygote. As stated this risk is very minor and we suggest inconsequential.

Of slightly greater risk are non-concordant alleles in a mixture. The risk depends on the expected (not the observed) heights of the non-concordant peaks. The risk is very minor if we can extrapolate the heights of the minor component from, say, the low molecular weight alleles and state that the expected height of these alleles at this locus is very low (preferably below threshold). If the expected height is above threshold and the alleles are non-concordant, then the risk is more considerable.

The only way to quantify the risk is the semi-continuous or continuous models.

Bias

There have been persistent allegations that the *LR* approach involves some significant risk of bias because it requires knowledge of the suspect's profile.[31,33,35,101,103,692] For example:

> Another difficulty, particularly with mixtures, is determining what allele constitutes a drop-in. In fact, these vagaries tend to create bias in deciding whether there is support for contamination.[31]
>
> Interpretation of the evidence profile contemporaneously with the reference profile is indicative of bias and is anathema to the objective nature of forensic science.[31]
>
> In the Budowle et al. (2) guidelines a locus is deemed inconclusive prior to the comparison, unlike the approach that seems to be advocated by Gill and Buckleton. It is vital to avoid interpretation bias based on the suspect's profile.[32]

These statements are some of the clearest indications that the nature of the model that we have previously explained has not initially been grasped by the critics and this is plausibly the cause of much of the discussion. Take an example of an epg showing two peaks a and b. If we are to model this as coming from a single donor with an aa genotype, then we need to model the b peak as a drop-in event. This is not to say that it is a drop-in event, nor has it been assigned as a drop-in event. For example, when the probability of this same epg is considered and the hypothesized genotype is ab, then there is no need to model the b peak as a drop-in. Hence the b peak is neither assigned as drop-in nor is it assigned as allelic. Simply the probabilities of obtaining this epg from different genotypes are modelled using the concepts of *drop-in*, *dropout* etc. In fact one of the benefits of the statistical model is that peaks do not need to be assigned as allelic, stutter or drop-in. We can see no bias in application of the model but rather see the release from the need to assign peaks as a great buffer against bias. It must be apparent that no method can actually decide whether a peak is a contaminant or not and hence it is very hard to see how the comments quoted above could arise.

Paradoxically, we have demonstrated that the suggestion to use the $2p$ rule without reference to the suspect profile may lead to substantial bias against the defendant.

The approach we advocate can be written down in a step-wise manner and is open to scrutiny. It can be, and has been, programmed.[108,114,686,688,693] It can be applied by different people to the same epgs and should give the same result. Therefore it would meet most tests for objectivity. There is some evidence of emerging consensus.[694]

8

Complex Profiles

John S. Buckleton, Duncan Taylor, Peter Gill,
James M. Curran and Jo-Anne Bright

Contents

Introduction

This chapter deals with the analysis of complex DNA profiles. We have defined these as any mixed sample, whether or not one or more components are at low template levels. The analysis of forensic stains will inevitably lead to mixtures of DNA from different individuals, as a result of the mixing of body fluids and secretions. The recognition, resolution and statistical evaluation of such mixtures are therefore integral and vital parts of forensic casework. The subject is relatively complex and requires experience and judgement. It is often treated as a separate competency by forensic organizations. Often scientists move to mixture interpretation after experience with simple stains. It is desirable that a formal training and testing programme be associated with this transition.

The typing of mixed samples may be undertaken using autosomal DNA or with Y chromosome or mitochondrial analysis. Each has advantages.[695]

Low template levels are known to lead to substantial changes to profile morphology such as greater peak imbalance, dropout and, at enhanced sensitivity, the almost unavoidable appearance of contaminant alleles.[99,100] In 1999 standard methods for interpretation appeared inadequate for some low template DNA (LTDNA) work and new methods and safeguards appeared desirable.[31–33,35,101–103,696,697]

Peaks from a heterozygote may be very imbalanced, with one or other of the alleles giving a much larger peak. This imbalance may be sufficiently extreme that the heterozygote appears to be a homozygote – usually this is termed *dropout*.

Such changes to profile morphology are likely to be due to sampling effects in the template.[98] While sampling is thought to be the main driver of stochastic effects, an early polymerase chain reaction 'event' such as a stutter in the first cycle when there are very few templates might theoretically have a large effect on subsequent peak heights.[98]

Heterozygote imbalance increases as the amount of DNA template is reduced.[104,632] A number of methods have been developed to facilitate the evaluation of evidence from mixed profiles. These methods include the following:

- Random man not excluded (RMNE) or cumulative probability of inclusion (CPI)
- Random match probability (RMP)
- Likelihood ratios (*LRs*)

Calculation of *LRs* dominates our own experience and rightly dominates the literature. Most of the rest of this chapter is devoted to calculating *LRs* that are accepted as being more powerful. However we will briefly introduce the other methods. For RMNE we largely follow Budowle[698] and for RMP we follow Bille et al.[699]

The Scientific Working Group on DNA Analysis Methods (SWGDAM) makes the following recommendation: '4.1. The laboratory must perform statistical analysis in support of any inclusion that is determined to be relevant in the context of a case, irrespective of the number of alleles detected and the quantitative value of the statistical analysis'.[106] When we first drafted this section, we added the simple phrase 'we agree'. However this position needs a rethink. The statement given by SWGDAM can be, and has been, interpreted as meaning that every positive association in a case needs a statistic. This is massive overkill and makes statements unreadable. Taken to the extreme, blood at the scene matching the deceased who is also at the scene would need a statistic. Our feeling is that selected highly probative samples in every case tending to inclusion of the person of interest (POI) should have a statistic. This might mean about three statistics in a complex case of hundreds of samples. These samples should be selected to answer the key questions likely to be of interest to the court.

The Sampling Formula

The addition of the subpopulation correction to mixtures is based on the application of the sampling formula.[358,455] It is useful to introduce the sampling formula for a simple single stain case first. Here we follow Harbison and Buckleton[700] who were assisted in their development by David Balding.

If x alleles are type a out of a total of n alleles sampled from the subpopulation, then the probability that the next allele observed will be of type a is

$$\frac{x\theta+(1-\theta)p_a}{1+(n-1)\theta} \qquad \text{(8.1) 'The sampling formula'}$$

where θ is the coancestry coefficient and p_a is the probability of allele a in the population. This is the basis for Equations 4.10 in the NRC II report and 4.20 in Evett and Weir.[176,257] For a stain at a scene that is typed as containing only the alleles a and b, matching a suspect of type ab, we require the probability that the unknown true offender is of type ab given that the suspect is of type ab. We write this as Pr (*offender is ab | suspect is ab*). In such a case, the LR

$$LR = \frac{1}{\Pr(\text{offender}=ab\,|\,\text{suspect}=ab)} = \frac{\Pr(\text{suspect}=ab)}{\Pr(\text{offender}=ab\,\&\,\text{suspect}=ab)},$$

which can be written as

$$LR = \frac{1}{\Pr(ab\,|\,ab)} = \frac{\Pr(ab)}{\Pr(ab\,\&\,ab)}$$

Application of the sampling formula follows from this last expression. Starting with the numerator we consider each allele in turn; the order is unimportant. Take allele a first. Application of the sampling formula gives $\frac{(1-\theta)p_a}{1-\theta} = p_a$ ($n=0$ and $x=0$; no alleles have previously been sampled and no alleles of type a have previously been seen). Next we take the allele b ($n=1$ and $x=0$; one allele has been sampled but no b alleles have yet been seen), which gives $\frac{(1-\theta)p_b}{1} = (1-\theta)p_b$. This gives the numerator as $2(1-\theta)P_aP_b$, a factor of 2 being included for each heterozygote.

A similar argument follows for the denominator. We have a factor of 4 because we are considering two heterozygotes. Turning to the alleles we consider the first a ($n=0$ and $x=0$), the first b ($n=1$ and $x=0$), the second a ($n=2$ and $x=1$) and the second b ($n=3$ and $x=1$) giving the denominator as

$$\frac{4(1-\theta)p_a(1-\theta)p_b[\theta+(1-\theta)p_a][\theta+(1-\theta)p_b]}{(1-\theta)(1)(1+\theta)(1+2\theta)} = \frac{4(1-\theta)p_ap_b[\theta+(1-\theta)p_a][\theta+(1-\theta)p_b]}{(1+\theta)(1+2\theta)}$$

Hence the LR follows by dividing the numerator by the denominator:

$$LR = \frac{(1+\theta)(1+2\theta)}{2[\theta+(1-\theta)p_a][\theta+(1-\theta)p_b]}$$

Most practising forensic scientists do not proceed in this manner. There are a number of shortcut rules that have been developed that allow the formulae to be written down directly.[701] These proceed from the conditional form of the probability. They can be seen to follow from the recursive formula given by Balding and Nichols.[455]

Shortcut Rules
Permutations
The number of permutations is the number of ways that the alleles can be arranged as pairs. In general the number of permutations at a locus exhibiting m_i copies of allele A_i is given by

$$\binom{2N}{m_1, m_2, ..., m_l} = \frac{2N!}{m_1! m_2! ... m_l!} = {}^{2N}P_{m_1, m_2, ..., m_l}$$

where $2N$ is the total number of alleles at the locus and m is the number of times each allele is seen at the locus. The exclamation point denotes a factorial. The factorial of a positive integer j, denoted by $j!$, is the product of all positive integers lower than or equal to j.

Shortcut Process
The shortcut rules are demonstrated by way of examples given below. These are not really formal derivations but are just a set of rules that allow the answer to be written down. With practice this method becomes second nature. We begin by writing the probability in the conditional form. In front of the conditioning bar we place the genotype(s) of the possible offender(s). Behind the bar we place the conditioning genotype(s). This should always include the suspect but in some circumstances other profiles may also be included. This has become an area of some debate which is covered in a short section later in the chapter.

Example 8.1: The Calculation of Pr($aa|aa$)

Although our purpose is to demonstrate the application of this process to mixed stains, it is easiest to start with a simple example of a case where the stain at the scene is unmixed and shows the genotype aa. The suspect is aa. Hence we see that the only genotype for possible offenders is aa and the only potential conditioning profile is that of the suspect, also aa. Accordingly in this example we consider the calculation of the conditional probability Pr($aa|aa$) shown figuratively in Figure 8.1. The following three steps are required to obtain the formula.

Apply a factor of ${}^2P_{1,1} = 2$ if the possible offender is heterozygous. The possible offender will be the term in front of the conditioning bar. In this example the possible offender is the homozygote aa, therefore no factor of 2 is required.

Counting from the back towards the front, label each allele as the first of this type seen, second of this type seen and so on. Replace each of the possible offender's alleles with the terms

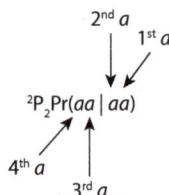

Figure 8.1 A diagrammatic representation to assist evaluation using the shortcut rules for a matching homozygote.

given in Table 8.1. It is necessary to proceed from one of the ends of the offender's genotype. For instance, in the calculation of $\Pr(aa|aa)$, we see that the homozygote aa in front of the conditioning bar is treated as the 3rd and 4th a alleles.

Divide by a correction term based on the number of alleles in front of and behind the conditioning bar as shown in Table 8.2.

This yields the familiar formula $\Pr(aa\,|\,aa) = \dfrac{(3\theta + (1-\theta)p_a)(2\theta + (1-\theta)p_a)}{(1+\theta)(1+2\theta)}$.

Example 8.2: The Calculation of Pr(ab|ab)

Consider the calculation of $\Pr(ab|ab)$ shown diagrammatically in Figure 8.2. Application of the rules leads quickly to the familiar formula.

$$\Pr(ab\,|\,ab) = \frac{2(\theta + (1-\theta)p_a)(\theta + (1-\theta)p_b)}{(1+\theta)(1+2\theta)}$$

Table 8.1	The Conversion of Terms Using the Shortcut Rules
1st allele a	$(1-\theta)p_a$
2nd allele a	$\theta + (1-\theta)p_a$
3rd allele a	$2\theta + (1-\theta)p_a$
4th allele a	$3\theta + (1-\theta)p_a$

Table 8.2	The Correction Terms
Two alleles in front, two behind	$(1+\theta)(1+2\theta)$
Two in front, four behind	$(1+3\theta)(1+4\theta)$
Two in front, six behind	$(1+5\theta)(1+6\theta)$
Four in front, two behind	$(1+\theta)(1+2\theta)(1+3\theta)(1+4\theta)$
Four in front, four behind	$(1+3\theta)(1+4\theta)(1+5\theta)(1+6\theta)$
Four in front, six behind	$(1+5\theta)(1+6\theta)(1+7\theta)(1+8\theta)$
N in front, M behind	$[1+(M-1)\theta]\ldots[1+(N+M-3)\theta][1+(N+M-2)\theta]$

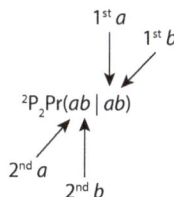

Figure 8.2   A diagrammatic representation to assist evaluation using the shortcut rules for a matching heterozygote.

Example 8.3 A Simple Mixture Example

As a more practical example consider the following where the complainant (of Race 1) has been genotyped as *ab*, the suspect (of Race 2) has been genotyped as *cc* and a semen-stained swab taken from the complainant after an alleged assault has been genotyped as *abc*. In the absence of any quantitative information the genotype of the offender could be *ac, bc* or *cc*.

Complainant	Race 1	Typed as *ab*
Suspect	Race 2	Typed as *cc*
Swab		Typed as *abc*

It is unreasonable to assume that the complainant and the suspect are from the same sub-population if they are of different races. This assumption follows from a rigid application of a hierarchical population/subpopulation approach. However subpopulations from different races could share alleles that are identical by descent by recent admixture, in which case this simplification may not be valid. Following the arguments of Nichols and Balding,[358] the suspect and offender are assumed to be from the same subpopulation.

The *LR* uses the probabilities of the offender's type conditional on the suspect's type (the complainant's type is ignored as having come from a different population):

$$LR = \frac{1}{{}^2P_{1,1}\Pr(ac\,|\,cc) + {}^2P_{1,1}\Pr(bc\,|\,cc) + {}^2P_2\Pr(cc\,|\,cc)}$$

since

$${}^2P_{1,1}\Pr(ac\,|\,cc) = \frac{2(1-\theta)p_a[2\theta+(1-\theta)p_c]}{(1+\theta)(1+2\theta)}$$

$${}^2P_{1,1}\Pr(bc\,|\,cc) = \frac{2(1-\theta)p_b[2\theta+(1-\theta)p_c]}{(1+\theta)(1+2\theta)}$$

$${}^2P_2\Pr(cc\,|\,cc) = \frac{[3\theta+(1-\theta)p_c][2\theta+(1-\theta)p_c]}{(1+\theta)(1+2\theta)}$$

$$LR = \frac{(1+\theta)(1+2\theta)}{(2\theta+(1-\theta)p_c)(3\theta+(1-\theta)(2p_a+2p_b+p_c))}$$

Substitution of $\theta = 0$ recovers the product rule formulae $LR = \dfrac{1}{p_c(2p_a+2p_b+p_c)}$, and provides a useful check.

When Should a Genotype Be Used in the Conditioning?[*]

The subpopulation model works best when those people who share the same subpopulation as the suspect are used in the conditioning. There are many complicating factors in this process, including the following:

- The subpopulation of the suspect may both undefinable and unknown.

- The subpopulation of any other typed person may be both undefinable and unknown.

---

[*] This matter was brought to our attention by a senior caseworker in New Zealand, Sue Vintiner. It has been constructively discussed in meetings in New Zealand and in conversations with Robert Goetz, Manager of the Forensic Biology Laboratory of the Division of Analytical Laboratories, NSW, Australia.

Clearly the suspect is a member of his or her own subpopulation whether or not we know that or can define it. However who else is? In many cases this question is unanswerable. The inclusion of additional genotypes in the conditioning if they are not members of the suspect's subpopulation essentially adds an unwelcome random element. Such an addition is not expected to improve the estimation process at all but rather adds variance about the true value. The addition of such people tends to give a more conservative *LR* when the person and the suspect share many alleles. It tends to give a less conservative *LR* when the person and the suspect share few or no alleles. It had been supposed that the addition of random persons was conservative *on average*. We are uncertain whether this is true but even if true it applies on average over a number of cases rather than in each case. Accordingly we consider that the addition of random genotypes to the conditioning set may make the *LR* more or less conservative but does not improve the probability assignment.

The effect of adding random genotypes is to randomize the answer.

As a first approximation, we suggest that only those persons *known* or *reasonably assumed* to share the subpopulation of the suspect should be added to the conditioning. This knowledge will very rarely be available in casework and hence most often only the suspect's genotype will appear behind the conditioning.

If the forensic scientist wishes to report the more conservative *LR*, we cannot think of anything better at this time than calculating the *LR* both ways and reporting the smaller.

The Number of Contributors to a Mixture

The number of contributors to a mixture is strictly unknown. This is also true for apparently single sourced DNA samples. It is at least theoretically possible that there is an additional contributor whose alleles are masked or dropped out at all loci.

Calculation of the minimum number of contributors is trivial if the minimum number of alleles, n, is known. It is simply the integer greater than $n/2$. Hence we come to the nub. How many alleles are there in the profile? This apparently trivial question may be slightly less trivial to answer. If one simply counted all peaks above some threshold, say 50 rfu, then one would include alleles, backward and forward stutters and some artefacts. What is usually done is to apply a set of heuristics such as the following:

Rule 1: If a peak is in a back stutter position and is less than $x\%$ of the peak upstream it may be assigned as stutter.

Rule 2: If heterozygote balance (Hb) for two peaks is outside a certain range they cannot be a heterozygote.

Rule 3: If a peak is in a forward stutter position and is less than $y\%$ of the peak downstream it may be assigned as stutter.

Rule 2 may need modification for the potential additive effect of stutter. Rules 1 and 3 may interact for an allelic position that is both in a backward and forward stutter position.

Heuristics such as Rules 1–3 present quite a conundrum. If the goal is to set limits outside which the statistic such as stutter ratio or Hb *never* varies, then they need to be set very wide. In fact they must be so wide that they will often misassign, say, alleles as stutters. How could one set a rule outside which something *never* varied? If the maximum in a set of n trials is taken, it is plausible that a larger maximum will be found in $2n$ trials. If we come to the view that a limit could be based on, say, the 99th percentile, then we get a more stable limit but we accept that the rule will misfire occasionally.

Trials with such rules suggest that it is not trivial to apply them consistently.

In some cases there may be genuine ambiguity as to the number of contributors. Workarounds to this include running the interpretation under a number of scenarios and plausibly offering the most conservative option. It should be recalled that there is no need for the number of contributors under H_p and H_d to be the same. The extension of 'offering the most conservative answer' to this situation is to vary the number of contributors under H_p and H_d separately and find the lowest LR. We begin to struggle to support this approach. There are multiple layers of conservatism creeping into the analysis when this is done and it is plausible that the results will be so conservative that they are a misrepresentation of the evidence. It also primes the case with a 'too easy' line of questioning where the bounds on the number of contributors are pushed to find the lowest possible LR. Recall that there is no absolute upper bound to the number of contributors. Hence the lowest possible LR will be 0.

Consider that ambiguity exists as to whether the profile (E) is reasonably assigned as a three or four ($N = 3$ or $N = 4$) person mixture. The number of contributors may simply be treated as a nuisance variable. Hence

$$LR = \frac{\Pr(E \mid N=3, H_p)\Pr(N=3 \mid H_p) + \Pr(E \mid N=4, H_p)\Pr(N=4 \mid H_p)}{\Pr(E \mid N=3, H_d)\Pr(N=3 \mid H_d) + \Pr(E \mid N=4, H_d)\Pr(N=4 \mid H_d)}$$

The terms $\Pr(N = 3|H_p)$, $\Pr(N = 4|H_p)$, $\Pr(N = 3|H_d)$ and $\Pr(N = 4|H_d)$ are needed but in the absence of strong evidence from H_p and H_d we feel subjectively comfortable with $\Pr(N = 3|H_p) = \Pr(N = 4|H_p) = \Pr(N = 3|H_d) = \Pr(N = 4|H_d)$ and hence $LR = \dfrac{\Pr(E \mid N=3, H_{1p}) + \Pr(E \mid N=4, H_p)}{\Pr(E \mid N=3, H_d) + \Pr(E \mid N=4, H_d)}$. This formula behaves very sensibly under uncertainty in the number of contributors.

The risk associated with the assignment of the number of contributors is expected to be different for different multiplexes. Misassignment using a very naive allele count method has been explored using simulation (see Table 8.3).

Recourse is usually taken to assigning a minimum number of contributors to a profile. This method is viewed by many commentators as a primary output of the DNA analysis and thought of as something that should be put in the report.[103]

The data in Table 8.3 are only part of the total question. In our experience the issue tends to relate to very small peaks and whether they are a trace contributor who is masked or dropped out at many allelic positions or whether such a peak is, for example, a large stutter, or a forward stutter. This question cannot be answered from such an analysis. Practically, a trace contributor if present is unlikely to have much effect on the profile and should not have much effect on the interpretation.

Recent court challenges have placed much emphasis on the possibility that the number of contributors used for analysis may be different from the 'true' number of contributors to the sample.

Q: What's your opinion about how likely it is that there are more than four contributors to this mixed DNA sample?

A: I have absolutely no idea and nor does [the prosecution witness]. The fact is that because we've got DNA peaks from people who are not there because they have dropped out, plus the fact that we have essentially all the peaks that are detectible anyway, it is not possible to say that you don't have more than four or more than five or more than six people.

This of course misses the point that for evidence samples the true number of contributors can never be known and is not required for LR calculations. It is also often forgotten that defence and prosecution have every right to nominate numbers of contributors in their own propositions, but have no jurisdiction over the other party's choice.

Likelihood methods are superior to allele counting.[704-706] These methods largely treat alleles as present or absent; that is they do not currently account for height. They estimate the probability

Table 8.3 Risks Associated with the Masking Effect When Assigning the Number of Contributors Using a Naive Allele Count Method

	Profiler Plus (9 Loci)[681]	SGM Plus (10 Loci)[681]	CODIS (13 Loci)[702]	CODIS (13 Loci) (Coble to Appear)[a] African-American Allele Probabilities Used	ESS (15 Loci)[703]	ESS + SE33 (16 Loci)[703]	Proposed CODIS without SE33 (Coble) (20 Loci)	GlobalFiler (21 Loci) (Coble)	Fusion (22 Loci) (Coble)
					Italian Allele Probabilities Used		African-American Allele Probabilities Used		
$2 \to 1$	5×10^{-7}	4×10^{-8}	1×10^{-8}	9×10^{-9}	1×10^{-11}	3×10^{-13}	2×10^{-14}	7×10^{-16}	1×10^{-16}
$3 \to 2$	0.064	0.033	0.053	0.043	5×10^{-3}	7×10^{-4}	2×10^{-3}	4×10^{-4}	3×10^{-4}
$4 \to 3$	0.758	0.663	0.764	0.697	0.430	0.163	0.408	0.216	0.216
$5 \to 4$				0.974			0.931	0.743	0.872
$6 \to 5$				0.999			0.998	0.938	0.994

CODIS, Combined DNA Index System; ESS, European Standard Set.

Note: $X \to Y$ means that an X contributor mixture presents as a Y contributor mixture on peak count alone.

[a] Uncertainty in the number of contributors in the proposed new CODIS set Michael D. Coble, Jo-Anne Bright, John Buckleton and James M. Curran. Forensic Science International: Genetics in press

of the observed alleles given various numbers of contributors and account for allele probabilities and the coancestry coefficient. NOCIt[707] adds a consideration of peak heights and as such is likely to be the most powerful tool.

It has been elegantly shown[708] that assigning probabilities to the number of contributors is superior to picking one value.

There is probably some sensible pragmatic limit to the complexity of a profile for which interpretation should be attempted. This limit is plausibly determined by the point when interpretation methods break down. Guersen[709] has suggested that 12 person mixtures should be attempted but we would disagree.

Excluded, Not Excluded and Included

This section raises a matter relating to the prevalent use of the words *excluded, not excluded* and *included*. The meaning of these words may seem obvious and it is likely that they are thought of as obvious by most practitioners in the legal system. The words *excluded* and *not excluded* look exclusive and exhaustive and linguistically they certainly are. *Non-excluded* also looks synonymous with *included* and again linguistically this would seem reasonable.

If we start with *excluded*, this plausibly means 'the person of interest is not a donor to the mixture'. This statement is clear linguistically and also scientifically. So what is *not excluded*? The opposite of the sentence given is 'the person of interest is a donor to the mixture'. This is not what is meant by *not excluded* at all.

We argue that the *excluded/not excluded* dichotomy, or worse the *excluded/included* dichotomy, is not useful and potentially hazardous. The issue is that in any profile of some complexity there is a continuous spectrum of evidence that cannot be adequately described by *excluded* or *included*. Consider a profile which shows a single *a* allele at height 301 rfu. If our limit from some data for a heterozygote showing only one allele is 300 rfu, then an *ab* donor is excluded. If we lower the height of the *a* peak to 299 rfu, then an *ab* donor is not excluded. What is a fair term for this? *Almost excluded*? Is *included* a fair representation of the evidence? Recall that it is quite a statement to say that a single peak at 301 is *impossible* from a heterozygote.

It is worth mentioning that the terms *excluded, not excluded, included* and *inconclusive* are pre-assessments of an evidentiary DNA profile, with respect to the potential contribution of DNA by an individual. The calculation of a *LR* does not require that this pre-assessment take place. The *LR* calculation simply considers the probability of obtaining the evidence given two competing propositions (typically one being inclusionary and the other exclusionary) and will give a numerical value to the ratio. In some labs in Australia these pre-assessment terms are no longer used. Rather the DNA reports state the two propositions and the numerical level of support the evidence lends to one or the other.

Exclusion Probabilities

In the mixture context the exclusion probability is defined as 'the probability that a random person would be excluded as a contributor to the observed DNA mixture'. When considered as a frequency it may be used to answer the question, 'How often would a random person be excluded?' This is the reason that it is often referred to as the *random man not excluded approach* or synonymously the *cumulative probability of inclusion*. The complement of the CPI is the cumulative probability of exclusion (CPE). It proceeds in two steps, an inclusion–exclusion phase followed by the calculation of a statistic. If the POI is not excluded, then we proceed to the next step. If the mixture has alleles $A_1 \ldots A_n$, then the exclusion probability at locus l (PE$_l$)

is PE$_l = 1 - \left(\sum_i p(A_i) \right)^2$ if Hardy–Weinberg equilibrium is assumed. By writing $\sum_i p(A_i) = p$ we

can obtain PE$_l = 1 - p^2$.

If Hardy–Weinberg equilibrium is not assumed, Budowle gives

$$PE_l = 1 - \left(\sum_i p(A_i) \right)^2 - \theta \sum_i p(A_i) \left(1 - \sum_i p(A_i) \right)$$

We can write this as PE$_l = 1 - p^2 - \theta p (1 - p)$. This expression follows from the use of

$$p(A_i A_i) = p_i^2 + \theta p_i (1 - p_i)$$
$$p(A_i A_j) = 2(1 - \theta) p_i p_j$$

The proof appears in Box 8.1 and was due to Professor Bruce Weir.

The use of the equivalent of NRC II Recommendation 4.1 leads to PE$_l = 1 - p^2 - \theta \sum_{i=1}^{n} p_i (1 - p_i)$,

which differs slightly from the expression based on Recommendation 4.2.

The PE across multiple loci (CPE) is calculated as

$$CPE = 1 - \prod_l (1 - PE_l)$$

The advantages of the exclusion probability approach are often cited as simplicity and the fact that the number of contributors need not be assumed. In Box 8.2 we give a well-worded argument for the use of this approach that was provided by Laszlo Szabo of the Tasmanian Forensic Science Laboratory.

NRC II comments on a similar exclusion approach (also advocated by NRC I), saying that the '… calculation is hard to justify, because it does not make use of some of the information available, namely, the genotype of the suspect'.

Weir[1] suggests, correctly, that exclusion probabilities 'often rob the items of any probative value'.

Brenner[710] gives a brilliant explanation of the shortcomings of the probability of exclusion. We follow him here. The evidence has two parts:

1. The blood types of the suspect.
2. The blood types of the mixed stain.

   Together this information would let us infer that
3. The suspect is not excluded.

   Brenner points out that 3 can be deduced from 1 and 2. However 1 cannot be deduced from 2 and 3, or from 1 and 3. Hence the use of 1 and 3 or 2 and 3 is a loss of information. The LR is a summary of the information in 1 and 2, whereas an exclusion probability is a summary of the evidence in 2 and 3. He concludes the following:

   > In … a mixed stain case the exclusion probability usually discards a lot of information compared to the correct, likelihood ratio, approach. But still the exclusion probability may be acceptable sometimes.

BOX 8.1   THE DERIVATION OF THE EQUATIONS FOR PE FOLLOWING NRC II RECOMMENDATION 4.1

Professor Bruce Weir

Consider a mixture that has alleles $A_1 \dots A_n$ present. We require the exclusion probability at locus l (PE$_l$). We start by considering the sum of all homozygotes and heterozygotes that are entirely within the mixture.

$$\text{Sum of the homozygotes } \sum_{i=1}^{n}\left(p_i^2+\theta p_i(1-p_i)\right)+\text{sum of the heterozygotes }\sum_{i\neq j}(1-\theta)p_i p_j$$

$$=\sum_{i=1}^{n}\left(p_i^2+\theta p_i(1-p_i)\right)+\sum_{i\neq j}(1-\theta)p_i p_j$$

$$=\sum_{i=1}^{n}p_i^2+\sum_{i\neq j}p_i p_j+\sum_{i=1}^{n}\theta p_i(1-p_i)-\sum_{i\neq j}\theta p_i p_j$$

$$=\left(\sum_{i=1}^{n}p_i\right)^2+\theta\sum_{i=1}^{n}p_i-\theta\left(\sum_{i=1}^{n}p_i^2+\sum_{i\neq j}p_i p_j\right)$$

$$=\left(\sum_{i=1}^{n}p_i\right)^2+\theta\sum_{i=1}^{n}p_i-\theta\left(\sum_{i=1}^{n}p_i\right)^2$$

Next we write $p=\sum_{i=1}^{n}p_i$, so the sum above becomes

$$= p^2 + \theta p - \theta p^2$$

$$= p^2 + \theta p (1 - p)$$

Since the exclusion probability

$$\text{PE}_l = 1 - \text{the sum of the homs + the sum of the hets}$$

$$\text{PE}_l = 1 - p^2 - \theta p (1 - p)$$

as given by Budowle.

However applying the rationale of NRC II Recommendation 4.1 gives the result as follows (also provided by Professor Weir).

$$\text{Sum of the homozygotes }\sum_{i=1}^{n}\left(p_i^2+\theta p_i(1-p_i)\right)+\text{ sum of the heterozygotes }\sum_{i\neq j}p_i p_j$$

$$=\sum_{i=1}^{n}\left(p_i^2+\theta p_i(1-p_i)\right)+\sum_{i\neq j}p_i p_j=p^2+\theta\sum_{i=1}^{n}p_i(1-p_i)$$

Hence

$$\text{PE}_l = 1 - p^2 - \theta\sum_{i=1}^{n}p_i(1-p_i)$$

BOX 8.2   ARGUMENTS FOR THE USE OF THE
RANDOM MAN NOT EXCLUDED APPROACH

Laszlo Szabo
Tasmania Forensic Science Laboratory

As the defendant has a right to silence, we will usually never know what the defence hypothesis is, and to impose one on the court from a myriad of likelihood ratio (*LR*) options may be unwarranted (it might be the wrong one).

Given that both the random man not excluded (RMNE) approach and *LR* are valid approaches to the mixture problem, the defendant may well prefer RMNE, as it is generally much more conservative than a *LR* for the same data. The difficulty here occurs when a forensic laboratory quotes the most compelling *LR* for a complex mixture (say around several billion), but does not report less impressive numbers (say around a million) for other *LR* scenarios (even though these calculations may appear in the case file), and the RMNE calculation comes in at 1 in 20,000 for the same data.

The RMNE approach allows the evidential value of a crime scene profile to be assigned without reference to a suspect's DNA profile. This is important in cases without a suspect, where the investigator can be given some indication as to the potential usefulness of the DNA evidence from the crime scene.

Similarly RMNE finds application in the Tasmanian DNA database, where all profiles (including partial and mixed crime scene profiles) have a calculation associated with them, so that we can see at a glance the strength of any DNA hits. So if we put a suspect on the DNA database and obtain a number of hits to complex crime scene mixtures, we can see immediately if these are 'good matches' or not. We also have a policy of not putting a mixture on the DNA database unless the RMNE calculation is at least as good as 1 in 50. These approaches require RMNE, which is independent of knowledge of the suspect's profile.

Intuitively RMNE is easier to explain to a jury and express in reports than a *LR*, and it is probably closer to what the court wants – e.g. the suspect matches the mixture, but if this is the wrong person then what is the probability that someone else in the population would also match the mixture (i.e. not be excluded as a contributor).

Generally worldwide the move is away from CPI towards *LR*s. We follow Buckleton and Curran.[711] The performance of the CPI method, in terms of reliable application, is dependent to a very significant extent on the exclusion or inclusion step. Some information used in the exclusion phase is not used in the calculation of the CPI statistic. For example, information on the potential number of contributors, the profiles of persons who can be safely assumed to be in the mixture and peak heights may, and should, be used in the exclusion phase. This information is typically not in the calculation phase. The genotype of the suspect is always used in the exclusion phase.

The mixed DNA profile must inform some issue of relevance to the court. This issue is often, but not always, the identity of the person who left the material from which the profile has been developed. The *LR* can be placed straightforwardly into a context where it can be used by the court to assess the probability of this issue given the scientific evidence. CPI does not have this direct relationship to the issue. CPI is a number between zero and one. A high value implies weaker evidence than a lower value. Proponents of *LR*s may argue that CPI is illogical because it cannot be placed in a formal logical construct.

The cry of illogicality is rather weak however. It is very unlikely that the court will use Bayes' theorem in their considerations. It has been shown that juries do not deal with any probabilistic evidence well and there is no reason to think that the agreed logical rigor of Bayes' theorem has any practical impact on judicial decision making. There is considerable evidence that *LRs* are harder to understand[195,196] and that they may be slightly more prone to the prosecutor's fallacy.[99,p. 50]

It would be wrong to leave this point here however. The fact that a jury may not understand *LRs* is no excuse for a scientist not to study them.

One day a senior pilot at CPI airlines walked in to the management office and stated, 'Planes are getting too complicated. I cannot understand all the new safety features. You must take these features out and simplify the planes so that I can still fly them without retraining'.

If *LRs* lead to better scientific decision making, then they should be used. Whether they are then presented to court is a secondary decision. It may be possible to present some disclosed and transparently simplified approach that is consistent with our best *LR* assignment.

It is accepted by both sides that the CPI statistic does not use some evidence. There is a general tendency for any wastage of evidence to be conservative if the suspect is a contributor and non-conservative if he is not. Proponents of CPI would argue that this wastage of evidence leads to a conservative statistic. This is true in the overwhelming majority of cases but only if care is taken at the exclusion stage to use the information present in peak heights, number of contributors and conditioning profiles to exclude wrongly implicated contributors. If this is done, then the number of instances where CPI is not conservative relative to the *LR* will be very small (see Box 8.3). These instances are confined to a few unlikely situations where the particular set of allele probabilities leads to non-conservatism of the CPI method and those instances where the evidence at one or a few loci is mildly supportive of the defence proposition but not sufficiently so to lead to an exclusion. Such instances include profiles where the peak heights are not a good fit under the assumption that the prosecution proposition is true.[99,p. 244]

Labs should leave out any locus that may have dropout. The following is the SWGDAM[106] recommendation:

> 4.6.3. When using CPE/CPI (with no assumptions of number of contributors) to calculate the probability that a randomly selected person would be excluded/included as a contributor to the mixture, loci with alleles below the stochastic threshold may not be used for statistical purposes to support an inclusion. In these instances the potential for allelic dropout raises the possibility of contributors having genotypes not encompassed by the interpreted alleles.

It may also be the recommendation of Budowle et al.[103] (plausibly at figure 16).

Taken literally this means the profile in Figure 8.3 on the left is interpretable at this locus, whereas the one on the right is not.

Both SWGDAM and Budowle et al. do mention that loci omitted for the statistic may still be used for exclusionary purposes but we would like the recommendation to go further. It is necessary to avoid the view that *not excluded* is synonymous with evidence for the presence of the POI. This is consistent with Butler.[258]

BOX 8.3   HAS THE USE OF CUMULATIVE PROBABILITY OF INCLUSION LED TO MAJOR INJUSTICE?

We have been critical of cumulative probability of inclusion largely because of the difficulty in making it scientifically robust especially when dropout is present and in the loss of power. However we feel that the chance of significant contribution to injustice is probably small.

In our trials using the more sophisticated system on old profiles the overwhelming trend is that previously inclusive samples get a large *LR* in the new system. Previously inconclusive samples can go either way or stay put. Previously excluded samples usually stay with a low or inconclusive *LR*.

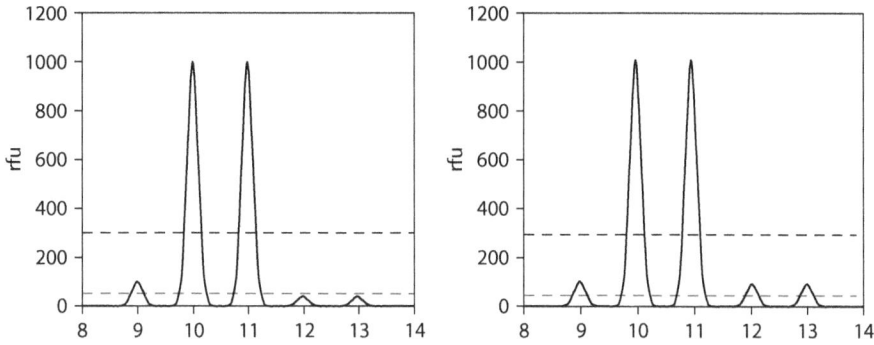

Figure 8.3   Mock electropherogram where the analytical threshold (AT) = 50 rfu and the stochastic threshold = 300 rfu. The minor peaks in the left electropherogram are below the AT and on the right above the AT.

The above rules may not be explicit enough and recently we, and SWGDAM, have moved to formalize them.

We propose, for discussion, a formalization of the rules used to implement CPI. This is in line with the spirit of the SWGDAM guidelines[106] and also with Butler's text.[258] The rules are called the *locus qualifying rule* and the *stutter rule*.

The principle is as follows:

P_1: Any locus that has a significant probability of dropout should be disqualified from use in the statistic.

The rules and guidance that follow are subservient to the principle. The rules never trump the principle. If the analyst at any point thinks that the rules suggest that the locus qualifies and the analyst thinks that dropout is plausible the locus should be disqualified.

R_1: *Locus qualifying rule.* Any locus where there is a reasonable probability of dropout is disqualified. Loci that are not disqualified qualify for use in the calculation of the statistic.

Guidance for R_1

G_1: Any locus with an allelic peak below the stochastic threshold (ST) and above the analytical threshold (AT) is disqualified.

G_2: Any locus with sub-threshold peaks below the AT that the analyst deems likely to be allelic is disqualified.

G_3: Any locus that has no allelic peaks below the ST or the AT but which looks likely to have an unseen contributor in the stochastic zone (below the ST) is disqualified.

Implementation of G_3. If there are minor peaks at other loci then a line could be drawn by, say, a ruler on the electropherogram (epg) between these peaks. This line should take into account locus effects. For example, if a locus consistently amplifies above or below the line, then the line should be adjusted to account for this. If the adjusted line passes through the stochastic region at the locus in question, then this locus is disqualified. We would suggest that a best fit adjusted line is created either by the human eye or mathematically. This line should be constrained to be flat or downwards with respect to molecular weight but never upwards.

Further, we suggest that the point where this line intersects a median allelic position at the locus in question be used to determine whether the line is in the stochastic region and hence whether this locus is disqualified. We recognize the limited buffer of conservancy in this rule. If insufficient minor peaks are available to draw a line, then we have no suggestion other than the judgment of the analyst.

R_2: *Stutter rule.* If the height of minor peaks at a locus is within a factor of 1/Hb (PHR) of the stutter peaks, then the stutter peaks should be included as potentially allelic in the calculation.

Guidance for R_2

G_2: If there are no minor peaks at a locus, then the expected height of the minor peaks should be assigned from peaks, if present, at other loci. The line approach suggested at G_3 could be applied except that the crucial position with respect to molecular weight is not defined as a median allele but at the actual stutter positions.

R_3: *Exception rule.* It is possible to reinstate some loci. If an assumption of one minor contributor can be made, then if both minor alleles can be seen the locus may be used.

G_3: The presence of both minor alleles can be verified by the presence of two minor peaks or in some case by other methods. Consider the locus TPOX showing an 8 allele at height 400 rfu and an 11 allele showing a height of 1000 rfu. This profile can be assumed to be a two person mixture in approximately a 2:1 ratio. The ST is 300 rfu. Plausible deconvolutions are 11,11:8,8 and 11,11:8,11. 11,11:8,Q (where Q is any allele other than 8 or 11) is excluded because the 8 is above the ST.

The practice of omitting loci is conservative only if the evidence at that locus has no exclusionary potential. Exclusionary potential would exist whenever the potentially dropped allele corresponds with one of the suspect alleles. We would advise that any locus that the scientist intends leaving out be critically examined for exclusionary potential, however mild, before the decision is made. It is likely that this paragraph will be misinterpreted as meaning 'examine the locus to see if it should really be an exclusion'. That is not what we are saying. There are many steps between inconclusive and a full exclusion, and the weight for all of this range is in the favour of the defendant. Omission of a locus with data in this range robs the defendant of the correct weight in his favour.

When peak heights and profile quality suggest that dropout is possible, it is possible to outline factors that should be assessed to ensure that ignoring a locus in the calculation of the statistic by CPI or *LR* will be reasonable. This should be done whether or not there is an allele in the suspect's profile that is not present in the crime profile.

In order to be reasonably confident that omitting a locus is safe, we require that one of the two situations appertain:

1. There are no non-concordant alleles (alleles in the POI's profile that are not present in the crime scene profile).

2. If there is a non-concordant allele, the peak height for any concordant alleles is low and there is an observable but non-reportable peak at the non-concordant position.

These conditions are in line with the recommendation of the DNA Commission of the International Society for Forensic Genetics (ISFG).[689] At this time it is difficult to be specific about exact numerical guidelines for the height of the concordant allele and the non-reportable peak at the non-concordant position. This is an area that warrants urgent experimental attention.

It is important not to leave the reader on this point with the impression that conservatism is a good thing. It is reasonable to concede true uncertainty to a suspect. However it is a dereliction of duty to give a low evidential value when no real uncertainty exists. Therefore if RMNE wastes reliable evidence and most often produces a conservative statistic, this would be a scientifically undesirable property.

The question then is whether there is true uncertainty in the information that is used in the *LR* calculation and that is not used in the CPI calculation. This will include the genotype of the suspect, the presence of any conditioning profiles and the number of contributors. As argued above much of this information is, and should be, used in the exclusion phase of the CPI calculation and therefore the difference between the two approaches is much less than may appear.

There can be very little argument that the genotype of the suspect is both relevant and reliable and should be used in the assessment. It is important that this genotype not be known to the analyst when he or she is making the more subjective judgements in mixture analysis. However after that phase it can and must be used.

It is very difficult to see why the matter of conditioning profiles is often cited as being contentious. If the sample is such that DNA from the victim can reasonably be expected to be present and a profile corresponding to the victim is present in the mixture, then it is unlikely to be contentious to assume that she is a contributor. It is unreasonable and unproductive to suggest that the victim is not the female component of her own vaginal swab.

The inclusion of a consensual partner of the victim is unlikely to be contentious and it is typically in the defence's interests to concede the presence of any contributor that is consistent with innocence. There may be cases where the proposed contributors are more contentious but strategies that explore a few possibilities seem to work completely adequately in practice. Long term practical use of *LRs* has not shown any real difficulties with proposition generation nor with conditioning profiles. The presence of conditioning profiles simplifies mixture interpretation markedly.

Not everyone would agree with us: Laszlo Szabo from Tasmania, Australia, has commented, 'LRs enter court with assumptions made by the scientist, and these assumptions, as reasonable as they often sound, may simply not be accepted by the defendant, and are often no more than guesses based on limited case information' (see Box 8.2). We would accept that information about case circumstances is often limited but if the information is useful and reliable then it should be used. This would occur at the exclusion phase for RMNE and at both the exclusion and calculation phases for *LRs*. The assumptions should be explicit, and this is the case in *LR* statements that we have seen but not in the CPI statements.

The number of contributors is a more serious matter. Studies have shown that early confidence in the assignment of this number was not warranted.[681,682] However it transpires that this uncertainty is not difficult to handle. It seems reasonable to allow the prosecution to select their proposition and this proposition also specifies a number of contributors. The scientist may also be allowed to optimize the defence choice and this typically, but not always, occurs with the minimum number of contributors required to explain the mixture. Again long term practical use of the technique has shown very few real difficulties. It is true that the defence may choose to alter their proposition at trial, but if the analyst has already chosen the optimal one for them, it is very unlikely that the defence will seek to force a suboptimal choice and it has never occurred in our experience.

Recall that CPI can, and should, use the number of contributors in the exclusion phase of the assessment. Therefore there seems to be little difference between the two methods in this regard.

The *LR* will change if the propositions are changed and this is viewed as a negative factor by some proponents of the CPI approach. As a matter of philosophy any statistic that does not change when the propositions change cannot distinguish between these propositions. We would be much more concerned about a statistic that did not change rather than one that did.

In fact the CPI approach can be coerced so that it does change with the propositions. Take the important matter of relatives as an example. An *LR* can be assigned for the defence proposition that the contributor is a brother of the accused. However we could also define an exclusion probability that a brother of the accused would not be excluded (cumulative probability of an included brother, CPBI).

$$\frac{1}{4}\left(1+2\frac{\left(2\theta+(1-\theta)p\right)}{1+\theta}+\frac{\left(2\theta+(1-\theta)p\right)\left(3\theta+(1-\theta)p\right)}{(1+\theta)(1+2\theta)}\right)$$

We have never heard of this statistic, CPBI, being used. The *LR* approach appears to force a completely reasonable focus on the fact that the propositions are important in the generation of the statistic. This appears to be masked with current use of CPI although this is not a necessity.

We dismiss the concept that *LR*s are too complex for trained forensic scientists. There are thousands of forensic scientists using them daily. Paternity analysts have used them routinely since the mid-twentieth century. What is real is that unfamiliarity with their use makes them appear more difficult than they are.

It is possible to modify the *LR* – but not the CPI – approach so that it operates in a reasonable manner whenever dropout is possible whether or not there are non-concordant alleles. We recommend these approaches in all cases as an alternative that is preferable to dropping a locus.

It may be worthwhile, for a moment, considering how we might ever know whether dropout is possible or not. In practice the determination as to whether dropout is possible is made by the observation of one or more low height peaks in a profile. It is then determined whether other alleles at this or other loci may have dropped out. Consideration is often given to the molecular weight of the loci with low peak heights. While this is a pragmatic solution, it cannot strictly be correct. Taken literally dropout is always possible. No matter how high a set of peaks is it would always be possible to postulate some additional very trace contributor, plausibly masked at some positions and not seen anywhere in the profile, which has dropped out. The finding that dropout is not possible is therefore confounded with some determination of the number of contributors. For example, if no more than four peaks are seen at any locus and all peak heights are high, then it may be assumed that there are two contributors and that no component of these two contributors has dropped out. We cannot see how to determine that dropout is not possible without going via some determination of the number of contributors. This has been previously noted.[711]

However it is certainly possible, if not trivial, to determine if dropout is possible for some alleles associated with the peaks observed. If one minor peak is present at a locus and that height is low, then it is possible that the partner of that peak may have dropped out. Similarly the partners of that peak at other loci, especially higher molecular weight loci, may have dropped out.

For profiles which have no chance of dropout at any locus, we advocate the use of an *LR* but accept the usage of CPI. This was the stance taken by the DNA Commission of the ISFG.[689] This stance is one of accepting parallel methods as long as both methods are sufficiently reliable, albeit one may be superior.

We are aware of an attempt to coerce the CPI statistic to handle dropout. Van Nieuwerburgh et al.[712] suggested a system that could be applied if the exact number of dropped alleles were known from the crime profile. While it is possible that their algebra is correct, it is impossible to know the number of dropped alleles.

More recently a viable extension to the CPI statistic has been made extending its ability to deal with dropout.[713] This extension does require an assignment of the number of contributors. In a widely circulated letter to the ISFG,[714] Evett warns:

> There is a school of thought that believes that in such cases we can indicate weight of evidence by quoting the RMNE probability. The reasoning behind this is that, in those cases where we can calculate a *LR*, it is generally the case that the RMNE approach will lead to a more conservative assessment of weight of evidence.
>
> In my opinion (a) the argument is fallacious and (b) the motivation behind it is prosecution biased.
>
> First the argument. Let us accept the premise (though I don't think that anyone has ever proved it) that in every case in which a numerical value can be assigned to a *LR* then the RMNE approach will yield a statistic that implies a more conservative assessment of weight of evidence. It is a fallacy to assert from this premise that RMNE must be conservative in any case in which

a numerical value cannot be assigned to the *LR*. If we do not have a value for the *LR* then we cannot possibly know that the RMNE statistic is conservative and it clearly is not possible to design any programme of research to investigate the truth of the assertion. This is not a fine academic point – it provides a sound basis for a defence challenge at court. Indeed I presented such a challenge in *R v Turner* (Newfoundland Supreme Court, 2001).

Second, the motivation behind the assertion is prosecution biased because it is the prosecution who will gain from the presentation of a numerical statistic, at least as far as UK courts are concerned. It lacks balance because it addresses only one of two key questions: it is an attempt to address the probability of the evidence given some kind of imprecisely stated defence proposition. We might convince ourselves that RMNE provides a conservative denominator but it tells us nothing about the probability of the evidence given the prosecution proposition. In a sense the prosecution hijacks the defence proposition – which would appear to be counter to Recommendation 5 of the ISFG report.

It is possible that the ISFG DNA Commission has not been exposed to the idea of using RMNE as a substitute for the *LR* in a case where a numerical value cannot be assigned to the latter. However there are some in the UK who think this way and the Commission would be doing a valuable service if they included a recommendation along the following lines:

Recommendation: in a case in which it is not possible to assign a numerical value to the *LR* it is neither logical nor balanced to use an RMNE statistic as an alternative.

Random Match Probability

The acknowledged wastage of information in the CPI approach has led to variants that try to make better use of this information within the general inclusion/exclusion paradigm favoured in the United States. Foremost among these is the RMP approach.

Let

N be the number of contributors

K be the genotypes of any individuals known or safely assumed to have contributed to the mixture

E be a vector or list of peak heights for each allele in the mixture

RMP answers the question, what is the probability a random donor would be included in this mixture given N, K and E?

Therefore the RMP calculation is the sum of the frequencies for all the genotypes that are possible contributors to a mixed DNA profile at a locus under the assumption of a defined number of contributors. First, exhaustively enumerate all sets of N genotypes that explain the mixture at locus l. Let us say that there are S sets. We collapse this $S \times N$ array of genotypes to the set of X of unique genotypes, G_{li} $i = 1...X$, that appear at least once in the $N \times S$ array. Then estimate $RMP = \sum_{i=1}^{X} \Pr(G_{li})$. For each G_i:

Assuming Hardy–Weinberg equilibrium we write

$$\Pr(G_i) = \begin{vmatrix} P_a^2 & G_i = aa \\ 2P_aP_b & G_i = ab \end{vmatrix} \qquad (8.2)$$

Applying Recommendation 4.1 of NRC II[176] we write

$$\Pr(G_i) = \begin{vmatrix} P_a^2 + P_a(1-P_a)\theta & G_i = aa \\ 2P_aP_b & G_i = ab \end{vmatrix} \qquad (8.3)$$

247

$$\Pr(G_i) = \begin{vmatrix} P_a\left(2 - P_a + (1 - P_a)\theta\right) \\ P_a\left(2 - P_a\right) & \qquad G_i = aF \\ 2P_a \end{vmatrix} \qquad (8.4)$$

Loci with potential dropout are usually interpreted with one or other variant of the $2p$ rule (Equation 8.4).

θ is the inbreeding coefficient often interpreted as the coancestry coefficient in the United States.

The RMP statistic is typically applied to single source DNA profiles. A 'modified RMP' can be applied to mixed DNA profiles after an assumption of the number of contributors is made.[106]

Bille et al.[284] were unable to predict the performance of the RMP method relative to RMNE and LR in full generality. They therefore covered the more common situations (see Table 8.4).

The RMP method when applied to two person mixed DNA profiles has been shown to result in an inverse of the restricted LR statistic in many but not all situations.

Likelihood Ratios

LR Models Employing Qualitative Approaches

Before the advent of automated fluorescent techniques (which provide quantitative data such as peak height and area), mixtures were interpreted without taking account of quantitative aspects of the data. The development of this qualitative style of interpretation commenced during the single locus probe era.[715] It is the method supported by NRC II, who said the '…correct approach (the LR approach), we believe, was described by Evett et al.'

This approach has also received judicial sanction in the United States. When Professor Weir presented the evidence regarding the mixed stains in the Bronco automobile during the trial of OJ Simpson he advocated the use of LRs. The defence preferred to argue for exclusion probabilities as suggested by NRC I. Judge Ito commented, 'I find that the analysis offered by Dr Weir is the more accurate and closest to what the evidence truly represents'. (Transcript page 33,345 quoted in Weir.[1,303])

The LR approach has been implemented in various guises ranging from use of the simple product rule to inclusion of sampling error and subpopulation corrections through to a refined treatment that accounts for all of these factors. In any manifestation it is superior to a probability of exclusion.

As with any Bayesian application a key step is the formulation of the propositions. In fact this is often the most difficult step; it relies on an understanding of the pertinent questions that are before the court and on what background information may be agreed upon.

One of the most important factors that may be decided from the circumstances of the case or by agreement between prosecution and defence is whether any persons may be assumed to be present in the mixture.

To put this into context consider a case in which fingernail clippings have been taken from a woman who has been assaulted and claims to have scratched her attacker. Suppose that a mixed DNA profile is obtained which appears to consist of DNA from two individuals and can be fully explained by the presence of DNA from both the woman and her suspected attacker. The expectations from this type of sample and the circumstances of the case suggest that DNA from the complainant is likely to be present irrespective of whether there is any DNA from her attacker.

Table 8.4   The CPI, RMP and *LR* Formulae for Some Common Situations

Sample epg	Genotype(s) of Known Contributors, POI and Possible Genotypes for the Unknown(s)	CPI, RMP and *LR*[a]
	K = 7,9 POI = 11,13 U = 11,13	$CPI = (P_7 + P_9 + P_{11} + P_{13})^2$ $RMP = 2P_{11}P_{13}$ $LR = \dfrac{1}{2P_{11}P_{13}}$
	K = 7,9 POI = 7,11 U = 7,11	$CPI = (P_7 + P_{11})^2$ $RMP = 2P_7P_{11}$ $LR = \dfrac{1}{2P_7P_{11}}$
	K = 7,9 POI = 7,11 U = 7,11 or 9,11 or 11,11	$CPI = (P_7 + P_9 + P_{11})^2$ $RMP_{4.1} = 2P_7P_{11} + 2P_9P_{11} + P_{11}^2$ $\qquad + P_{11}(1 - P_{11})\theta$ $LR_{4.1} = \dfrac{1}{2P_7P_{11} + 2P_9P_{11} + P_{11}^2}$ $\qquad + P_{11}(1 - P_{11})\theta$
	K = 7,7 POI = 7,9 U = 7,9	$CPI = (P_7 + P_9)^2$ $RMP = 2P_7P_9$ $LR = \dfrac{1}{2P_7P_9}$
	K = 7,7 POI = 7,9 U = 7,9 or 9,9	$CPI = (P_7 + P_9)^2$ $RMP_{4.1} = 2P_7P_9 + P_9^2$ $\qquad + P_9(1 - P_9)\theta$ $LR_{4.1} = \dfrac{1}{2P_7P_9 + P_9^2}$ $\qquad + P_9(1 - P_9)\theta$

(Continued)

249

Table 8.4 *(Continued)* The CPI, RMP and *LR* Formulae for Some Common Situations

Sample epg	Genotype(s) of Known Contributors, POI and Possible Genotypes for the Unknown(s)	CPI, RMP and *LR*[a]
	K = 7,7 POI = 7,7 U = 7,7	CPI = $(P_7)^2$ $RMP_{4.1} = P_7^2 + P_7(1-P_7)\theta$ $LR_{4.1} = \dfrac{1}{P_7^2 + P_7(1-P_7)\theta}$
	K = 7,9 POI = 7,11 U = 7,11 or 9,11 or 11,11 or 11,Q	CPI not applicable. $RMP_{4.1} = P_{11}[2+\theta-(1+\theta)P_{11}]$ $LR_{4.1} = \dfrac{1}{P_{11}\left[2+\theta-(1+\theta)P_{11}\right]}$
	K = 7,9 POI = 7,13 U = 7,11 or 9,11 or 11,11 or 11,Q	CPI not applicable. This is a non-concordance. It would typically be interpreted as below but care must be taken as there is a risk of non-conservativeness. See text for a discussion. $RMP_{4.1} = P_{11}[2+\theta-(1+\theta)P_{11}]$ $LR_{4.1} = \dfrac{1}{P_{11}\left[2+\theta-(1+\theta)P_{11}\right]}$
	K = 7,7 POI = 7,9 U = 7,9 or 9,9 or 9,Q	CPI not applicable. $RMP_{4.1} = P_9[2+\theta-(1+\theta)P_9]$ $LR_{4.1} = \dfrac{1}{P_9\left[2+\theta-(1+\theta)P_9\right]}$
	K = 7,7 POI = 7,7 U = F,F	CPI not applicable. $RMP_{4.1} = 1$ $LR_{4.1} = 1$

(Continued)

Table 8.4 *(Continued)* The CPI, RMP and *LR* Formulae for Some Common Situations

Sample epg	Genotype(s) of Known Contributors, POI and Possible Genotypes for the Unknown(s)	CPI, RMP and *LR*[a]
	POI = 11,13 U_1:U_2 = 7,9:11,13 7,11:9,13 7,13:9,11	$CPI = (P_7 + P_9 + P_{11} + P_{13})^2$ $RMP = 2P_7P_9 + 2P_7P_{11} + 2P_7P_{13}$ $\quad\quad + 2P_9P_{11} + 2P_9P_{13} + 2P_{11}P_{13}$ $LR = \dfrac{1}{12P_{11}P_{13}}$
	POI = 11,13 U_1 = 7,9 U_2 = 11,13	$CPI = (P_7 + P_9 + P_{11} + P_{13})^2$ $RMP = 2P_7P_9 + 2P_{11}P_{13}$ $LR = \dfrac{1}{2P_{11}P_{13}}$
	POI = 7,11 U_1:U_2 = 7,7:9,11 or 7,11:9,9 or 7,9:11,11	$CPI = (P_7 + P_9 + P_{11})^2$ $RMP_{4.1} = (P_7 + P_9 + P_{11})^2$ $\quad\quad\quad \begin{bmatrix} P_7(1-P_7) + P_9(1-P_9) \\ +P_{11}(1-P_{11}) \end{bmatrix}\theta$ $LR_{4.1} =$ $\dfrac{P_9 + (1-P_9)\theta}{4P_7P_{11}\big[3\theta + (1-\theta)(P_7 + P_9 + P_{11})\big]}$
	POI = 7,11 U_1:U_2 = 7,7:9,11 or 7,9:7,11	$CPI = (P_7 + P_9 + P_{11})^2$ $RMP_{4.1} = P_7\begin{bmatrix} P_7 + (1-P_7)\theta \\ + 2(P_9 + P_{11}) \end{bmatrix} + 2P_9P_{11}$ $LR_{4.1} = \dfrac{1}{2P_{11}[\theta + (3-\theta)P_7]}$

(Continued)

251

Table 8.4 *(Continued)*   The CPI, RMP and *LR* Formulae for Some Common Situations

Sample epg	Genotype(s) of Known Contributors, POI and Possible Genotypes for the Unknown(s)	CPI, RMP and *LR*[a]
	POI = 7,7 $U_1:U_2$ = 7,7:9,9 or 7,9:7,9	$CPI = (P_7 + P_9)^2$ $RMP_{4.1} = P_7 (2P_9 + P_7 + (1 - P_7)\theta)$ $\qquad + P_9 (P_9 + (1 - P_9)\theta)$ $LR_{4.1} = \dfrac{P_9 + (1 - P_9)\theta}{2P_7P_9\left[\dfrac{2P_7 + [P_7 + (1 - P_7)\theta]}{[P_9 + (1 - P_9)\theta]}\right]}$

CPI, cumulative probability of inclusion; RMP, random match probability; *LR*, likelihood ratio; K, known contributors; U, unknown contributors; POI, person of interest; Q, any allele other than those specified; F, al allele.

[a] For RMP and *LR* we use the NRC II recommendation to comport with US usage rather than our preferred Balding and Nichols equations.

Furthermore, the assumption seems wholly justified as there is *prima facie* evidence, from the mixed profile itself, of a contribution of DNA from the donor herself. Therefore it may not be in contention that the profile of the complainant is present. Under these circumstances it seems reasonable to form the following two propositions:

H_p: The nail clippings contain the DNA of the complainant and the POI.

H_d: The nail clippings contain the DNA of the complainant and an unknown person unrelated to the POI or complainant.

The presence of DNA from the complainant under both propositions effectively allows the scientist to 'condition' on the presence of her DNA. In practical terms this allows much or all the profile of the other contributor to be deduced straightforwardly. Those alleles that are not attributable to the complainant must be from the other contributor.

At this point it will be noted that the resolution of the mixture has assumed that there were exactly two contributors. This assumption is unnecessary and the formulation can be generalized to any number of contributors under H_p or H_d with an associated significant increase in complexity. However it simplifies the manual analysis appreciably if one can make this assumption. Under many circumstances this type of assumption can be strongly justified. If each locus in a highly discriminating multiplex has only one to four alleles, it seems very likely that there are only two contributors.[*] One could state that there is no evidence to indicate a contribution of DNA from a third individual and, given the context of the case, there is no need to invoke the presence of DNA from a third individual to explain the observed result. The argument regarding this assumption is in fact no different from that involving an apparently single source stain. Strictly, that profile may be a mixture of DNA from two individuals but the scientist assumes, justifiably, that it emanates from a single individual.

---

[*] Strictly this statement is a transposition. A more correct statement would be that we can infer that most of the posterior density lies on those propositions which have two contributors.

If we call the evidence of the alleles in the stain E and the genotypes of the complainant and the POI G_v and G_s, respectively,* we require

$$LR = \frac{\Pr(E\,|\,G_s,G_v,H_p)}{\Pr(E\,|\,G_s,G_v,H_d)}$$

If we assume that E is independent of G_s under H_d (this is in effect the assumption of Hardy–Weinberg and linkage equilibrium), then

$$LR = \frac{\Pr(E\,|\,G_s,G_v,H_p)}{\Pr(E\,|\,G_v,H_d)}$$

Weir et al.[716] give a general approach that allows calculation of the LR for any mixture in those cases where peak area or height data are ignored and dropout is not possible at any locus. The nomenclature is provided in Table 8.5.
The LR is

$$LR = \frac{\Pr(E\,|\,H_p)}{\Pr(E\,|\,H_d)} = \frac{P_x(U_1\,|\,E,H_p)}{P_x(U_2\,|\,E,H_d)}$$

where $P_x(U\,|\,E,H) = T_0^{2x} - \sum_j T_{1;j}^{2x} + \sum_{j,k} T_{2;j,k}^{2x} - \sum_{j,k,l} T_{3;j,k,l}^{2x} + \dots$

Mortera at al.[717] give an elegant implementation of this approach for any number of known or unknown contributors.

Table 8.5	Nomenclature for the General Formulation of Weir et al. for a Mixture Likelihood Ratio without Accounting for Peak Area, Peak Height or Subpopulation Effects
E	The set of alleles in the crime stain.
H	A shorthand simply to avoid writing H_p or H_d.
x	The number of unknown contributors to the stain under H.
U	The set of alleles in E not carried by the known contributors under H.
ϕ	The empty set. This may be necessary if there are no alleles in U not carried by the known contributors.
$P_x(U\|E,H)$	The probability that x unknown contributors carry the alleles in U but no alleles outside E under H. We differ from Weir et al. here by specifying the proposition. This was implicit in the original publication. The difference is pedantic and cosmetic.
T_0	The sum of all allele probabilities in E.
$T_{1;j}$	The sum of all allele probabilities in E except the jth allele in U.
$T_{2;j,k}$	The sum of all allele probabilities in E except the jth and kth allele in U.

---

* General usage is to use the terms 'victim' and 'suspect' here, hence G_V and G_S. However the word 'victim' has implications that may be unwarranted. For example, the defence may be that the sex was consensual or indeed the matter may be a 'false complaint' altogether in which case it would be interesting to argue who the victim is. We will attempt to use the word 'complainant' in the text. However we have persisted with G_V in the equations to avoid the potential confusion with G_s, which we have already used for crime stain and to keep aligned with previous publications.

Curran et al.[718] extended the general formula of Weir et al.[716] to allow calculation of the LR in those cases where peak area or height data are ignored but subpopulation effects are to be considered. This approach has been applied in Melbourne, Australia, and is taught in lectures by some commentators in the United States. It can also be used to calculate the LR for those cases where peak area or height data are ignored and subpopulation effects are also ignored.

We outline the use of the Curran general formula (nomenclature is summarized in Table 8.6). Consider the crime profile. It has C_g distinct alleles. Since we are not considering area or height, each of these alleles may have originated from one, two or more contributors and may have come from heterozygotes or homozygotes. Each proposition H_p and H_d declares some people to be contributors, some to be non-contributors and may require some unknown contributors. For example, H_p is likely to declare that the POI is a contributor whereas H_d is likely to declare him or her to be a non-contributor. Both H_p and H_d may declare the complainant to be a contributor. H_d is likely to have at least one unknown contributor, the 'random man' who replaces the POI as a contributor. However both H_p and H_d may require unknown contributors in cases of, say, multiple rape when one suspect has been developed.

The alleles from people declared to be non-contributors may appear irrelevant however they do appear in the conditioning and affect the result if the subpopulation correction is applied.

Sometimes it will help to refer to the propositions H_p and H_d as H simply to avoid writing 'H_p or H_d'.

Each proposition therefore declares a total number of contributors to the stain, C. Let this be n_C, and hence the total number of alleles in the stain is $2n_C$. These $2n_C$ alleles may not be distinct since contributors may share alleles or may be homozygotes. Consider one particular allele A_i from the set C_g of alleles in the stain. There may be one, two or more copies of this allele declared to be present. Let the number of copies of A_i be c_i. We can count the number of copies of A_i contributed by the declared contributors. However there may be additional copies of A_i contributed from the unknown contributors.

At least one of the propositions and possibly both will require unknown contributors. The unknown contributors must carry those alleles in the crime stain that are unaccounted for by the declared contributors. Beyond this constraint the remaining alleles of the unknown contributors may be any of the alleles in the set C_g (recall that we are not accounting for area or height). These unassigned alleles are free and may be assigned to any of the alleles in the set C_g. We need to permute these unassigned alleles over all possibilities by assigning each possible number r_i of them to each allele A_i and sum the result. We need to account for the possible ways of ordering the alleles into genotypes and keep track of the factors of 2 for the heterozygotes. Using the product rule and specifying x unknown contributors this leads to

$$P_x(T,U,V \mid C_g) = \sum_{r_1=0}^{r} \sum_{r_2=0}^{r-r_1} \cdots \sum_{r_{c-1}=0}^{r-r_1-\ldots r_{c-2}} \frac{2^{h_T+h_V} n_T!(2x)!n_V!}{\prod_i u_i!} \prod_{i=1}^{c} p_i^{t_i+u_i+v_i}$$

To introduce the subpopulation correction we replace $\prod_{i=1}^{c} p_i^{t_i+u_i+v_i}$ with

$$\frac{\Gamma(\gamma.)}{\Gamma(\gamma.+2n_T+2x+2n_V)} \prod_{i=1}^{c} \frac{\Gamma(\gamma_i+t_i+u_i+v_i)}{\Gamma(\gamma_i)}$$

where $\gamma_i = \dfrac{(1-\theta)p_i}{\theta}$ and $\gamma. = \displaystyle\sum_{i=1}^{c} \gamma_i$

The LR is evaluated by calculating this probability under H_p and H_d and dividing the two results. When this is done we note that the number of typed individuals and the alleles that they

Table 8.6   Notation for Mixture Calculations

Alleles in the Evidence Sample

C	The set of alleles in the evidence profile, comparable to E in Table 8.5
C_g	The set of distinct alleles in the evidence profile
n_C	The known number of contributors to C
h_C	The unknown number of heterozygous contributors
C	The known number of distinct alleles in C_g
c_i	The unknown number of copies of allele A_i in C $1 \le c_i \le 2n_c, \sum_{i=1}^{c} c_i = 2n_c$

Alleles from Typed People That H Declares to Be Contributors

T	The set of alleles carried by the declared contributors to C
T_g	The set of distinct alleles carried by the declared contributors
n_T	The known number of declared contributors to C
h_T	The known number of heterozygous declared contributors
T	The known number of distinct alleles in T_g carried by n_T declared contributors
t_i	The known number of copies of allele A_i in T $1 \le t_i \le 2n_c, \sum_{i=1}^{c} t_i = 2n_T$

Alleles from Unknown People That H Declares to Be Contributors

U	The sets of alleles carried by the unknown contributors to C, also U in Table 8.5
X	The specified number of unknown contributors to C: $n_C = n_T + x$, also x in Table 8.5
$c - t$	The known number of alleles that are required to be in U
R	The known number of alleles in U that can be any allele in C_g, $r = 2x - (c - t)$
n_x	The number of different sets of alleles U, $\dfrac{(c+r-1)!}{(c-1)!r!}$
r_i	The unknown number of copies of A_i among the r unconstrained alleles in U. $0 \le r_i \le r, \sum_{i=1}^{c} r_i = r$
u_i	The unknown number of copies of A_i in U. $c_i = t_i + u_i, \sum_{i=1}^{c} u_i = 2x.$ If A_i is in C_g but not in T_g: $u_i = r_i + 1$. If A_i is in C_g and also in T_g: $u_i = r_i$.

Alleles from Typed People That H Declares to Be Non-Contributors

V	The set of alleles carried by typed people declared not to be contributors to C
n_V	The known number of people declared not to be contributors to C
h_V	The known number of heterozygous declared non-contributors
v_i	The known number of copies of A_i in V: $\sum_i v_i = 2n_V$

Source: Reproduced in amended form from Curran, J.M., et al., *Journal of Forensic Sciences*, 44(5), 987–995, 1999 ©1999 ASTM International. Reprinted with permission.

carry are the same under each proposition. Hence the term $2^{h_T + h_V}$ will cancel as will portions of the terms in the products.

Beecham and Weir[576] later added a confidence interval.

In the original paper Weir et al.[716] gave a warning that applies to the Curran et al. and Beecham and Weir extensions equally. The method cannot handle silent alleles (*null* was the word used in those days). Perhaps the warning was not explicit enough because the method was applied to profiles where dropout was possible as late as 2010. Perhaps the connection between the warning about silent alleles and dropout was not obvious. We draw the conclusion that such methods are 'tools and like all tools may be misused with the potential to cause great harm' Gavin Turbett 2012. The solution is to understand the tool, its strengths and limitations. There is no potential to procedurize forensic science so that it may be applied by untrained and cheaply paid employees and we support no effort in that direction.

Example 8.4: *R v Donnelly*

This was an alleged rape case in which it was to the defence's advantage to demonstrate the presence of complainant DNA on a blanket. This tended to support the accused's version of events. A segment of the evidence offered by G is reproduced below. The profile was a low-level four person mixture. The case allows the illustration of a number of important points.

John Buckleton

Sample		Comp		Joe		Blanket Female Fraction						Female A		Likelihood Ratio
	Site													
1	D8	10,	12	13,	14	10	12	13	14	15	.16	14,	15	6.74
2	D21	30,	32.2	30,	31.2	28	30	31	31.2	32.2		28,	31	4.44
3	D7	11,	11	9,	9	9	11					11,	11	6.64
4	CSF	11,	11	12,	13	10	11	12	13			10,	10	1.36
5	D3	16,	17	16,	16	14	.15	16	17	18		14,	18	2.91
6	THO1	7,	8	6,	9.3	6	7	8	9.3			6,	9.3	5.91
7	D13	8,	11	11,	11	8	9	11	12			9,	11	4.04
8	D16	11,	12	13,	13	9	.10	11	12	13		9,	12	1.87
9	D2	16,	17	19,	20	16	17	19	20	21		16,	21	4.38
10	D19	12,	15.2	13,	16.2	12	13	14	15.2	16.2		13,	14	22.44
11	vWA	17,	19	16,	19	14	16	17	18	19		14,	18	1.72
12	TPOX	8,	11	8,	11	8	9	11				8,	9	1.18
13	D18	12,	14	16,	17	12	14	15	16	17		15,	16	7.09
	Amel	X	X	X	Y	3XY : 7XX						X	X	
14	D5	12,	12	11,	13	10	11	12	13			10,	12	1.15
15	FGA	20,	24	19,	23	19	20	22	23	24		22,	24	4.08
														234,293,525

Un-highlighted peaks are uniformative (because they are shared)

Peaks that distinguish the complainant from Joe & female A

Peaks that distinguish Joe from the complainant and female A

Peaks that distinguish female A from Joe and the complainant

Unidentified trace DNA

256

COLOUR CODING

I question the colour coding in the G table. I feel that this leads too strongly to the inference that the coloured alleles come from the nominated source.

ERRORS AND CHECKING

There are four-allele probability input errors and one mathematical error in the sheet produced and checked by G and T (G&T sheet). Below is a section of the G&T sheet.

	Allele	Asian 0.0637	Cauc 0.7117	EP 0.17	WP 0.055	Allele	Asian 0.064	Cauc 0.712	EP 0.1698	WP 0.0548
	16	0.785	0.252	0.315	0.348	17	0.205	0.194	0.217	0.224
D3	14	0.041	0.129	0.046	0.014	18	0.073	0.14	0.085	0.098
	15	0.349	0.268	0.328	0.308					
	7	0.304	0.189	3.08	0.4	8	0.069	0.103	0.062	0.137
THO1	6	0.128	0.224	0.252	0.145	9.3	0.076	0.334	0.293	0.2
	12	0.04	0.072	0.035	0.05	15.2	0.152	0.039	0.201	0.007
D19	13	0.28	0.241	0.183	0.25	14	0.24	0.353	0.257	0.16
	16	0.017	0.051	0.017	0.007	14.2	0.099	0.023	0.081	0.164

The cells marked with yellow were incorrectly input. Note the allele probability of 3.08, which is bigger than 1, and the 0.785, which adds with alleles nearby to greater than 1. This error is rather careless and we were assured in statement and testimony that it had been checked. The other two errors (0.152 and 0.007) are less obviously wrong but are incorrect nonetheless.

The mathematical error occurs at D3, where the spreadsheet values add the allele probabilities for 16, 14, 18 and 17 but omits 15.

Allele Frequencies						
16	14	18	17			15
0.3019	0.103	0.1241	0.2003			0.2855
HO		x	1		U	15
TO	0.7293		TO²ˣ	0.53188		
T1;15	0.4438		T1;15²ˣ	0.03879		
			Numerator	0.49309		

METHOD

However lamentable the matters given above are, the main point of this example is that G and T applied the method of Weir et al.[716] (the method in PopStats) to a profile where dropout is possible.

The propositions under consideration were as follows:

H_p: Complainant, POI, female A and unknown
H_d: POI, female A and two unknowns.

If we look at D7 for example, the Weir et al. method compels the unknowns to have genotypes 9,9 or 9,11 or 11,11. If dropout is possible other possibilities exist and should be considered. Failure to consider them makes the probabilities much smaller. The Weir et al. method cannot be used when dropout is possible. This is 1997 technology (actually developed in 1995 for the OJ Simpson case) being used in 2010 and then used inappropriately.

Models Employing Quantitative and Qualitative Data

In order to facilitate discussion of these methods, it is necessary to digress slightly and introduce various notations, nomenclature and naming conventions peculiar to the analysis of mixed stains and quantitative data.

A mixture can contain DNA from any number of contributors, N, and N may be 1.

A concept in mixture analysis (at least where the quantitative aspects of the data are being considered using the binary approach) is the mixing proportion (M_x; see Table 8.7). For a two person mixture, this can take any value between 0 and 1. Practitioners often prefer to use a mixture ratio as this is intuitively easier to estimate from a visual inspection of the profile. In this text we will use mixture proportions as the mathematics flows more easily.

Where the mixing proportion is such that in the judgement of the scientist the unambiguous profile of one of the contributors is discernible from the others, then practitioners generally refer to this as a major component of the profile. The remaining component(s) are referred to as minor component(s). In artificially created two person mixtures, a good estimate of the mixing proportion is known in advance. In forensic stains, however, it is not, and the scientist may attempt to deduce this from the electropherogram. Necessarily this will be conditional on which particular genotypes are being considered.

Third, when peak area data (or height) are being considered, the symbol ϕ is used to denote this area.

A warning[197] has been given of the potential in court to use an unassigned minor peak to foster doubt in the mind of a jury by postulating that the unknown minor represents the true assailant. This seems a timely warning to us and suggests that full mixture analysis may be warranted more often than we had previously considered.

The Evett et al.[715] paper was the progenitor of what we now term the *binary model*. In these manual methods the scientist uses expert judgement, together with a number of numerical parameters, to decide which, if any, of all the possible genotype combinations at a locus can be excluded. Effectively this method assigns a probability of 1 or 0 to the profile given each of the genotypes based on whether the analyst considers the profile possible or impossible given these genotypes. This decision is based on expert judgement or whether the quantitative information falls within certain predefined parameters for the multiplex system. Strictly, partitioning of all possible contributing genotypes as included (weight 1) or excluded (weight 0) will never lead to the correct *LR* since all possible contributing genotypes should have some weight between 0 and 1. This situation has naturally led to the development of alternative continuous probability models. These approaches attempt to take account of the need to weight all of the possible genotypes but generally require software support, as they are computationally intensive. Foremost among these is the model that is based on treating peak areas as random variables and determining the probability of these peak areas for any given set of contributing genotypes.[719] These probabilities can be shown to act as the weights discussed above.

We will first discuss the binary model at some length here as it is the practice currently implemented in many laboratories internationally and then, more briefly, the continuous models. The binary model can be applied with or without a subpopulation correction.

Quantitative Data – Peak Areas or Heights?

Automated sequencers display quantitative information giving both allele peak height and peak area. The question of the use of peak height or area has arisen although little has been published on this matter. Theoretical considerations would tend to favour area as more accurately

Table 8.7 Mixture Nomenclature

Term	Definition
M_R The true but unknown mixture ratio	We assume this to be a pre-amplification term. Under many circumstances it will be possible to assume that it is constant across all loci pre-amplification. Such a circumstance would be when we have a large number of undegraded diploid cells in the template, and sampling effects in the pre-amplification stage may be ignored.
$\hat{M}_R^l \mid ab : cd$ The estimated post-amplification mixture ratio at locus l, conditional on the genotypes being ab and cd	The estimated ratio of the components post-amplification at locus l in the mixture postulated to be ab and cd. We explicitly allow $\hat{M}_R^l \mid ab : cd$ to vary across loci. Whether or not the mixing ratio is constant across loci pre-amplification, there is no requirement for it to be constant post-amplification. For instance, $\hat{M}_R^l \mid ab : cd = 1$ means that the mixture is comprised of a 1:1 mix of two components ab and cd at locus l, $\hat{M}_R^l \mid ab : cd = 2$ means that the mixture is comprised of a 2:1 mix of two components ab and cd at locus l, and $\hat{M}_R^l \mid ab : cd = \frac{1}{2}$ means that the mixture is comprised of a 1:2 mix of two components ab and cd at locus l. Hence we expect $\hat{M}_R^l \mid ab : cd = \dfrac{1}{\hat{M}_R^l \mid cd : ab}$.
$\hat{M}_R$ Estimated mixture ratio abbreviation	For brevity we may drop the conditioning on the genotypes and the nomination of locus. However strictly the mixture ratio can only be estimated if the genotypes are known. The ratio post-amplification is likely to vary across loci even if it is constant pre-amplification.
M_x The true but unknown mixture proportion	Again we assume this to be a pre-amplification term.
$\hat{M}_x^l \mid ab : cd$ The estimated post-amplification mixture proportion of the genotype ab in the mixture of ab and cd at locus l	The estimated post-amplification proportion of one component in the mixture at locus l. This will usually be taken to be the minor component; however this distinction is not necessary. For instance, $\hat{M}_x^l \mid ab : cd = 0.5$ means that genotype ab is estimated to represent 50% of the total area in the epg. $\hat{M}_x^l \mid ab : cd = 0.33$ means that genotype ab is estimated to represent 33% of the total area in the epg.
$\hat{M}_x$ The estimated mixture proportion abbreviation	For brevity we may drop the conditioning on the genotypes and the nomination of the locus. However strictly the mixture proportion can only be estimated if the genotypes are known. The ratio post-amplification is likely to vary across loci even if it is constant pre-amplification.
a, b, c etc.	The name of the allelic peak present in the mixture.
Φ_a	The area of peak a.
$\Phi_{a\&b}$	An abbreviation for $\Phi_a + \Phi_b$.
p_a	The allele probability for allele a in some relevant population.

epg, electropherogram.

reflecting the amount of DNA present. This is most likely to be true if peaks have differing shapes, as peak area should more accurately adjust for differing peak morphology. For instance, the higher molecular weight alleles might be broader and squatter.

Due to the fact that peaks are approximately triangular one would not expect to see a doubling of height to equate to a doubling of area (a doubling of height should lead to a quadrupling of area if the shape remains the same and is triangular). On the other hand, when peak heights are low, apparently arbitrary decisions by the software as to where to delineate the boundaries of a peak can lead to the baseline contributing to the total peak area – the so-called plinth effect. Thus when peaks are low, height may be preferable to area. These theoretical considerations aside, limited trials by the authors on Hb suggest that area has no practical advantage or disadvantage over height. No preference is given here although consistency is important.

The Binary Model

The binary method is a method for the resolution of mixtures. It relies upon the experience of the expert together with the application of a number of numerical guidelines. The rationale was outlined by Clayton et al.[720]

The name *binary model* refers to the fact that the profile (E) is designated as either possible or impossible given a certain genotype combination S_i. This probably warrants some expansion. Imagine a two person mixture. We could imagine a number of pairs of genotypes G_1, G_2 that might potentially explain the mixture. It is convenient to refer to each pair as a set. So we may have genotype sets S_1, S_2, ... If we think the profile is impossible given a certain set we assign $\Pr(E|S_i) = 0$. It is sustainable but unwise to refer to the genotype set as impossible given the profile. Strictly we can infer that if $\Pr(E|S_i) = 0$ then $\Pr(S_i|E)$ is also 0 but such a statement invites us to reverse our thinking from the probability of the profile to the probability of the genotypes. Profiles deemed possible given a genotype set are assigned $\Pr(E|S_i) = 1$. This should make it clear why the reversal is unwise. Clearly $(S_i|E)$ is not necessarily 1. The 1 is arbitrary and any positive number will do. The occurrences of 1 and 0 are the origin of the term *binary*.

Before interpreting a potential mixture, it is important to have knowledge of the behaviour of the multiplex system of interest. It is necessary to have an appreciation for the following:

- The normal variation in peak height between the two alleles of a known heterozygote (termed *heterozygote balance*, Hb, in Europe and Australasia and *PHR* in North America)

- The size of stutter peaks by marker and locus

- The variation of mixture proportion across loci

Heterozygote balance and stutter are discussed in Chapters 1 and 7. There are a few terms that are particularly useful when considering mixtures. These are set out in Table 8.7.

Typically we have found that forensic caseworkers prefer to work with the mixture ratio, whereas the mathematics flows slightly better working with the mixture proportion. A simple relationship exists between the two parameters (but not necessarily their estimates)

$$M_x = \frac{M_R}{1 + M_R}, \quad M_R = \frac{M_x}{1 - M_x}$$

The mixture proportion can range from the contributors being approximately equal to each other, to one being in great excess.

It has been demonstrated that if DNA templates are mixed, then this ratio will be approximately, but not exactly, preserved throughout all loci.[721] For SGM Plus at 28 cycles Kirkham[722] observed that the estimated mixture proportion at some loci could differ by as much as 0.35 from the known mixture proportion.

The variability across loci in mixture proportion is typically expressed as $D = \left| M_x^l - M_x \right|$ where M_x^l is the estimate of mixture proportion at a locus and M_x is the average across loci. We now, subsequently, regret using the absolute value. $D = M_x^l - M_x$ is likely to be more informative.

The average peak height of the active alleles, APH, was defined previously[118] and is reproduced in Table 8.8 for two person mixtures. For single source DNA samples, APH is the simple average of the two allele heights. When assessing mixtures, this depends on the pattern of allelic overlap.

In Figures 8.4 and 8.5 we plot D versus APH from data obtained from mixed DNA profiles from casework samples and data from mixtures artificially constructed from laboratory controls, respectively.

Table 8.8   The Form of the Equations for Estimation of the Mixture Proportion (M_x^l) and Average Peak Height (APH) at Individual Locus Styles

Locus Style	APH
ab single source	$\dfrac{\phi_a + \phi_b}{2}$
ab:aa *aa:ab*	$\dfrac{\phi_a + \phi_b}{4}$
ab:ac	$\dfrac{\phi_b + \phi_c}{2}$
aa:bb	$\dfrac{\phi_a + \phi_b}{4}$
aa:bc	$\dfrac{\phi_a + \phi_b + \phi_c}{4}$
ab:cd	$\dfrac{\phi_a + \phi_b + \phi_c + \phi_d}{4}$

Note: ϕ_a, ϕ_b, ϕ_c and ϕ_d represent the heights of alleles *a*, *b*, *c* and *d*, respectively. Locus style is given as Contributor 1:Contributor 2.

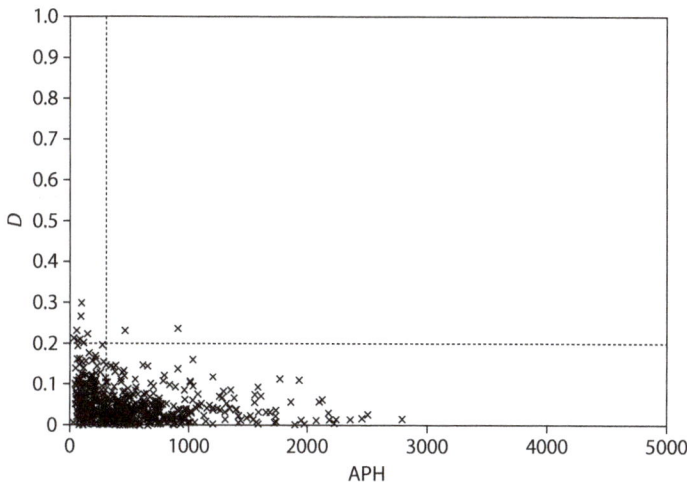

Figure 8.4   *D* from mixed DNA profiles from casework samples (*N* = 622) versus average peak height (APH). The horizontal dotted line is at *D* = 0.2 and the vertical dotted line is at APH = 300 rfu.

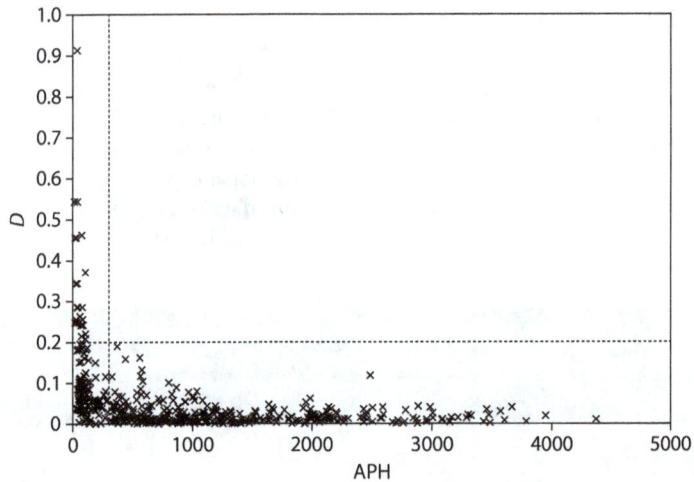

Figure 8.5 D from mixed DNA profiles from artificially constructed mixtures ($N = 873$) versus average peak height (APH). The horizontal dotted line is at $D = 0.2$ and the vertical dotted line is at APH = 300 rfu.

Table 8.9	A Useful Classification Scheme for Mixtures	
Classification	**Description**	**Approximate Definition**
Type A	No clearly defined major contributor	$0.33 \le \hat{M}_x \le 0.67$ $0.5 \le \hat{M}_R \le 2$
Type B	Clearly defined major and minor contributors	$0.13 \le \hat{M}_x \le 0.33$ $0.15 \le \hat{M}_R \le 0.5$
Type C	A mixture containing a low-level minor	Strictly this is any mixture where the minor is sufficiently low that it could be confused with an artefact such as a stutter
Type D	The majority of peaks are below 150 rfu in height	

Bearing in mind that the human eye is drawn to outliers when examining graphical data, it is plausible that there is a broad similarity of distribution with slightly more outliers in the data derived from casework samples. A guideline[118] for D of 0.2 at APH above 300 rfu appears supportable from these data.

It is helpful to classify the mixture as shown in Table 8.9.

Either the mixture proportion or the ratio can be estimated relatively easily when there are no shared alleles (Figure 8.6).

Consider the profile of D18S51 in Figure 8.6. It is possible to pair the alleles into the minor contributor (14,15) and the major contributor (16,18). The mixture proportion can be estimated from peak heights (ϕ):

$$\hat{M}_x = \frac{\phi_a + \phi_b}{\phi_a + \phi_b + \phi_c + \phi_d} = \frac{1375 + 1465}{1375 + 1465 + 2867 + 2281} = \frac{2840}{7988} = 0.36$$

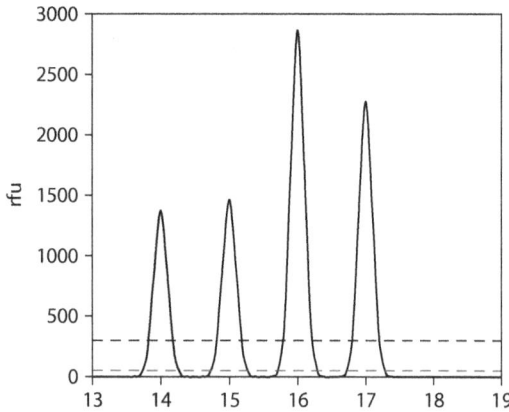

Figure 8.6   A stylized electropherogram of D18S51 showing a mixed profile from two different heterozygotic individuals.

$$1 - \hat{M}_x = \frac{\phi_c + \phi_d}{\phi_a + \phi_b + \phi_c + \phi_d} = 0.64$$

Alternatively a mixture ratio can be estimated as

$$\hat{M}_R = \frac{\phi_a + \phi_b}{\phi_c + \phi_d} \cong 0.55$$

which we may write as approximately 1:2.

Note however the conditional nature of this estimate in that it is based upon the genotypes of the contributors being 16,18 and 14,15, respectively. The formulae required are outlined in Table 8.10.

There has been some argument that the mixture proportion (M_x) cannot be estimated. This idea appears to be a misunderstanding of the conditional nature of the mixing proportion estimate. It is indeed correct that the true mixing proportion is unknown, but this is also true of almost any other parameter in DNA or any other statistical problem. In addition the process of estimating a mixture proportion requires knowledge of the genotypes, and hence any mixture proportion estimate is always conditioned on the genotypes. This means that different combinations of genotypes will result in different mixture proportion estimates. This is an integral part of the theory.

Further criticism has been levelled when M_x is subsequently used to help decide which genotypes are present at a locus on the basis that there is a circularity to the argument. That is, the assumed genotypes are used to estimate M_x and then M_x is used to decide the genotypes. We accept this criticism of the circularity in this argument but in essence the binary model procedure simultaneously estimates those genotypes and mixing proportions that jointly have high support.

Once the mixture proportion or ratio has been estimated it is then possible to calculate the expected peak areas (or heights) for any given genotype combination.

It is possible to automate the process of M_x estimation using a software algorithm based on the concept of least residuals. This has been programmed at the FSS into a software package called *PENDULUM*.

Consideration of All Possible Genotype Combinations

Having obtained an estimate of M_x from one or more loci, the next step is to enumerate all possible genotype combinations for the locus under consideration and generate a list of every

Table 8.10 Estimating the Mixture Proportion and Mixture Ratio for Two Person Mixtures

Proposed Genotype Combination			$\hat{M}_x$	$\hat{M}_R$
Four-Allele Loci	1,2	3,4	$\hat{M}_x = \dfrac{\phi_1 + \phi_2}{\phi_1 + \phi_2 + \phi_3 + \phi_4}$	$\hat{M}_R = \dfrac{\phi_1 + \phi_2}{\phi_3 + \phi_4}$
Three-Allele Loci	1,1	2,3	$\hat{M}_x = \dfrac{\phi_1}{\phi_1 + \phi_2 + \phi_3}$	$\hat{M}_R = \dfrac{\phi_1}{\phi_2 + \phi_3}$
	2,3	1,1	$\hat{M}_x = \dfrac{\phi_2 + \phi_3}{\phi_1 + \phi_2 + \phi_3}$	$\hat{M}_R = \dfrac{\phi_2 + \phi_3}{\phi_1}$
	1,2	1,3	$\hat{M}_x = \dfrac{\phi_2}{\phi_2 + \phi_3}$	$\hat{M}_R = \dfrac{\phi_2}{\phi_s}$
Two-Allele Loci	1,1	2,2	$\hat{M}_x = \dfrac{\phi_1}{\phi_1 + \phi_2}$	$\hat{M}_R = \dfrac{\phi_1}{\phi_2}$
	1,2	2,2	$\hat{M}_x = \dfrac{2\phi_1}{\phi_1 + \phi_2}$	$\hat{M}_R = \dfrac{2\phi_1}{\phi_2 - \phi_1}$
	1,1	1,2	$\hat{M}_x = \dfrac{\phi_1 - \phi_2}{\phi_1 + \phi_2}$	$\hat{M}_R = \dfrac{\phi_2 - \phi_1}{2\phi_2}$
	1,2	1,2	No information is present	
One-Allele Loci	1,1	1,1	No information is present	

possible combination. The number will vary according to whether the allele pattern has four, three, two or just one allele. These combinations are given in Table 8.11.

Taking each locus separately, every genotype in the list is then considered in turn. Two parameters are then estimated – Hb and mixture proportion, M_x. First, the Hb guidelines are applied. These are written as a set of mathematical rules and appear in Table 8.11. These 'rules' need to be applied with care as no simple mathematical rule can match human judgement.

Second, M_x should be similar at each locus of the mixture and so should show consistency with the previously estimated mixture proportion.

Those combinations that are not supported on the basis of the guidelines are considered very unlikely* and are removed. In this way the list may be reduced to leave only those allelic combinations that are well supported by the quantitative data.

Compare Reference Samples

Once a list of all the well-supported genotypes has been generated and recorded, a comparison is made with the reference samples. If the genotype of an individual is such that he or she matches one of the well-supported combinations at each locus, then there is evidence that may support the suggestion that this person has contributed to the mixture and a statistical evaluation of that evidence may be warranted. Conversely, if at one or more loci the individual either lacks one or other or both alleles for either combination, then this is evidence supporting non-contribution. Even if the individual possesses the necessary alleles but that combination was excluded during application of the rules, then this evidence also may support non-contribution.

---

* Again strictly this is a transposition. A better term would be to consider these combinations to have a *low posterior probability*.

Table 8.11   Allele Combinations for Differing Loci and Hb Rules

Four-Peak Locus 6 Combinations

Individual 1	Individual 2	Guideline
ab	cd	
ac	bd	
ad	bc	All hets in this table may be checked using the simple het guideline
bc	ad	
bd	ac	
cd	ab	

Three-Peak Locus 12 Combinations

Individual 1		Individual 2	
aa	No test	bc	Simple het
ab	Shared het	ac	Shared het
ab	Shared het	bc	Shared het
ab	Simple het	cc	No test
ac	Simple het	bb	No test
ac	Shared het	bc	Shared het
bc	Simple het	aa	No test
ac	Shared het	ab	Shared het
bc	Shared het	ab	Shared het
cc	No test	ab	Simple het
bb	No test	ac	Simple het
bc	Shared het	ac	Shared het

Two-Peak Locus 7 Combinations

Individual 1		Individual 2	
aa	Het hom	ab	Het hom
aa	No test	bb	No test
ab	Het hom	bb	Het hom
ab	Het hom	aa	Het hom
bb	No test	aa	No test
bb	Het hom	ab	Het hom

(Continued)

Table 8.11 *(Continued)* Allele Combinations for Differing Loci and Hb Rules			
One-Peak Locus 1 Combinations			
Individual 1		**Individual 2**	
ab	Simple het	*ab*	Simple het
aa		*aa*	

Hb, heterozygote balance; het, heterozygote; hom, homozygote.

Note: H_b is the accepted heterozygote balance level, say 0.6.

Simple het guideline $H_b \leq \dfrac{\phi_2}{\phi_1} \leq \dfrac{1}{Hb}$ where peaks 1 and 2 are the low and high molecular weight peaks of the heterozygote, respectively.

Shared het guideline $H_b \leq \dfrac{\phi_s}{\phi_1 + \phi_2} \leq \dfrac{1}{Hb}$ where s is the shared peak and peaks 1 and 2 are the peaks of the different heterozygotes.

Het hom guideline $Hb\phi_s \geq \phi_1$

Note that all calculations are conditional on the proposed genotypes.

Assumptions of the Binary Model

The binary model makes a number of assumptions. These include the following:

- The mixture proportion is approximately constant across loci.

- The peak height is proportional to the amount of DNA.

- The height of 'shared' peaks is the sum of the contribution of the two contributing individuals.

Allowing for Stutters

In some cases it will not be possible to decide whether or not a minor peak in a stutter position is composed entirely of area (or height) derived from stuttering or whether it does contain an allelic contribution. It is, however, possible to proceed on the basis that the peak may or may not be in part allelic.

In the example shown in Figure 8.7, Peak 11 is in a stutter position. If this is a two-person mixture, the genotype of the minor contributor could therefore be 10,10; 10,11; 10,12 or 10,13 if the peak at Position 11 could be stutter or stutter and allele.

Gill et al.[723] consider interpreting such a electropherogram in a circumstance where, say, the victim is the major 12,13 genotype and the POI corresponds with the minor. They suggested a bound for the *LR*:

$$LR \geq \frac{1}{\Pr(10,10\,|\,X) + 2\Pr(10,11\,|\,X) + 2\Pr(10,12\,|\,X) + 2\Pr(10,13\,|\,X)}$$

This bound was suggested in 1998 and still looks supportable at time of writing, although now superseded by continuous methods.

F and Q Models

This method seeks to extend the binary model to complex two to four person mixtures where dropout is possible but where there are no non-concordances.[724] It is wasteful of information and significantly understates the *LR* if there are many unknowns or considerable ambiguity

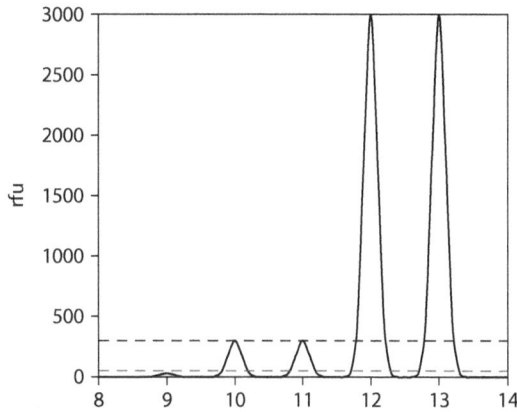

Figure 8.7 This diagram shows a stylized rendition of an electropherogram.

in the allelic vector. It is likely that two or more unknowns under H_p renders the approach too conservative. The method is readily extended to allow for substructure using the Balding and Nichols equations[358] but we cannot see how to incorporate NRC II Recommendation 4.1 easily. In order to understand this section reprising some statistical and biological principals is helpful.

Conversion of the Observed Peaks to Observed Alleles
Using heuristics such as those discussed in Tables 8.10 and 8.11, it is often possible to infer the minimum number of copies of each type of each allele from the observed peaks at a locus. At a minimum there is one copy of each allele observed above the designated limit of detection but often it is possible to infer the existence of extra copies of these alleles. When converting peaks into alleles, a number of contributing factors are taken into account including number of assumed contributors to a DNA profile, peak height ratio, average mixture proportion and known conditioning profiles if available and applicable.

Consider the example in Figure 8.8a. If we assume this profile is a two person mixture, then the 11 peak exceeds the threshold, T, where dropout is deemed possible. This indicates the presence of two 11 alleles. The allelic vector becomes (10,11,11,12).

Note that the allelic vector may be different under the prosecution (H_p) and the defence (H_d) propositions since the known profiles differ by at least the POI and may also differ in the number of contributors, N.

Ambiguity in the Allelic Vector
In certain circumstances it may not be possible to infer a unique vector of alleles, but there might be a limited number of possibilities. Consider, for example, the example in Figure 8.8b.

This is an idealized example of a two person mixture with three peaks of equal height above T. We can infer that there is one more copy of the 13, 14 or 15 allele but we cannot tell which allele is duplicated. The possible allelic vectors are therefore (13,13,14,15), (13,14,14,15) and (13,14,15,15).

Assigning the Allelic Designation for a Locus
We assume that the observed peaks have been converted into observed alleles for a mixed profile with N contributors, and the total number of observed alleles at that locus is $\leq 2N$. In some instances where dropout may have occurred a 'placeholder' is required. We use the F designation to signify that an allele may have dropped. F designations are added until there are $2N$ entries in the allelic vector. Alleles in this vector are either observed alleles or F alleles and add to $2N$.

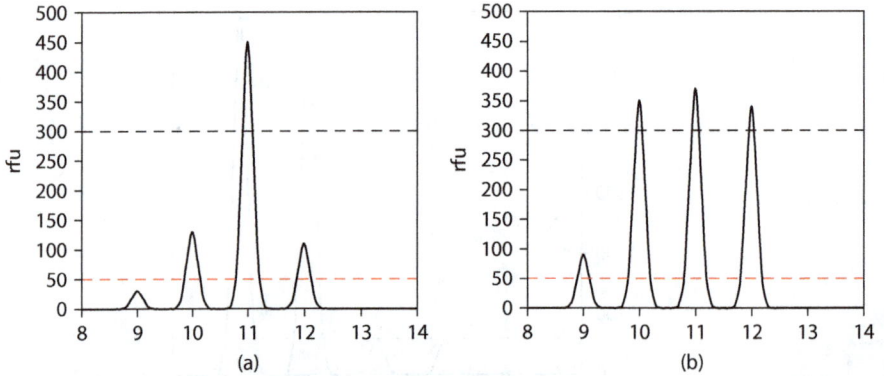

Figure 8.8 (a) Example of a three-peak locus, with one peak above and two below the homozygote threshold, T. (b) Example of a three-peak locus, with three peaks above the homozygote threshold, T.

Assigning a Probability Using the F Model

Recall that the number of permutations of the alleles A_1, ..., A_l is $^{2N}P_{m_1,m_2,...m_l} = \dfrac{2N!}{m_1!m_2!...m_l!}$.

For an allelic vector with alleles A_i, $i = 1 ... l$ each with m_i copies we assign the probability as

$$^{2N}P_{m_1,m_2,...m_l} \Pr(A_1,...,A_l \mid X)$$

where X is a set of conditioning alleles. The F alleles are used in the term $\dfrac{2N!}{m_1!m_2!...m_l!}$ and are then dropped from the allelic vector.

Assigning a Probability Using the Q Model

The Q model is slightly less wasteful of evidential value than the F model. For an allelic vector with alleles A_i, $i = 1 ... l$ with m_F F alleles we form all allelic vectors with the F alleles permuted to all options of the observed alleles plus the F alleles as either an observed allele or an allele Q which signifies all alleles outside the observed set of alleles. We assign the probability of the allelic vector as the sum of these permuted allelic vectors.

We reiterate that neither the F nor the Q model is capable of dealing with profiles that show a non-concordance. The formulae for some common situations are available in Kelly et al.[724] as supplementary tables.

A Semi-Continuous Model

Since we accept that LTDNA profiles can be affected by dropout, the appearance of spurious alleles (termed *drop-in*), high levels of heterozygote imbalance and stuttering, a belief developed in 1999 that they suit a different method of interpretation. The passage of time has taught us that this method is applicable quite broadly and that a coherent approach may be applied to all DNA evidence.

With LTDNA samples it may be unrealistic to unambiguously assign a genotype to a sample. Most especially it may be difficult to unambiguously determine if the genotype is a homozygote or a heterozygote with a dropped allele. It may, in fact, be very difficult to determine whether the evidence supports the presence of one or more contributors. Rather than try to assign genotypes from the sample, we are better served to consider the probability of the epg *given* various genotypes. In the following section we outline one approach to this that has gained some support in the United Kingdom, Europe and the United States. However the reporting officer must be warned that not only will the evidence take greater skill to interpret and explain but also the very concept that the scene profile and the genotype of the suspect may differ will undoubtedly be a source of questioning in court. The key to interpreting and understanding this type of evidence is to think of the probability of the evidence *given* a genotype, not the other way around. This approach has been given considerable support by the DNA Commission of the ISFG[685,689] and the provision of uncontrolled software.[108,122,684] The term *probabilistic method* has been coined to cover these methods which include the semi- and fully continuous methods.

Uncertain Allele Calls

Balding and Buckleton[113] suggested an extension of previous work to deal with uncertain stutter, masking and near-threshold allele calls. In current practice the scientist makes a judgment call from an epg to designate peaks as stutter, masking or allelic. The alternative, which is highly realistic but subjective, is to accept some uncertainty in such calls. Consider a peak in a stutter position that is 18% of the parent peak. While this may be stutter it is also plausible that it is, in part, allelic. If we could assign probabilities to the chance that this peak is stutter or partly allelic the problem could be solved. It is this assignment of probabilities that is difficult. It is much easier to comment on the probability that a peak of this height would occur *if* it were stutter. This is different from the probability that the peak is stutter.

It is possible to treat uncertain peaks as neither allelic nor stutter (and therefore ambiguous). The method was taught to us by Keith Inman and we have checked that it can be applied to both LRmix and Lab Retriever. A profile is constructed that includes all the ambiguous peaks. This may have 0, 1, 2 ... peaks per locus. This profile is set up as a known contributor. The effect is to treat the peak as either allelic or not in the mathematics.

LR for Multiple Contributors, One Unknown

We follow Balding and Buckleton[113] but omit some smaller terms that they used that relate to less likely contributors, the Mj. This omission is unnecessary and should not be done if software is being developed, but it allows simplification of some complex formulae for visualization by eye.

Consider a two person mixed profile. We assume a profile, v, typically the victim, that may be accepted by both prosecution and defence to be a contributor and one unknown profile that is the profile of interest. The alleles from v can mask alleles from the profile of interest either directly or via stutter peaks. Initially we ignore stutter.

CSP = ABc s = cd

Consider a crime scene profile (CSP) with major peaks A and B and one minor peak at c in the one and only replicate. We will use the upper- and lowercase letters to signify major and minor components. The suspect is cd. It will be convenient to denote the set of masking alleles M. We obtain

$$LR = \frac{D\bar{D}}{\bar{D}_2 P_{cc|cd} + 2D\bar{D}P_{cx|cd} + 2\bar{D}P_{cM|cd}} \tag{8.5}$$

where x is any allele other than a, b or c. The *LR* tends to zero in Equation 8.5 as $D \to 0$ and, if $\alpha < 1$, as $D \to 1$.

CSP = ABc s = cc

Consider a CSP with major peaks A and B and one minor peak at c in the one and only replicate. We will use the upper- and lowercase letters to signify major and minor components. The suspect is cc. It will be convenient to denote the set of masking alleles M. We obtain

$$LR = \frac{\bar{D}_2}{\bar{D}_2 P_{cc|cc} + 2D\bar{D}P_{aQ|cc} + 2\bar{D}P_{cM|cc}} \tag{8.6}$$

$CSP = ABcd \; s = cd$

$$LR = \frac{\bar{D}^2\bar{C}}{2\bar{D}^2\bar{C}P_{cd|cd} + (\bar{D}_2 P_{cc|cd} + 2\bar{D}P_{cM|cd})CP_d + (\bar{D}_2 P_{dd|cd} + 2\bar{D}P_{dM|cd})CP_c} \tag{8.7}$$

$CSP = AB \; s = cd$

The effect of masking can be very important when the minor component CSP is null, especially if D is small. Please recall we are dropping some terms.

$$LR = \frac{D^2}{P_{MM|cd} + DP_{Mx|cd}} \tag{8.8}$$

$CSP = AB \; s = cc$

$$LR = \frac{D_2}{P_{MM|cd} + DP_{Mx|cd}} \tag{8.9}$$

In either case, Equations 8.8 and 8.9 favour the defence proposition when there are masking alleles, strongly so unless D is large.

Multiple Unknown Contributors

These principles extend readily to multiple unknown contributors. The denominator involves summations over the possible genotypes for each unknown contributor. The result can be approximated by averaging over repeated simulations of their genotypes, which can reduce the computational burden at the cost of some approximation. However, for one or two unknown contributors, the exact value is fast to compute and so simulation-based approximation is not necessary.

Extending the Semi-Continuous Model

In a strict application the semi-continuous models do not directly use peak height although this may inform the probability of dropout. Consider the classical two person mixture in Figure 8.7 with a clear major and minor and no known contributors. The POI matches the minor component.

With no consideration of peak height the genotypes could be, for example, 10,12 and 11,13. An effective method to interpret the minor profile was taught to us by Carlos Baeza-Richer. We have confirmed that this method works for LRmix and Lab Retriever. Construct a profile with all the major alleles and make this a known contributor. This will mean that the minor is interpreted correctly except that the factor of 2 issue is overlooked (the answer will be too big by a factor of 2).

Highlighting Risk Situations for the Binary and Consensus Models

When Buckleton and Gill initially developed the semi-continuous model their goal was to highlight those areas where the binary and consensus models may be unfair to defendants. A set of the tables were developed, initially called the *alert sheet*. In some situations it is obvious that some non-probabilistic methods need review. These situations are where the suspect has an allele not present in one or more of the replicates, defined as a *non-concordant allele*. If this allele does not appear at all in any replicate, then current practice may be seriously unfair to defendants. If the allele appears in some replicates or has significant sub-threshold peaks, then the situation is much alleviated.

As a general rule if the POI's genotype is also the best fit to the evidence, then non-probabilistic methods are either

1. Conservative, or

2. Very mildly non-conservative for some, usually extreme, values of C and D

It was pleasing to note that this aligned strongly with intuition.

It may be possible to look at this in a general way. There are a very large number of various genotype combinations that may explain the replicates, some of which are very poor at explaining the evidence. Let these genotype combinations be C_i, $i = 1 \ldots \infty$. Each C_i may consist of one, two or more genotypes. For example, $C_1 = \{ab;cd\}$, meaning that it is composed from two genotypes, one an ab and the other a cd. This formulation may be theoretically extended to absorb the uncertainty in the number of contributors but, for simplicity, we make no effort to do so here. We let the particular combination defined under H_p be C_1 and consider that there is only one combination under H_2 this is also one of the combinations under H_d. We consider the evidence, E, to consist of replicates R_i, $i = 1 \ldots M$, then we can consider the fit of the combination to the replicates $F_i = \Pr(E|C_i)$, $i = 1 \ldots \infty$. The LR will be

$$LR = \frac{F_1 \Pr(C_1 | H_p)}{F_1 \Pr(C_1 | H_d) + \displaystyle\sum_{i=2}^{\infty} F_i \Pr(C_i | H_d)} \tag{8.10}$$

We now consider the approximation

$$LR = \frac{\Pr(C_1 | H_p)}{\displaystyle\sum_{i=1}^{N} \Pr(C_i | H_d)} \tag{8.11}$$

The summation will not be across an infinite number of genotype combinations but rather some smaller set, N, which represents all the C_i with significant F_i.

It is helpful to rewrite Equation 8.10 as

$$LR = \frac{\Pr(C_1 | H_p)}{\Pr(C_1 | H_d) + \displaystyle\sum_{i=2}^{\infty} \frac{F_i}{F_1} \Pr(C_i | H_d)} \tag{8.12}$$

This allows us to compare the denominators of Equation 8.11 with Equation 8.12.

The difference between the denominators (subtracting the denominator of Equation 8.11 from that in Equation 8.12) is

$$\sum_{i=2}^{N} \left(\frac{F_i - F_1}{F_1} \right) \Pr(C_i | H_d) + \sum_{i=N+1}^{\infty} \frac{F_i}{F_1} \Pr(C_i | H_d).$$

Now let us consider that the combination under H_p is the one that best explains the profile; hence F_1 is the largest of the F terms. Then $F_i - F_1$ is negative and $\dfrac{F_i - F_1}{F_1}$ may be close to -1. The terms $\dfrac{F_i}{F_1}$ are positive but small. Given these considerations it seems very likely that

$$\sum_{i=2}^{N} \left(\frac{F_i - F_1}{F_1} \right) \Pr(C_i | H_d) + \sum_{i=N+1}^{\infty} \frac{F_i}{F_1} \Pr(C_i | H_d)$$ is negative. This implies that as long as all C_i with significant F_i are incorporated and F_1 is the largest of the F terms, then the approximation $LR = \dfrac{\Pr(C_1 | H_p)}{\displaystyle\sum_{i=1}^{N} \Pr(C_i | H_d)}$ is likely to be conservative or at worst mildly non-conservative.

In attempting to nurse the biological model along we were responding to reluctance by case-workers, and indeed ourselves, to embrace the considerable complexity of developing formulae for the semi-continuous model. In many situations there are more than two replicates, and in mixture situations development of the formulae can be quite challenging. More often than not the profile was considered to be uninterpretable. However reflection and practice suggested that the concept of alerting analysts to situations where current practice had risk was not going to work. This was because it was very unclear what we were suggesting analysts should do if, for example, they had 13 'no risk' loci and 2 'risk' loci. Ignoring the risk loci is not acceptable, as these loci may be mildly or seriously exculpatory. For LTDNA profiles, situations such as this are common.

We initially pursued heuristics that suggested when the risk was minimal, such heuristics are plausible. Consider, for example, the $2p$ rule situation, which is the most common risk situation. Let the suspect be ab and the stochastic threshold (MIT) be 200 rfu. If a peak is at 199 rfu and there is absolutely no sub-threshold peak at the b position, then there is a serious risk that the $2p$ rule is non-conservative.

Contrast this with a peak at 51 rfu and a sub-threshold b peak at 49 rfu. On the face of it, this seems worse evidence since the peak is smaller. However there is almost no risk that the $2p$ rule is non-conservative. At this point we cannot quantify the value of the sub-threshold peak. However the height of a peak affects the value of D and via that the risk associated with use of the $2p$ rule.

When we thought of the task of explaining and defending in court the binary or consensus model using heuristics and considering the subjective and in some instances non-quantified aspects of this, we were forced to the conclusion that we may be better served by changing to the semi-continuous or continuous model. This is now what we begin to advocate. Some effort has been put into providing software and training and some research effort was needed to establish values for D and C. However the final result is much more objective, more defensible and is a better representation of the evidence. There is very encouraging evidence that this policy has paid dividends.[725]

Assessing the Probability of Dropout

Empirical trials suggest rather obviously that the probability of dropout, D, is affected by the amount of DNA. However, in casework, the amount of DNA is not known for certain. A quantification result will often be available but at low levels often unreliable. We have argued, elsewhere, that the profile itself may be the best indicator of the amount of DNA. This is consistent with empirical findings. Low-level profiles, in terms of the height of the peaks, clearly are more susceptible to dropout. Perhaps, then, the best indicator of the total amount of DNA is some function of the peak heights. This leads us to the logistical regression method introduced by Tvedebrink et al.[726-728]

Logistic regression is a type of regression analysis that can be used to predict the probability of a binary event, based on one or more explanatory variables. In the context of a DNA profile the best explanatory variable to predict the probability of dropout would be the true, but unknown, template available at each locus for amplification. This introduces the concept that the available template at each locus differs.

Often epgs arising from casework exhibit a decrease in allelic peak height as the molecular weight (M_a) of the alleles increases. This is variously described as the *degradation slope* or the *ski slope*.[729,730] Effective modelling of degradation is likely to provide the most effective explanatory variable for dropout.

Following Tvedebrink et al.[726-728] we could envisage that the average peak height, $\hat{H}$, serves as a proxy for template pre-amplification and is thought to be constant at every allelic position. We introduce the term *mass* and denote it $\hat{H}_a$, to subsume the concepts of template number and degradation. Hence $\hat{H}_a$ serves as the proxy at allelic position a.

If the degradation of the DNA strand were random with respect to location, then we would anticipate that the expected height of peak a, E_a, would be exponentially related to molecular weight, M_a, and to whether the peak was a heterozygote or homozygote. Let X_a be the count of allele a. $X_a = 1$ for a heterozygote with a and $X_a = 2$ for a homozygote a. The expected height, E_a, of peak a is therefore modelled as

$$E_a = \hat{H}_a X_a$$
$$\hat{H}_a = \alpha_0\, e^{\alpha_1 M_a}$$

A decreasing exponential relationship between allele height and molecular weight was described by Tvedebrink et al.[728] in relation to models for allelic dropout and has been confirmed at least once empirically.

Experience in casework has also suggested that there is a locus effect in addition to a general downward slope. As an example, in one report three loci within the Identifiler™ multiplex were preferentially inhibited to varying extents in the presence of a laboratory cleaning agent.[731] Inhibitors co-extracted with the sample could affect certain loci more than others. The cameras used to detect the fluorescence have been shown to differ in their response to the different dyes used in detection and it is likely that the camera response changes as the camera ages. Collectively these factors suggest that loci may be above or below the trendline and that whether a specific locus is above or below may change from time to time or even sample to sample.

Three models have been suggested by Tvedebrink et al.[726–728] for the probability of dropout of a single allele D_a and of a homozygote, D_{2a}, as

$$D_a = \frac{e^{(l_{i0}+\beta_0)+(l_{i1}+\beta_1)\ln \hat{H}}}{1+e^{(l_{i0}+\beta_0)+(l_{i1}+\beta_1)\ln \hat{H}}}, \quad D_{2a} = \frac{e^{(l_{i0}+\beta_0)+(l_{i1}+\beta_1)\ln 2\hat{H}}}{1+e^{(l_{i0}+\beta_0)+(l_{i1}+\beta_1)\ln 2\hat{H}}} \qquad \text{(for locus } i\text{)} \qquad \text{T}_1 \text{ model}$$

$$D_a = \frac{e^{(l_{i0}+\beta_0)+(l_{i1}+\beta_1)\ln \hat{H}_a}}{1+e^{(l_{i0}+\beta_0)+(l_{i1}+\beta_1)\ln \hat{H}_a}} \qquad \text{(for locus } i\text{)} \qquad \text{T}_2 \text{ model}$$

$$D_a = \frac{e^{\beta_0+\beta_1 \ln \hat{H}_a}}{1+e^{\beta_0+\beta_1 \ln \hat{H}_a}} \qquad \text{T}_2' \text{ model}$$

The first model (T$_1$), published by Tvedebrink et al.[726] in 2009, uses an average of peak heights across a full profile, $\bar{H}$, as a proxy for mass. A logistic model was fitted, allowing separate logistic parameters β_0 and β_1 for each locus. Tvedebrink et al.[728] subsequently published a second model (T$_2$) that, correctly, models mass as an exponential function of molecular weight, $\hat{H}_a$. This model also allows separate β_0 and β_1 for each locus. Therefore in model T$_1$ one DNA proxy is used for all loci, whereas in T$_2$ the DNA proxy variable is locus-dependent. However the instability of locus effects over time suggests that tuning a model for these effects at one time is likely to be counterproductive to their use at a subsequent time. Therefore the use of an exponential degradation curve but without locus effects, model T$_2'$, appears to be the best compromise.

Different curves may be applied to each contributor in a profile.

Lab Retriever[108] uses a variant of T$_1$

$$D_a = \frac{e^{\beta_0+\beta_1 \hat{H}}}{1+e^{\beta_0+\beta_1 \hat{H}}}, \quad D_{2a} = \frac{e^{\beta_0+\beta_1 2\hat{H}}}{1+e^{\beta_0+\beta_1 2\hat{H}}} \qquad \text{Lohmueller and Rudin (L\&R) model}$$

Note that this differs in having no degradation and no locus effect and not using the log of height. In limited trials by the authors the performance of T$_1$ was slightly better than L&R. In these same limited trials we used the quantification value instead of peak height. In our hands this was very ineffective.

The LRmix software allows multiple dropout probabilities to be assigned, one for each contributor. The dropout probability for the minor is varied a range and then a conservative assignment is taken.

Balding in LikeLTD allows different dropout probabilities for each contributor and adopts a degradation model. The parameters of the degradation curve are assigned by maximum likelihood estimation.

By dealing with separate dropout probabilities for each contributor and locus these software recapture some of the information present in peak heights.

An approach initially brought to our attention by Balding is to treat the probability of dropout (or the true mass of DNA of the contributor, M) as a nuisance variable and integrate it out. This avoids the criticism that the explanatory variable is a function of the data and is then used to assess the probability of the data. This slight circularity is probably not serious but best avoided. If the true mass of DNA were known at each allelic position, then it is possible to try a model consistent with the observations that the distribution of peak heights appears to be approximately lognormal with variance proportional to $\frac{1}{M}$. Since M is unknown we should integrate it out. Later we will describe one Markov chain Monte Carlo approach to do this. For the purposes of a simple comparison with the T_1, T_2, T_2' and L&R models, we can take the tail area assuming a lognormal distribution with mean M and variance proportional to $\frac{1}{M}$ (this is marked *STRmix*™ in Figure 8.9). There is little difference between the curves and it will take a lot of empirical data to choose between them. However limited trials by the authors suggest that the STRmix model is less tolerant when M is high and dropout has occurred. This is the same observation as noting that the STRmix model approaches $D = 0$ more rapidly. Greater tolerance of dropout at moderate template is likely to add robustness to an application.

Relatives

The matter of relatives should be dominant in the interpretation of single source stains analyzed with modern multiplexes. This is because the current systems are so powerful that there is almost no posterior probability (probability after analysis) on unrelated donors. Most of the posterior probability resides on relatives of a matching accused. This is true whether or not there is any particular reason to suspect a relative. All that is required is the possibility that a relative could be the donor.

The same issue presents in mixtures. No new theory is required but implementation requires some attention to detail[732] and might be best done with validated software. A feel

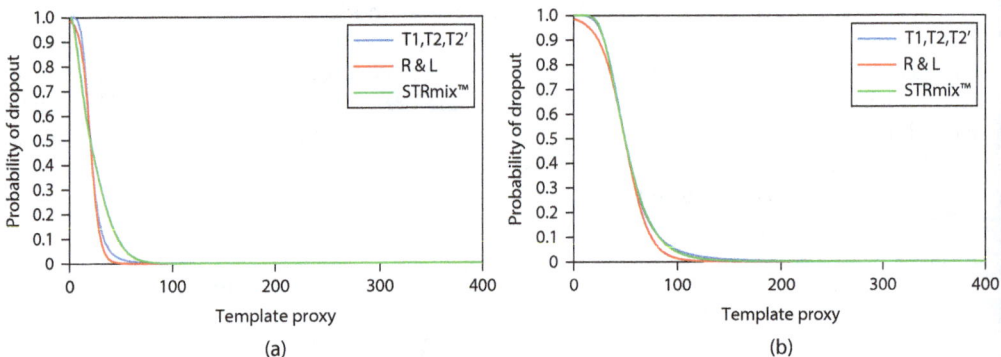

Figure 8.9 Plot of the performance of difference models of dropout. The template proxy is in rfu. The threshold is taken arbitrarily as (a) 20 rfu and (b) 50 rfu. T_1, T_2, T_2' and L&R are constrained to pass through (20,0.5) and (50,0.5), respectively.

Table 8.12 Likelihood Ratios for Unrelated and Related Propositions Given a Number of Different Mixture Scenarios

N	Knowns	POI Matches	Unrelated	Sibling	Parent/ Child	Half-Siblings Grandparent/ Grandchild Uncle–Aunt/ Niece–Nephew	First Cousin
1	0		8×10^{43}	2×10^{10}	8×10^{23}	6×10^{28}	1×10^{33}
3	0	One of two equal minors	2×10^{11}	4×10^{4}	2×10^{6}	1×10^{8}	2×10^{9}
2	1	Minor	1×10^{20}	3×10^{6}	4×10^{10}	3×10^{13}	5×10^{15}
1	0		2×10^{19}	1×10^{8}	5×10^{12}	2×10^{15}	1×10^{17}
3	2	Trace	7×10^{7}	5×10^{2}	3×10^{3}	9×10^{4}	1×10^{6}

POI, person of interest.

for the magnitude of the resulting *LR*s is given for five single source samples or mixtures in Table 8.12.

Mixtures and the Factor of 2

We have written previously on this subject with little effect possibly because of an excessively complex approach.[733] In this section we try to describe the matter in a 'back to the basics' manner.

Consider a clear major/minor stain. The genotype of the major is G_1. There is plausibly ambiguity in the genotype of the minor so let us consider that the genotype of the minor is G_2, or $G_3 \ldots G_N$. We assign the probability of the major by some model as p_1 and the minor $p_2 + p_3 + \ldots + p_N = p_m$.

We imagine that the police produce one POI, S_1 and that the other contributor to the stain is unknown, U_1. Before we look at the profiles at all, we would consider this evidence if the suspect matched the major or any of the minor possibilities. Reasonable propositions seem to be as follows:

Pair A:

H_p: The donors to the stain are S_1 and U_1.

H_d: The donors to the stain are U_1 and U_2.

Now we examine the comparison to the profile. If the POI matches the major the *LR* is $\frac{1}{2p_1}$, and if he matches the minor it is $\frac{1}{2p_m}$. It is the factor of 2 that causes concern but not to Whittaker,[734] Evett,[735] Aitken,[736] Evett and Weir,[257,737] Triggs and Buckleton,[738] Dawid,[242] Meester and Sjerps[241] and Gittelson et al.[739,740]

Consider the POI matching the major. We need an unknown matching the minor with probability p_m. However, if we have a major minor profile from two contributors, then the POI could have been the major or the minor. If we give these probability 1/2 each, then the factor of 2 arises naturally

$$LR = \frac{\frac{1}{2}p_m}{p_1 p_m} = \frac{1}{2p_1}$$

Another pair of propositions could be Pair B:

H_p: The donor of the major stain is S_1.

H_d: The donor of the major stain is U_1.

which gives $LR = \dfrac{1}{p_1}$.

How can there be two different LRs for the same evidence? Pair B can only be formed by having a peep at the evidence and noting that the POI matches the major. In effect some of the findings are used when forming the proposition. We also glance at Pair A and see that it is a two person mix but we do not need to know the genotype of the POI when forming our propositions.

The matter is possibly not that vital. We assume that prior odds alter in balance. For example for proposition Pair A, the prior would be formed from the concept that the accused was one of two contributors to the stain. By contrast for Pair B the prior would be formed from the concept that the accused is the single contributor to the major fraction of the stain. This would suggest a compensating factor of 2.

We believe, however, that the prevalence of clear major/minor stains is much exaggerated. In reality we believe that many forensic scientists when applying the binary approach take an (admirably) conservative stance by 'allowing' a large number of combinations at each locus and between loci. By doing this, however, they do not treat the mixture as a clear major/minor. In such cases the question of whether there should be a factor of 2 or not is very complex.

If a DNA profile is partially resolved, then the difference between the LR produced from proposition Pair A (LR_A) and the LR produced from proposition pair B (LR_B) will be less than 2. Taken to its extreme a profile that is completely unresolved will result in $LR_A = LR_B$.

Note that the same theory extends to numbers of contributors greater than 2. The maximum possible correction required will depend on the number of ways in which contributors can be ordered. For a three person mixture we could order contributors as 123, 132, 213, 231, 312, 321 so that a factor of 2 would become a factor of 6. In general the factor will be $N!$ for an N person mixture, although in many instances the true correction required (as a result of the number of references compared and the level of resolution between contributors) will be much less than this theoretical maximum. We continue to use the 'factor of 2' terminology due to its use in the literature but note that it is in fact a 'factor of $N!$'.

9

The Continuous Model

Duncan Taylor, Jo-Anne Bright and John S. Buckleton

Contents

Introduction

The key point of difference of a continuous model[741-744] is that it considers the peak heights as a continuous variable. This chapter describes the biological models and statistics behind STRmix™, one such continuous model.

Let the genotype of person i be G_i. The genotype of the person of interest is G_p. To form the likelihood ratio (LR) we consider two propositions H_p and H_d, chosen to align with the prosecution and the defence, respectively. We consider a mixture assigned as coming from two people although the principle is quite general. The two propositions H_i therefore each define one or many sets of two genotypes G_i and G_j as the proposed contributors. These may or may not include the person of interest (POI). Typically the POI is included in all sets under H_p, but not under H_d. There may or may not be genotypes from other persons known or reasonably assumed to be part of the mixture.

We seek

$$LR = \frac{p(G_C \mid H_p, G_p, I)}{p(G_C \mid H_d, G_p, I)}$$

For simplicity we drop the background information I from the conditioning henceforth and use p for a probability density and Pr for a probability. It is convenient from here on to consider terms of the type $p(G_C \mid S_k, G_p)$. Let H_i specify the sets of pairs of genotypes S_k $k = 1 \ldots M$, then

$$p(G_C \mid H_i, G_p) = \sum_{k=1}^{M} p(G_C \mid S_k, G_p) \Pr(S_k \mid H_i, G_p)$$

The binary model assigns the terms $p(G_C \mid S_k, G_p)$ the value 0 or 1 depending on whether the crime profile is deemed possible or impossible if it originated from the genotypes specified by S_k.

If one sample is run multiple times the results will not always be the same. Both the absolute and relative peak heights may vary within and between loci.[118,745] What the binary model is doing is assigning the values 0 and 1 based on very reasonable methods that approximate the relative values of $p(G_C \mid S_k, G_p)$. In essence $p(G_C \mid S_k, G_p)$ is assigned as 0 if it is thought that this probability density is very small relative to the other probability densities. It is assigned a value of 1 if it is thought that this value is relatively large. As such it is an approximation.

This method has served well for a number of years and in a great many cases. However all approximations suffer from some loss of information.

A fully continuous model for DNA interpretation is one which assigns a value to the probability density $p(G_C \mid S_k, G_p)$ based on treating the peak heights as a continuous variable.

Such models may require some preprocessing, say of stutter peaks, or may be fully automated. These methods have the potential to handle any type of non-concordance and may assess any number of replicates without heuristic preprocessing and the consequent loss of information. Continuous methods are likely to require models for the variability in peak heights and potentially stutter.

Many of the qualitative or subjective decisions that the scientist has traditionally handled – such as the designation of peaks as alleles, the allocation of stutters and possible allelic combinations – may be removed. Instead the model takes the quantitative information from the electropherogram (epg), such as peak heights, and uses this information to calculate the probability of the peak heights given all possible genotype combinations.

Profile Information

As described in this book the DNA profile evidence is typically assessed in the framework of an LR. LRs have the general form

$$LR = \frac{\sum_i w_i \Pr\left(S_i \mid H_p\right)}{\sum_j w_j \Pr\left(S_j \mid H_d\right)}$$

where w_x is a weight for a set of explanatory genotypes (S_x). In Chapter 8 we showed how the weights can be a list of ones or zeros in a binary system or dropout and drop-in probabilities in a semi-continuous system. Both these systems summarize the DNA profile data in some way. In the case of a binary system the summary comes in the form of interpretational thresholds. Peaks are summarized by grouping them into binary categories of either passing or failing a threshold-based test. For example, a dropout threshold (ST) will group single-peaked loci either as originating from a homozygote or potentially having a dropped-out partner peak. Semi-continuous systems summarize the data in that they use the DNA profile to develop probabilities for dropout or drop-in that are applied to all peaks and all posited contributing genotypes. Semi-continuous systems may also have a secondary system for screening out potential contributing genotypes based on stutter or heterozygote balance (Hb) thresholds.

The more correct and relevant information a system is able to make use of, the better its ability will be to differentiate true from false donors.[746] Figure 9.1 shows diagrammatically that as more information is provided to a DNA profile analysis system (either with more DNA, more polymerase chain reaction [PCR] replicates, simpler profiles or more information about assumed contributors) the ability to distinguish true from false hypotheses is increased.

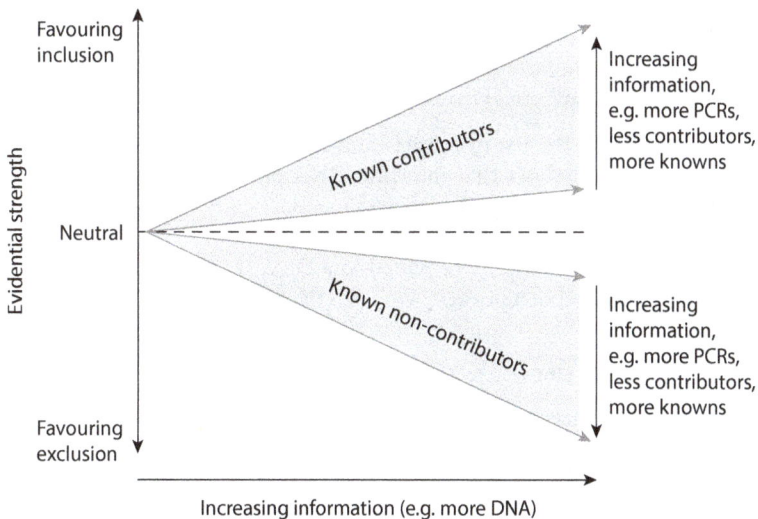

Figure 9.1   Demonstration of the effect that information has on the ability to distinguish true from false hypotheses.

This same thinking can apply to the system being used to interpret a DNA profile, i.e. the more relevant information that is provided, the better the system will be able to distinguish true from false hypotheses. In simple terms true contributors will have more support for their inclusion to a profile and non-contributors will be excluded more often or with more strength. This situation then leads to the question, what information exists within a DNA profile?

On face value the observable data are as follows:

- Peak heights
- Molecular weights
- Allelic designations (which broadly represent underlying DNA sequences)

However there is further information that can be provided to an interpretation system that is not directly obtained from the DNA profile:

- How peak heights are related to template DNA amount
- How DNA profiles degrade
- How loci amplify at differing efficiencies
- How peak heights have a level of variability
- Information about the generation of artefacts during PCR (i.e. stuttering or drop-in)
- How replicate amplifications of the sample extract behave

All of these are termed *models*. There is a further class of information that could be described as *calibration data*. This will typically be specific for a set of laboratory hardware and a method of profile generation:

- How much a specific allele and locus combination is expected to stutter
- How much peak heights are expected to vary (both allelic and stutter)
- How much peak height balance is expected between loci
- How much drop-in is expected
- When a capillary electrophoresis instrument is expected to reach fluorescent saturation
- Below what level a laboratory is not prepared to read information (typically referred to as a baseline or analytical threshold)

It is apparent that both the list of models and the calibration data list is typically the type of information learnt by analysts that interpret DNA profiles. Their knowledge of these DNA profile behaviours and laboratory performances has classically been used in their assessment of DNA profiles prior to interpretation in an analytical system.

The final set of data that could be provided to a DNA interpretation system would relate to specifics of a DNA profile being analyzed. We term these the *unknowables* as in reality their true value can never be known:

- The number of contributors to a profile (N)
- DNA amounts of each contributor (t_n)
- The degradation of each contributor (d_n)
- The amplification efficiency of each locus (A^l)
- Replicate amplification strength (R_r)
- The level of peak height variability within the sample

There are two points to note here. First there is typically a model that describes the behaviour of each of the unknowables. Second again in classic DNA profile interpretation an analyst would be trialling different combination of these factors (perhaps unknowingly) in their assessment of potential contributing genotypes.

Continuous DNA profile analysis systems seek to make use of all the observable data using models and calibration data and even the unknowable information in order to deconvolute a profile into a list of genotype sets (S, a set of N individual genotypes) each with an associated weight that in general terms describes how well the observed data is described by that particular genotype set.

STRmix

There are at least four implementations of the continuous approach of which we are aware.[110,111,743,747] For a good summary of the programmes and their abilities we direct the reader to Ref. 462. While it would clearly be more balanced to discuss the various continuous approaches available at this time, we are unable to do justice to three of them due to a lack of in-depth understanding and in some cases suggestions of potential litigation. We therefore concentrate on the one with which we are most familiar.

STRmix uses standard mathematics and a model for peak and stutter height. Total allelic product modelling assumes a degradation curve that is exponential but allows each contributor to a mixture to have different curves. Individual loci are allowed a limited liberty to be above or below this curve. The total allelic product is split into stutter and allelic peaks using allele-specific stutter ratios developed from empirical data. The contribution to a peak from different allelic or stutter sources is assumed to be additive. The variability about the expected peak height is modelled on empirical data and the relative variance is large for small peaks and small for large peaks. This variance is allowed some limited flexibility within the system so that it can adapt slightly for good or bad profiles. Independence is assumed across peaks at a locus and between loci.

The model for the peak and stutter heights and other assumptions results in a probability density for the profile given a set of input parameters for such things as template and degradation. These input parameters are unknown.

To deal with these unknown inputs STRmix uses Markov chain Monte Carlo (MCMC) and the Metropolis–Hastings algorithm. These terms will be unfamiliar to most forensic biologists but appear to be teachable. MCMC is close to a 'hot and cold' game.

It is likely that continuous methods will supersede all other methods. At this stage we suspect that STRmix has a slightly higher false exclusion rate than the semi-continuous models and a much lower false inclusion rate. The false exclusions for STRmix are usually caused by unusual PCR behaviour.

The software has improved the number of interpretable volume crime cases in New Zealand by 17%.

Mass Parameters

We may consider the evidence of the crime stain G_c to consist of a vector of observed peak heights $\mathbf{O}$ made up of a number of individual observed peak heights O_{ar}^l for allele a at locus l for replicate r. Let there be R replicates and L loci.

To describe these observed peaks we must consider various values for the unknown parameters. We introduce parameters to describe the true template level. Experience and empirical studies suggest that the height of peaks from a single contributor are approximately constant across the profile but generally have a downtrend with increasing molecular weight. Given this general downtrend individual loci may still be above or below the trend. In addition the slope of the downtrend trend may vary from one contributor to another. The product from the amplification of an allele is dominated by correct copies at the allelic position and back stutter at one repeat shorter than the allele. There are a number of other more minor products ignored in this treatment. We term the sum of the allelic and back stutter product *total allelic product*. We require a term for the true but unknown template level available at a locus for amplification. This is a function of the input DNA and any degradation or inhibition effects. Since template is described by weight, usually in picograms, we coin the term *mass* to subsume the concepts of template, degradation, inhibition and any other effect that determines the expected total allelic product at a locus.

Hence the mass of an allele at a locus is modelled as a function of various parameters which we collectively term the *mass parameters*. These are as follows:

1. A constant t_n, for each of the n contributors that may usefully be thought of as template amount.

2. A constant d_n, which models the decay with respect to molecular weight (m) of template for each of the contributors to genotype set S_j. This may usefully be thought of as a measure of degradation.

3. A locus offset at each locus, A^l, to allow for the observed amplification levels of each locus.

4. A replicate multiplier R_r. This effectively scales all peaks up or down between replicates.

We write the mass variables $\{d_n: n = 1, ..., N\}$ and $\{t_n: n = 1, ..., N\}$ as **D** and **T**, respectively, $\{A^l: l = 1, ..., L\}$ as **A** and $\{R_n: n = 1, ..., R\}$ as **R**. The variables **D**, **A**, **R** and **T** are written collectively as **M**.

Template

The heights (or areas) of the peaks within the epg are approximately proportional to the amount of undegraded template DNA.[748–751] Therefore when building a picture of an expected profile the amount of DNA for each contributor will directly relate to the peak heights of contributors. We show this empirically by calculating the average peak height for GlobalFiler™ (Thermo Fisher Scientific, Waltham, MA) profiles generated using varying amounts of DNA (Figure 9.2).

As expected there exists some stochastic variation in average peak heights; however a clear linear relationship can be seen between input DNA and fluorescence.

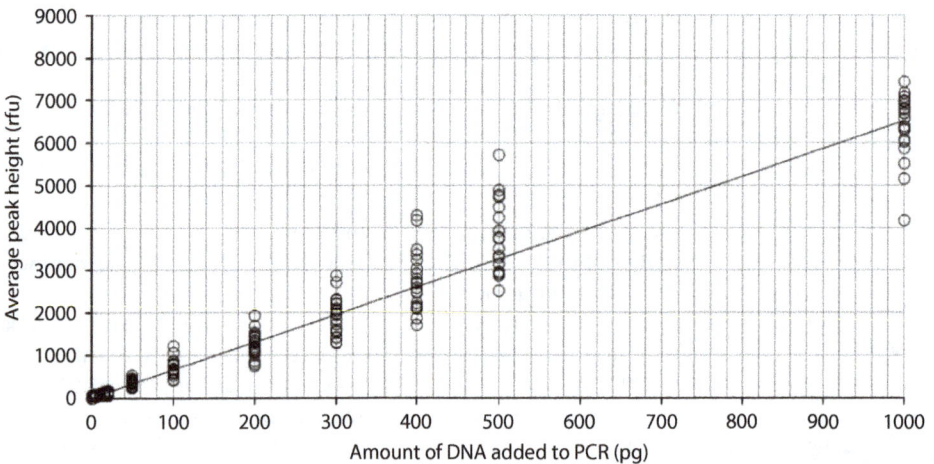

Figure 9.2 Average peak height for GlobalFiler profiles produced on a 3130*xl* with varying amount of input DNA.

It is also expected that peak heights are additive; i.e. if there are multiple sources of a single allele, the height of that allele will equal the sum of the individual expected heights from each source. This is termed *stacking* in the United States. This additivity is assumed to hold true whether the sources are all allelic or whether they are a combination of stutter and allele.

Degradation

The heights (or areas) of the peaks within the epg are approximately proportional to the amount of undegraded template DNA.[748–751] However this relationship is affected by a number of systematic factors. Notable among these factors is the molecular weight (m_a) of an allele, a.

A typical epg has a downward trend with increasing molecular weight. This is variously described as the degradation slope or the 'ski slope'.[729,752,753] The term *degradation slope* alludes to a suggested cause, degradation of the DNA. There are many chemical, physical and biological insults which are believed to contribute to DNA degradation or inhibition of a profile. Environmental factors such as humidity,[754] bacteria[753] or other forces such as ultraviolet light break down the DNA, destroying some fraction of the initial template.[755] Although the cause of the slope may not be known, we will refer to this ski slope effect as *degradation* to comport with common usage. Of interest is that fresh buccal scrapes processed immediately show a degradation slope.

It is important to understand how degradation affects these models. The simplest model is linear. That is, the expected peak height declines constantly with respect to molecular weight. This can be demonstrated crudely by taking a paper epg and drawing a downward sloping straight line across the apex of the heterozygote peaks from the lowest molecular weight locus to the highest molecular weight locus.[120]

If the breakdown of the DNA strand was random with respect to location, then we would expect that the observed height of peak a, O_a, would be exponentially related to molecular weight.[728]

Amplification Efficiency

When template DNA amount, degradation, fluorescence and peak height variation are taken into account using the models described thus far, the variation in peak heights between loci is still more variable than predicted. This additional variability arises from differences in amplification efficiencies between loci. These differences appear to vary with time and maybe even sample to sample. They may be affected by, at least, co-extracted materials that affect the PCR process. Imagine, initially, that we allow a locus-specific amplification efficiency, A^l (LSAE), at each locus. Consider the profile in Figure 9.3.

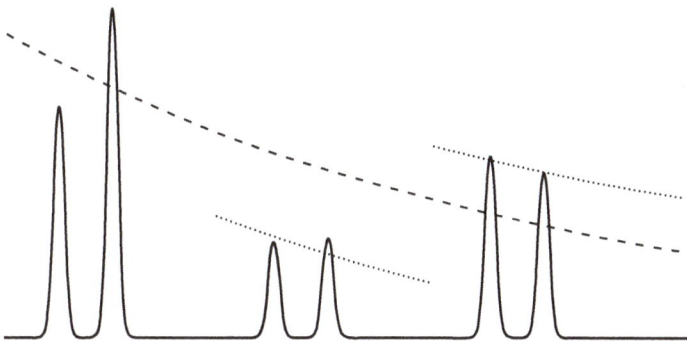

Figure 9.3 Profile showing expected heights at a whole profile level with the dashed line and the adjustment made by locus-specific amplification efficiency if it were completely free to take any value.

If we allow the A^l variables to be free, we will model the mass of template at each locus according to the dotted lines in Figure 9.3. Look now at the heterozygotic loci. If one allele is above the mass line then the other is always below. In fact if one is x rfu above then the other is x rfu below. They are fully correlated. This is because the mass has been overfitted to the data. How could we fit at the correct level, neither over nor underfitted?

Consider the question, how high is peak b? It would be helpful to know the height of peak a, the partner allele of b from a heterozygote. Let us say peak a is height 400 rfu. It would make sense to guess that peak b was also about 400 rfu. However further imagine that you were told that peak a was a bit high relative to the true template at this locus. In fact the true template at this locus suggests that peak a should be of height 350 rfu and in this case it must have varied upwards. Given this knowledge, we would guess that peak b would be about 350 rfu. What this suggests is that if we know the true template at a locus then the height of peak a is not further information regarding the height of peak b. Another useful way to think of this is that the two peaks of a heterozygote should scatter around the true template and if one goes up that does not imply the other one will. This gives us a diagnostic to find the true template. It is that value where the two peaks of a heterozygote are uncorrelated when we consider their variation from this value.

To obtain this value we cannot allow the A^l values to be free. If we did they would overfit.

The continuous method with which we are most familiar is STRmix. We would write in more generality if we knew better what the other implementations do. However it is very likely that the principles are the same. The method applied in STRmix to find the true template at a locus allows the A^l values some limited freedom to fit to the data. The amplification efficiency at each locus is modelled by a lognormal distribution with a mean of zero and a fixed, but optimized, variance determined from laboratory calibration data:

$$\log_{10}\left(\frac{O\{A^l\}}{E\{A^l\}}\right) \sim N\left(0, \sigma_A^2\right)$$

where $O\{A^l\}$ is the observed amplification efficiency for locus l. Note that $E\{A^l\}$ is the expected amplification efficiencies, which we expect to be 1, giving $\log_{10}\left(A^l\right) \sim N\left(0, \sigma_A^2\right)$ where we have just used A^l to signify the observed amplification efficiency for locus l.

By applying this penalty (strictly a prior distribution) there is a pull back towards the mean. This acts against peak height variability like rubber bands pulling the expected heights for the locus back towards the expected level for the whole profile (Figure 9.4 shows this process diagrammatically).

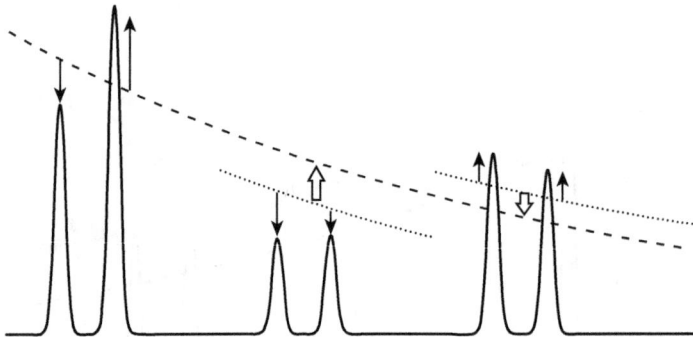

Figure 9.4   Profile showing expected heights at a whole profile level with a dashed line, the influence of peak height variability (solid arrows) pushing the locus-specific expected height (dotted lines) towards the observed heights and the effect of locus-specific amplification efficiency (A^l) (hollow arrows) pulling the locus-specific expected heights back towards the whole profile-expected heights.

Replicate Amplification Strength

Replicate amplification efficiencies are used in the calculation of total allelic product and scale all peaks up or down relative to one another. This allows the inclusion of multiple PCR replicates into a single analysis even if different amounts of template DNA have been added to the PCRs, as long as they originate from the same DNA extract.

The simplest model for replicate amplification efficiencies makes the assumption that the DNA profiles will contain the same individuals with the same degradation, the same relative DNA amounts and the same locus amplification efficiencies.

Note that the replicate amplification terms should be scaled by their logs. In other words, if two replicates were used in an analysis and one was four times the intensity of the other, then the appropriate replicate amplification efficiencies (to prevent differences when considering the two PCRs in different orders) would be 50% and 200% rather than 100% and 400%.

Generating Weights

In order to generate the weights we start with the observed evidence ($\mathbf{O}$), which will be a number of peaks at a number of alleles (a), across a number of loci (l) and replicate amplifications (r). Individually each peak can be referred to by $O_{a,r}^{l}$. We seek the following:

$$\Pr(\mathbf{O}|I) = \Pr\left(O_{1,1}^{1} \ldots O_{A,R}^{L} \mid I\right)$$

where I is all the background information the system has about DNA profile behaviour and laboratory calibration. From this point on we omit the I term but recognize that it is important to the calculation. To progress this further we require information about the mass parameters. These of course are unknowable for a DNA profile and so it appears initially as though an impasse has been reached. However in order to consider the effect of mass parameters on the probability of the evidence we need not know their value, rather just the effect that each of the mass parameters has on the probability of the observed data. This allows them to be considered 'nuisance' parameters and integrated over without ever knowing their true value. Box 9.1 explains the concept of integrating out a nuisance parameter.

BOX 9.1 INTEGRATING OUT A NUISANCE PARAMETER

Imagine that we were interested in the average foot size within a population of people. However this information was not readily obtained by records and measuring foot size was impractical. Records were however present for the distribution of height in the population and additionally studies had been carried out on the link between foot size and height.

We define some terms:

F = foot size

H = height

We create a model linking foot size to height:

$$F = E[F|H = h]$$

We seek the average foot size. We could initially consider a simplified model where the average height was calculated ($\bar{h}$) and then calculate the foot size by the following:

$$\hat{F} = E\left[F|H = \bar{h}\right]$$

Doing this makes a number of simplifying assumptions about the distribution of heights and the model linking foot size and height. If we wanted to take the distribution heights into account (and use a model that better described reality) we could start splitting height into brackets, for example if it were split into two brackets around 150 cm, and take the average of each bracket ($\bar{h}_{>150\,cm}$ and $\bar{h}_{<150\,cm}$):

$$\hat{F} = E\left[F \mid H = \bar{h}_{>150\,cm}\right]\Pr(H > 150\ cm) + E\left[F \mid H = \bar{h}_{<150\,cm}\right]\Pr(H < 150\ cm)$$

We could continue to break apart the height into ever smaller discrete brackets (h_i), multiplying by the probability of obtaining an individual within that bracket and summing across

$$\hat{F} = \sum_i E\left[F \mid H = \bar{h}_i\right]\Pr(h_i)$$

Ultimately the discrete brackets are reduced to a point where they approximate a smooth continuous distribution. This continuous equivalent is integration and expressed as follows:

$$\hat{F} = \int_i E\left[F \mid H = \bar{h}_i\right]\Pr(h_i)dh_i$$

In words this is explained as the foot size integrated across the distribution of height. It treats height as a nuisance parameter, as we aren't really interested in the height of people but must consider it to calculate the value of interest, in this case foot size.

Each parameter (p) in the analysis can then be treated in this manner to obtain the following:

$$\int_{p_1}\ldots\int_{p_D} \Pr\left(O^1_{1,1}\ldots O^L_{A,R} \mid p_1 \ldots p_D\right)\prod_{i=1}^{D}\Pr(p_i \mid p_{i+1}\ldots p_D)dp_1\ldots dp_D$$

where D is the number of parameters (or dimensionality) in the analysis. This rather daunting formula is visually simplified by referring to all parameters as M (for mass parameters):

$$\int_M \Pr\left(O^1_{1,1}\ldots O^L_{A,R} \mid M\right)\Pr(M)dM$$

We must now also recognize that genotype sets (S_i) themselves are treated as nuisance parameters within the LR calculation. That is, we don't really care what their value takes; however we must consider them in order to calculate the probability of the evidence. If we add mass parameters into the above equation we obtain the following:

$$\sum_i \Pr(S_i)\int_M \Pr(O \mid M, S_i)\Pr(M)dM$$

In theory it is possible to have different mass parameters for each hypothesis but, since the only factors affecting their values are the genotypes, this is unnecessary. Hence they will cancel out in numerator and denominator of the LR so that from the equation above:

$$w_i \propto \int_M \Pr(O \mid M, S_i)\Pr(M)dM$$

We then obtain a term that looks very much like the denominator and numerator terms of the LR at the beginning of this chapter. Note that there are no locus terms in this equation, and this is because it is considering the whole profile at once. There are mathematical advantages to considering the data in this manner, but many disadvantages in the required computer power and comprehensibility of results. Some simplifying assumptions can be made to make the problem tractable:

Assumption 1: Peak heights are assumed to be conditionally independent given S_j and M:

$$\Pr\left(O \mid S_j, M\right) = \Pr\left(O^1_{1,1}\ldots O^L_{AR} \mid S_j, M\right) = \prod_a \prod_r \Pr\left(O^l_{ar} \mid S_j, M\right)$$

And considering the observed data across loci and treating mass parameters as a nuisance the model becomes

$$w'_j = \int_M \prod_l \prod_a \prod_r \Pr(O^l_{ar} \mid S_j, M)\Pr(M)dM$$

Assumption 2: The weight across a profile is the product of the weights at each locus

$$w_j = \prod_l w^l_j$$

which gives

$$w'_j = \prod_l \int_M \prod_a \prod_r \Pr\left(O^l_{ar} \mid S_j, M\right)\Pr(M)dM$$

In other words the weight of a genotype set at a locus is the probability of obtaining the observed data if that genotype set had given rise to it, integrating across all mass parameters. The full profile weight is the product of the weights of the individual loci.

Even with modern computers it is prohibitively complicated to enumerate this complex multiple integral completely. In order to overcome this limitation the use of methods such as MCMC is employed.

MCMC and Profile Building

DNA profile problems can be highly complex – so complex that even with modern computers it would be impossible to test every possible combination of all parameters. Instead the computer can use a process similar to a game of hot and cold with the DNA profile. This mathematical process is called *MCMC* and allows the computation of complex problems with standard computers.

Figure 9.5 shows a diagrammatic representation of the hot and cold analogy of MCMC. Imagine that each square on the board represents a possible answer to some problem. One possible way to find the best answer would be to start at the top left and work down each possible answer in each row and column and then at the end to choose the answer that gave the

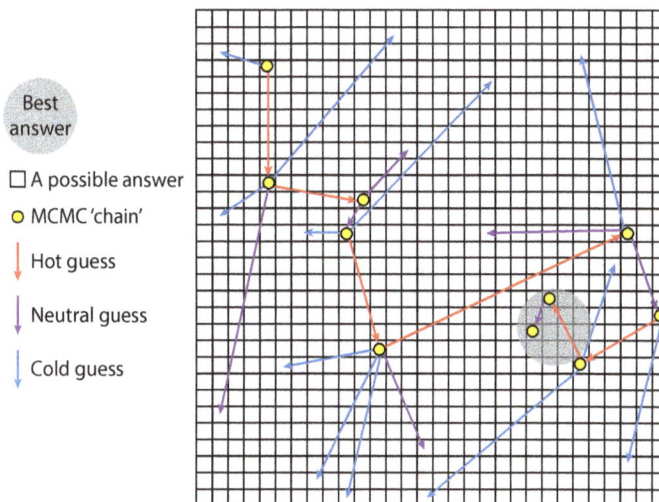

Figure 9.5 Diagrammatic representation of a Markov chain Monte Carlo process as a game of hot and cold.

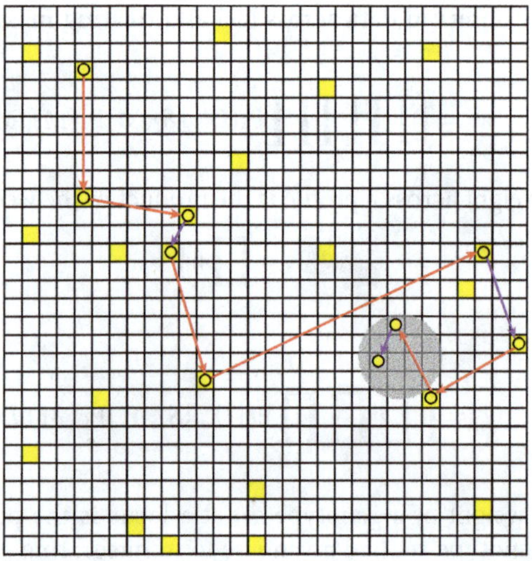

Figure 9.6   Squares landed on (highlighted) in the hot and cold game shown in Figure 9.5.

best solution. Doing this would highlight the solutions that occupy the grey circle on the diagram, but it would take some time as each possible solution would need to be assessed.

Now instead we are going to try and find the good solutions by playing hot and cold. A random point on the board is chosen (in the example below this is near the top left) and the goodness of fit calculated. Next a nearby square is randomly chosen and the goodness of fit calculated. If it is better than the current position it will be adopted and we will 'move' the new position. If the position is much worse than we would be very unlikely to move to it and if it is neutral, then there is a chance we will move there some of the time.

Figure 9.5 shows a series of guesses, some hot, some neutral and some cold, and the eventual path taken by the MCMC chain over the course of 10 moves.

Figure 9.6 shows the answer board, where we have highlighted all the possible solutions that were considered in the journey from starting position to the best answers. It can be seen from Figure 9.6 that only a very small percentage of all possible answers needed to be considered. This is the power of MCMC, its ability to find good answers, or in MCMC parlance 'good sample space', in problems that are very complex, without having to consider every combination of every parameter value in the model.

MCMC Robot

MCMC Robot is available from http://web.uconn.edu/gogarten/bioinf/mcrobot.html or as an application for Apple devices from https://itunes.apple.com/nz/app/mcmc-robot/id454055791?mt=8. This is a useful teaching tool.

Figure 9.7 gives screen grabs from MCMC Robot. The blue circles are a probability 'hill'. We can usefully think of this as a contour map. The starting position of the MCMC chain is a blue dot.

In the second screen grab the starting position of the MCMC chain and the first 10 steps are visible.

In the third grab the robot has taken 1000 steps.

In the last grab, in addition to the 1000 accepted steps, the failed steps have been added (in purple).

At the end of these 1000 steps the robot is at the top of the hill and is wandering around. This 1000-step phase is the burn-in. These results are then discarded and the real count begins from the position that was arrived at the end of burn-in. This is to get rid of the 'bad' steps early in the process.

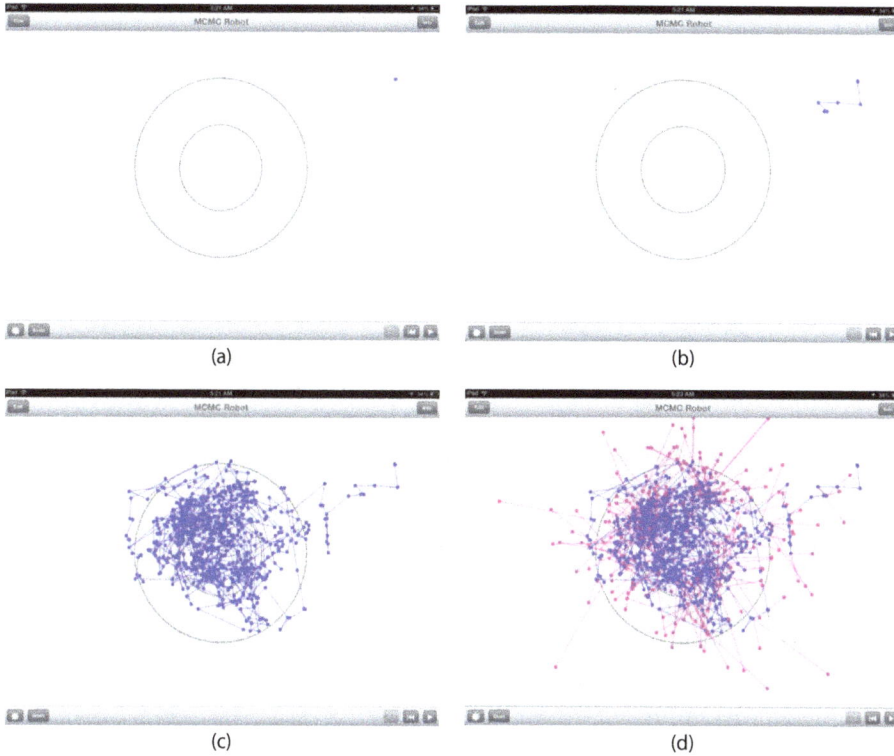

Figure 9.7 Four screen grabs from the MCMC Robot programme. (a) before any steps have been taken, (b) after a small number of steps have been taken, (c) after many steps have been taken and (d) after many steps have been taken and also showing rejected steps.

The Metropolis–Hastings Algorithm

The basis of an MCMC chain is that it steps from one state to another in some sensible way so that it will preferentially sample from the high probability density portion of the sample space. In STRmix the stepping is done using the Metropolis–Hastings algorithm (MHA). MHA compares two states, the current state and the proposed state. The algorithm considers whether to step to the proposed state or stay at the current state. If the proposed state has a higher probability density the chain always steps. If it has a lower probability density it will step some of the time.

It is useful to think of the probability density as a landscape with a hill in it. The objective is to find the top of the hill. The MHA always steps uphill if that is proposed. If the proposal is downhill it does this sometimes. After a while the chain will get to the top of the hill and then wander around sometimes going a way down the slopes.

If the MCMC is sitting at iteration $(y-1)$ and the probability of this current state is $\Pr(y-1)$, the proposed state is y with probability $\Pr(y)$. The MHA will accept the proposed state if $\Pr(y) \geq \Pr(y-1)$ or if a randomly chosen value from $U[0,1] < \dfrac{\Pr(y)}{\Pr(y-1)}$.

Burn-In

When an MCMC starts it is guessing. Mass parameter values are chosen at random and it will be accepting explanations of the observed data that have a very low probability. As the process continues the MCMC will start accepting more and more likely descriptions of the observed data until it has reached an equilibrium state where a small distribution of values for mass parameters and a limited number of genotype sets are being regularly chosen in accordance with how

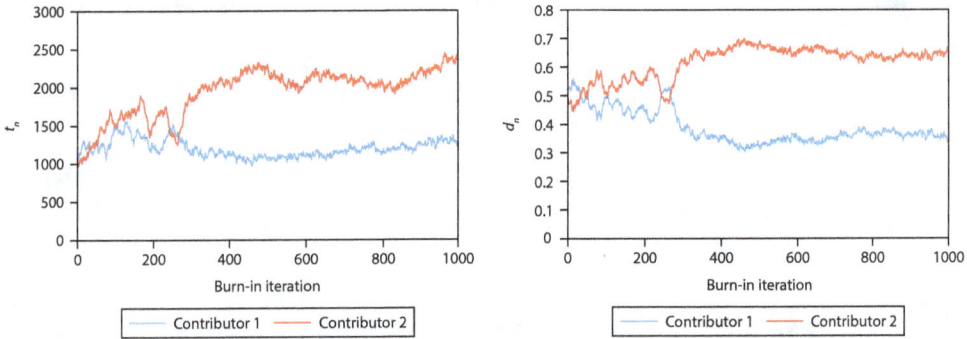

Figure 9.8   Burn-in values for a two person mixture, t_n on left and d_n on right.

well they describe the observed data. The time between when the MCMC starts and when the equilibrium state is reached is termed the *burn-in phase*. In essence it is the time when the MCMC goes from complete randomness to some sensible position.

The first n steps in the MCMC chain are termed *burn-in*, where n is set by the user. These steps are used to get the chain to a reasonable position and the data from these first n steps are discarded. The real count is then started.

The penalty in the first 1/4 of the burn-in for peak heights is $\log(O/E) \sim N(0,0.04)$ and after that it reverts instantly to

$$\log(O/E) \sim N\left(0, \frac{S_a^l c^2}{O_{a+1}^l} + \frac{A_a^l k^2}{E_a^l} \right)$$

The initial constant variance allows the MCMC to find the genotypes more quickly. Figure 9.8 shows two figures giving the t_n and d_n values for a two-person 2:1 mix using a short burn-in of 1000 steps.

Note the resolution of the template amounts for the two contributors. From this output we can tell that the profile must have clearly distinguishable major and minor components. The degradation values for both contributors are very low and do not show any resolution; this is fine. Unlike template amounts the degradation values do not have influence over each other, i.e. just because one degradation value increases does not mean that the other will decrease.

MCMC General

MCMC is a widely used technique outside forensic science and is considered mainstream. It has been used in predicting weather, betting, computational biology, computational linguistics, genetics, code breaking, engineering, physics, aeronautics, stock market and social science.

MCMC is based on a random number generation process. Typically a model will be proposed to describe some data that contains a number of parameters of unknown value. The MCMC trials numerous combinations of parameter values to describe the observed data and ultimately generates posterior distributions for each parameter in the model.

The parameters in the model are the mass parameters (those that are integrated across as nuisance parameters in the previous section). The information supplied by the user is the stutter ratio, the number of contributors and some parameter priors. The data is the observed profile. To picture how the MCMC works for DNA profile interpretation consider the process of building a picture of an expected profile from mass parameters and ultimately comparing it to the observed profile data to calculate a likelihood.

In the following section we show an example of an expected profile being generated from a set of posited parameter values. Note that although the example shows this occurring in a step-wise manner the actual calculations will often occur all together. This means that the order in

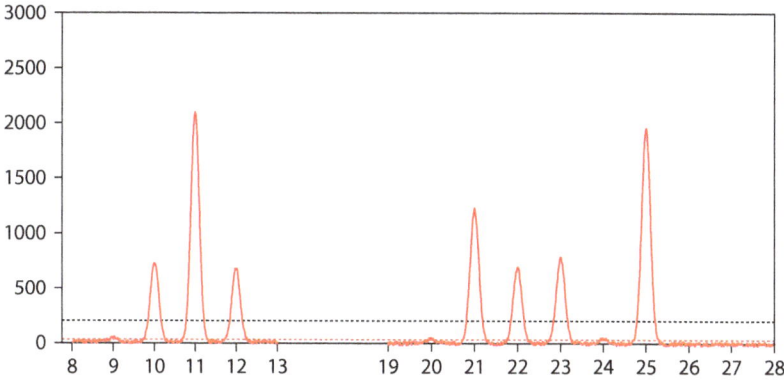

Figure 9.9   An observed two locus profile. Locus 1 has alleles 8 to 13 and locus 2 alleles 19 to 28.

which the various components of the example below occur can easily be changed and would be equally valid.

In Figure 9.9 is an example of an observed two locus profile being analyzed as a two person mixture. Figure 9.10 shows how STRmix builds up an expected profile.

STRmix now has a complete two locus expected DNA profile that it can compare to an observed profile (Figure 9.11).

Converting Mass Parameters to Peak Heights

The peaks in the early stages of Figure 9.10 (before stutter is taken into account) are the total allelic product (T). This is the sum of the allele and the stutter peak. If there are additional replicates they are allowed to scale up or down by a constant factor, R_r. This allows the whole epg to scale but requires the same relative mixture proportions and degradation. The final formula for total allelic product is

$$T^l_{anr} = R_r A^l t_n e^{d_n \times f(m^l_a)} X^l_{an}$$

The terms R_r, A^l, t_n and d_n are termed *mass variables*, M, as they are used to calculate the mass, or total allelic product, of an allele. In the example shown in Figure 9.10 some genotypes were heterozygote and other homozygote. For the homozygote the height is doubled for that individual. This is termed *dose*, X^l_{an}, i.e. the count of allele a at locus l in contributor n. $X^l_{an} = 1$ for a heterozygote with a and $X^l_{an} = 2$ for a homozygote a. The degradation affects peak heights with a dependence on their molecular weight. The term $f(m^l_a)$ is a function of molecular weight and can be as simple as $f(m^l_a) = m^l_a$ or can utilize an offset if the desired behaviour of the model is to begin degradation at some minimum molecular weight.

The next step is to introduce stuttering. The back stutter ratio ($N - 1$ repeat), SR, is a function of the sequence (LUS). Hence, different alleles have slightly different stutter ratios. FS is the forward stutter ratio ($N + 1$). T can be apportioned to stutter and allele using the following equations where SR and FS are determined from a model:

$$E^l_{(a-1)} = SR^l_a O^l_a, \qquad E^l_{(a+1)} = FS^l_a O^l_a, \qquad E^l_{an} = \frac{T^l_{an}}{1 + SR^l_a + FS^l_a},$$

where:
$E^l_{(a-1)}$ is the expected back stutter peak height of the ath allele at locus l
$E^l_{(a+1)}$ is the expected forward stutter peak height of the ath allele at locus l

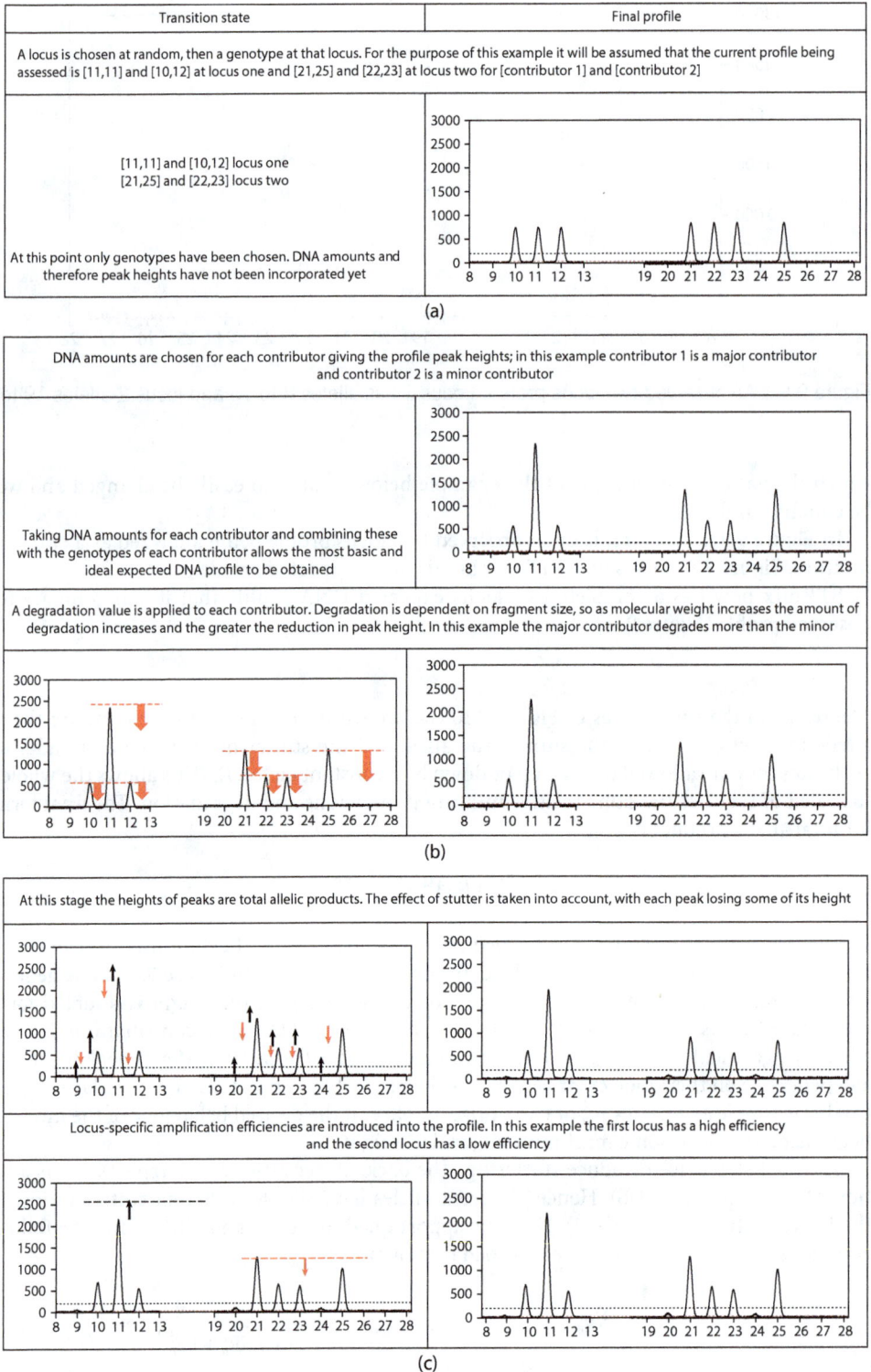

Transition state	Final profile
A locus is chosen at random, then a genotype at that locus. For the purpose of this example it will be assumed that the current profile being assessed is [11,11] and [10,12] at locus one and [21,25] and [22,23] at locus two for [contributor 1] and [contributor 2]	

(a)

(b)

(c)

Figure 9.10   Example of building up an expected profile from mass parameters. (a) Choice of genotypes, (b) Development of TAP, and (c) Development of allele and stutter heights.

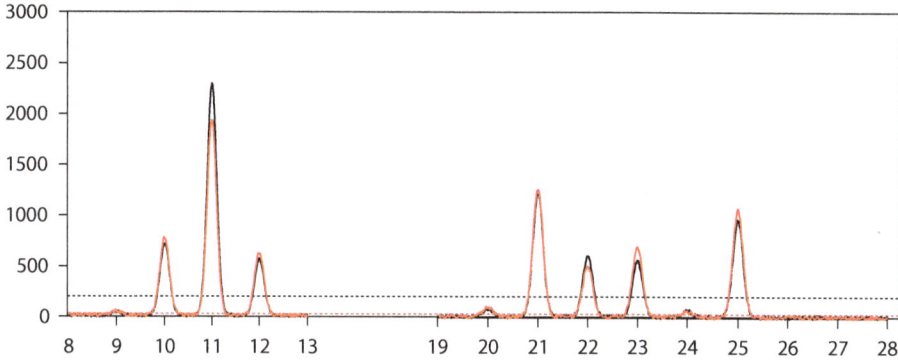

Figure 9.11 Two person mixture expected profile (black) built up from mass parameters overlaying the observed profile (red).

E_{an}^l is the expected allelic peak height of the ath allele for the nth contributor at locus l

O_a^l is the observed height of the ath allele at locus l

T_{an}^l is the total allelic product of the ath allele for the nth contributor at locus l

SR_a^l is the back stutter ratio of the ath allele at locus l

FS_a^l is the forward stutter ratio of the ath allele at locus l

For the Markov chain we will need $f(O_{ar}^l \mid S_q, M)$, which is read as the probability density of the peak at position a given that we know the genotypes and the true template at that allelic position and the one upstream. The modelling above has given the expected heights given that we know the genotypes and the true template at that allelic position. Empirical trials suggest that the relative variance of small peaks is large and that of large peaks is small. The data fit the curve:

$$\text{var}\left[\log_{10}\left(\frac{O}{E}\right)\right] = \frac{c^2}{E},$$ where c^2 is an empirically determined constant. This indicates that the variance of the log of observed over expected heights is inversely proportional to the expected peak height. Most forensic biologists are more familiar with the standard deviation. This is the square root of the variance and is modelled as $\frac{c}{\sqrt{E}}$.

Database Searches Using Continuous Systems

Traditionally, single source profiles or single contributor profiles which have been unambiguously resolved from a mixture have been considered to reach this standard and be suitable for entry into a crime sample database. Single source profiles are relatively simple to interpret, with standard methods generally agreed on and accepted worldwide. Profiles from crime scenes however are frequently compromised in quality. Stochastic events such as heterozygote imbalance, allelic dropout, locus dropout and allelic drop-in can complicate interpretation.[36,37,120] In addition in many cases crime scene samples may be mixed where DNA from more than one individual is present. Stutter, a by-product of the PCR process, can further complicate profile interpretation whenever stutter peaks are of a similar height to the minor allelic peaks in mixed DNA profiles.

Interpretation of these profiles using a continuous model may result in improved profile information and therefore permit database entry. Unless the weight for any given genotype combination is 1, assessing the 'quality' of a profile for its suitability for comparison to a database is not straightforward. A guideline for database entry based on some assessment of the risks of loading an incorrectly inferred profile may be employed where the genotype combination of a contributor is ambiguous, such as $w_i > 0.99$. If an individual's profile cannot be reasonably

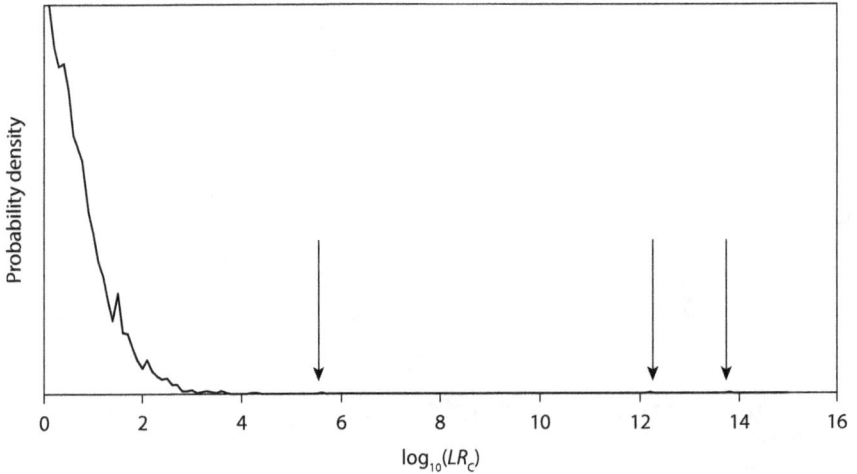

Figure 9.12   Distribution of likelihood ratios (*LR*s) shown on a logarithmic scale, when considering known non-contributing individuals as contributors to a complex three person mixed DNA profile. Only values of *LR* > 1 are shown. Arrows show the *LR* for the three individuals known to make up the mixture. The maximum value for the *LR* when comparing a known non-contributor was 20,348 ($\log_{10} (LR_c) = 4.3$).

inferred from a DNA mixture, regardless of the interpretation method, then it is unsuitable for entry to a database using traditional database methods.

If there is no interpretable single profile from the mixture then a search of the mixture itself should be performed. Comparison of profiles to profiles in a database, where there are multiple possible genotype combinations at one or more loci for matching against known individuals, can be undertaken using the output of a continuous method of interpretation with a modified search algorithm using an *LR* framework.

Each of the individuals on a database can be considered a potential contributor in turn under the following two hypotheses (or others if desired):

H_p: Database individual and $N - 1$ unknown contributors

H_d: N unknown contributors

where N was the number of contributors under consideration. This will provide an *LR* for each individual in the database, compared to the relevant mixture. A cut-off value is then used to reduce the list to a manageable size and remove the most likely potential adventitious matches.

Figure 9.12 shows the results of considering 57,612 individuals as potential contributors to a complex three-person Identifiler® (Thermo Fisher Scientific) profile. Of these 57,612 individuals, 3 were known contributors and 57,609 were known non-contributors.

Of the 57,612 individuals, 4000 gave an *LR* in favour of H_p and as Figure 9.12 shows the majority of these were below an *LR* of 100. In contrast the known contributors gave *LR*s of greater than 400,000 and were clearly distinguishable from the non-contributors.

Continuous *LR*s in Practice

Artificial two and three person mixed DNA profiles with known contributors were amplified with an Applied Biosystems NGM SElect™ multiplex (Invitrogen, Carlsbad, CA) and separated on an Applied Biosystems 3130*xl* capillary electrophoresis instrument.

The *LR* was calculated for each contributor to each of the four two-person and six three-person mixed DNA profiles using both a binary method and the continuous method of interpretation discussed in this paper. The hypotheses considered are as follows:

H_p: The DNA came from P_1 and unknown people up to the number of contributors.

H_d: The DNA came from all unknown people.

LR_B was calculated in MS Excel following the 'F model' as described in Kelly et al.[724]

Table 9.1 shows the *LR* produced from the continuous method as described above and implemented through Java software and a binary method for the same set of mixtures of known source calculated in Excel following the F model described in Kelly et al.[724] Profiles were of reasonable quality to allow assessment by the binary method. Table 9.1 shows the information gain by using a continuous system. In the two person scenarios where the individual profiles can be well resolved the information obtained from the two methods are similar. For three person mixtures, the results of the two systems diverged. LR_B was markedly lower or unable to be determined for three person mixtures, whereas LR_C continued to produce *LR*s consistently much greater than 1.

Table 9.1 shows a mild increase in *LR*s when using the continuous system for simpler two person mixtures, but the real strength comes when three person mixtures are considered. The wastefulness of the binary system is highlighted when complex profiles are analyzed based only on the presence or absence of peaks and do not make use of their height.

There has been a view that peak heights are of limited value at low template. To investigate this concept a cut-down version of STRmix (STRmix™ lite) that ignored heights was tested against the full STRmix version. The full version outperformed STRmix lite in a limited trial both for true and false donors even at very low template (see Figure 9.13 and Table 9.2).

Table 9.1 Likelihood Ratio Results of Continuous vs Binary Method for Assessing Two- and Three-Person Profiles

Continuous		Binary	
Mixed DNA Profiles from Two Contributors			
Person 1	**Person 2**	**Person 1**	**Person 2**
6.1×10^{15}	3.2×10^{16}	1.2×10^{16}	3.8×10^{15}
1.9×10^{19}	6.4×10^{19}	9.5×10^{17}	1.9×10^{19}
2.4×10^{19}	4.9×10^{19}	2.1×10^{18}	9.6×10^{18}
3.0×10^{17}	1.3×10^{20}	4.0×10^{14}	1.3×10^{20}

Mixed DNA Profiles from Three Contributors					
Person 1	**Person 2**	**Person 3**	**Person 1**	**Person 2**	**Person 3**
2.7×10^8	4.7×10^{11}	3.8×10^{13}	NC	226	1.39×10^6
9.1×10^8	4.2×10^{11}	2.8×10^{13}	NC	3	14,261
8.4×10^{19}	4.7×10^{11}	6.0×10^{18}	57	<1	331
4.5×10^{12}	5.7×10^{12}	7.20×10^{14}	<1	<1	846
9.6×10^7	1.2×10^{20}	1.1×10^{20}	NC	65	317
7.7×10^{18}	3.1×10^{19}	1,254	23	356	NC

NC, non-concordance (and therefore a statistic was not calculated).

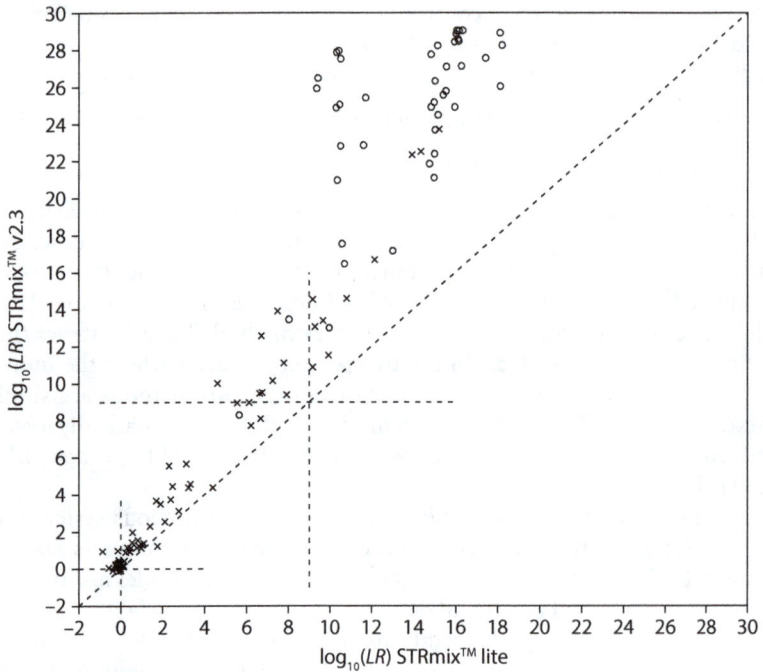

Figure 9.13 $Log_{10}(LR)$ for STRmix™ lite and STRmix™ v2.3. The diagonal dashed line is $x = y$. Circles represent values that were derived from greater than 50 pg of total input DNA and crosses those less than 50 pg.

Table 9.2 Results of H_d True Tests for a Four-Person 0.25:0.25:0.25:0.25 Mix at 50 pg Total Input Template		STRmix™ v2.3	STRmix™ Lite
Number of simulations		12,000,000	10,000,000
H_p True LR		374,104	207
H_d True	p ('1 in')	3,000,000	11,947
	$LR = 0$	99.958%	94.491%
	$LR > 1$	0.0173%	0.0472%
	Average LR	1.005	1.078

LR, likelihood ratio.
Note: Average peak height for the profile was 89 rfu.

In this trial three of the four contributors were input as *knowns*. The *LRs* for both STRmix v2.3 and STRmix lite would be lower if there were fewer knowns. However, for the trial shown the effect is higher *LRs* for true donors and lower ones for false donors.

Comparison with Human Interpretations
A continuous model for DNA interpretations should produce results that are intuitively correct to a trained scientist. We would therefore expect to see a relationship between LR_C and human interpretations.

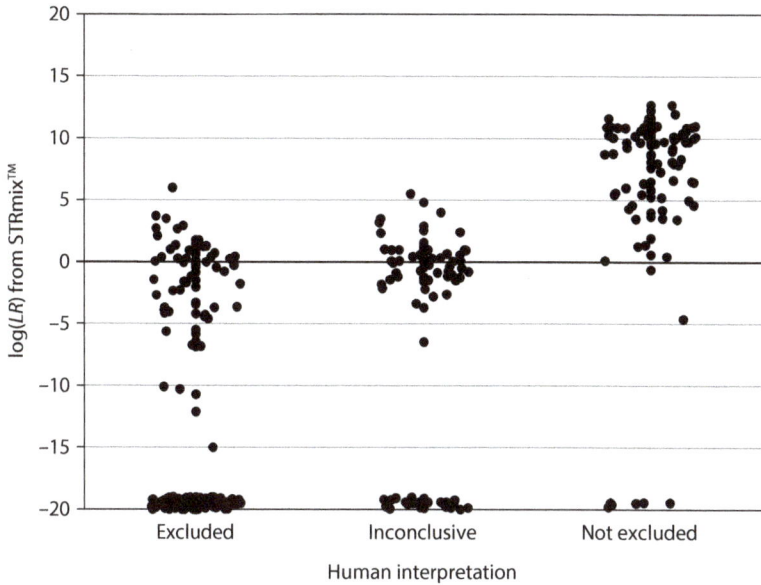

Figure 9.14   Comparison of likelihood ratios (*LR*s) produced using a continuous system with human interpretation. The line at 0 represents neutrality, i.e. the probability of obtaining the profile is the same under propositions of exclusion or inclusion. Results above the 0 line favour inclusion and results below the line favour exclusion. When $LR_C = 0$ (when G_P did not feature in the Markov chain Monte Carlo at any point) the result has been plotted at the bottom of the graph against the *y*-axis label '$LR_C = 0$'.

To test this concept, previously reported casework Profiler Plus® profiles were reanalyzed using the continuous model described. The samples in this study resulted in 39, 274, 207 and 50 comparisons to single source, two, three and four person mixed profiles, respectively. LR_C produced by the model were compared with the human interpretation for the same result (Figure 9.14). The propositions considered were as follows:

H_p: The DNA came from the POI and unknown people up to the number of contributors.

H_d: The DNA came from all unknown people.

Human interpretations were sorted into three categories: *not excluded*, *inconclusive* and *excluded*.

Inspection of the graph shows a broad alignment of human- and model-based interpretation except that on average human interpretations were more conservative.

Use on Profiles of Varying Quality

Specificity and sensitivity are not trivial to define when we talk of a software system for DNA profile interpretation. In Ref. 756, Taylor and Buckleton clone a drop model and show that STRmix extracts useful and correct information from very low level DNA results beyond what would be expected by systems not using peak height (any of the drop models).

To answer the question of sensitivity most directly we suggest that the work described in Ref. 746 and reproduced below in Figures 9.15 through 9.19 might be useful. The *LR* distributions for H_p true and H_d true are very well separated at high template for two person mixtures. As the number of contributors increases and the template lowers the two distributions converge on log(*LR*) = 0. This is the correct result. What it means is that the performance of the software is most dependent on the sample (see Box 9.2). At high template, STRmix correctly and reliably

BOX 9.2   PERFORMANCE OF STRmix ON VOLUME CRIME

The Institute of Environmental Science and Research Limited (New Zealand) adopted the continuous interpretation software STRmix™ in August 2012. Since then they have been using it for the interpretation of mixtures and the calculation of likelihood ratios for all casework. Within the plot below are the success rates for a number of different sample types submitted for analysis to volume crime team. Success was defined as the ability to obtain a profile suitable for entry to the New Zealand DNA Profile Databank.

The plot shows data for two financial years. The only change in process between the 2011–2012 and 2012–2013 financial years was the introduction of STRmix. The improvement in loading rates is attributable to STRmix's ability to interpret more profiles (data provided by Sarah Scott).

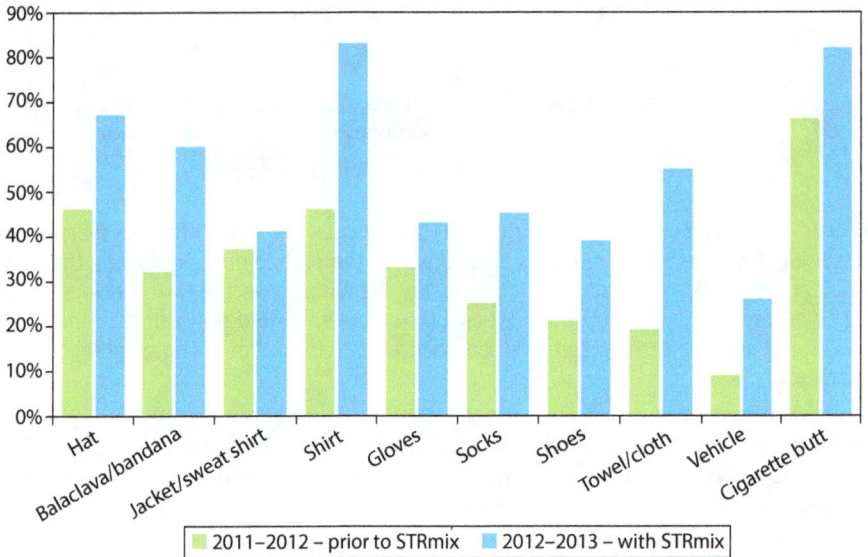

gives a high *LR* for true contributors and a low *LR* for false contributors. At low template or high contributor number, STRmix correctly and reliably reports that the analysis of the sample tends towards uninformative or inconclusive.

Figure 9.20 has been reproduced for Identifiler Plus™ data (courtesy of Erie County Department of Public Safety, Erie County, NY). The laboratory generated 22 four-person mixed DNA profiles. Ten of the profiles were in the approximate proportions of 4:3:2:1. The amount of DNA corresponding to the smallest contributor ranged from 100 pg to 0.625 pg. Twelve of the profiles were in equal proportions (1:1:1:1), where the amount of DNA from each contributor ranged from 400 pg to 1.25 pg. Three and two contributor profiles were prepared similarly. These profiles represent the 'worst' types of profiles likely to be encountered by the laboratory. Each profile was interpreted in STRmix and compared to the four known contributors and 200 known non-contributors. The non-contributors were generated artificially using a Caucasian allele frequency database.[502] A plot of the log(*LR*) versus DNA per contributor (pg) for each dataset is provided in Figure 9.20. The per-contributor amount for H_d true contributors was taken as the average of the known contributors.

Inspection of Figure 9.20 shows the separation of the *LR* distributions for H_p and H_d true propositions is less for Identifiler Plus profiles than for GlobalFiler profiles. Identifiler Plus has six fewer loci used within the *LR* calculation which explains the lower discrimination.

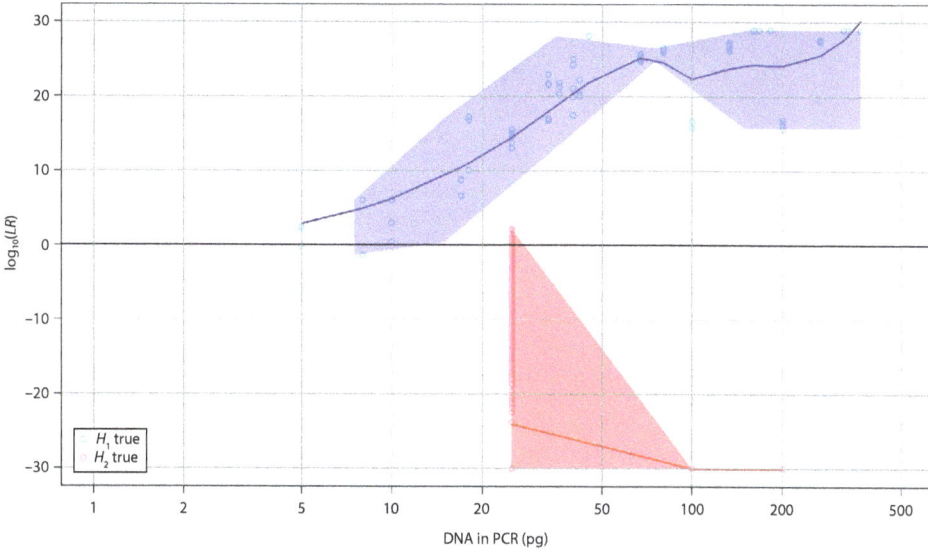

Figure 9.15   Likelihood ratios produced for two person mixtures, with LOWESS lines and polygons showing coverage of scatterplot points.

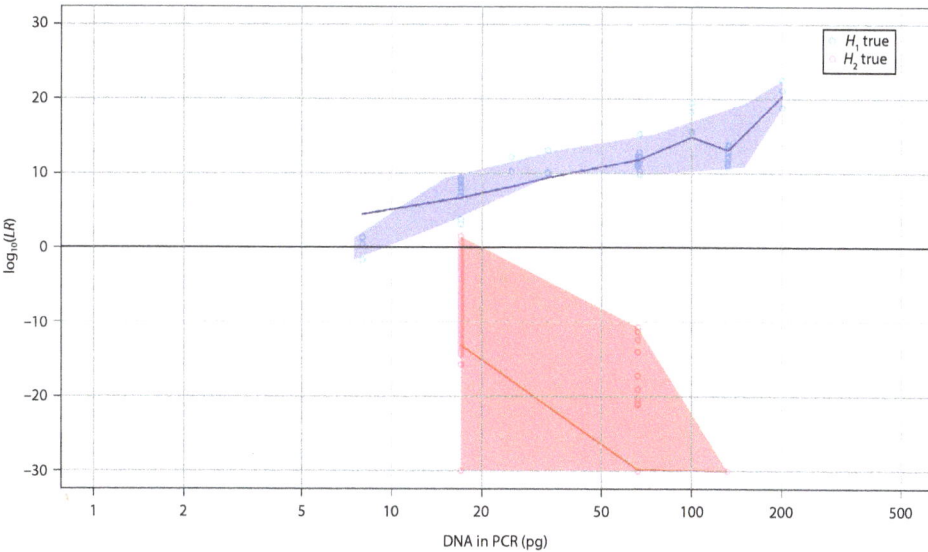

Figure 9.16   Likelihood ratios produced for three person mixtures, with LOWESS lines and polygons showing coverage of scatterplot points.

Results from Bille et al.[699] are given in Figure 9.21 below for a number of trials on true donors. The broad conclusion is that a continuous approach gives better performance for true donors across a range of mixture ratios and template.

Diagnostics for Continuous Systems

Ground truth comparisons should produce a large *LR* when the prosecution proposition is true and a low one when the defence proposition is true. Any results in the opposite direction should have a detectable cause, such as very poor PCR amplification of the known contributors.

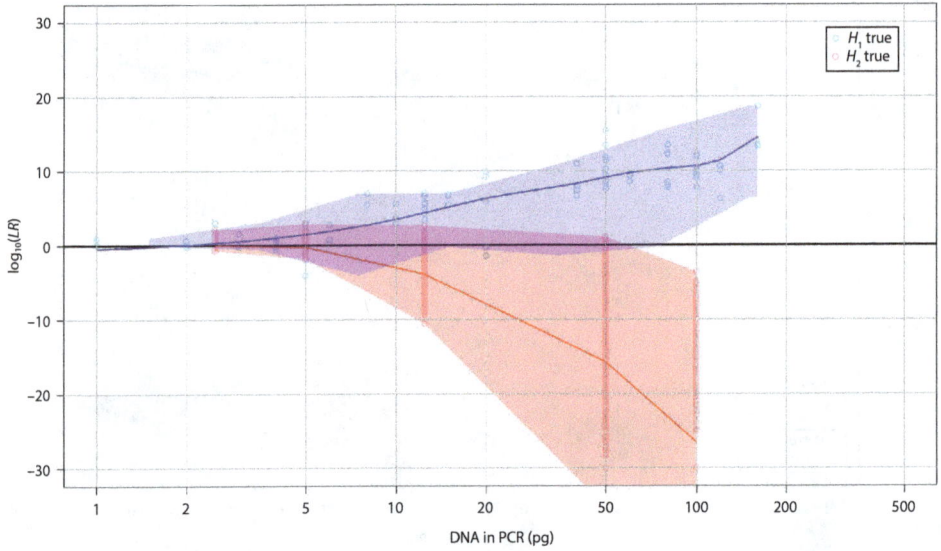

Figure 9.17   Likelihood ratios produced for four person mixtures, with LOWESS lines and polygons showing coverage of scatterplot points.

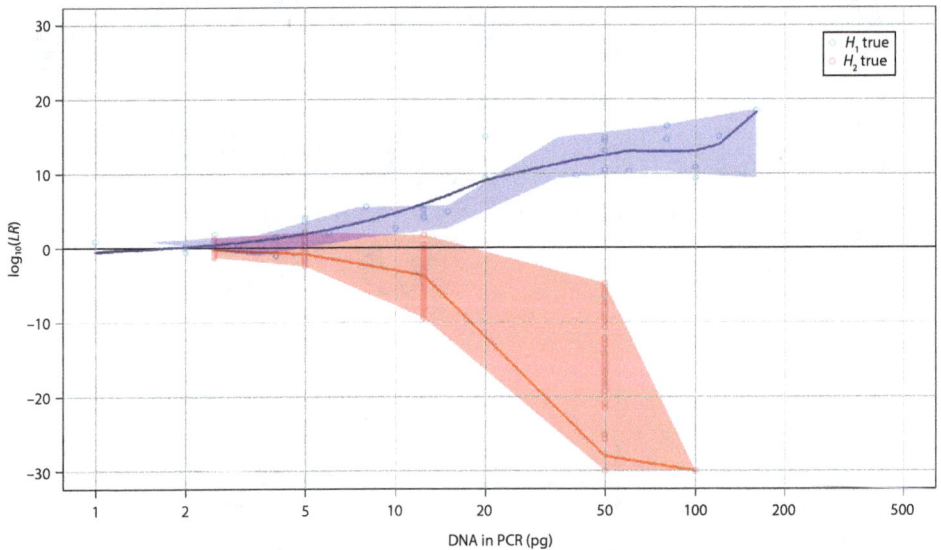

Figure 9.18   Likelihood ratios produced for four person mixtures using three replicate amplifications, with LOWESS lines and polygons showing coverage of scatterplot points.

Equally, occasionally a false contributor may give a high *LR*. This is termed an *adventitious match*. Such tests give little guidance as to whether the *LR* is too large or not large enough but sensible limits may be placed. For example, a two person mix cannot exceed the expected result that would have occurred if it was fully resolvable.

A large number of mixtures where the ground truth is known have been run in STRmix and published in peer-reviewed journals. H_p true trials are comparisons to the known contributor to a profile. H_d true trials are comparisons to known *non-contributors* (i.e. individuals who have

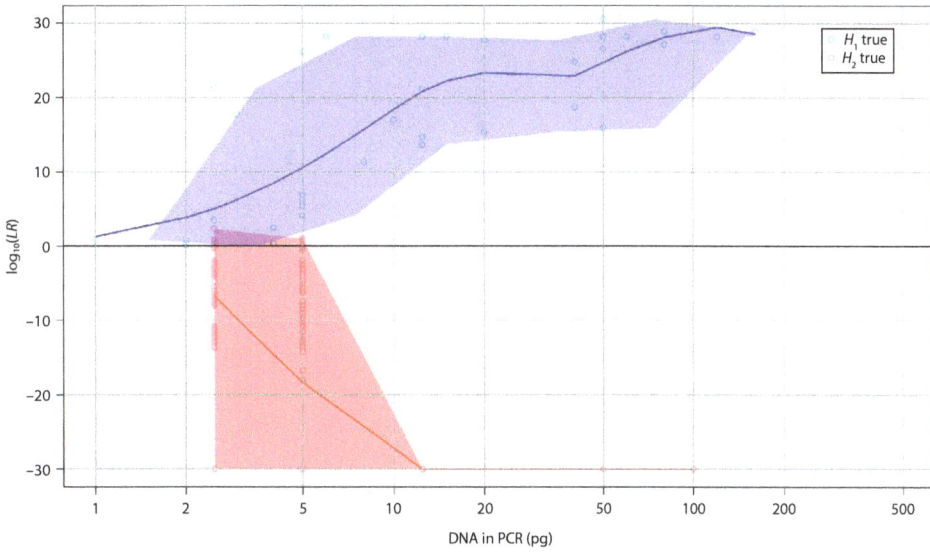

Figure 9.19 Likelihood ratios produced for four person mixtures using three replicate amplifications and assuming three out of the four known contributors in each analysis, with LOWESS lines and polygons showing coverage of scatterplot points.

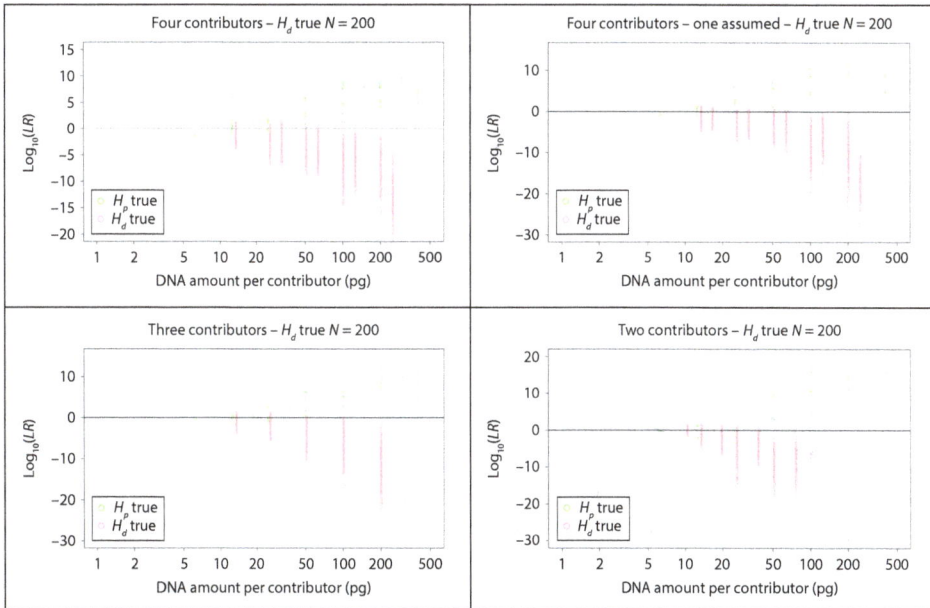

Figure 9.20 Likelihood ratios produced for four, three and two person mixtures from Erie County, PA, NY.

not contributed DNA to the profile). We expect high *LR*s for the true contributors and low *LR*s for the false ones.[746,757]

Turin showed that the average *LR* for the H_d true tests should be 1 (quoted in Good[250]).

Following from this we can state: 'The probability (p) of observing a likelihood ratio of LR_{POI} or larger from an unrelated non-donor is less than 1 in LR_{POI}'.

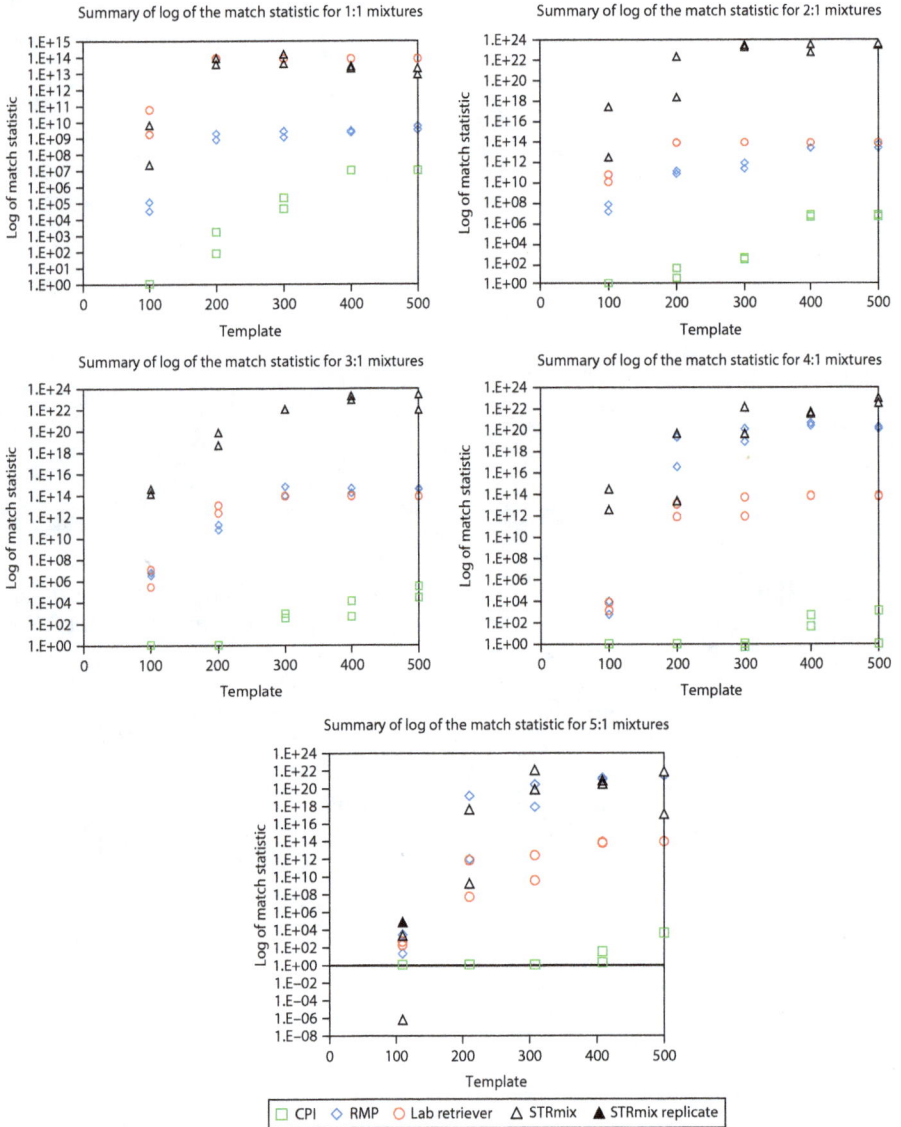

Figure 9.21 A summary of some comparisons. (From Bille, T.W., et al.: Comparison of the performance of different models for the interpretation of low level mixed DNA profiles. *Electrophoresis*. 2014. 35(21–22). 3125–3133. Copyright Wiley-VCH Verlag GmbH & Co. KGaA. Reproduced with permission.)

This gives a frequentist-sounding interpretation to the *LR* but is actually a statement that follows from the laws of probability.

Below we reproduce some examples of these principles generated from in vitro profiles and STRmix. The false donors were simulated using the product rule.

Other published ground truth known tests include the following:

1. GlobalFiler: 264 H_p true; 17,406 H_d true[746]

2. Identifiler: 57 H_p true; 1,902,524 H_d true[757]

3. Identifiler: 54 H_p true; 54,000 H_d true[758]

4. Varying multiplexes: 21 H_p true; 123,230,000 H_d true[759] (results appear in Table 9.3)

Table 9.3   Results of Comparisons of Simulated Random References

Experiment	Number of Contributors	Simulations	Number of H_d True with $LR = 0$	Average H_d True LR	H_p True LR(s)	p, '1 in'
1	4	12,000,000	11,994,959	1.0046	374,104	3,000,000
2	4	10,000	0	0.977	9	44
3	4	120,000	0	0.927	4	29
					7	56
					5	34
					6	49
4	1	80,000,000	79,998,779	1.001	312,325	6,666,666
5	1	100,000	99,618	1.022	215	262
6	2	10,000,000	9,898,155	1.017	278	4,163
					12,557	78,125
7	3	1,000,000	922,585	0.906	234,738	>1,000,000
					2,530	17,241
					43	2,262
8	1	10,000,000	9,999,960	0.872	218,070	250,000
9	1	10,000,000	9,274,620	1.003	14	14

LR, likelihood ratio.
Note: Multiple results, where shown, are due to multiple unknown contributors under H_d.

Gelman–Rubin Convergence Diagnostic $\hat{R}$

This statistic gives an indication of whether the chains have converged. It compares the within-chain variance (W) and between-chain variance (B) for M chains each of n measurements. This means that more than one chain must be run in order to use this method. To visualize the effect imagine that the chains have each chosen one corner of the space. Then the between-chain variance might be high and the within-chain low. This is a symptom of non-convergence. If the chains are all intertwined across similar space then the within- and between-chain variances are similar:

$$\hat{R} = \sqrt{1 - \frac{1}{n}\left(1 - \frac{B}{W}\right)}$$

If we set the between-chain variance, B, approximately equal to the within-chain variance, W, we can see that $\hat{R}$ tends to 1. If $\hat{R} > 1.2$ (approximately) then the chains may not have properly converged. In practice, the performance of the Gelman–Rubin Convergence Diagnostic is not to the expected level.

Effective Sample Size

The successive states from an MCMC chain are correlated.

If you were to look at each set of adjacent points compared to the mean, they would be correlated (both above or both below): A, both *above*; B, both *below*; C, *changed*.

If the points in Figure 9.22 were independent then we would expect equal numbers of As and Bs and twice as many Cs. If they are correlated then As and Bs will outnumber Cs. Figure 9.22 shows 15 As, 19 Bs and 5 Cs; therefore the points in this MCMC separated by one iteration are correlated.

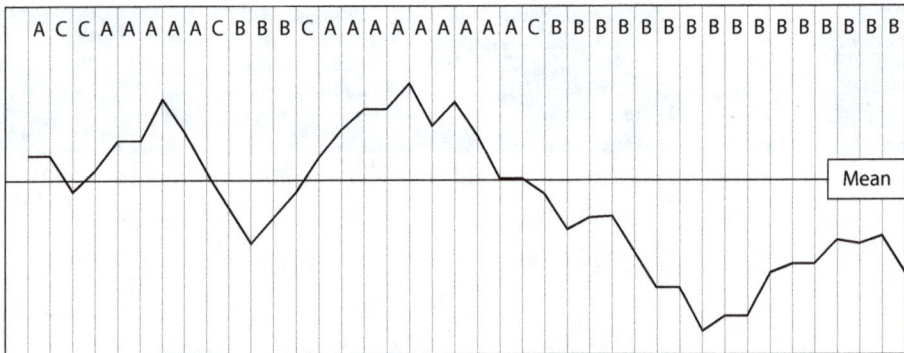

Figure 9.22   Tracking of a Markov chain Monte Carlo property over a number of iterations.

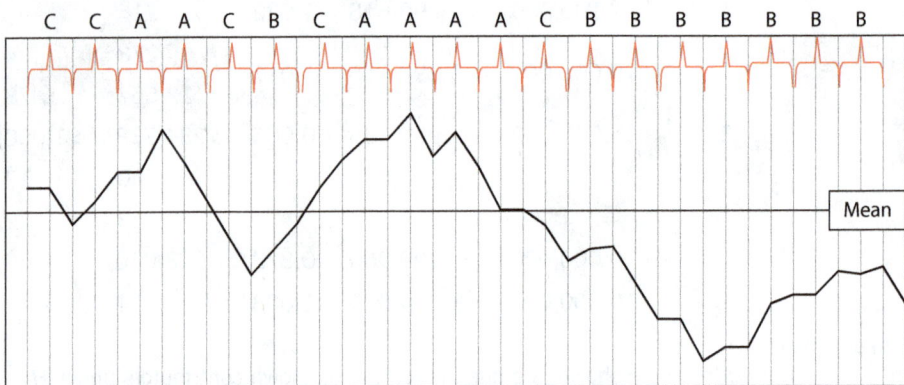

Figure 9.23   Tracking of a Markov chain Monte Carlo property over a number of iterations, looking at pairs of values separated by two iterations.

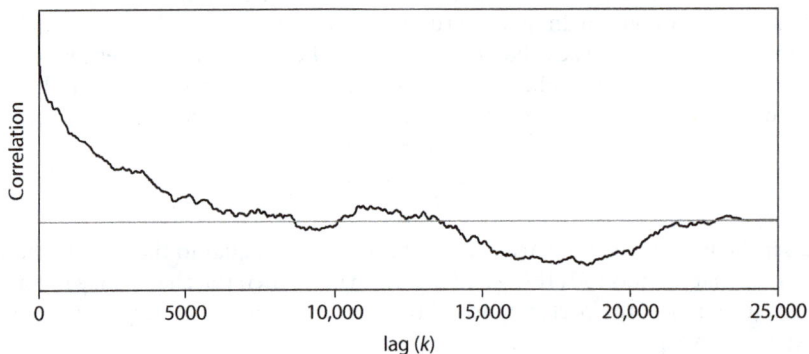

Figure 9.24   Correlation at lag *k* for an STRmix™ calculation.

The next step tries points that are separated by two iterations, as shown in Figure 9.23.

Figure 9.23 shows 6 As, 8 Bs and 5 Cs and the data are therefore still correlated. This process continues until the correlation is 0. This is called the *correlation at lag* k. Figure 9.24 shows the correlation for a real STRmix calculation at lag 0 to 25,000. In this example the correlation is not 0 until examining values are separated by approximately 8000 iterations.

Once we know how correlated the data are, we can determine how many *independent* samples the MCMC has run for. This is called the *effective sample size* (ESS) of the MCMC. We can then use the effective sample size and the weights to calculate the effective count, i.e. the number of independent counts that genotype set S_j was the focus of the MCMC.

Getting the Number of Contributors Wrong

STRmix requires the assignment of a number of contributors (hereafter N) that have donated to those alleles showing peaks above the selected analytical threshold (AT). However N is never known with certainty. It may be useful to start the thought process from first principles.

$$LR = \frac{\sum_n \Pr(E \mid N=n, H_p)\Pr(N=n \mid H_p)}{\sum_m \Pr(E \mid N=m, H_d)\Pr(N=m \mid H_d)} \qquad (9.1)$$

We remind ourselves that what is behind the bar is assumed to be true and what is in front of the bar is unknown. This informs us that we do not determine N from E, the evidence. The rationale for our current process is that we assume $\Pr(N = n \mid H_p) = \Pr(N = m \mid H_d) =$ constant for all n and m. This assumption may be motivated by the observation that the information in H_p and H_d seldom informs N strongly. Hence

$$LR = \frac{\sum_n \Pr(E \mid N=n, H_p)}{\sum_m \Pr(E \mid N=m, H_d)} \qquad (9.2)$$

There is no need for the distributions of m and n to be the same in the numerator and denominator. However we are cognizant both of the reality of and perception of bias and of fitting the profile to the POI. So, initially at least, we will constrain n to equal m. This is also a current technical limitation of STRmix up to v2.3.

$$LR = \frac{\sum_n \Pr(E \mid N=n, H_p)}{\sum_n \Pr(E \mid N=n, H_d)} \qquad (9.3)$$

The summation in the denominator is usually dominated by one term. This term is when n is the number that best explains the profile. Given the constraints above, this should also return on average not only the best approximation to Equation 9.2 but one that is fair and reasonable to the defence.

Assigning N. Recall before we start that N is unknown and unknowable. We have plausibly added to confusion by suggesting that N should be determined. A much better word would be *assigned*. In most cases an N that optimizes $\Pr(E \mid N = n, H_d)$ is obvious. It is only rarely to the advantage of the defence to posit an additional unknown beyond that required to explain the profile. These situations tend to occur for high order mixtures and are discussed later. Recall that we seek to maximize $\Pr(E \mid N = n, H_d)$, not minimize the LR. The LR can always be minimized to at least 1 if that was the goal.

For STRmix, E is composed of those peaks above AT. Therefore we seek a reasonable maximization of $\Pr(E|N = n,H_d)$ where E is confined to those peaks above AT. This is usually obtained by the minimum N that is needed to explain E and would usefully consider peak heights and balances. We will term this assigned number N_{Hd}^E.

What Happens If We 'Add One'?

In our experience if N is set to one larger than N_{Hd}^E one of a number of things happens:

1. STRmix splits the smallest contributor.

2. STRmix adds a trace that is scattered widely among genotypes including dropped alleles.

Behaviour 1 tends to happen if there is no evidence in E to suggest another contributor (termed *situation 1*). Behaviour 2 tends to happen if there is some evidence in E to suggest a trace contributor (termed *situation 2*). However we are unable to guarantee that this list is completely exhaustive.

Where uncertainty exists in the number of contributors a routine policy of the 'addition of one' is not recommended. It is advised that replication by PCR of the profile is attempted to help inform the decision. The addition of one when there is little or no evidence in E to do so increases the risk of adventitious hits.[757,758] This effect is highly undesirable.

What about Sub-Threshold Peaks?

Imagine that situation 1 holds but that there are considerable indications of an additional contributor below AT. We will term this E_{sub}. First it is essential to note that modern multiplexes show a range of artefacts, including but not limited to forward stutter, double backward stutter and for SE33 –2bp stutter. All of these may appear in the sub-threshold region if a large allelic peak is present.

Four potential policies come to mind:

1. Rework (re-PCR) the profile in order to help confirm the number of contributors.

2. 'Add one'.

3. Lower the AT.

4. Deem the profile uninterpretable after checking for exclusionary potential.

In all cases where sub-threshold peaks suggest uncertainty in the number of contributors, replication should be the first option. Of the other options STRmix is likely to cope best with the third policy. This will allow STRmix to 'see' the same information as the operator is using.

To implement this approach it is necessary that validation and especially investigation of the drop-in parameters have been done to at least as low as the AT will be lowered.

The risks of the 'add one' option were discussed above.

When Is $\Pr(E|N = n,H_d)$ Maximized?

It is relatively easy to find the N that maximizes $\Pr(E|N = n,H_d)$ if peak heights are ignored; however this is not useful for continuous systems that use height information. STRmix itself does not provide access to this information and minimizing the LR across N does not achieve this.

We can construct profiles where an $N = 4$ mixture looks exactly like an $N = 3$ mixture and NIST 13 case 5 is one of these.[760] In such a case it is the lower N not the higher that optimizes $\Pr(E|N = n,H_d)$. The choice of an N that is lower than the true (but unknown) runs an increased risk of false exclusion, not false inclusion.

We do not have experience of a situation where an N greater than that needed would optimize $\Pr(E|N = n,H_d)$; however it is not clear to us how we would have known that such a situation had occurred. It seems likely to us that the safest policy is to set N to the lowest number that effectively explains the profile when considering peak heights. We accept the subjectivity inherent in this statement. It is possible that for very high order mixtures this assessment is very difficult. These profiles may be uninterpretable with current technology.

What If the POI Does Not Fit for the Assigned *N* under Pr(*E*|*N = n*,*H$_d$*)?

It is possible that under N^E_{Hd} the POI is excluded but under $N^E_{Hd} + 1$ he or she is not. To examine this it is helpful to go back to Equation 9.2:

$$LR = \frac{\sum_n \Pr(E \mid N = n, H_p)}{\sum_m \Pr(E \mid N = m, H_d)}$$

In the case described it is likely that the best approximation to Equation 9.2 is achieved by

$$LR = \frac{\Pr(E \mid N = N^E_{Hd} + 1, H_p)}{\Pr(E \mid N = N^E_{Hd}, H_d)}$$

Versions of STRmix up to v2.3 cannot implement this and it is unlikely that

$$LR = \frac{\Pr(E \mid N = N^E_{Hd} + 1, H_p)}{\Pr(E \mid N = N^E_{Hd} + 1, H_d)}$$

is a fair and reasonable assessment.

Empirical Trials

The effect of the uncertainty in the number of contributors has been reported for a number of profiles with *N* and *N* + 1 assumed contributors, where *N* is the known number of contributors.[757,758] The inclusion of an additional contributor beyond that present in the profile most often had the effect of lowering the *LR* for trace contributors within the profile. STRmix most often adds the additional (unseen) profile at trace levels which interacts with the known trace contribution, diffusing the genotype weights and lowering the *LR*. There was no significant effect on the *LR* of the major or minor contributor within the profiles.

Addition of One Contributor

A selection of one, two and three person mixtures was interpreted as two, three and four person profiles, respectively. The *LR* was calculated for both the known contributors and 200 known non-contributors. A summary of the *LR*s assuming the correct and one additional contributor is given in Table 9.4.

Most of the time the *LR*s for the known contributors were affected very little. The four largest changes downwards are shown in bold. This means that the wrong assumption leads to a lower *LR*. The five largest changes upwards are shown in red. In these cases the wrong assumption leads to a larger *LR*.

For the 200 or more known non-contributors the distribution of *LR*s is given in Figures 9.25 through 9.27.

Subtraction of One Contributor

A two contributor profile was adjusted by artificially adding a third contributor. The third contributor was constructed as a child of the two known contributors and therefore shared alleles at all loci. In this way it was possible to confuse the true number of contributors. The child was added in the varying average heights 50 rfu, 100 rfu and 200 rfu. At higher amounts the evidence of a third contributor would be clear. Each artificially constructed three person profile

Table 9.4 Summary of the Likelihood Ratio for Profiles Assuming the Correct and One Additional Contributor

Known Ground Truth	Likelihood Ratio			
	Assumed Number of Contributors			
	1	2	3	4
Single-source samples	4.19×10^{20}	4.19×10^{20}		
	4.19×10^{20}	4.19×10^{20}		
	2.65×10^{23}	2.65×10^{23}		
	2.65×10^{23}	2.65×10^{23}		
	6.81×10^{19}	6.81×10^{19}		
Two-person mixtures		6.31×10^{17}	5.01×10^{17}	
		2.51×10^{16}	2.51×10^{16}	
		6.31×10^{19}	7.94×10^{19}	
		2.51×10^{16}	2.51×10^{16}	
		3.98×10^{22}	3.98×10^{22}	
		2.00×10^{15}	1.58×10^{12}	
		3.98×10^{22}	3.98×10^{22}	
		7.94×10^{14}	3.98×10^{14}	
		3.98×10^{22}	3.98×10^{22}	
		2.51×10^{9}	1.00×10^{9}	
		3.98×10^{22}	3.98×10^{22}	
		3.16×10^{9}	7.94×10^{6}	
		3.98×10^{22}	3.98×10^{22}	
		7.94×10^{15}	6.31×10^{15}	
		3.98×10^{22}	3.98×10^{22}	
		6.31×10^{15}	5.01×10^{15}	
Three-person mixtures			9.77×10^{12}	1.05×10^{13}
			3.09×10^{21}	2.75×10^{21}
			5.37×10^{12}	5.89×10^{12}
			4.79×10^{12}	2.24×10^{13}
			1.86×10^{21}	2.09×10^{21}
			5.01×10^{12}	2.40×10^{13}
			2.75×10^{3}	2.24×10^{3}
			2.34×10^{24}	2.34×10^{24}
			1.86×10^{3}	7.24×10^{2}
			26.3	15.8

(Continued)

Table 9.4 *(Continued)* Summary of the Likelihood Ratio for Profiles Assuming the Correct and One Additional Contributor

Known Ground Truth	Likelihood Ratio			
	Assumed Number of Contributors			
	1	2	3	4
			2.34×10^{24}	2.34×10^{24}
			6.17	4.57
			2.69×10^{3}	5.25×10^{3}
			2.34×10^{24}	2.34×10^{24}
			7.94×10^{10}	4.37×10^{9}
			4.79×10^{9}	1.12×10^{10}
			3.63×10^{13}	1.17×10^{15}
			6.76×10^{11}	5.13×10^{12}
			4.79×10^{9}	5.62×10^{9}
			6.61×10^{12}	2.51×10^{13}
			1.74×10^{9}	4.07×10^{9}
			5.13×10^{16}	**3.09×10^{12}**
			3.09×10^{13}	**9.12×10^{10}**
			9.77×10^{9}	**9.33×10^{7}**
			2.51×10^{20}	2.51×10^{20}
			2.57×10^{14}	**3.55×10^{12}**
			24.5	60.3

Note: Bold text represents the four largest downward changes; red text represents the five largest upward changes.

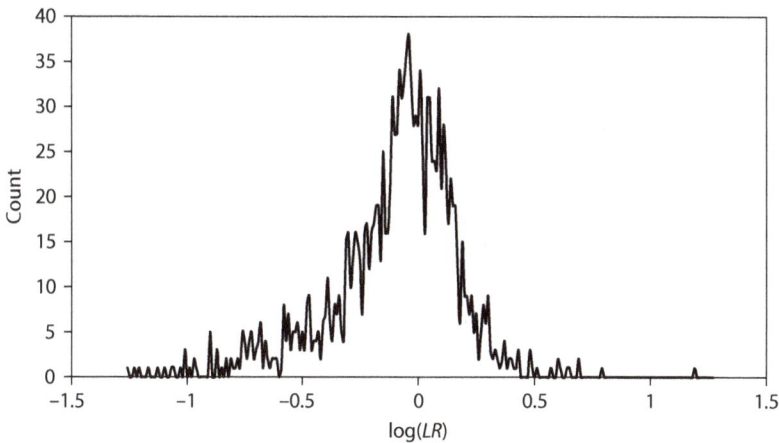

Figure 9.25 Distribution of adventitious link likelihood ratios for single source profiles interpreted as two person mixtures.

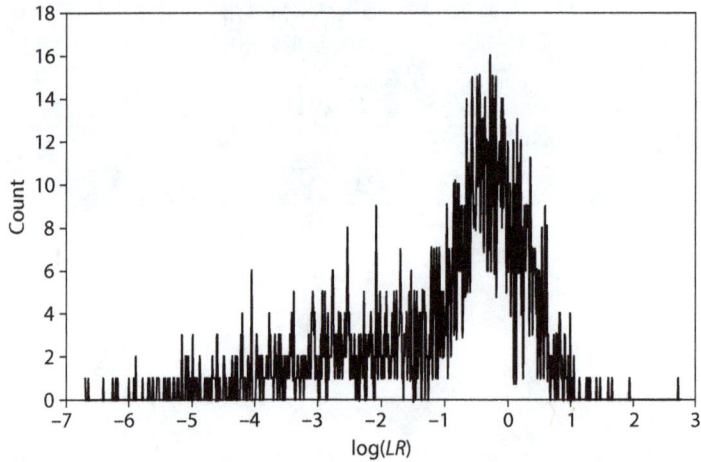

Figure 9.26   Distribution of adventitious link likelihood ratios for two person mixtures interpreted as three person mixtures.

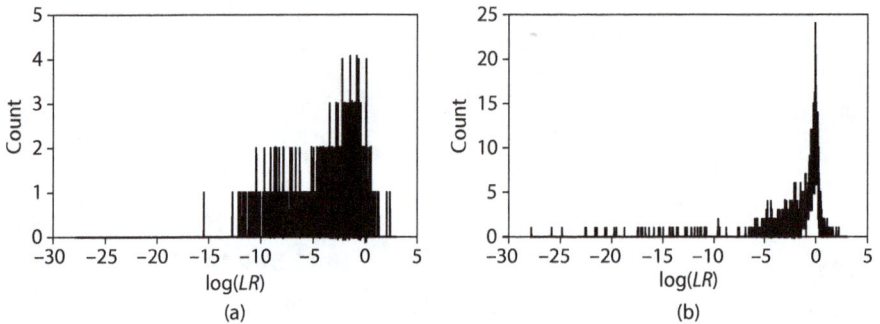

Figure 9.27   Distribution of adventitious link likelihood ratios for three person mixtures assuming three (a) and four (b) contributors.

was interpreted assuming two contributors and compared with the three known contributors and 200 non-contributors.

The LR of the two contributors was not affected in any of the trials. For all trials 216 known non-donors all returned $LR = 0$.

TH01 9.3,10

In some circumstances where 9.3 and 10 at TH01 are present in the same mixture one can end up as an unresolved shoulder on the other. In some circumstances this will cause a false exclusion. The diagnostic is $LR_{TH01} = 0$ and $LR > 1$ elsewhere. The recommended action is to check for exclusionary potential at TH01 and if none exists to exclude the locus. We have no instances of it occurring but by analogy this problem is likely for all 0.1 and 0.3 variants at tetra allelic repeat loci, 0.1 and 0.4 at penta allelic repeat loci, and 0.1 and 0.2 at triallelic repeat loci.

Very Significantly Overloaded Samples

STRmix has a function for overloaded profiles. This function allows the examination of some overloaded profiles. However in some circumstances false exclusions eventuate. This has occurred for very significantly overloaded profiles of the order of 3 ng amplified. It is highly preferable to avoid significantly overloaded profiles.

Triallelic Loci

STRmix has no modelling currently for triallelic loci. If a reference is triallelic (either type I or II) and is present in significant proportion, a false exclusion is possible. The diagnostic is $LR = 0$ for the triallelic locus and $LR > 1$ elsewhere. The recommended action is to check for exclusionary potential at the triallelic locus and if none exists to exclude the locus. The action should appear in the report.

Use and Acceptance of Continuous Systems in Courts

The Frye standard[761] arises from the case *Frye v United States*, 293 F. 1013 (D.C. Cir. 1923) in which the court gave the following opinion:

> Just when a scientific principle or discovery crosses the line between the experimental and demonstrable stages is difficult to define. Somewhere in this twilight zone the evidential force of the principle must be recognized, and while the courts will go a long way in admitting experimental testimony deduced from a well-recognized scientific principle or discovery, the thing from which the deduction is made *must be sufficiently established to have gained general acceptance* in the particular field in which it belongs.

This passage emphasizes that the deduction must proceed from a well-recognized scientific principle or discovery. Moving to software this would appear to mean that the software must implement accepted scientific principles. We would not read this as meaning that the software itself must be in prevalent use but that the principles upon which it is based must be generally accepted. This is thoroughly sensible. Obviously when any software first appears it will be in limited use but it may be very soundly programmed from well-accepted principles. The court clearly envisages that the standard is that the principles are sound, not some sort of vote about how often the software is used.

Any developer should outline the principles upon which the software is based and ensure that these meet the standard. We outline these for the STRmix software in Table 9.5.

Agreement in science proceeds by the peer-reviewed literature. We have surveyed the literature using the Scopus online search tool. We searched for the keywords 'forensic and DNA and interpretation' for the time period from 2012 to January 2015 and obtained 150 references. These were scored as being for the use of probabilistic genotyping, against or irrelevant. We obtained 39 references for, 1 against[764] and 110 that were not relevant. A key phrase from the one scored as against probabilistic genotyping was, 'The variance of heterozygote balance was more expanded in two person mixtures than in one-person samples. Therefore it is not suitable to use allelic peak heights/areas for estimating the genotypes of the contributors such as the quantitative analysis'.

Table 9.5 Evidence of Acceptance for Some Principles Underlying the STRmix™ Software	
Principle	**Evidence of Acceptance**
Markov chain Monte Carlo	This is very standard mathematics employed in many areas of science. Searching the term *Markov chain Monte Carlo* in Scopus returns more than 22,000 records. Scopus is an online bibliographic database containing abstracts and citations for 20,000 peer-reviewed academic journal articles.
Stutter and peak heights and the variance about them can be predicted from empirical models	Studies of stutter and allele peak heights are now quite numerous and have appeared in the peer-reviewed literature.[120,762,763]
The probability of a multilocus genotype can be estimated from allele probabilities and the coancestry coefficient	For STRmix the model follows Balding and Nichols.[358] This model is based on published literature and appears as NRC II Recommendation 4.2. It is the most conservative of the methods in common forensic use.[365]

The right to confront adverse witnesses is ancient. It appears in the Acts of the Apostles 25:16, when Roman governor Porcius Festus states when discussing the proper treatment of Paul: 'I answered them that it is not the custom of the Romans to hand over any man before the accused meets his accusers face to face, and has an opportunity to make his defense against the charges' (New American Standard 1977). It is also cited in Shakespeare's *Richard II*: 'Then call them to our presence; face to face, And frowning brow to brow, ourselves will hear The accuser and the accused freely speak'.

The European Court of Human Rights, Article 6(3), provides that 'everyone charged with a criminal offence' has the right to 'examine or have examined witnesses against him'. This basically means that the accused, or his or her lawyer, should have a chance to put questions to adverse witnesses. The Sixth Amendment to the Constitution of the United States provides that a person accused of a crime has the right to confront a witness against him or her in a criminal action. This includes the right to be present at the trial as well as the right to cross-examine the prosecution's witnesses. It is therefore essential that the witness can represent the evidence and meet the needs of cross-examination. No analyst can be expected to understand the mathematics and computer programme to the extent that they could recreate the system, except the developers themselves. However it is an expectation that analysts at least understand the workings of any system they use to be able to understand and explain the results.

In *R v Noll* (1999, 3 VR 704) the witness acknowledged that although his evidence was based on accepted scientific theory he himself could not describe that theory. At appeal it was submitted that this meant the witness was incapable of giving the DNA evidence and should have been excluded. The court found that although the witness was unable to explain the technical aspects of the theory, he was entitled to rely on other expert opinion. Addressing this issue specifically Justice Ormiston explains:

> Professional people in the guise of experts can no longer be polymaths; they must, in this modern era, rely on others to provide much of their acquired expertise. Their particular talent is that they know where to go to acquire that knowledge in a reliable form.

It has yet to be established in either the scientific or legal frames what level of comprehension is required of a witness giving testimony based on probabilistic methods. However it is clear that this must at least meet minimum levels that ensure that inappropriate testimony is not given. In this document we will attempt to progress the establishment of such standards.

Of note, the International Society for Forensic Genetics (ISFG) *2012 Guidelines* recommend probabilistic methods. In the United States, both the Scientific Working Group on DNA Analysis Methods and the Organization of Scientific Area Committees DNA Analysis 2 subcommittee are working on guidelines for assessing probabilistic genotyping software tools. In addition a considerable number of modern probabilistic genotyping software programmes have been or are being developed by researchers or academics, often with very strong mathematical or statistical backgrounds.[107,108,110,111,686,693,725,742,743,747]

Open Source

Open source software (OSS) is computer software with its source code made available with a license in which the copyright holder provides the rights to study, change and distribute the software to anyone and for any purpose.

In the forensic DNA field several programmes involved in the interpretation of DNA are open source. This is supported by the ISFG. There are however clear pros and cons to this approach. The goal of OSS was, in part, to invite collaborative development. We are aware of only one attempt at this and that was the development of Lab Retriever[108] from LikeLTD.[109,114,462]

This initiative did not meaningfully improve LikeLTD except in the area of interface at the cost of introducing two new errors into the software.*

Both Lab Retriever and LikeLTD maintain a variant population genetic model regrettably introduced by Balding and Buckleton.[114] We lament the addition of another variant in the forensic field as it further fragments practice.

Balding reports that the reprogramming of LikeLTD into Lab Retriever did result in a number of minor bugs being noticed in the original software and this is clearly beneficial. Only one of these affected the math. Balding reports that it did not affect any casework. However with open source it is difficult to know exactly who has used the software in which cases and therefore hard to inform them of a bug in previously used versions. LikeLTD maintains a mailing list and Lab Retriever reports bugs on their website.

Collaborative development is easy to achieve without recourse to OSS. In the STRmix instance Professor James Curran has proposed many useful additions or amendments to the code that have improved runtime performance greatly. In fact a great many scientific collaborations proceed every day without the use of open source.

Probably the primary perceived benefit was openness. The placement of the code in the public domain allowed open scrutiny of the code. In our own work we have never discovered a bug by examination of the code. This has always occurred either by examination of intermediate results in the process or observation of an aberrant result in testing. The two bugs described for Lab Retriever were discovered by the authors, not from the code but by repeating simple calculations.

There have been applications, unsuccessful to date, by defence to access code from closed source software.† A summary of known applications is provided below.

1. A request for the source code of the Office of the Chief Medical Examiner's (OCME, New York) Forensic Statistical Tool (FST) was denied by New York County Supreme Court Justice Carruthers in his May 2, 2012 decision in *People v William Rodriquez*, Indictment No. 5471/2009. The court declined to sign a judicial *subpoena duces tecum* compelling the OCME to produce the source code of the FST.

2. Kings County Supreme Court Justice Dwyer similarly denied a request by defence to compel the OCME to disclose FST's source code in *People v Collins*, Indictment No. 8077/2010 and *People v Peaks*, Indictment No. 7689/2010.

3. In *Commonwealth of Virginia v Brady*, an oral decision on July 26, 2013, Honourable W. Allan Sharrett denied the request for True Allele's source code, ruling that 'validation studies are the best tests of the reliability of source codes. In this case validation studies have been performed, and they have been performed with positive results. [The validation studies] have shown, in fact, that it has been proven to be reliable'.

4. In *Commonwealth of Pennsylvania v Foley*, an appellate court ruled in February 2012 that the True Allele methodology was not novel (testimony at trial provided by Dr Mark Perlin) and further rejected the defendant's claim for the source code – 'scientists can validate the reliability of a computerized process even if the "source code" underlying that process is not available to the public'.

5. Defence attorneys invoked the Confrontation Clause in support of their argument that the FST source code is necessary to confront witnesses at trial. However, in New York State it is firmly established that evidence representing DNA testing procedures and results is non-testimonial in nature. See *People v Brown*, 2009 NY Slip OP 8475 (NY 2009), *People v Freycinet* 2008 NY Slip OP 5776 (NY 2008), *People v Rawlins*, 2008 NY Slip Op 1420 (NY 2008).

---

* These errors were reported in the document 'Release notes for version 2.2.1' in the notes in the section titled 'Version 1.2.4 released May 18, 2014' at http://scieg.org/lab_retriever.html.
† We gratefully acknowledge that much of this was provided by Melissa Mourges.

We suspect that a request for the code is not intended to obtain the code but rather to get a refusal, which can in itself be used as evidence. STRmix is looking at ways to disclose the code and still mitigate the commercial risk.

Suppliers of commercial code are reticent to risk disclosure. What realistic testing could someone do with the code other than compile it and run it? However there is a real risk of commercial damage. It is clear that defence should have meaningful access to a method for checking software. Would not an executable version be better? In fact an executable version that outputs intermediate values and access to the formulae is much more useful, in our opinion, than the code. We note the risk of variants of OSS proliferating and fragmenting the community. We already have Lab Retriever and LikeLTD as differing variants evolving separately from the same origin and introducing errors. Chris Steele makes the perfectly valid point that fragmentation has actually occurred without any assistance from OSS. There are now quite a number of independently created software packages. He goes on to argue, rationally, that this might lead to useful natural selection.

Ranked Lists of Weights: A Courtroom Discussion

Genotype	Weight
9,10	38.30%
8,9	24.66%
9,9	13.94%
7,9	6.67%
8,10	5.36%
10,10	5.23%
8,8	2.35%
7,10	1.29%
7,8	1.01%
Q,9	0.67%
Q,10	0.19%
7,7	0.13%
Q,8	0.11%
Q,7	0.10%

STRmix can give a ranked list of the weights for different genotype combinations. A hypothetical one is given above. We discuss here an argument we have met with in Australia: 'The POI is a 10,10 and he is not even in the top five possibilities'. We assume that this comment is made to suggest that the weight of evidence should be downgraded. The weight for 10,10 in this list is 0.0523. This will appear in the numerator of the LR for this locus. The smaller it is, the lower the LR for this locus. The evidential weight is being downgraded for this locus by the use of this term in the numerator. There is no need for any further adjustment. We assume that the comment about the placement in the list either arises from misunderstanding or the wish to create misunderstanding.

As a technical point the weight is the probability of the evidence given the genotype, not the probability of the genotype given the evidence. It is incorrect to call the 9,10 in this list the most probable genotype. If a description is needed, the best one is that the 9,10 is the genotype with the highest likelihood.

10

Non-Autosomal Forensic Markers*

*Michael Coble, Mikkel Meyer Andersen, John S. Buckleton,
Duncan Taylor and Jo-Anne Bright[†]*

Contents

---

* Certain commercial equipment, instruments, or materials are identified in this paper to foster understanding. Such identification does not imply recommendation or endorsement by the National Institute of Standards and Technology, nor does it imply that the materials or equipment identified are necessarily the best available for the purpose.

† Based on earlier work by John Buckleton, Simon Walsh and Sally Ann Harbison.

Introduction

In this chapter we describe some of the molecular biology and the inheritance and interpretation models relevant to the forensic analysis of non-autosomal markers. Specifically we will discuss the DNA profiling of mitochondrial DNA (mtDNA) and the two gonosomes; the X and Y chromosomes. Since the first edition of this book it has become apparent that one of the crucial aspects of Y chromosome typing is that it is often used when autosomal typing has failed. Because of this it is often applied to low template, mixed or degraded samples.

Forensic Mitochondrial DNA Typing

The analysis of mtDNA is of considerable use in forensic science, and it has been extensively used in archaeology[765,766] and anthropology.[767–773] The increased copy number and stability of mtDNA provided by the additional protective mitochondrial membrane layers and closed circular double-stranded DNA structure leads to increased success in the analysis of samples from old and otherwise compromised samples. An example of this is the successful recovery of mtDNA from the Pleistocene skeletal remains of an indigenous Australian Aboriginal, putatively dating the skeleton beyond 60,000 years before the present.[774] The matrilineal inheritance of mtDNA coupled with its enhanced stability has been used extensively in anthropological studies and has been used to estimate, for example, that New Zealand was settled by a founding population that included a mere 56 women.[775] Analysis of mtDNA is also used increasingly in the investigation of victims of mass disasters[776] and mass graves.[777]

In forensic science mtDNA analysis is often used to provide evidence where nuclear DNA fails to give a result or when distant relatives must be used as reference samples. Typically tissue almost devoid of nuclear DNA is utilized. This may be because there was little nuclear DNA present originally, for example in bone and hair shafts, or because the sample has been subjected to such severe environmental insult that the mtDNA has survived but the nuclear DNA did not, for example in burnt remains. The prevalent approach involves the determination of sequence variants, and there are a number of approaches to achieve this, ranging from conventional polymerase chain reaction (PCR) and sequencing technology based on the chain termination method originally described by Sanger et al.,[778] denaturing high performance liquid chromatography,[779,780] mass spectrometric base composition[781,782] and more recently massive parallel sequencing technologies.[783,784] Hallmark cases have included the identification of the last Russian Tsar, Nicholas II, and his family,[785–787] the exclusion of Anna Anderson as Grand Duchess Anastasia,[788,789] the identification of Air Force 1st Lt. Michael Blassie as the soldier buried in the Vietnam Tomb of the Unknown Soldier[790] and the identification of the remains of Jesse James[791] and Martin Bormann.[792]

Mitochondria are the remnants of symbiotic α-purple bacteria that were ingested by a eukaryotic cell with no cell wall. The existence of separate DNA in the mitochondrion was first suspected because the inheritance of some mitochondrial genes was non-Mendelian. It is now understood that mitochondria contain their own DNA which, in common with bacteria, is a double-stranded closed circular molecule. There is evidence that some of the genes from the ancestral bacteria have been transferred to the nuclear DNA; however about 16,569 bases remain within the mitochondrion. The molecule contains coding and non-coding areas. The coding regions code for the 37 remaining genes of the mitochondria, which comprise 22 transfer RNAs, 2 ribosomal RNAs and 13 protein enzymes. Deletions, duplications and substitutions in this region have been linked to diseases.[793]

Of greatest forensic interest is the control region, also termed the *D-loop* (displacement loop), a structure visible by electron microscopy during replication. The control region is 1122 bases long and flanks the origin of replication. It is non-coding, although it does contain the light (L-) and heavy (H-) strand promoters, transcriptional regulatory elements, binding sites for mitochondrial transcription factors, the origin of H-strand replication and the termination associated sequence.[794–806] These elements would be expected to be under greater selective pressure than areas with no known function, although the lack of functionality of non-coding areas is coming under increasing scrutiny.

Two portions of the control region have been found to be the most variable between individuals, termed *hypervariable regions 1 and 2* (HV I and HV II, respectively). HV I extends from Position 16,024 to 16,365. HV II extends from approximately Position 73 to approximately 340. A third region, HV III, has been added to this pair. This region shows less polymorphism than HV I and II but may resolve some cases where additional discrimination is desired.[807–809] An excellent review is given by Tully et al.[810] We follow them here.*

Matrilineal Inheritance and Recombination

Varying degrees of uniparental inheritance have been suggested for both chloroplasts and mitochondria[811] and 'strict uniparental inheritance is probably not as common as is generally believed. The inheritance of mtDNA in interspecific crosses of mice was believed to be strictly uniparental until a more sensitive technique (PCR amplification) was used to detect low levels of paternal mtDNA'. It is supposed that the ancient mechanism of inheritance in the first mitochondria carrying cells was biparental and that uniparental inheritance has arisen subsequently. Mechanisms leading to full or partial uniparental inheritance are thought to vary. They may be as simple as fixation of the more populous maternal mtDNA; however it does appear that there may be more complex and effective mechanisms, for instance in mammals.[793] The mitochondria reside in the sperm midpiece. In the majority of mammals, including humans, the entire sperm with head, midpiece and tail enter the egg and can be seen for several cell divisions. The only known exception is the Chinese hamster.[812]

Species-specific exclusion of sperm DNA has been observed in mice.[813] Experimental injection of liver and sperm mtDNA suggests that the mechanism is specific to sperm mtDNA.[814] Recognition of sperm mitochondria by embryonic cells and inhibition of the inheritance of paternal mtDNA have been reported.[815] Possible mechanisms[816] include ubiquitination. This is a process by which a protein is thought to bind to sperm mitochondria and mark them for subsequent degradation by the 26S proteasome.

Failure of the mechanism has been reported in abnormal embryos[817] but persists following intracytoplasmic sperm injection.[818] A possible replicative advantage for deleteriously mutated mtDNA has also been reported[819] and may be a factor in increasing the fraction of paternal mtDNA in some human cases.[793,819,820] Over 20 cases of clear-cut mixed ancestry for the mtDNA have been reported.[821]

Uni- or biparental inheritance and recombination are different things and should not be confused. Because there are numerous organelles in each cell, it is possible for there to be biparental inheritance with no recombination. In this process different organelles contain copies of the DNA from only one parent but the total population contains examples of each parent. Recombination of chloroplasts has been noted in fungi[822–825] and slime mould.[826] In contrast, no recombinants were noted in screens of blue mussel even though both genomes 'have been present in the fertilized egg and germ line cells of embryos in every generation for over five million years'.[811] The disequilibrium in human and chimpanzee mtDNA declines as a function of distance between sites. The most plausible explanation is recombination either with other mtDNA or with mitochondrial sequences in the nucleosome.[827]

Maternal passage of mtDNA in humans has been demonstrated through multiple extended lineages with rare evidence of paternal contribution.[828,829] Recent papers have suggested that

---

* Sections that are reproduced in full from Tully et al.[810] appear with permission from Elsevier (Copyright 1999).

there may be some biparental inheritance and recombination leading to hybrid mtDNA molecules in humans.[827,830] Some of this evidence was based on a dataset with multiple errors[816] and the evidence is much weaker when these errors are corrected. Sykes[767] goes to some effort to rebut the claims of recombination in humans in his popular science book *The Seven Daughters of Eve*. The consensus appears to be emerging that recombination in humans is either minimal or does not occur[831] (for excellent reviews see Birky[816] or Holland and Parsons[793]). For practical purposes in identification cases maternal inheritance alone is usually assumed, and we will follow that practice here.

The consequences of a lack of recombination are quite marked. First the entire mtDNA genome is treated as a haplotype. This means that the whole DNA sequence is treated as a unit not as the sum of its parts. Frequency estimates are typically made by counting the number of occurrences of this haplotype in a database rather than by recourse to population genetic models. The mtDNA is expected to be under severe selection. Any deleterious mutation cannot be repaired and cannot be masked by a dominant gene on a homologous chromosome (since there is none). Since the segments do not recombine, deleterious or advantageous mutations are always linked to the positions that we are investigating forensically. Hence, even if we consider the D-loop as selectively neutral, we must consider the whole mtDNA haplotype to be under selection. However, since we do not invoke either the Hardy–Weinberg or linkage equilibrium assumption there is no requirement for selective neutrality and accordingly this selection has no implications for the interpretation.

Mutations and Heteroplasmy

mtDNA has a much higher mutation rate than nuclear DNA, about 20-fold higher according to one estimate, although arguments persist as to the exact rate (for a review see Ref. 832). The estimates of mutation rate from short pedigrees or mother–child pairs appear to be higher than that obtained from phylogenetic studies. An explanation for this is still required but such discrepancies have also been noted for the Y chromosome. A modest effect of purifying selection has been confirmed for mtDNA.[833] Mutations and heteroplasmy are relatively common occurrences. The reasons advanced for the higher mutation rate include the relatively high turnover both in mitotic and post-mitotic cells and the susceptibility of mitochondrial structures to oxidative stress.[834] The functioning of the mitochondrion produces the superoxide anion, O_2^-, that is implicated in the promotion of mutation. However the female germline mitochondria are present in the eggs of females that have undergone a mere 24 divisions early in embryonic development. There is also evidence that the mitochondria of ova have been 'shut down' and that these cells are respiring anaerobically. This helps to preserve the mtDNA of the female germline (recall that the male germline does not pass on its mtDNA).

The most common types of mutation found within the forensically significant D-loop region are single-base substitutions with transitions outnumbering transversions by approximately 40:1. Small insertions and deletions are common in the two homopolymeric polycytosine (poly(C)) regions between positions 302 and 310 and between positions 16,183 and 16,194. Insertions and deletions can hinder the interpretation of both single source and mixed samples as the sequence of the contributing individuals is thrown out of register. The chance of observing insertions and deletions at homopolymeric regions increases as the length of the uninterrupted homopolymer stretch increases. Other alterations include large deletions and short duplications.[834]

Stability varies along the mtDNA genome as some base positions appear to be very stable while others are highly mutable.[793,835–842] Furthermore, some body tissues, such as hairs, tend to show more variability in their mtDNA sequence.[843] This could be due to differential segregation of pre-existing heteroplasmic variants to the accumulation of new somatic mutations or to a combination of both phenomena. There is still some debate over whether the number of point mutations increases with age or whether or not it is implicated in the ageing process.[834] Mutations are passed between generations in varying ratios and segregate during development and later life. Mutations also accumulate and segregate during the lifetime of an individual.[793]

This results in mixtures of mtDNA molecules that characteristically differ from each other at one or more bases. This is known as *heteroplasmy* (reviewed in Ref. 844).

Heteroplasmy can be either sequence- or length-based. It can occur in an individual in essentially three different ways.[780]

A single tissue type from an individual may have more than one mtDNA type, or different tissues from the same person may exhibit different mtDNA types or some tissues may have more than one mtDNA type but another tissue from the same person only one mtDNA type. Heteroplasmy probably exists in all individuals, although it is often at such a low level that it cannot always be detected by the routine sequencing techniques presently used. In order for a mutation to be detected above background by sequencing, it must currently be present at a level approaching 20%. In addition the chance of detection of heteroplasmy is dependent upon the sequencing chemistry used. Detection may be more efficient at certain nucleotide positions than at others, and differences in detection may be also observed between the two DNA strands. Massive parallel sequencing techniques hold the promise of substantially higher detection of heteroplasmy compared to Sanger sequencing.[783,845] There is an interrelationship between observation of heteroplasmy and amplification strategy.[846]

The location of heteroplasmy should correlate with sites of high variation.[847,848] Evidence[849,793] for this was found by direct comparison of new mutations which occur at both hot-spot and novel sites.[850] Length heteroplasmy is a particular concern in the poly(C) stretches of both HV I (between 16183 and 16194) and HV II (between 302 and 310).[793]

Once a mutation has led to significant heteroplasmy in the germ line, the offspring will either be heteroplasmic or fixation on one mitotype will have occurred, so that heteroplasmy can no longer be detected. This suggests that heteroplasmy may be an intermediate state in the evolution from one mitotype to another. There is evidence that suggests that the mitochondria are reduced in number during oogenesis.[793] This bottleneck has the potential to alter the ratio of heteroplasmic variants or to lead to fixation on one mitotype. An interesting investigation of this looked at 180 twin pairs and found matching heteroplasmy in four instances. Analysis of other family members showed differing ratios of the heteroplasmic variants. Various authors have estimated the size of the bottleneck and these estimates vary widely.

There is some residual debate as to whether or not mutations accumulate during an individual's lifetime. For example, Calloway et al.[851] investigated the variation of heteroplasmy with tissue and age. They found the highest levels in muscle and found that heteroplasmy increased with age. Bai et al.[852] presented supporting data from a study of a large deletion that is associated with ageing and deafness. Lagerstrom-Fermer et al.[853] presented limited data that would support the opposite conclusion. Review articles strongly favour the former position.[793,810]

A consequence for forensic science of the presence of an elevated mutation rate and heteroplasmy is that the evidential (crime) sample and reference samples may exhibit sequence differences even when the two are, in reality, from the same individual or lineage. This strongly suggests use of the logical interpretation approach that will be discussed later.

mtDNA variation is reported by reference to the revised Cambridge reference sequence, rCRS (NC001807),[854] which corrects errors in the first published sequence,[855] referred to as the *Anderson sequence*. The rCRS resides in a peripheral European haplogroup H2a2a1. Because of this there have been understandable suggestions to move the reference to a position nearer the root of the mtDNA phylogeny, the RCRS[856,857] and the rRCRS.[858] These more ancient and non-existent mitotypes have been inferred by reference to chimpanzee, bonobo, Neanderthal and *Homo Sapiens Altai* and lie between haplogroups L0 and L1'2'3'4'5'6. The change has been likened to shifting the thought process about the solar system from the Earth at the centre to the sun at the centre. Concerns about the potential negative consequences of a conversion have been expressed and the forensic reference remains the rCRS.[859]

Forensic Y Chromosome Analysis
Introduction

Each male has only one Y chromosome, a condition known as *hemizygosity*. The human Y chromosome represents about 2% of the total human genome and is approximately 60 Mb in length. It emerged from a severely degenerate X chromosome.[860] This arose when an ancestral mammal developed a sex-determining gene on one X chromosome. It is assumed that prior to that event sex had been determined by factors such as temperature, mechanisms that persist in reptiles and many other animal orders. The male determining gene (SRY gene) resides in the male-specific (MSY) or non-recombining (NRY) region near the distal end of the short arm.

For about 95% of the length of the Y chromosome no X–Y crossover occurs.[861] This region is known as the *non-recombining region*.[862] Recombination occurs only at the distal portions of the short and long arms of the chromosome, the pseudoautosomal regions (PAR 1 and 2).[863] The recombination between the ends of the Y chromosome and the X chromosome has been observed down the microscope and is part of the original evidence that identified these as a pair.

There is growing evidence that the MSY region of the Y chromosome may have some tendency to recombine within itself.[864] Large segments of DNA are repeated in reverse along the length of the Y chromosome. These sequences are termed *palindromes*, as they read the same forward or reverse, and they may have some ability to recombine (perhaps more appropriately termed *gene conversion*). This ability is very different from normal recombination with a homologous chromosome but may have some implications for DNA repair in the Y chromosome. There is also extensive evidence that such gene shuffling is implicated in massive deletions and infertility.

The lack of ability to recombine is thought to be the reason that there are few functional genes on the Y chromosome. There are 78 protein coding sequences in the MSY that encode 27 distinct proteins. This is a low density of genes compared with the autosomes. Any deleterious mutation that 'knocks out' a gene has little chance of repair and cannot be removed by recombination. High population frequencies have been observed for some deleterious mutations[865,866] and are supposed to be the result of repetitive recreation by mutation or support from advantageous mutations elsewhere on the Y chromosome. It is generally expected that all functional genes on the Y chromosome will slowly be deactivated by mutation including eventually the male-determining switch. Unless these genes have relocated elsewhere they will be lost.[14]

The MSY contains repetitive sequences, called *amplicons*, comprising long intra-chromosomal repetitive sequences, each of which possessed little sequence variation.[861,867] However these small sequence variations were used to determine a physical map of the MSY[868] that has now been developed into the complete DNA sequence. The unusual chromosomal structure of the Y chromosome coupled with a lack of crossover and high apparent rate of gene conversion suggests that Y chromosome sequence variation might differ markedly from other chromosomes.

There is a large array of different polymorphisms that are suitable for PCR-based analysis including single nucleotide polymorphisms (SNPs), microsatellites and minisatellites (see Figure 10.1). It is estimated that thousands of base substitutions probably exist in the contemporary human population.[869]

The characteristics of a high degree of polymorphism, the ability to multiplex using PCR and the ease of analysis make the analysis of short tandem repeats (STRs) the current method of choice for forensic DNA profiling favoured over SNPs. The first use of STR on the Y chromosome occurred in 1992[870] and this STR is now known as DYS19. Since then the potential use of Y-STR analysis for forensic casework has been recognized and well documented.[87,871–877] Y-STR typing is useful when there is a low level of male DNA in comparison to the amount of female DNA present in a sample or when a study of family relationships is needed.

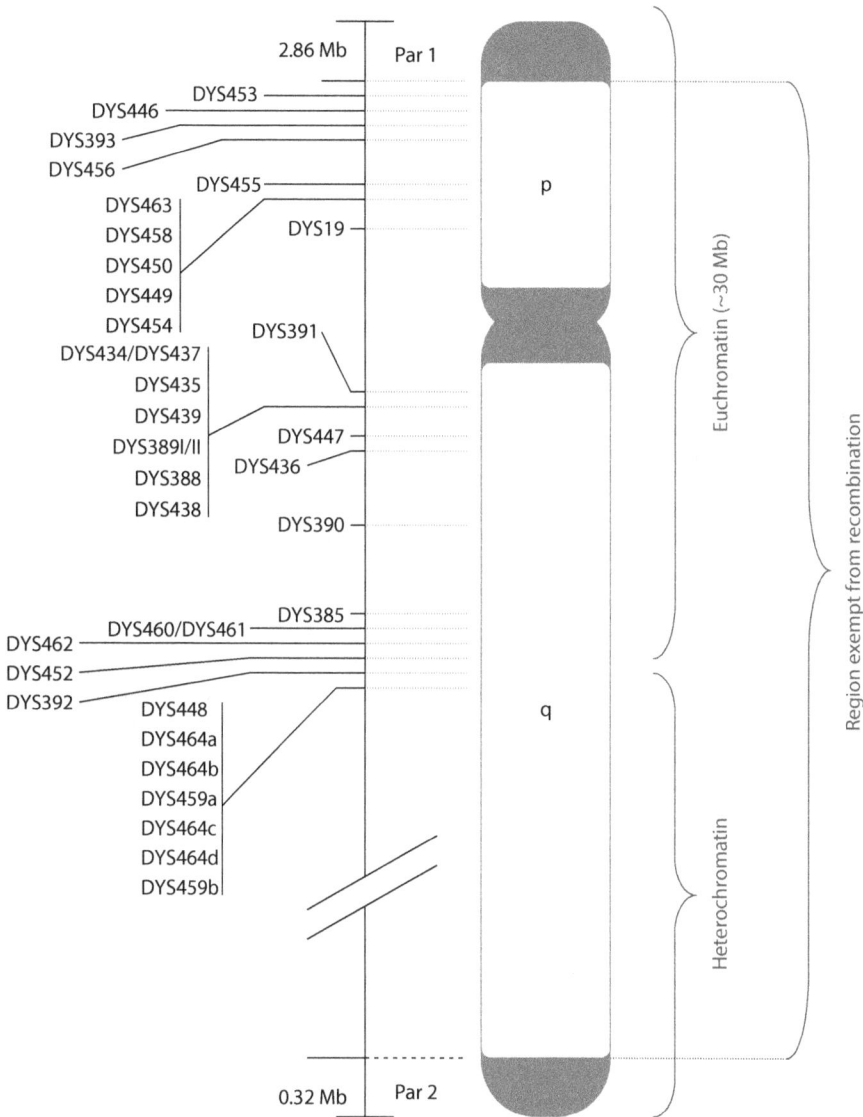

Figure 10.1 A schematic of the Y chromosome showing approximate locations of microsatellite loci (not drawn to scale).

Recently there have been reports of foetal microchimerism. This describes a situation where foetal cells become established in the mother and give rise to chimerism. Potentially a female could contain cell lines derived from a male child and hence this female could give rise to a weak Y chromosome typing result. This issue was investigated[878] and it was found that no interference was likely under normal template and amplification conditions.

Specific sets of loci, often referred to as *minimum haplotypes,* have been chosen by groups in Europe[879] and the United States (Scientific Working Group on DNA Analysis Methods, SWGDAM) to encourage the standardization of population data. This objective was helped by the construction of large databases including the YHRD (Y chromosome Haplotype Reference Database; see http://www.yhrd.org/) and the US YSTR database.[880] Over 114,000 haplotypes are compiled on YHRD and are available online for researchers and caseworkers.[881,882] There is an ongoing search for suitable Y-STRs with novel markers identified and validated regularly.[883–886] These STRs are occasionally duplicated, triplicated or quadrupled,[887] giving rise to two, three or four amplification products.

There are a variety of commercially available multiplexes now produced for forensic Y chromosome applications. For example, ReliaGene Technologies (New Orleans, LA) produced the first Y-STR multiplex: Y-plex 6,[888] followed by the Y-plex 5 and Y-plex 12, a kit that contained the European minimal haplotype and the two SWGDAM-recommended loci along with amelogenin.[889] ReliaGene no longer manufacture Y-STR kits.

The PowerPlex Y kit[890] (Promega Corporation, Madison, WI) included the core European and SWGDAM loci and one additional marker. Applied Biosystems (Foster City, CA) produced the Yfiler kit that incorporated 17 Y-STR loci, including all of the markers in the PowerPlex Y kit[891]. Y-STR profiling kits containing additional loci are available from both the Promega Corporation and Life Technologies (previously Applied Biosystems), who offer PowerPlex Y23 and Yfiler Plus, respectively.

Y-STR analysis is undertaken in the same way as autosomal STR analysis using the same equipment and methods.[892] Homologous regions with varying regions of conservation are present on the X and Y chromosomes.[892] This means that supposedly Y-chromosome-specific primers may sometimes amplify similar products from the X chromosome. An example of such non-specific amplification was described by the initial set of primers chosen for DYS391.[893] Since the Y chromosome does not recombine, it is treated as a haplotype in much the same way as mtDNA. Again the forensic loci will be linked to any deleterious or advantageous mutation. Even if our forensic loci are selectively neutral, and there is little evidence either way, we must expect selection to be active on the whole haplotype including, by linkage, our forensic loci. For example, spermatogenic ability is thought to vary in differing Y lineages.[894] Hallmark studies have included the investigation of whether Thomas Jefferson fathered a child by one of his slaves (the evidence supports that he did)[895] and the finding that approximately 8% of all males in Asia may be descended from Genghis Khan.[87]

Y Chromosome Mutation

Y chromosomes evolve along paternal lineages accumulating diversity only by mutational processes. The lineages are distributed in a clustered manner among human populations supposedly because of genetic and cultural factors.[896] The patrilineage of Y chromosome haplotypes reduces their diversity in the general population.[896] To this effect is added a smaller effective population size and hence more rapid drift. The effective population size of the Y chromosome is one-quarter that of the autosomes and one-third that of the X chromosome* but is the same as the mtDNA. The time to the most recent common ancestor for the Y chromosome is currently thought to be about 90,000 years, whereas it is about 240,000 years for mtDNA. Both of these estimates have considerable uncertainty. The shallower nature of the Y chromosome tree may be explained by men having a higher variance in reproductive success, by higher rates of migration or by selection. There is some evidence in support of each of these.

This loss of diversity and a more structured population may be seen as disadvantages given the high discriminating power that forensic scientists are accustomed to from multilocus autosomal profiles. However this feature affords significant advantages as well, particularly for the study of population genetics and human evolution. The lower mutation rates for base substitutions make them extremely valuable in tree building. They tend to give a reliable coarse structure to the tree. However a sufficient number are needed.[875,897,898] Microsatellites are more rapidly evolving and tend to be useful to investigate the fine structure of trees.

---

* Consider a male–female pair of individuals. They have four autosomes, three X and one Y chromosomes between them. This suggests that the autosomes have an effective population size four times that of the Y. The X chromosome has an effective population size three times that of the Y.

Some Y-STRs originate from a duplicated tandem repeat array, additional alleles arising by insertion polymorphisms of the larger chromosomal region including the STR locus followed by a mutational change in the number of repeats within the STR locus. Locus multiplication (the multiplication of the amplicon including both forward and reverse primer binding sites) has been reported for several Y-STR loci, including the following:

- DYS19[87,870,876]
- DYS385[879,899–901]
- DYS390[886]
- DYS435[87]

These can be explained as a result of insertion polymorphism of a larger chromosomal region (or replicative transposition)[861] followed by a mutational change in the number of repeats within the STR locus. This produces two, three or four peaks of similar size if two, three or four PCR products are produced. Using standard PCR methods, assignment of the alleles to loci cannot be done.[879] This means that a haplotype a_1a_2 as a duplicated locus may have either allele at either locus and could not be differentiated with standard technology. There is no effect on the interpretation.

There has been a deliberate search for rapidly mutating Y-STR markers to increase discrimination even within a pedigree.[902]

Mutation rates vary by at least two orders of magnitude, one large study[903] giving a plausible range from 3.81×10^{-4} to 7.73×10^{-2}. There was a very slight and not significant excess of repeat loss over repeat gain. The repeat step transitions are given in Table 10.1.

Mutation rates rise with the length of homogenous repeats plus any non-variable repeats adjacent. Large alleles have a propensity to loss and small alleles to gain a repeat. The repeat complexity, repeat length and father's age also contributed to increase mutation rate.

A very valid call for improved data recording and reporting has been made.[904] Data on the frequency and type of mutations but most especially the number of non-mutation events needs to be recorded.

The YHRD maintains an extensive and continuously updated compilation of mutation rate publications (http://www.yhrd.org/Research/Loci).

Y Chromosome STR Marker Artefacts

Back Stutter

Y-STR loci are thought to be structurally the same as autosomal STR loci and hence it is likely that the same models may apply. Only limited studies have been published on the subject of quantifying artefacts at Y-STR loci.[905] It was suggested[906] that the log of stutter ratio for each allele, a, at each locus, l, $(SR_{l,a})$, is linearly related to longest uninterrupted stretch for that allele and locus $(LUS_{l,a})$ as in autosomal work: $\log(SR_{l,a}) = \beta_{l0} + \beta_{l1}LUS_{l,a}$.

The test set however could not differentiate this model from one using allele designation[905] only since all STRs in the test set were simple repeats. The compound repeat DYS390 is not well described by the Bright et al. model[906] and appears to have two populations of data. Sequencing

Table 10.1 The Relative Frequencies of Repeat Change in Mutations Observed in Ballantyne et al.

Repeat Change	1	2	3	4	5
Relative frequency	96.19%	3.18%	0.38%	0.13%	0.13%

Source: Ballantyne, K.N. et al., *American Journal of Human Genetics*, 87(3), 341–353, 2010.

of a sample of these alleles would be helpful to investigate their LUS values and inform the model. The pentanucleotide repeat locus DYS438 did not stutter significantly in comparison with other loci within the multiplex. Pentanucleotide repeat loci are known to have reduced rates of stutter.[907]

Forward Stutter
Forward stutter has been noted for the Y-STR with observed rates[906] of forward stutter in the range of 0.9–3.6%. The triallelic repeat locus DYS392 had the highest rate of observed forward stutter peaks.

Double Back Stutter
Double back stutter peaks (peaks two repeat units shorter than the parent allele) were observed[906] at varying rates for different loci up to 2.1% of samples.

DYS19 Artefact
An artefact of two nucleotides smaller than the parent allele was observed at locus DYS19. The two base pair variant allele was observed often (407 of the 461 profiles analyzed). The height of this peak was proportional to the height of the parent allele just like other stutters.

DYS385 Artefact
An artefact nine nucleotides smaller than the parent allele was observed at locus DYS385. The height of this peak was also proportional to the height of the parent allele.

DYS385 is at least duplicated on the Y chromosome.[908] The single set of primers results in two amplicons, where the two alleles are typically labelled *a* and *b*. Less frequently the locus is replicated three or four times.[908] In the current dataset, locus DYS385 was triplicated in 23 of the 461 profiles (allele *c*). Increased observations of triplication of the DYS385 locus have been reported in Polynesian populations.[909]

The Promega PowerPlex Y Technical Manual reports low level *a* + 0.2 artefacts at DYS19 and amplification products in the *a* − 0.2 and *a* + 0.2 positions (two bases below and above the true allele peak, respectively), at DYS389II.[910] None of these artefacts were observed by Bright et al.[906]

The Interpretation of Single Source Lineage Marker Matches
A clear single source match of a lineage marker presents, on the surface, the simplest problem in forensic science. It would seem that a simple count of other matching profiles in a relevant database would provide a complete interpretation. This superficial simplicity is deceptive and treats the problem as simply a statistical one. Doing so overlooks the considerable understanding from evolutionary models that allows inferences about the current state in the population.

Interpretation: The Likelihood Ratio Approach
The various options for interpretation that were discussed in Chapter 2 are equally applicable to lineage markers, except that there are some situations where the logical approach has very considerable additional advantages.

Before progressing to a discussion of matches and exclusions it is best to set up the logical framework. This departs from the approach taken in previous chapters where the frequentist approach was given first. The reason for this is that the terms *match* and *exclusion* can be ambiguous in lineage marker work. The correct line of thinking is best laid down before approaching these complexities. We move to the development of two propositions. As always care must be taken. We consider that we have typed a crime stain or material, C, and produced its haplotype G_C. The prosecution allege that this stain or material comes from a person, POI. If this person, or a sample from him (we consistently use *him* for simplicity), is available we may have the haplotype for the POI, G_P. It is unnecessary to assume that the haplotype is a single sequence. It may be two or more if the samples are showing heteroplasmy.

Often we may not have a sample from the POI and may be using as a reference material from a relative, K, with haplotype G_K. Consider two alternative source-level propositions:

H_p: The evidential sample, C, originates from the POI.

H_d: The evidential sample, C, originates from an individual other than the POI.

We need to differentiate the situations where the haplotype from the POI is available and where it is not. Let us begin with the situation where we have the haplotype for the POI. As usual, following the logical approach, we require

$$LR = \frac{\Pr(G_C \mid G_P, H_p)}{\Pr(G_C \mid G_P, H_d)}$$

having made the assumption that $\Pr(G_P \mid H_p) = \Pr(G_P \mid H_d)$.

If, and only if, we assume that the haplotype from two samples from the same person will always be the same, then it would be possible to write $\Pr(G_C \mid G_P, H_p) = 1$. However it may be necessary to consider somatic variations such as heteroplasmy. If so it may not always be possible to assume that two samples from the same person, but from different tissues or at different times, will give the same haplotype. Equally, if the haplotype is a combination of two or more sequences these may appear in differing ratios from sample to sample, even when they are from the same source. What is needed is a probabilistic model to assess the joint probability of two samples, or the probability of one sample conditional on another when both have come from the same individual. This would be a profitable area for interpretation research.

Next consider that we may not have the POI available and are working with a reference sample from K. We have available the background information, I, which includes the information on the relationship between K and S.

Following the logical approach we require

$$LR = \frac{\Pr(G_C \mid G_K, H_p, I)}{\Pr(G_C \mid G_K, H_d, I)}$$

having made the assumption that $\Pr(G_K \mid H_p, I) = \Pr(G_K \mid H_d, I)$.

Now we need to consider whether or not the haplotype from two samples from the two different people related by I will always be the same. If they were always the same then $\Pr(G_C \mid G_K, H_p, I) = 1$. However it necessary to consider mutation between generations and somatic variation especially with the newer marker sets. Again what is needed is a probabilistic model to assess the joint or conditional probability.

The value of $\Pr(G_C \mid G_K, H_p, I)$ taking into account the mutation rate will depend on the number of meioses between the POI and K. This can be done also taking into account the step size of the mutation (as shown in Table 10.1) but at a simplistic level. Figure 10.2 shows the effect a profile-wide mutation rate of μ will have on the probability of relatives sharing a common haplotype. Figure 10.2 also ignores the possibility of back-mutation to a previous state.

It is well established that the mutation rate for mtDNA is substantially higher than that encountered with nuclear DNA. Consequently it is not uncommon for differences to be observed in the DNA sequence when comparing close maternal relatives (such as a mother and a child).[828] Substitution has also been observed in somatic tissues, presumably due to the segregation of existing heteroplasmy within the individual. This means that differences may be observed between different hairs or tissues within an individual.[843,851,911] Consequently, if there are mismatches between G_C and G_p or G_K, this does not automatically exclude the hypothesis that C and POI are from the same individual or that C and K are matrilineally related.[780]

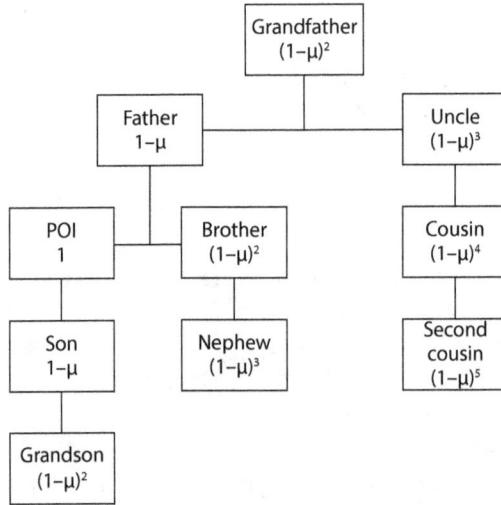

Figure 10.2   Pedigree showing male relatives of the person of interest (POI) and the probability that they will share a haplotype with the POI.

This is also true for Y chromosome haplotypes especially when the new highly mutable markers are in use.

If C and P or K do not match, the strength of the evidence will be dependent upon the inherent mutability of that base or locus.

Y chromosomal mutation rates have been reported for most markers in use.

The current level of knowledge regarding substitution rates at each position within the mtDNA non-coding region has also been investigated. Estimation of substitution rates in the control region is assisted by the following:

- Observations of both heteroplasmy and substitutions from germline and intra-individual mutation studies[39,793,828,843,851,911–915]

- Observations of the occurrence of heteroplasmy in casework and research

- Inferences from phylogenetic studies[835–842]

For example, long poly(C) stretches (between positions 302 and 310 and between 16,183 and 16,194) are extremely mutable. At the opposite end of the spectrum, Position 73 is thought to be relatively stable.[840] Thus a difference at Position 73 may provide stronger evidence for exclusion of K as the matrilineal origin of C than two base differences between K and C if these are at positions 309.2 (homopolymeric region) and 16,093 (an apparent mutation 'hotspot' that has been observed to vary in studies from several laboratories).[915]

However, despite such estimates, precise values for substitution rates are difficult to determine for the following reasons:

- Segregation of mutations will occur at different rates in different tissues.

- There may be sequence context-specific variations in substitution rates.

- Paternal inheritance and recombination, if they occur at appreciable rates, may bias inference from phylogenetic studies.

In applying a likelihood ratio (LR) approach (for example as given by Holland and Parsons[793]) the assessment of the term $\Pr(G_C \mid G_K, H_p, I)$ is informed by these considerations. If there are many differences between G_C and G_K, the probability $\Pr(G_C \,|\, G_K, H_p, I)$ is effectively 0, and hence an exclusion can be reported. Conversely, if G_C and G_K share no differences, the probability $\Pr(G_C \,|\, G_K, H_p, I)$ approaches, but does not quite reach, 1. In the case of sequences that differ at one or two base positions, the value of the numerator term, $\Pr(G_C \,|\, G_K, H_p, I)$, is intermediate but likely to be low.

This may be the correct time to return to the subject of the words *match* and *exclusion*. Because of germline mutation, somatic mutation and heteroplasmy, two samples from the same person or the same lineage may not be identical in sequence. This makes the words *match* and *exclusion* problematic both because they may not describe the situation well but more importantly because they reinforce in the mind of lawyers the incorrect view that there are only two states.

Interpretation: The Frequentist Approach

The logical approach does not require a statement of inclusion or exclusion. The nearest equivalent to these terms would be an *LR* greater or less than 1, respectively. The frequentist approach to interpreting this evidence, however, does require such a definition. An inclusion is usually defined by nominating the maximum number of bases or alleles at which two samples may differ and yet be deemed to match. An exclusion is the converse, sometimes with an inconclusive zone. Logically this should relate to whether the reference sample is alleged to be the same person (POI) or a relative (*K*), and if a maternal relative then it should be conditional on the pedigree information (*I*). As described above this criterion should also consider exactly which bases differ. This is because different mutation rates can be expected for different sequence positions. However in practice the criterion usually specifies simply the number of bases that are allowed to differ. There is less official guidance than one might expect.

The SWGDAM guidelines on mtDNA typing[916] give the following recommendations:

3.1.1 Exclusion: If samples differ at two or more nucleotide positions (excluding length heteroplasmy), they can be excluded as coming from the same source or maternal lineage.

3.1.2 Inconclusive: The comparison should be reported as inconclusive if samples differ:
   a. at a single position only (whether or not they share a common length variant between positions 302–310)
   b. only by not sharing a common length variant between positions 302–310 (all other positions are concordant)

3.1.3 Cannot Exclude: If samples have the same sequence, or are concordant (sharing a common DNA base at every nucleotide position, including common length variants), they cannot be excluded as coming from the same source or maternal lineage.

The 2009 SWGDAM Y-chromosome Short Tandem Repeat (Y-STR) Interpretation Guidelines[917] give the following recommendations:

4. Conclusions and Reporting
4.1. The laboratory should prepare guidelines for formulating conclusions resulting from comparisons of evidentiary samples and known reference samples.
4.1.1. General categories of conclusions are *inclusion match, exclusion or nonmatch, inconclusive or uninterpretable*, and *no results.*
4.1.2. Comparison of haplotypes cannot distinguish between males from the same paternal lineage; therefore, inclusions need to be qualified.

Significantly insightful recommendations came early from the International Society of Forensic Genetics (ISFG).[918]

If the sequences are the same, then the reference sample and evidence cannot be excluded as potentially being from the same source.

In cases where the same heteroplasmy is observed in both the questioned sample and the known sample, its presence may increase the strength of the evidence.

If heteroplasmy is observed in the questioned sample but not the known sample or vice versa, a common maternal lineage cannot be excluded.

If the questioned and known samples differ by a single nucleotide and no evidence of heteroplasmy is present, the interpretation may be that the results are inconclusive. However one nucleotide difference between two samples may, on occasion, provide evidence against the samples originating from the same source or maternal lineage; in particular, where both the questioned sample and known sample are a tissue such as blood, a single nucleotide difference points towards exclusion of a common maternal origin.

In cases where more than a single nucleotide difference exists between the evidence and known sequences, careful analysis of the sequences which differ will determine the proper interpretation of the comparison. The sources of the tissues investigated should be taken into consideration, because differences in mtDNA sequences due to mutations seem to be more likely between e.g. hair and blood than between two blood samples taken from the same individual. Moreover, the knowledge of mutation rates is presently limited and may not allow precise estimates but should be taken into consideration. In general, however, the larger the number of differences between samples, the smaller the chance of them being from the same source or having the same maternal origin.

—Reprinted from Carracedo et al.[918] (With permission from Elsevier.)

The 2014 SWGDAM Y chromosome guidelines[919] and the DNA commission of the ISFG mtDNA guidelines[920] do not comment.

We have some considerable concern about the situation where one or two differences exist but a failure to exclude is declared. We would feel that it is inappropriate to then proceed to produce and report a count of the matching features.

In the first edition of this book we equivocated about an *LR* or frequentist approach. However with the advent of rapidly mutating Y chromosome maxrkers and the general progress of science it is time to state that the frequentist approach has no place in interpreting lineage marker comparisons across generations. It also has no place in the interpretation of samples alleged to come from the same person if there is any difference between the samples, such as a length variant in a c-stretch in mtDNA analysis.

The frequentist approach is probably still viable for exactly matching samples alleged to come from the same person. This is because the frequentist approach has some claim to equal validity with the *LR* when the numerator of the *LR* is 1. For exactly matching profiles the numerator is not 1 but is likely to be close to 1. When considering matches across generations or samples with any difference the numerator is unlikely to be very close to 1.

In the case of matching profiles alleged to come from the same person the frequency reported should be calculated as the sum of the frequencies of all sequences that would be deemed to be not excluded. This is not the normal procedure.

If the sequence of interest has not been observed in the database, it is incumbent on the forensic scientist to ensure that the court is not left with the impression that the sequence could be as rare as an autosomal STR profile.

Statistical and Genetic Sampling

To begin with let us consider that the haplotype is inherited as an intact copy of genetic material in one parent (either the mother in the case of mtDNA or the father in the case of the Y chromosome). We have a database of N haplotypes and in the case in question the person of interest has haplotype G_{POI}, which corresponds with the haplotype of a sample reliably associated with the offender, G_O. We assume initially that $G_{POI} = G_O$, meaning that the two haplotypes are equivalent and we term this haplotype A.

For a mtDNA or Y chromosome haplotype of type A, the match and profile probabilities for a specific subpopulation are both equal to p_A^*, the profile frequency in that subpopulation. If there was a sample available from that subpopulation it would furnish an estimate of this quantity although, as described in the following section, care is needed if the profile is not present in the sample or if the sample is not only from the subpopulation of interest.

If a sample is not available from the relevant subpopulation, then an estimate of p_A^* is not available. Instead we work with a sample estimate $\tilde{p}_A$ of the frequency p_A, the average over all subpopulations assembled from the database where the subpopulation is undefined or unknown. We need to take into account the variation among subpopulations, i.e. population structure. With population structure, match and profile probabilities are no longer the same and the expected value of the match probability $\left(p_A^*\right)^2$ is needed. Assuming a particular population genetic model, namely the Balding–Nichols model, it can be shown that this expectation is $p_A^2 + p_A(1-p_A)\theta$, so that the match probability is

$$\Pr(A\,|\,A) = \theta + (1-\theta)p_A. \tag{10.1}$$

This can be given a numerical value if reasonable estimates of p_A (e.g. $\tilde{p}_A$) and θ are available. Note that the match probability within a particular subpopulation is greater than the haplotype frequency in the whole population since $\theta + (1-\theta)p_A \geq p_A$ and $\theta + (1-\theta)p_A \geq \theta$. On average, two haplotypes are more likely to be the same when they are taken from the same subpopulation than when they are taken randomly from the whole population.

Normally our reference databases are from a population that consists of subpopulations. This is often referred to as a *population with substructure*. We do not have information about these subpopulations (which individuals belong to which subpopulations). The problem with this situation is that we would normally want to consider the case where the suspect and culprit are assumed to belong to the same subpopulation. Had we known that particular subpopulation, we could have used this information. Instead we take an expected value, which leads to Equation 10.1.

Example 10.1: Using a Danish Reference Database to Interpret a Crime in Denmark

Assuming no population substructure:

H_d: A random Dane left the Y chromosome DNA in the crime sample.

Use a Danish reference database to estimate the population probability p_A. Make no θ correction.

Example 10.2: Using a Danish Reference Database to Interpret a Crime in Denmark

Assume population substructure:

H_d: A random Dane from the same (unknown) subpopulation as the POI left the Y chromosome DNA in the crime sample.

Use a Danish reference database to estimate the population probability p_A. Make a θ correction (Equation 10.1) with a θ value developed from Danish subpopulations.

Example 10.3: Using a Bornholmian* Reference Database to Interpret a Crime on Bornholm

Assuming no population substructure:

H_d: A random Bornholmian left the Y chromosome DNA in the crime sample.

Use a Bornholmian reference database and estimate the population probability p_A. Make no θ correction.

---

* Bornholm is a small Danish island.

Example 10.4: Using a European Reference Database to Interpret a Crime in Denmark

Assuming population substructure:

H_d: A random Dane left the Y chromosome DNA in the crime sample.

Use a European reference database and estimate the population probability p_A. Make a θ correction with a θ value developed from European subpopulations (at a level corresponding to countries).

In Figure 10.3 we give the results of a not-very-scientific experiment. The markers show the locations of the close male relatives of Mikkel Meyer Andersen and two colleagues. Does this experiment suggest subpopulation effects? It would certainly be nicer to have more extensive data for larger pedigrees. In the figure we can see a cluster of the Andersen haplotype in the village of Hjallerup (the set of four orange markers). The remaining markers are fairly spread out across Denmark and Norway but from a European perspective would be considered quite clustered. We hope to be able to report a better experiment soon.

If haplotype A is seen x times in a sample of N haplotypes, the sample estimator $\tilde{p}_A = \dfrac{x}{N}$ is an unbiased estimator as long as the requirements for binomial sampling are fulfilled, i.e. sampling is at random and every sampled haplotype has the same probability of being of type A. We expect that these assumptions are close but not quite met. The estimator does not perform well near the tails (i.e. for true values close to 0 or 1) and various variations have been proposed. Despite this, the estimator is traditionally considered and it is called the *counting method*. Note that with this method we implicitly assume that we have observed all possible haplotypes, as the sum of $\tilde{p}_A$ for all haplotypes in the database is 1. Hence, by using this estimator, we leave no probability mass for the haplotypes that we haven't yet observed. This would suggest that this estimator assigns too much probability mass to the observed haplotypes (we overestimate the haplotype frequency) and too little to the unobserved. This is also what is seen in various simulation studies.

A sensible Bayesian estimator[570] is

$$\hat{p} = \frac{x+1+\alpha}{N+1+\alpha+\beta}$$

where x is the number of matching samples in that database and N is the total number of samples in the database. This arises as the standard beta-binomial solution after we have added the

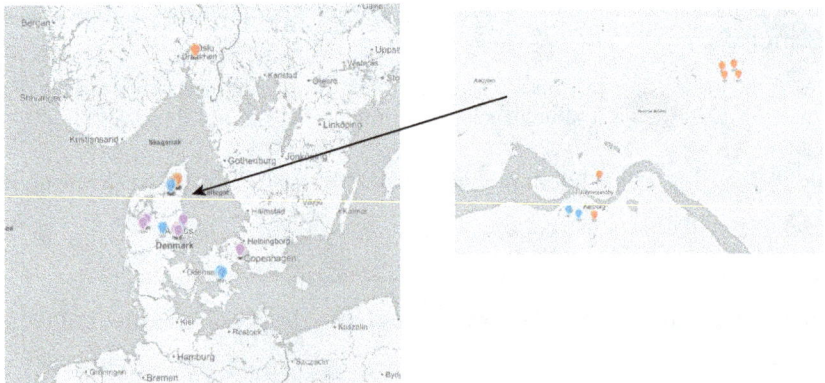

Figure 10.3   The known male relatives of Mikkel Meyer Andersen and two colleagues.

POI to the database and asked the question, what is the chance of a second copy of the POI's haplotype? α and β have historically both been assigned the values of 1 giving

$$\hat{p} = \frac{x+2}{N+3}$$

which differs from the formula given in, say, the ISFG recommendations.[920] We will call this the *Bayesian estimator*. Balding never said that $\alpha = \beta = 1$ was anything more than a convenient and conservative choice. A beta distribution with these parameters is just a continuous uniform distribution from 0 to 1. This corresponds to *a priori* (before seeing the database and the haplotype in question) stating that the haplotype frequencies are uniformly distributed between 0 and 1. That is, we have no more reason to believe that haplotypes are rare than to believe that they are common. It seems likely that $\alpha = 1/k$ and $\beta = 1-1/k$ is better where k is some large integer. This puts probability mass closer to 0 meaning that we have more reason to believe *a priori* that a haplotype is rare than it is common.

The counting method, the Bayesian estimator and the kappa method could be called purely statistical methods. This is a little unfair. The Bayesian and kappa methods do contain information about the spread of haplotypes in the population. However they seem to be eclipsed by methods that take direct inference from the known behaviour of haplotypes. As described, the counting method uses all probability mass on the observed haplotypes. The Bayesian estimator and the kappa method deflate the count estimates in different ways, meaning that they leave some probability mass for the unobserved haplotypes (see Boxes 10.1, 10.2, 10.3 and 10.4 for some extended discussion). However neither of the methods describes how it must be distributed to the unobserved haplotypes, only that there are haplotypes out there that we have yet to observe.

BOX 10.1   WHY NOT ADD THE PERSON OF INTEREST AND OFFENDER?

There is quite a common belief that the person of interest (POI) and the offender should be added when modelling the probability under H_d. Careful thought about how the third law works with multiple events clarifies this. Let us have the database, D, the haplotype of the POI, G_P, and the haplotype of the offender, G_O. We require

$$LR = \frac{\Pr(G_O, G_P, D \mid H_p)}{\Pr(G_O, G_P, D \mid H_d)}$$

$$LR = \frac{\Pr(G_O \mid G_P, D, H_p)\, \Pr(G_P, D \mid H_p)}{\Pr(G_O \mid G_P, D, H_d)\, \Pr(G_P, D \mid H_d)}$$

assuming

$$\Pr(G_P, D \mid H_p) = \Pr(G_P, D \mid H_d)$$

gives

$$LR = \frac{\Pr(G_O \mid G_P, D, H_p)}{\Pr(G_O \mid G_P, D, H_d)}$$

Looking at the denominator term and noting that you 'know' the events behind the bar when assessing the event in front of the bar, the addition of one copy is apparent. But please do not stop here. Recall that the Bayesian estimator includes the terms α and β. Hence

$$\Pr(G_O \mid G_P, D, H_d) \hat{=} \frac{x+1+\alpha}{N+1+\alpha+\beta}$$

BOX 10.2   BRENNER'S KAPPA METHOD

John Buckleton

If a highly discriminating Y chromosome multiplex is used or if the database is small, many haplotypes will not have been observed in the database. This shows that there are a great many unobserved haplotypes. Furthermore, it ensures that haplotypes that are observed in the database are on average rarer in the population than their sample frequency. Brenner[309] very reasonably adds the person of interest haplotype to the database and shows that statistically the overstatement is on average a factor of $1/(1 - \kappa)$, where κ is the fraction of haplotypes observed once (*singletons* in Brenner's nomenclature) in the database of size $N - 1$.

Next we ask the question, what is the chance of a second copy of this haplotype?

Deciding whether the overstatement applies equally for singletons, doubletons, tripletons etc. of the database, as opposed to the overstatement perhaps being more concentrated in some of those categories at the expense of others, requires going beyond mere statistics and taking into account population genetic theory and evolution. If all categories are equally over-represented – which holds for e.g. Ewens' 'infinite alleles' model – then:

$$\Pr(\text{match} \mid \text{haplotype previously observed } X \text{ times}) \approx (X + 1)(1 - \kappa)/N.$$

That general result is hard to verify or refute for real populations. According to Brenner's analysis, though, for haplotype populations reasonably expected to occur in nature, the singletons do overestimate their population frequency by about the expected factor anyway, giving

$$\Pr(\text{match}|\text{haplotype previously unobserved}) \approx (1 - \kappa)/N$$

as the probability for a coincidental match by a non-donor to a crime scene type.

Brenner[155] also suggests a Bayesian solution with a $\beta(0,\theta)$ prior. θ is not the usual population genetic term but is some large number. This gives a posterior for the singletons of $\dfrac{1}{N+\theta}$. If we set $\theta = \dfrac{N\kappa}{1-\kappa}$ then $\Pr(\text{match}|\text{haplotype previously unobserved}) = (1 - \kappa)/N$ as given above.

Having received some tuition from Brenner, for which I thank him, I believe that the kappa method is suitable at least for singletons and naturally occurring populations of highly discriminating multiplexes.

The kappa method is available on the Y-HRD website.

The inheritance and mutation patterns of lineage markers are reasonably well understood. We can draw two conclusions from these understandings:

1. The frequencies of haplotypes that are evolutionarily close are likely to be correlated.

2. The distribution of haplotypes is likely to be highly structured along ethnic or geographical lines.

The inference that evolutionarily close haplotypes should be correlated has been used in interesting and almost certainly valid estimation procedures[881,892,921–927] that should outperform any simply statistical method.

In Figure 10.4 we give the performance of the counting method, the kappa method and the discrete Laplace method (see Box 10.3) in estimating haplotype probabilities against a simulated population that is undergoing mutation and drift. Perfect estimation would have all data on the $x = y$ line. To our eyes the counting method and the kappa method show no real correlation to the line. The counting method is typically conservative with respect to this line, often by orders of magnitude. The kappa method may be conservative or non-conservative again by

BOX 10.3   THE DISCRETE LAPLACE METHOD

There is considerable evidence developing that the most robust method for estimating haplotype probabilities is the discrete Laplace method.[921,923–925,928] This method uses the following genetic assumptions to model a probability distribution:

1. That a population of haplotypes is composed from clades of haplotypes.
2. Each clade has arisen from one ancestral haplotype by stepwise mutation.
3. Mutations occur independently of each other.

Given these assumptions it is possible to multiply probabilities of allele differences from a central haplotype across loci within the haplotype clade to assign a probability to a full haplotype in that clade. Hence, given the clade (or within the clade), the loci are assumed independent, though it is not the actual allele probabilities that are used, but instead probabilities of allele difference to a central haplotype (in the given clade). The probability of the haplotype in the full population is assigned by weighting the assignment from each clade by the estimated contribution of that clade to the total population.

This recovers the significantly useful ability to model a multilocus haplotype by multiplication across loci, whereas such a multiplication is not permissible unless the population has been devolved to its constituent clades.

This method can estimate haplotype probabilities for all haplotypes. It has the advantage of being able to estimate haplotype probabilities for haplotypes that have not been observed yet. This can for example be used for mixture separation.[929]

The best description of the method appears in Andersen et al.[930] The method is available from the Y-HRD website and in the R package disclapmix.

BOX 10.4   COALESCENCE THEORY

More accurately this is described as 'coalescent-based estimation of haplotype match probability'. It stems from the same idea as the discrete Laplace approach in that there was some ancient state of a population where a single haplotype existed and that all current haplotype diversity is from mutations of that ancient state haplotype. By constructing phylogenetic trees from the haplotypes observed in a database, the coalescence of haplotypes (taking the difference between each haplotype that could be accounted for by mutation) can be considered back through the generations until at the root of the tree exists the ancient haplotype that all modern haplotypes have coalesced to.

The theory was described by Kingman[931] and subsequently expanded to more of a forensic context.[932] Also included were generalizations that allowed population size changes over time. To obtain a coalescent-based estimation of haplotype match probability a large number of trees are simulated from the haplotypes in a database (including the person of interest haplotype). The evidence haplotype is trialled in different positions in each tree and linked to its neighbour in that position by a common ancestor who existed at t time in the past. The match probability for that tree is then the probability that the common ancestor could have mutated to the evidence haplotype in time t.

This method is implemented using a Markov chain Monte Carlo approach in the programme BATWING (available free online and as R equivalents) and from simulations appears to estimate haplotype frequencies well for small databases with few loci.[921] The main drawback at this stage is the long computing time required to generate match probabilities. This limits its practical use for all but small databases with few loci.

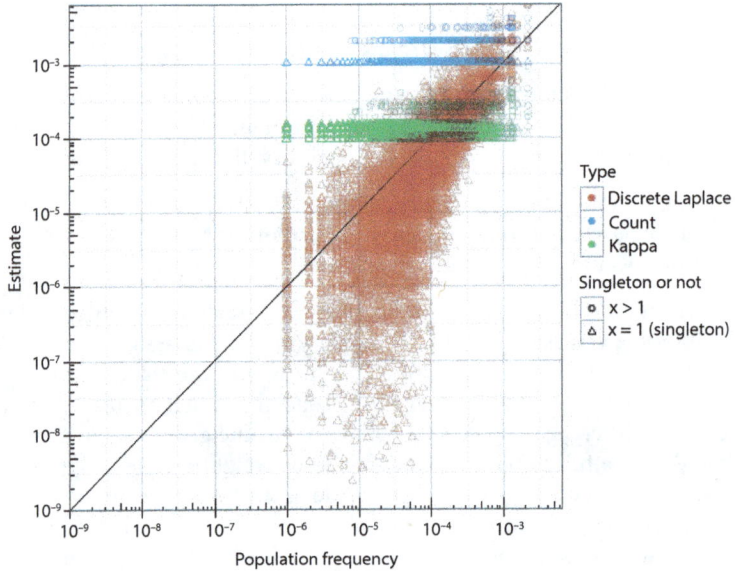

Figure 10.4   A plot of the estimates using the discrete Laplace method, counting method and the kappa method versus the frequency in a simulated population. Description of the simulation: at $t = 0$: there are one million seven locus haplotypes all the same. Generation $t + 1$ is created by selecting at random and with replacement from generation t. Each haplotype mutates either +1 or −1 step with an equal mutation rate (0.0015). After $t = 400$, 10 databases are taken from this population, each of size 1000. The various estimates are applied to these databases.

orders of magnitude. The Laplace does show a good correlation to the line. The cloud of points for the discrete Laplace method to the right of the line and at low frequency in the population all have an estimated probability that is too low. Work trying to improve this aspect is in progress. However, if a θ value is used then the suggested value from the SWGDAM guidelines is 0.003 in many cases for such a seven-locus profile. This would remove any risk of underestimation (in this experiment) using the discrete Laplace or kappa methods.

Estimating θ

Geographical structuring of haplotypes has been demonstrated empirically. This geographical structuring has been shown in older populations such as Europe and in more recently settled populations such as the United States. Structuring can be observed geographically and may be quite short range. It is also likely that structuring may exist in local populations if, for example, cultural factors lead to restriction of marriage choice.[892]

To give Equation 10.1 a numerical value, valid estimates of p_A and θ are required. We have discussed estimating p_A above. For autosomal markers the value assigned for θ is usually selected subjectively at the upper end of the plausible range after some data analysis. The upper end of the plausible range is usually selected because there has developed a forensic tradition that a conservative estimate is judged to be good. *Conservative* in this sense tends to mean an estimate that on average is larger than the median estimate. Without sanctioning this value judgement we discuss practical implementation for the Y chromosome.

Following Bhatia et al.[539] for a set of n_i haplotypes from subpopulation i, let $\tilde{M}_{Wi}$ be the proportion of pairs of haplotypes that match within that subpopulation. If there are n_{iu} haplotypes of type u in subpopulation i, then

$$\tilde{M}_{Wi} = \frac{1}{n_i(n_i - 1)} \sum_u n_{iu}(n_{iu} - 1)$$

It is unnecessary to calculate and use the n_{iu}; all that is needed is the number of matching pairs, m_i, since

$$\tilde{M}_{Wi} = \frac{2m_i}{n_i(1-n_i)}$$

For subpopulations i and j let

$$\tilde{M}_{Bij} = \frac{1}{n_i n_j} \sum_u n_{iu} n_{ju}$$

This may be the most straightforward computing formula, but it can also be expressed in terms of sample haplotype proportions $\tilde{p}_{iu} = \dfrac{n_{iu}}{n_i}$ as

$$\tilde{M}_{Wi} = \frac{n_i \left(\displaystyle\sum_u \tilde{p}_{iu}^2 - 1/n_i \right)}{n_i - 1}$$

Alternatively the proportion of pairs of haplotypes that match may be found without keeping track of the counts of each different haplotype. There is also a matching proportion $\tilde{M}_{Bij}$ for pairs of haplotypes, one from each of subpopulations i and j. In terms of haplotype counts,

$$\tilde{M}_{Bij} = \frac{\displaystyle\sum_u n_{iu} n_{ju}}{n_i n_j}$$

For a set of r subpopulations, the sample matching proportions within and between subpopulations are

$$\tilde{M}_W = \frac{1}{r} \sum_i \tilde{M}_{Wi} \text{ and } \tilde{M}_B = \frac{1}{r(r-1)} \sum_{i \neq j} \tilde{M}_{Bj}$$

and the quantity of interest is

$$\hat{\beta}_W = \frac{\frac{r-1}{r} \frac{\tilde{M}_W - \tilde{M}_B}{1 - \tilde{M}_B}}{1 - \frac{1}{r} \frac{\tilde{M}_W - \tilde{M}_B}{1 - \tilde{M}_B}}$$

It is $\hat{\beta}_W$ that may be used as an estimate of θ in the match probability equations. This formulation has been described by Weir and it has the benefit of making explicit the need to consider the increase of matching within subpopulations over that between subpopulations and in the population as a whole. If every haplotype is unique across all subpopulations, there is no matching and $\hat{\beta}_W$ is 0.

Testing the Model by *Steven Myers, Bruce Weir and John Buckleton*

Using the model incorporating a θ value, the predicted match probability for haplotype u in subpopulation i is $M_{Wiu} = \theta_{Wi} + (1-\theta_{Wi})p_u$, where p_u is the expected haplotype frequency averaged across all subpopulations. Summing over haplotypes gives

$$M_{Wi} = \theta_{Wi} + (1-\theta_{Wi}) \sum_u p_u^2$$

Averaging over subpopulations

$$M_W = \theta_W + (1-\theta_W) \sum_u p_u^2$$

The only available information about the population haplotype frequency p_u comes from the sample haplotype frequency $\tilde{p}_u$. This suggests an estimate of M_W as

$$\hat{M}_W = \hat{\beta} + (1-\hat{\beta})\sum_u \tilde{p}_u^2$$

In this section we test whether a subpopulation correction is necessary and if needed whether the method of Bhatia et al. provides a suitable estimate. A dataset of 12,727 published haplotypes from 91 European subpopulations was analyzed at seven Y-STR loci.[933] These haplotypes were initially condensed to 45 meta populations following Roewer et al.[933] Each subpopulation was divided in half randomly to provide two sets of 45 subpopulations (each with a smaller sample size). We seek to test initially whether the average matching within a subpopulation is greater than the average in the full population. This goal is achieved by simply developing the proportion of haplotypes which match within each subpopulation $\tilde{M}_{Wi}$ and averaging across the r subpopulations, $\tilde{M}_W = \dfrac{1}{r}\sum_i \tilde{M}_{Wi}$. This can be compared with the matching proportion in the full population. If these two matching proportions differ, then we seek to determine whether Equation 10.1 informed by data from one half of the dataset can make useful predictions about the other half. We therefore use one half of the data to estimate $\hat{M}_W = \hat{\beta} + (1-\hat{\beta})\sum_u \tilde{p}_u^2$ and compare it with the other half.

Roewer et al. noted an east–west cline in haplotype frequencies across Europe and proposed a division into Eastern Eurasian and Western Eurasian. We repeat the above experiments using a two-level hierarchy which treats Europeans as divided into eastern and western and then into the appropriate subpopulations.

In Table 10.2 we give some results for the experiments. The average matching within the populations (observed M_w) was often higher than the prediction ignoring substructure, $\sum_u \tilde{p}_u^2$. The predictions using a subpopulation correction, $\hat{M}_W = \hat{\beta} + (1-\hat{\beta})\sum_u \tilde{p}_u^2$, are much better. When examining the table it may be useful to take the prediction for a studied set, say the first half, and compare it with the other set. This would mimic the situation where we had predicted the subpopulation match probability using one set of data and wished to apply it to an unstudied situation.

The match probability in a subpopulation is often greater than in the population as a whole. This is expected. Predictions of this match probability using a subpopulation correction appear better; compare the columns with and without $\hat{\beta}$ correction with the observed. The method of Bhatia et al.[539] appears useful at least for these seven locus haplotypes.

Propositions
We rediscuss propositions here because of a persistent misconception. Recall that the prosecution proposition aligns with the prosecution view and the defence with any proposition consistent with exoneration.

The propositions for much lineage marker work at the sub-source level should be of the following form (Pair 1):

H_p: The POI is the source of the DNA.

H_d: A random person is the source of the DNA.

We have seen the pair (Pair 2)

H_p: The POI or a close maternal/paternal relative is the source of the DNA.

H_d: A random person not a close maternal/paternal relative is the source of the DNA.

Table 10.2   The Results of Experiments Predicting the Match Probability

		$\hat{\beta}_W = \dfrac{\frac{r-1}{r}\frac{\bar{M}_W - \bar{M}_B}{1 - \bar{M}_B}}{1 - \frac{1}{r}\frac{\bar{M}_W - \bar{M}_B}{1 - \bar{M}_B}}$	Predicted Match Rate with No $\hat{\beta}$ $\sum_u \tilde{p}_u^2$	Observed Match Rate M_W	Predicted Match Rate with $\hat{\beta}$ $\hat{M}_W = \hat{\beta} + (1 - \hat{\beta})\sum_u \tilde{p}_u^2$
45 European meta populations	First half	0.0085	0.0073	0.0161	0.0157
	Second half	0.0085	0.0076	0.0156	0.0160
2 Subpopulations, Eastern and Western	First half	0.0064	0.0101	0.0156	0.0164
	Second half	0.0056	0.0086	0.0135	0.0142
Belorussia, Kiev, Ljubljana, Moscow, Novgorod, Poland, Riga, Vilnius, Zagreb	First half	0.0009	0.0115	0.0110	0.0124
	Second half	0.0051	0.0113	0.0160	0.0164
Emilia-Romagna, London, Portugal, Pyrenees, South Holland, Southern Ireland, Spain, Strasbourg	First half	0.0040	0.0174	0.0275	0.0213
	Second half	0.0029	0.0261	0.0263	0.0289

Pair 2 arise from the wish to use and expose to the court the fact that close relatives are likely to have the same haplotype. We agree that this should be disclosed, and we suggest that it should be done in the statement not the propositions. Putting this in the propositions is significantly counterproductive.

1. It is the POI on trial and H_p should align with the prosecution position.
2. With many loci and highly mutating markers it is not necessarily true that close paternal relatives will have the same haplotype.
3. We cannot think how to inform $\Pr(E|H_d)$ for Pair 2. This needs a survey of non-relatives. We would need to examine all matches in the database and check if they were a relative. If they were, we would remove them.
4. Theory suggests that $\Pr(E|H_d)$ for Pair 2 might be 0, all or nearly all matches being relatives in some sense.

Confidence or Probability Intervals

The recommended method for an upper confidence interval on a haplotype probability p_0 follows the method of Clopper and Pearson.[934] p_0 is the solution to the equation

$$\sum_{k=0}^{x} \binom{N}{k} p_0^k \left(1 - p_0\right)^{N-k} = \alpha$$

for a sample of size N haplotypes with x of the haplotype of interest. α is the level of confidence: $\alpha = 0.05$ gives a 95% confidence limit.

This is described as 'should be calculated' by the SWGDAM[916,919] working groups for Y and mtDNA and is described as 'an extremely conservative approach' in the ISFG mtDNA recommendations.[920] We cannot locate any ISFG recommendation for a confidence interval for the Y chromosome haplotype. The method applies to the counting method only and would not extend to mixtures.

The Bayesian highest posterior density (HPD) method (see Chapter 6) gives the same answers as Clopper and Pearson and is used in Australasia.

Statement Wording

There is some interest in a wording that may be used in reporting results. Assuming that two matching haplotypes have been obtained and that a statistical weighting has been generated for this match, perhaps the simplest method of reporting a result is to state the number of observations of that haplotype in a database, e.g.: 'The haplotype was observed x times in a database comprising of N individuals of ancestry z'.

A statement such as this is a factual statement of an observation and, given that the database has been constructed correctly, should be relatively safe from any challenge. For a majority of haplotypes, x will be zero and so the statement of zero observations in the database may not give the court an appreciation of the significance of the result. In the minds of the jury, zero observations may be equated to very strong evidence.

To apply a statistical weighting to a haplotype that is unobserved in the database, a population frequency (discussed above) can be estimated that seeks to find how common the haplotype could be in the population. Let the estimated frequency in the population be $\frac{1}{y}$. A frequency estimate of $\frac{1}{y}$ could therefore be reported along with the statement above: 'The expected frequency of this haplotype in the population is estimated as 1 in every y unrelated individuals'.

Because of the mode of inheritance of lineage markers a statement about relatives is commonly included with the statements above: 'All paternal/maternal relatives will possess the same haplotype unless a mutation event has occurred'.

The above reporting style provides a frequentist statement regarding haplotype frequency. A framework that is more consistent with statistical weightings provided for autosomal data would be to provide an LR. The structure of the LR would remain the same as for autosomal DNA evidence in that it would still be considering the evidence given the two competing hypotheses:

H_p: The POI is the source of the DNA.

H_d: A random unrelated individual from the same population as the POI is the source of the DNA.

So the statement for matching evidence and reference haplotypes would be: 'The evidence is y times more likely to have been obtained if the POI is the source of DNA rather than an unrelated individual'.

When assessing mixed haplotypic profiles the use of the LR becomes more important as a meaningful frequentist extension to the single contributor example given above is lacking.

We would suggest that an appendix should be attached plausibly along the lines:

The value for y is estimated using a population genetic model using a co-ancestry coefficient developed from empirical data using the method of Z. Sampling uncertainty has been assessed using the method of (either Clopper and Pearson, the Bayesian HPD or X). A one-sided 99% confidence interval (for Clopper and Pearson, or a one-sided 99% probability interval for the HPD) has been estimated.

For the information of court reporting scientists, if asked, the correct wording for a confidence interval is, '99% of confidence intervals calculated in this way are expected to contain the true value'. For a Bayesian HPD the correct wording is, 'with 99% probability the true value is greater than y'. It is incorrect to use the word probability in the confidence interval statement.

Heteroplasmy

If both the crime and reference samples have the same degree of heteroplasmy, it will increase the strength of the evidence.[793] This occurs because the denominator term $\Pr(G_C \mid G_K, H_d, I)$ is low, since the occurrence of a certain heteroplasmic mitotype is expected to be low.[935] This is mentioned in the ISFG 2000 mtDNA recommendations.[918]

Holland and Parsons[793] discuss the situation where a blood sample from a suspect is known to exhibit heteroplasmy. A single hair alleged to be from this person is examined and found to exhibit a homoplasmic sequence for one of the types present in the blood. Clearly if multiple hairs from the suspect could be examined, a probabilistic approach could be taken. Imagine that a fraction x of hairs exhibited a matching homoplasmic mitotype. Then the numerator of the LR is x. The denominator of the LR may be taken as the population frequency of the homoplasmic variant. However Holland and Parsons point out that this detailed knowledge of the fraction of hairs with this variant would seldom be available.

Examples of the Logical Approach in Practice

Although the current data regarding mtDNA substitution rates and population genetics are limited, the general LR formulation is a useful framework upon which an assessment of evidential significance can be made. Examples of how this framework could be used in commonly encountered situations are given below. In each, the LR framework is used to assess the evidence.

Example 10.5: Matching POI and C Haplotypes

The POI, P, and questioned, C, sequences match exactly. There are no observations of the same or similar sequences in the database. Under H_p the samples are alleged to have come from the same person. H_d alleges that they come from different people. We seek to assess

$$LR = \frac{\Pr(G_C \mid G_P, H_p)}{\Pr(G_C \mid G_P, H_d)}$$

The numerator term $\Pr(G_C \mid G_P, H_p)$ relates to the chance of obtaining a matching sample from the same person as the reference. Hence issues such as the type of bodily samples used for questioned and known profiles and somatic mosaicism are relevant. However this term is likely to be close to 1. The denominator term $\Pr(G_C \mid G_P, H_d)$ relates to the chance of obtaining a matching sample from a different person to the reference sample. An assigned probability informed by one of the methods described above and considering sampling uncertainty and population subdivision could be used for this term.

Example 10.6: Matching K and C Haplotypes

The known, K (relative of POI), and questioned, C, sequences match exactly and there are no observations of the same or similar sequences in the database. Under H_p the samples, C, are alleged to have come from a person P who is not available. However his grandparent, K, has provided a sample. H_d alleges the samples, C, have come from a different person to P and hence are not necessarily related to K. We seek to assess

$$LR = \frac{\Pr(G_C \mid G_K, H_p, I)}{\Pr(G_C \mid G_K, H_d, I)}$$

The numerator term $\Pr(G_C \,|\, G_K, H_P, I)$ relates to the chance of obtaining a matching sample from a person who is the grandchild of the donor of the reference sample. Hence issues such as, 'what is the chance of no mutations in two generations?' and 'what body samples were used to obtain the questioned and known profiles?' are relevant. Somatic mosaicism must also be considered. Once again this term is likely to be near to 1. The denominator term $\Pr(G_C \,|\, G_K, H_d)$ relates to the chance of obtaining a matching sample from a different person to the grandchild of the donor of the reference sample. Again an assigned probability informed by some method and considering sampling uncertainty and population subdivision could be used for this term.

Example 10.7: Haplotypes *K* and *C* Differ by a Single Base or Locus

The known, *K*, and questioned, *C*, sequences differ by a single base or locus that is known to mutate frequently. Neither sequence has been observed previously in the database, but there are other sequences in the database differing by a single base. Under H_p the samples, *C*, are alleged to have come from a person, *P*, who is not available. We have a sample from his grandparent, *K*. H_d alleges that the samples, *C*, have come from a different person from *P*. As usual we seek to assess

$$LR = \frac{\Pr(G_C \,|\, G_K, H_p, I)}{\Pr(G_C \,|\, G_K, H_d, I)}$$

The numerator term $\Pr(G_C \,|\, G_K, H_p, I)$ relates to the chance of obtaining a matching sample from a person who is the grandchild of the donor of the reference sample. Hence issues such as 'What is the chance of this particular mutation at this site in two generations?' must be assessed. This term is likely to be small but non-zero. The denominator term $\Pr(G_C \,|\, G_K, H_d)$ relates to the chance of obtaining a sample matching *C* from a different person to the grandson of the donor of the reference sample. Again the same sensible method could be used to inform an assignment of this term.

Each case should, of course, be treated on its own merits, using all available data regarding the frequency of the haplotypes in question, mutation rates, somatic mosaicism and the structure of the relevant populations. In instances where population structure has been well studied, differences between sequences are at well-characterized nucleotide positions and sizeable frequency databases for the relevant population are available, the *LR* estimate may be sufficiently accurate to warrant a numerical statement. In other cases this may not be true.

Example 10.8: *R v Aytugrul*

In this example we discuss an actual case that highlights some of these issues.

Ms Sveda Bayrak had met Mr Yusuf Aytugrul in 2002 through their children who attended the same school. They had a relationship, which Ms Bayrak ended in 2003. The Crown alleged that Mr Aytugrul was never able to accept that the relationship was ended and wrote poetry and undertook intimidation-type activities. Ms Bayrak was found dead in her home in 2005.

The forensic evidence centred around the mtDNA sequence of a hair found under the fingernails of the deceased. The hair associated with the deceased, Ms Bayrak, and a saliva sample from Mr Aytugrul show a close correspondence, differing only in the C stretch with Mr Aytugrul having one more C. Ms Pineda of ReliaGene described this as *not excluded* following the then-current SWGDAM guidelines. (The 2013 SWGDAM guidelines,[916] we think, would call this *inconclusive*.) Pineda initially reported *no matches* to the profile of the hair in 4839 profiles in the SWGDAM database. This was described as a typographic error in court, presumably having passed peer review, but could also occur by searching Mr Aytugrul's profile without allowing for ambiguity in the C stretch.

Clearly if our goal is to provide a frequency of not-excluded individuals and we intend to include all persons who correspond in mtDNA except for the C stretch we should ignore C stretch differences when searching. A facility is included in the search for this.

However, is this a match or not? This highlights the problem in describing close but differing mtDNA haplotypes using a *match/non-match* nomenclature. Mr Chris Maxwell, for the Crown, argued aggressively but wrongly that there were two states, *match* and *non-match*. He would not countenance any more sophisticated treatment of close mismatches.

By the time of appeal[936] the difference between the haplotypes was forgotten: 'Gina Pineda gave evidence that the appellant had a particular DNA profile (a "mitochondrial haplotype"). She also gave evidence that the same mitochondrial haplotype was detected in a hair found under a nail of the deceased when she was discovered in her new apartment, which the appellant was said never to have visited. And she gave evidence that one in 1600 persons could be expected to have the same mitochondrial haplotype as was detected in that hair'.

There are other issues in the case, such as whether the US mtDNA database can reliably inform probabilities in Sydney, Australia, but of most importance is the poor treatment of close mismatches and the disinterest of the prosecution in advancing standards.

Structuring Lineage Marker Databases

Defining Ethnicity

Databases for the interpretation of autosomal markers are usually created along ethnic lines. Individuals are assigned to an ethnic database based on self-declaration, surname analysis or the declaration of the person taking the sample. The ethnic databases tend to be relatively broad, such as African-American, Hispanic from the southwestern United States, Hispanic from the southeastern United States and European ancestry.

The structured distribution of lineage markers has raised two possible changes. First, lineage marker databases might be constructed on a finer scale than autosomal databases and, second, the result from a lineage marker analysis might be used to verify or change both the assignment to a lineage marker ethnic database or the assignment of an individual profile to an autosomal database.

This debate is emerging and has not been argued extensively in the literature.

We would identify the following issues:

1. Do we intend to combine lineage and autosomal estimates?

2. How strong an inference about autosomal markers can be drawn from lineage markers?

3. What do we intend to do with the separate estimates for the separate ethnic databases?

4. What do we do when different profiling techniques lead to different interpretations? For example consider an autosomal profile that appears to originate from a single individual, but shows two individuals when profiled with lineage markers.

A recent study[937] showed that only approximately one-quarter of individuals who self-declared as Aboriginal Australians carry an ancestral Y chromosome of that ethnicity. This brings in to question what the correct composition of a lineage marker database should be, those that identify themselves as a particular ethnicity or those that are known to contain a lineage marker that corresponds to the ethnicity of interest.

To place this in focus we could envisage two structures for the database and two parallel statements arising from this. If structure 1 was composed of self-declared Aboriginals and structure 2 was composed of haplotypes inferred to be Aboriginal, most probably from an SNP analysis, then the parallel statements would be

1. The haplotype was observed in x_1 of N_1 self-declared Aboriginals.

2. The haplotype was observed in x_2 of N_2 haplotypes inferred to be Aboriginal.

We are unaware of any debate on the relative merits of these approaches but we suspect that fact finders may react in a similar way to the two options.

Random Sampling or Exclude Relatives

To ensure representative statistics it is desirable that sampling for the database be random or nearly so[938] and relatively free from error.[859,939] There are two sampling regimes that we are aware of that depart from these guidelines:

1. Sampling by avoiding the same surname or known relatives

2. The inadvertent sampling of clusters of relatives by deliberate sampling of, say, a sub-group in one location

Either regime should be avoided where possible.

The avoidance of known relatives or individuals with the same surname has some logic and it may be worthwhile briefly discussing why this should be opposed if two relatives are sampled randomly. Imagine a population of 1000 individuals, 991 of which are named Smith and the remaining 9 of which are named Bright, Taylor, Buckleton, Coble, Butler, Brenner, Roewer, Parson and Weir. All the Smiths have the same haplotype, whereas the other 9 individuals are all the only representative of their haplotype. The correct frequency of the Smiths' haplotype is 0.991. If we avoid any second instances of Smith we get 0.1.

We are fully aware that truly random sampling is impossible and we accept that a pragmatic balance of the factors discussed above must be reached.

> The presence of maternally related donors in a 'random' population sample has so far not been as thoroughly addressed in quality control as other aspects of mtDNA analysis and databasing. The simple practical approach presented here helps to detect the 'clear and easy' cases of close maternal kinship between donors in a sample set: following the procedure described, these samples can be identified and subsequently excluded. If appreciated, this additional tool will contribute towards better random mtDNA population samples representative for their population, for the benefit of all research applying mtDNA as a genetic marker.[938]

This will not lead to a representative sample.

Interpretation of Low Level Y Chromosome Profiles

Y chromosome work is often used after an autosomal analysis has failed to detect any male DNA or has given partial results. The methods employed often involve PCR at elevated cycle numbers, e.g. 30 or 32. This means that Y chromosome profiles are often produced from limited template. The resulting profiles are often partial and may be from multiple contributors. Some considerable experience has been developed in the interpretation of low template autosomal profiles (LTDNA). The principles inherent in the interpretation of autosomal LTDNA appear to translate to the Y chromosome with little adaption required. A Y chromosome profile is developed at a number of markers, usually simultaneously in a multiplex. Most typically a profile from one individual will show one allele at each marker. More rarely this individual will show zero, two or more alleles due to a deletion or locus replication. In an analogy with autosomal work the markers are termed *loci*; however strictly if gene duplication has occurred these are not one locus but two loci that are amplified with the same primers for a given marker.

Partial Samples

At each marker a Y chromosome is expected to show one allele, but copy number variation resulting from deletion, duplication or other events can lead to other numbers. Since one allele is the most common situation we restrict discussion here to that situation, although the principle extends straightforwardly.

The semicontinuous model[114] currently applied to autosomal DNA may also be applied to the Y chromosome. This usage is not implemented in any jurisdiction of which we are aware but SWGDAM is experimenting with it under the guidance of Steven Myers. Current practice is often along the lines of searching a database for haplotypes that match at the loci where an allele is observed. We believe that current practice will be robust as long as certain caveats are observed. We highlight the following:

- If the locus shows no allele, the POI shows one or more alleles and the locus is ignored in the calculation, there is a mild overstatement of the value of the evidence since a haplotype with no alleles at this locus is more favoured by the evidence. This overstatement is smallest if the probability of dropout is substantial and haplotypes with no alleles at this locus are rare.

- If the locus shows one allele, the POI shows two or more alleles and a frequency is obtained for all haplotypes showing this allele and any others, then there is a mild overstatement of the value of the evidence since a haplotype with this allele only at this locus is more favoured by the evidence. This overstatement of the evidence is smallest if the probability of dropout is substantial. However haplotypes with one allele at this locus are likely to be reasonably common and if the probability of dropout is not substantial then the overstatement may be considerable. Ignoring the locus may not be neutral or conservative if the probability of dropout is small.

Y Chromosome Mixed Samples

There have been some publications describing basic methods to interpret multiple-contributor samples using lineage markers. However these methods require extension for practical situations especially at low template.[99,940,941]

In this section we consider the question of Y chromosome mixtures. This follows from an insightful inquiry and discussion with Oscar García of the Basque Country Forensic Genetics Laboratory, Spain.

The interpretation of mixtures of DNA from males using Y chromosome analysis differs from the interpretation of autosomal DNA mixtures in at least two respects. First many Y chromosome loci are represented by a single allele at each locus. This means that the complications of heterozygote imbalance are eliminated for these loci. Some loci are duplicated, triplicated or quadrupled such that two, three or four amplicons are produced. For these loci the term *heterozygote imbalance* is inappropriate; each of these 'linked' alleles exists in a different sequence environment to others attributed to the same locus such that amplification efficiency may differ for each one and they may not appear 'balanced'.

Second, the Y chromosome is treated as a haplotype and this must be accounted for when considering Y chromosome mixtures.

Male/male mixtures have been successfully resolved at ratios of 10:1[87] and even 50:1 where no minor alleles were in stutter positions.[942] There are no reports of major and minor proportions changing significantly across loci and we have not observed this in our laboratory.

Like autosomal STRs, Y chromosome STR profiles from mixed samples can be affected by the presence of stutter peaks and this needs to be taken into consideration when interpreting profiles from mixed samples. Stutter ratios for Y-STR loci appear to be of a similar magnitude to those for autosomal STRs.[87,942,943] Similar rules need to be developed by each laboratory to determine how to interpret a peak in a stutter position.

Likelihood Ratios
No Possibility of Dropout

It is quite hard, but not impossible, to develop rules about when dropout is not possible for Y chromosome mixtures since the locus to locus variability is considerable. Consider the possible rule that if two alleles have been seen for a two person mixture, then dropout is not possible. It is still conceivable that the minor haplotype had a duplicated allele not visualized at this locus. Probabilistic genotyping is almost mandatory for Y chromosome mixtures. However, initially we consider mixtures where dropout is deemed so unlikely that it is designated as not possible.

Consider a simplified Y chromosome mixture with just three loci, 1, 2 and 3. We term the DNA type of this mixture S. At each locus there is a clear major contributor and a clear minor contributor. The two alleles at a locus are labelled 1 and 2. Hence the alleles at Locus 1 are A_1^1 and A_2^1, where we label the A_1^1 allele to be from the major contributor. Clearly, then, this is a mixture of a major with haplotype $H_1 = A_1^1 A_1^2 A_1^3$ and a minor with haplotype $H_2 = A_2^1 A_2^2 A_2^3$. We assume a scenario such as a double-rape where the two hypotheses may be as follows:

H_p: The contributors are Suspect 1, S_1, of haplotype H_1 and Suspect 2, S_2, of haplotype H_2.

H_d: The contributors are two random men.

Under this scenario, assuming independence between random men,

$$\Pr(S \mid H_p) \approx \frac{1}{2}$$

$$\Pr(S \mid H_d) \approx \Pr(H_1)\Pr(H_2)$$

$$LR = \frac{1}{2\Pr(H_1)\Pr(H_2)}$$

or

$$LR \approx \frac{(1+\theta)(1+2\theta)}{2(\theta+(1-\theta)\Pr(H_1))(\theta+(1-\theta)\Pr(H_2))} \tag{10.2}$$

Next we consider the masking effect. This follows similar principles to mixtures of autosomal DNA. Consider a mixture where the major appears to be $H_1 = A_2^1 A_2^2 A_1^3$. There are minor peaks at loci 1 and 2, $A_2^1 A_2^2$. At Locus 3 we see only the major peak.

In such a case, as long as we are confident that the minor allele has not dropped out we can assume that the allele of the minor contributor must be A_1^3 and that $H_2 = A_2^1 A_2^2 A_1^3$. The suspect has the haplotype H_2. This suggests

$$LR \approx \frac{1}{2\Pr(H_1)\Pr(H_2)}$$

or

$$\approx \frac{(1+\theta)(1+2\theta)}{2(\theta+(1-\theta)\Pr(H_1))(\theta+(1-\theta)\Pr(H_2))}$$

If we suspect that the minor allele may have dropped out, we need to consider all haplotypes that match at the remaining loci. We could write $H_2 = A_2^1 A_2^2 *$, where the asterisk (*) is meant to indicate that any allele may be present. To estimate this we can simply count those haplotypes in the database that possess the pair of alleles $A_2^1 A_2^2$.

Consider the case where a peak is present in a stutter position and we cannot conclude whether it is allelic or not. If the minor is sufficiently small that it may be the peak in the stutter position, then we need to consider two possibilities: the minor allele may be masked by the major peak or it could be the peak in the stutter position.

Let the stutter peak be at position A_2^3. Possible donors could have the haplotypes $H_2 = A_2^1 A_2^2 A_2^3$ or $H_7 = A_2^1 A_2^2 A_1^3$.

The suspect, again, has the haplotype $H_2 = A_2^1 A_2^2 A_2^3$. This would suggest

$$LR \approx \frac{1}{2\Pr(H_1)\{\Pr(H_2)+\Pr(H_7)\}}$$

or

$$\approx \frac{(1+\theta)(1+2\theta)}{2(\theta+(1-\theta)\Pr(H_1))(\theta+(1-\theta)[\Pr(H_2)+\Pr(H_7)])}$$

Ge and Budowle have supported this approach. The formulae differ and this caused some discussion. We condition on both people in the mixture and they conditioned on the POI only. Both methods are sustainable logically.[940,944]

Last we come to the situation where peak area information suggests two approximately equal contributors or is unreliable for some reason. Hence the stain shows alleles $A_1^1 A_2^1$ at Locus 1, $A_1^2 A_2^2$ at Locus 2 and $A_1^3 A_2^3$ at Locus 3. We cannot tell which alleles originated from one or other of the contributors.

There are eight combinations of haplotypes possible for these three loci. These combinations come as four pairs. For example, we could have H_1 and H_8 or H_8 and H_1.

Let

$$H_1 = A_1^1 A_1^2 A_1^3 \qquad H_2 = A_1^1 A_1^2 A_2^3 \qquad H_3 = A_1^1 A_2^2 A_1^3 \qquad H_4 = A_1^1 A_2^2 A_2^3$$

$$H_8 = A_2^1 A_2^2 A_2^3 \qquad H_7 = A_2^1 A_2^2 A_1^3 \qquad H_6 = A_2^1 A_1^2 A_2^3 \qquad H_5 = A_2^1 A_1^2 A_1^3$$

Recall that Suspect 1 has haplotype H_1 and Suspect 2 has haplotype H_8.

Dropout Possible

For mixed samples with the possibility of dropout, probabilistic genotyping is the only method we can recommend. Either the semi-continuous or continuous approach should work. The only implementation we are aware of is by Steven Myers working on behalf of the SWGDAM Y Chromosome Working Group. It implements the approach given in Box 10.5.

Combining Autosomal and Lineage Marker Results

Theta Values

In 2007 Walsh et al.[945] published an elegant method for combining lineage and autosomal marker results that proceeded by a small upward revision of the θ value for the autosomal result followed by multiplication of the individual results. SWGDAM[917] recommends combination by multiplication without any further adjustment.

Speaking on paternity ISFG[946] recommend multiplication with caution for mtDNA and autosomal markers. 'The weight of the genetic evidence of mtDNA markers shall be combined with the genetic weight from independent, autosomal genetic markers by multiplication of

---

BOX 10.5   THE MYERS SEMI-CONTINUOUS MODEL FOR THE Y CHROMOSOME

$$LR = \frac{\Pr(G_c \mid G_p, G_k, H_p)}{\Pr(G_c \mid G_p, G_k, H_d)}$$

G_c is the crime scene profile.
G_p is the haplotype of the person of interest (POI).
G_k are the haplotypes of any individuals assumed to be present in the mixture.

$$LR = \frac{\sum\limits_{u} \Pr(G_c \mid G_p, G_k, S_u, H_p)\Pr(S_u \mid G_p, G_k, H_p)}{\sum\limits_{v} \Pr(G_c \mid G_p, G_k, S_v, H_d)\Pr(S_v \mid G_p, G_k, H_d)}$$

S_U is a set of haplotypes G_W of the M unknown contributors, each of which is modelled as

- $\dfrac{x}{N+1}$, where x is the count after a database search if $G_U \neq G_p$.

- $\theta + (1-\theta)\dfrac{x+1}{N+1}$ if $G_U = G_p$.

- The probability of the set S_U is modelled as the product of the probabilities of the constituent haplotypes.

$$\Pr(G_c \mid G_p, G_k, S_u, H_x) = C^a (1-C)^{l-a} \left(\prod_i D_i^{b_i} (1-D_i)^{n_i - b_i} \right)$$

$$\times \prod_{i,k \neq i} \left[(D_i D_k)^{f_{ik}} (1 - D_i D_k)^{n_{ik} - f_{ik}} \right] \prod_{j=1}^{a} p_j$$

where
a is the number of alleles modelled as drop-in
b_i is the number of unstacked alleles of contributor i modelled as dropout
C is the probability that an allele drops in
D_i is the probability of dropout of an allele of contributor i
f_{ik} is the number of stacked alleles of contributors i and k modelled as dropout
l is the number of loci
n_i is the number of unstacked alleles of contributor i
n_{ik} is the number of stacked alleles of contributors i and k
p_j is the probability of allele j, where $j = 1 \dots a$ are the alleles modelled as drop-in

---

contributions to the likelihood ratio. Independence is key here, and caution is warranted in simple multiplication based on the grounds of population substructure'. However no warning exists in the same paper about combining autosomal and Y chromosome markers. 'The weight of the genetic evidence of Y chromosome markers shall be combined with the genetic weight from independent autosomal markers'. Other than the unusual term *genetic weight*, having qualitatively different recommendations about combining mtDNA and the Y chromosome with autosomal DNA is not sustainable and we are unable to see how to proceed 'with caution'.

Recently Amorim[947] raised the issue of whether *LR*s calculated from lineage and autosomal markers may be multiplied in order to obtain a single measure of the genetic evidence in a given case. Amorim challenged the practice of *LR* multiplication mainly on the grounds that lineage markers are not individual-specific but are instead shared by the suspect's whole lineage. He argued for replacing the following:

H_p: The suspect is the source of the stain.

H_d: The suspect is not the source of the stain.

Amorim suggested that when lineage markers are employed for genetic analysis the prosecution and defence hypotheses should instead read as follows:

H_p^*: The suspect or somebody from their lineage is the source of the stain.

H_d^*: Neither the suspect nor anybody from their lineage is the source of the stain.

Amorim concluded that 'the combination of likelihood ratios from the two sources of data should be avoided'.

Unless the circumstances of an individual case suggest differently, however, there seems to be neither a logical nor legal basis for changing the prosecution hypothesis from H_p to H_p^*. Moreover, if the possibility of mutation is neglected, then the likelihoods of the two hypotheses, H_p and H_p^*, would be identical for lineage markers anyway.

The shift between H_d and H_d^* is more subtle. $\Pr(E|H_d)$ will be larger, possibly much larger, than $\Pr(E|H_d^*)$. However, again there seems to be neither a logical nor a legal basis for changing the defence hypothesis. The data required to inform $\Pr(E|H_d^*)$ would need to be reprocessed for each case subtracting from the database those persons of the same lineage as the POI. This is an almost insurmountable challenge complicated by the impossible task of defining same lineage. On the other hand $\Pr(E|H_d)$ may be reasonably informed by a simple sample from the relevant population, incorporating relatives if they come into the sample by chance. The change to H_d^* appears to produce neither practical not logical benefit.

We believe that the concern was partly motivated by what we hope is the now-defunct practice of sampling lineages rather than sampling at random. Under such regimes, people with the same surname would be deliberately avoided when constructing a frequency database, which in turn would lead to biased haplotype frequency estimates. We reiterate that databases underlying match probabilities need to be representative of the population(s) of interest and are best constructed by as close to random sampling as is possible.

In summary we support or extend the recommendation of Walsh et al.[945]

The autosomal co-ancestry coefficient θ_A is usually assigned in what is believed to be a conservative manner. This assignment is often informed by studies of the differences between populations thought to be diverging primarily by drift. While informed by these studies, the assigned value is usually a round number believed to be near the top of the plausible range and not the actual estimate. Since this is an assigned value rather than an estimated value, we cannot expect it to have a direct relationship with values derived theoretically from the effective population size and mutation rates.

Extending the work of Walsh et al.,[945] Buckleton and Myers[948] obtain

$$\theta_{A|Y} = \sum_{t=1}^{\infty} \frac{(1-\lambda)^{t-1} v_Y^t}{\sum\limits_{t=1}^{\infty}(1-\lambda)^{t-1} v_Y^t} \left[v_A^t \frac{1+F_A}{2^{2t+1}} + \left(1-\frac{2}{2^{2t+1}}\right)\theta_A \right] \tag{10.3}$$

where $\theta_{A|Y}$ is the adjusted value for the autosomal locus given the observation of a Y haplotype match. Equation 10.3 represents very little change from the equations outlined by Walsh et al.[945] It differs in that mutation is considered for the autosomal locus and that the background co-ancestry coefficients F_A and θ_A appear explicitly rather than via modification of the size of the effective population of males, N_M.

The modified θ_A value given in Equation 10.3 includes a contribution from first- and second-order relatives and assumes all relationships are unilineal, half-siblings and half-cousins in this case. In routine forensic work these relationships are usually assigned a separate match probability and many relationships are bilineal. Let x be the fraction of relationships that are bilinear. This would suggest that

$$\theta_{A|Y} = \sum_{t=3}^{\infty} \frac{(1-\lambda)^{t-1} v_Y^t}{\sum_{t=1}^{\infty}(1-\lambda)^{t-1} v_Y^t}\left[(1+x)v_A^t \frac{1+F_A}{2^{2t+1}} + \left(1 - \frac{2(1+x)}{2^{2t+1}}\right)\theta_A\right] \tag{10.4}$$

may be more appropriate for the unrelated statistic (often assumed to exclude first- and second-order relatives). As observed in Table 10.3, the increase in $\theta_{A|Y}$ is modest and fairly insensitive to N_M when applying Equation 10.4.

Table 10.3 Modified θ_{AY} Values Applying Equation 10.4 to Various Commercial Multiplexes, N_M, and θ_A

Multiplex Loci (l)		PPY 11	Yfiler 16	PowerPlex Y23 22	Yfiler Plus 25
$\mu_{ave.}$		0.00210	0.00256	0.00354	0.00566
θ_A	N_Y	$\theta_{A|Y}$	$\theta_{A|Y}$	$\theta_{A|Y}$	$\theta_{A|Y}$
0.001	100	0.002	0.003	0.004	0.006
	1,000	0.002	0.002	0.004	0.005
	10,000	0.002	0.002	0.004	0.005
	100,000	0.002	0.002	0.004	0.005
0.01	100	0.011	0.012	0.013	0.014
	1,000	0.011	0.011	0.013	0.014
	10,000	0.011	0.011	0.013	0.014
	100,000	0.011	0.011	0.013	0.014
0.03	100	0.031	0.032	0.033	0.034
	1,000	0.031	0.031	0.033	0.034
	10,000	0.031	0.031	0.033	0.034
	100,000	0.031	0.031	0.033	0.034

Notes: The proportion of full siblings (x), 0.88, assumed an average of two children per family[949] and 12% of children having half-siblings.[950] The μ_A was 0.0025. F_A was assumed to equal θ_A. The duplicated locus DYS385 was counted as one locus for l.

The maximum cumulative difference across all loci of an Identifiler profile was less than a factor of 2.2, a change of limited practical import given the overall low probability estimates. This factor was for the most common alleles. The factor would be larger for rare alleles but the overall match probability would be smaller.

The match probabilities for siblings and first cousins also contain a $\theta_{A|Y}$. There is no effect on $\theta_{A|Y}$ for a Y chromosome match for two brothers, nor for two cousins whose parents included brothers. For cousins whose parents included sisters or a brother/sister pair there is an effect.

Formulae appear in Buckleton and Myers.[948]

The values of $\theta_{A|Y}$ are not much larger than θ_A and a coherent argument could be made that any adjustment is unnecessary.

Sampling Uncertainty

We can envisage three relatively straightforward ways of assessing sampling uncertainty for a combined result: the Taylor expansion method, the bootstrap and a Bayesian approach. We describe the Taylor expansion for single source but cannot readily extend it to more complex situations. We also describe the Bayesian method and this can be used for single source and more complex situations. The bootstrap is readily applicable to all situations and is not described here.

Taylor Expansion (Duncan Taylor)

For the autosomal loci a confidence interval may be assigned using the asymptotic normality of the logarithm method. Since the United States uses a different population genetic model to Europe and Australasia, we direct the reader to the NRC II report, either equations 5.8a through c (p. 146) for those using NRC II[176] Recommendation 4.1 (the United States) or p. 147 in the footnote for those using NRC II Recommendation 4.2 (Europe and Australasia).

For a lineage marker with an LR designated by LR_L:

$$\mathrm{Var}\left[\ln(LR_L)\right]=\left(\frac{\partial\ln(LR_L)}{\partial f_G}\right)^2\mathrm{Var}(f_G)=\left(\frac{1}{LR_L}\times\frac{\partial LR_L}{\partial f_G}\right)^2\mathrm{Var}(f_G)$$

where f_G is the haplotype frequency. Using the example of a single sourced haplotype with a matching reference, the simplest form of the LR can be expressed as $LR_L=\dfrac{1}{f_G}$, and assuming

$$\mathrm{Var}(f_G)=\frac{f_G(1-f_G)(1+\theta)}{2n}$$

gives

$$\mathrm{Var}\left[\ln(LR_L)\right]=\frac{(1-f_G)(1+\theta)}{2nf_G}$$

Assuming no correlation between autosomal and lineage markers, the confidence interval for the combined LR can then be given by

$$\exp\left[\ln(LR_A\times LR_L)\pm Z\sqrt{\mathrm{Var}\left[\ln(LR_A)\right]+\mathrm{Var}\left[\ln(LR_L)\right]}\right]$$

The extension of this method for lineage markers from multiple contributors is complex as it requires covariances for each pairwise comparison of potential haplotypes; therefore we have not attempted it.

Using the Bayesian Approach

For the autosomal loci, at locus l we observe allele counts x_1, x_2, ..., x_k on the k possible alleles. Assuming a k-dimensional Dirichlet prior with parameters $\alpha_i = \dfrac{1}{k}, i = 1, \ldots, k$, multinomial sampling yields a Dirichlet posterior on the allele probabilities, such that

$$p_1, p_2, \ldots, p_k \sim \mathrm{Dir}\left(\alpha_1', \alpha_2', \ldots, \alpha_k'\right)$$

where

$$\alpha_i' = x_i + \frac{1}{k}$$

For the lineage marker we have suggested a plausible prior $\beta(1/k, 1-1/k)$.

The posterior distribution of any function across the combined autosomal and lineage markers may be formed by taking the quantiles from repeated realizations of this formulation from samples from this distribution.

To generate samples from a Dirichlet it may be expedient to proceed from the gamma distribution. A randomly sampled allele frequency for allele p_i using a gamma distribution would then be

$$p_i = \frac{g_i}{\displaystyle\sum_{i=1}^{k} g_i} \quad g_i \sim \Gamma(\alpha_i', 1)$$

To obtain the LR value corresponding to the quantile of interest of the combined marker types, y resamplings of the databases are carried out and used to calculate LRs:

$$LR_y = \left(\prod_l LR_{Ay}^l\right) LR_{Ly}$$

where LR_{Ay}^l is the LR for the autosomal data at locus l in resampling y and LR_{Ly} is the LR for the lineage haplotype in resampling y.

The $C\%$, S-sided probability interval is then the $\left[\dfrac{y}{S}\left(1 - \dfrac{C}{100}\right)\right]$th LR value in the list of y LRs, sorted in ascending order.

Forensic X Chromosome Analysis

Most human females possess two X chromosomes that are present as a homologous pair. This is often written as XX. It is thought that one of this pair is inactivated[951,952] and reduced to a Barr body. This explains why X chromosome monosomies, trisomies and polysomies are not ubiquitously fatal. Complete and partial monosomies have been observed and are associated with Ullrich–Turner syndrome. The X chromosomes recombine in the female.

Normal males possess one X and one Y chromosome. This is often written as *XY*. However syndromes do exist whereby XY individuals present as the female phenotype. In such cases it is thought that the sex-determining gene is either absent or inactive on the Y.

The genome database (www.gdb.org), now defunct, listed 26 tri- and 90 tetra-nucleotide repeat polymorphisms on the X chromosome. The VNTR locus DXS52 as well as 18 tetra- and 3 tri-nucleotide repeat loci are in common forensic use.[951] X chromosome markers have advantages in deficient paternity cases, for example when a biological sample is not available from the putative father and samples from paternal relatives are used instead. When females have the same father, they also share the same paternal X chromosome. This can be used to investigate, for instance, half-sisters (if they have four alleles between them, then they are not half-siblings). If two close relatives are suspects in a paternity case, the X chromosome may have advantages over autosomal markers. Szibor et al.[951] consider a father/son pair. These two cannot have X chromosomes that are identical by descent (IBD). This may assist in determining the paternity of a female child. Pinto et al.[953] have examined multiple scenarios where X chromosome testing can provide additional information.

X chromosome mutation rates would not be expected to be markedly different from autosomal rates; however data are sparse (see Table 10.4 for some reported mutation rates).

Using both physical and genetic mapping methods, the relative locations of some X chromosome STRs of practical interest were investigated. This resulted in the map shown in

Table 10.4 X Chromosome STR Mutation Rates as Estimated from Tests of Trios			
STR	Mutations/Meioses	$\mu \times 10^{-3}$	95% CI
DXS6807	0/440	0.00	0.00–8.38
DXS9895	0/761	0.00	0.00–4.85
DXS8378	1/308	3.25	0.08–18.09
DXS9902	0/304	0.00	0.00–12.13
DXS7132	1/260	3.85	0.09–21.43
ARA	4/562	4.92	1.01–14.37
DXS6800	0/440	0.00	0.00–8.38
DXS9898	0/754	0.00	0.00–4.89
DXS6789	0/752	0.00	0.00–4.91
DXS101	0/440	0.00	0.00–8.38
DXS7424	0/440	0.00	0.00–9.22
DXS7133	0/263	0.00	0.00–14.03
GATA172D04	0/370	0.00	0.00–9.97
HPRTB	3/610	4.92	1.01–14.37
DXS7423	2/234	8.55	1.03–30.87
DXS8377	5/760	6.58	2.13–15.35
CUMULATIVE	16/658	2.09	1.25–3.32

STR, short tandem repeat; CI, confidence interval.
Source: Szibor, R., et al., *International Journal of Legal Medicine*, 117, 67–74, 2003.

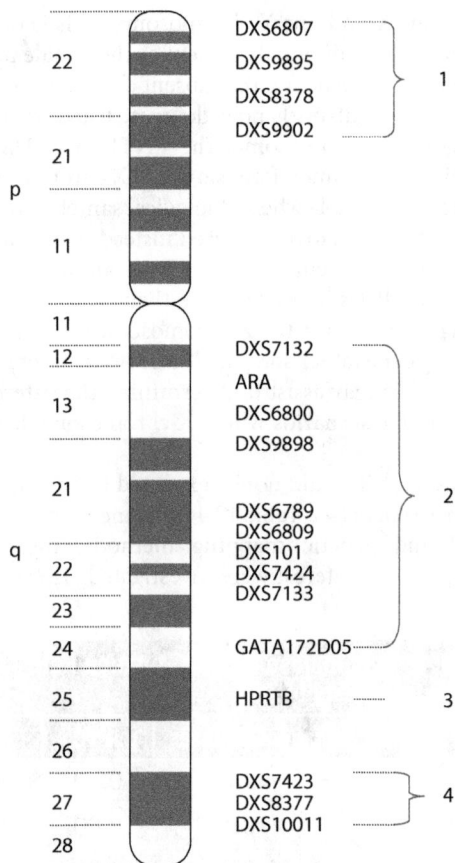

Figure 10.5   A diagrammatic map of the human X chromosome showing the approximate location of microsatellite loci used in forensic analyses. The numbers 1 to 4 represent four known linkage groups. (This figure draws heavily from a more detailed description provided from Szibor, R., et al., *International Journal of Legal Medicine*, 117, 67–74, 2003.)

Figure 10.5. Linkage disequilibrium was observed only for DXS101 and DXS7424 based on the investigation of 210 male DNA samples.[951]

We discuss the effect of linkage in paternity testing in Chapter 11, but in brief there are no implications in this context unless there are two meioses (for example, two children) or the phase of the mother is known from other data, such as the typing of the X chromosome of her father.

11

Parentage Testing

*John S. Buckleton, Duncan Taylor and Jo-Anne Bright**

Contents

---

* Based on earlier work by John Buckleton, Tim Clayton and Chris Triggs.

Introduction

Familial investigation features prominently in forensic science within both the criminal and civil jurisdictions.[954,955] This chapter reviews the application of autosomal short tandem repeat (STR) evidence to parentage testing and discusses the issues associated with mutation, null alleles and genetic anomalies. Application of both X- and Y-linked markers[951] to these purposes is also briefly reviewed. Single nucleotide polymorphisms (SNPs) are in use but are not discussed here.[956]

This chapter concentrates on pedigrees involving one or two alleged parents and one or more children. In Chapter 12 we consider the application of familial testing to more complex pedigrees.

In a criminal context such testing can be required following sexual assaults, for example to identify the father of a child conceived as a result of an alleged assault. Likewise, familial testing can be used to support the assertion that two individuals are genetically related in order to support charges arising from entrance into a proscribed (incestuous) sexual relationship. In cases involving concealed births, abandoned children or infanticide it may be necessary to prove a genetic relationship to either ensure the rightful return of an infant or to support criminal charges.

During civil litigation familial investigation can be used to substantiate claims by an estranged partner for financial support and maintenance of a child. Similarly, in the field of wills and probate, disputes over inheritances can be informed by the application of genetic testing. Familial testing is also now being widely applied by governmental bodies to adjudicate in cases of immigration and naturalization. The identification of bodies for legal purposes can also be effected using familial testing.

Paternity and familial identification can provide evidence in either civil or criminal proceedings, and a forensic scientist has a different responsibility in these two settings. In criminal cases it is customary to concede reasonable doubt to the defendant. However in civil cases there is no direction in which doubt may be conceded. This removes the oft-used prop of conservatism.

Testing Diverse Sample Types

Other than those samples taken from bodily remains, most samples for testing paternity will be pristine reference samples. These are presented either as venous blood samples, as samples of buccal mucosa (in the form of scrapes and oral rinses) or as samples of plucked hair. Consequently, these types of samples present few difficulties during the extraction of DNA. However a number of sample types are sometimes encountered that do pose significant technical challenges.

Termination Products

In many countries it is common for the scientist to be presented with samples from a pregnancy termination procedure.[957] In the United Kingdom terminations can be performed legally up to the 24th week of gestation. Clinically, those terminations performed up to about the 12th week of gestation use a technique known as vacuum aspiration. This results in the severe fragmentation of the foetus and subsequent mixing of those fragments with maternal tissues. Care must be taken to identify foetal structures among the largely maternal tissues in the termination products in these cases. The earlier in the gestation period the termination, the more technically difficult this is to achieve. Failure to identify sufficient foetal tissue will result in a solely maternal profile being obtained. Alternatively, if both maternal and foetal tissues are present, a mixture will be obtained in which the ratio of the mixture will be governed by the relative proportions of maternal and foetal cells. There is a maximum of three peaks per locus due to the maternal relationship. In theory (if the maternal profile is known) such a mixture can be substantially resolved using the principles outlined in Chapters 7 through 9, to yield the foetal profile.

Preserved Histology Samples

In some criminal cases, the complaints are retrospective and the only samples from a foetus may be in the form of archival histology samples. The most common form of tissue preservation used by histopathology laboratories is a procedure that involves a transient immersion of the tissue in formal saline, followed by embedding in blocks of molten paraffin wax. This presents additional technical difficulties. First, sectioning from the block is required to produce thin slices with large surface areas to facilitate efficient removal of the wax. Second, the wax in each slice must be dissolved using xylene. The xylene must then be removed by washing with ethanol. The tissue is then air dried to volatilize the ethanol remnants before digestion of the nascent tissue can begin. Third, the formalin used as preservative is known to have effects deleterious to the DNA. Depending upon the severity of the fixation treatment prior to embedding, the DNA can be rendered unamplifiable. Similarly, 'wet' preserved samples stored in formalin solution have been demonstrated to be highly refractory to polymerase chain reaction (PCR) analysis.

Principles of Mendelian Inheritance

The year 1900 marks the beginning of the modern period in the study of heredity. Despite the fact that there had been some development of the idea that a living organism is an aggregation of characters in (the) form (of) units of some description, there had been no attempts to ascertain by experiment, how such supposed units might behave in the offspring of a cross. In the year above mentioned the papers of Gregor Mendel came to light, being quoted almost simultaneously in the scientific correspondence of three European botanists, de Vries in Holland, Correns in Germany, and von Tschermak in Austria. Of Mendel's two papers, the important one in this connection, is entitled 'Experiments in Plant Hybridisation', and was read at the meetings of the Natural History Society of Bruun in Bohemia at the sessions of February 8 and March 8, 1865. This paper had passed entirely unnoticed by the scientific circles of Europe, although it appeared in 1866 in the Transactions of the Society. From its publication until 1900, Mendel's paper appears to have been completely overlooked, except for the citation in Focke's 'Pflanzenmischlinge'. And the single citation of Hoffmann....[958]

Two laws of heredity have been developed from Mendel's work. In modern times they are often phrased with the benefit of hindsight. We now know the chromosomal basis of inheritance associated with meiosis. However, at the time that Mendel wrote, none of this was known. An elegant phrasing of Mendel's laws without over-reliance on modern terminology is given by Thompson.[496] We follow her treatment here.

1. *The law of segregation.* Each individual has two 'factors' controlling a given characteristic, one being a copy of a corresponding factor in the father of the individual and one being a copy of the corresponding factor in the mother of the individual. Further, a randomly selected copy of one of the two factors is copied to each child, independently for different children and independently of the factor contributed by the spouse.

2. *The law of independent assortment.* The factor copied from one pair is independent of the factor copied from another factor pair.

Modern molecular biology allows us to see the basis for these laws in the segregation of chromosomes and their recombination into a zygote. The human genome is diploid. It has a normal complement of 46 chromosomes arranged into 22 pairs of autosomes and a single pair of sex chromosomes (XY). The somatic cells divide mitotically to maintain their diploid status, whereas the sex cells (gametes) are produced by meiotic divisions and are haploid. During meiosis one of each of the pairs of the homologous chromosomes is randomly partitioned to the ovum or spermatozoon. In addition there are recombination events that 'shuffle' the genetic material further still. At fertilization the union of an ovum and a single spermatozoon restores the diploid chromosomal constitution and in doing so ensures that the embryo receives a random assortment of genes, half provided by one biological parent and the remaining half from the other biological parent (see Figure 11.1). Mendel's laws form the basis of familial testing.

An exception to the usual Mendelian inheritance pattern occurs for loci that are physically close on the same chromosome. If two loci are close enough, they tend to be inherited together. This phenomenon was discussed in Chapter 3 and is known as *linkage*.

Typically, the STR loci selected as forensic markers for familial analysis are situated on different chromosomes to ensure that they assort randomly and are inherited in a Mendelian fashion (the law of independent assortment). However there are cases, for instance in the Combined DNA Index System (CODIS) set, where two loci are resident on the same chromosome. As long as they are separated by sufficient genetic distance to guarantee an intervening recombination event there are no potential consequences. As discussed in Chapter 1 there are some pairs of loci that are close enough that some linkage effects are expected. This situation will become more frequent as more loci are added to forensic sets, or when we move to SNPs. We include a small section later in this chapter on the consequences of linkage which has not been extensively reported in the forensic literature.

The Mendelian inheritance pattern is most easily represented in the format of a family tree (Figure 11.2). If one locus is considered and the two paternal alleles are represented as P_1, P_2 and the maternal alleles as M_1, M_2, then there are four combinations for the offspring: P_1M_1, P_1M_2, P_2M_1 and P_2M_2. By Mendel's first law each combination is equally probable, occurring with probability 1/4.

More recently the non-autosomal DNA in the mitochondrion and the X and Y chromosomes have begun to play an important part in familial testing. For most of its length, the Y chromosome

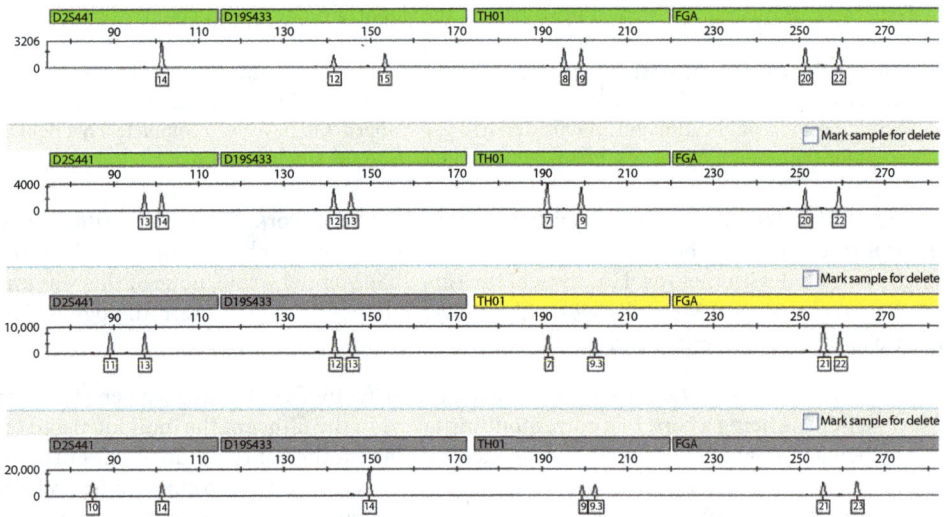

Figure 11.1 Profiles of mother, child, the true father and a putative father at four autosomal STR loci.

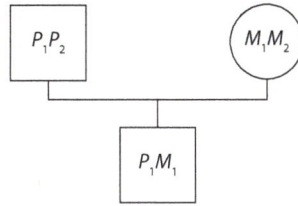

Figure 11.2   Pedigree for simple paternity trio.

does not recombine and is patrilinearly inherited. Y-STR markers therefore form a 'haplotype' that, barring mutation, will be passed down the male line. This pattern of inheritance can be useful in certain cases where there is a shortage of relatives (so-called deficiency cases) or where there are large generational gaps.

The X chromosome can recombine in the female but not the male. As discussed in Chapter 10 individual loci of forensic interest may be linked. The major advantages of markers on the X chromosome again arise in deficient paternity cases, when a biological sample is not available from the putative father and samples from paternal relatives are used instead. When females have the same father they also share the same paternal X chromosome.[951]

Mitochondrial DNA was also discussed in Chapter 10. It is assumed to be exclusively inherited matrilineally with no recombination in mammals. Its uses strongly mirror those of the Y chromosome for paternity cases, especially when there is a shortage of relatives.

Evaluation of Evidence

Three methods have been offered for the evaluation of parentage testing results. These are the paternity index (PI), the probability of paternity and an exclusion probability.[959,960] These methods all have strong parallels to concepts used elsewhere in this book. Every interpretation method assumes correct typing of the biological samples.

Exclusion Probability

Consider the most common case of parentage testing, where we have a mother (M), child (C) and a man alleged to be the father (AF). These three persons have been typed and found to have the genotypes G_M, G_C and G_{AF}, respectively. The genotypes of the mother and the child define one (or in some cases one of two) paternal alleles at each locus.

An exclusion probability may be defined as 'that fraction of men who do not possess the paternal allele or alleles'. As such it is strongly akin to the exclusion probability in mixtures evaluation.

If the possible paternal alleles at a locus are $A_1 \ldots A_n$ (often there is only one possible paternal allele), then the exclusion probability at this locus (PE_l) is

$$PE_l = \left(1 - \sum_{i=1}^{n} Pr(A_i)\right)^2$$

assuming Hardy–Weinberg equilibrium. The PE across multiple loci (PE) is calculated as

$$PE = 1 - \prod_l (1 - PE_l)$$

For an extension to the consideration of relatives see Fung et al.[961]

We have previously discussed Dr Charles Brenner's[710] explanation of the shortcomings of the probability of exclusion. We follow his treatment again here.

Let us describe the evidence as follows:

1. The blood type of the mother.

2. The blood type of the child.

3. The blood type of the alleged father.

From this information we can infer that

4. The alleged father is not excluded.

Brenner points out that, although Statement 4 can be deduced from Statements 1, 2 and 3, Statement 3 cannot be deduced from 1, 2 and 4. Hence the use of Statement 4 represents a loss of information. The exclusion probability is a summary of the evidence in 1, 2 and 4.

Paternity Index

PI is a specialist term used in paternity testing to describe the likelihood ratio. Its structure is exactly as described for the likelihood ratio in Chapter 2 but it has been used in paternity testing for longer than in other areas of forensic biology.[229]

Consider the following two hypotheses:

H_1: The alleged father is the true father.

H_2: The alleged father is the not the true father.

Hypothesis H_1 represents one side of the allegation. In many paternity cases the action will be civil and it may not be appropriate to view this as the 'prosecution' hypothesis. Hypothesis H_2 represents the other side of the allegation; similarly it may not be appropriate to view this as the 'defence' hypothesis.

If we consider some evidence, E, typically the genotypes of a child, the alleged father and possibly the mother, then Bayes' theorem informs us that

$$\frac{\Pr(H_1|E)}{\Pr(H_2|E)} = \frac{\Pr(E|H_1)}{\Pr(E|H_2)} \times \frac{\Pr(H_1)}{\Pr(H_2)}$$

The likelihood ratio term $\dfrac{\Pr(E|H_1)}{\Pr(E|H_2)}$ is usually written as PI and is the central term calculated under this approach.

Probability of Paternity

Recall that Bayes' theorem states that

$$\frac{\Pr(H_1|E)}{\Pr(H_2|E)} = PI \times \frac{\Pr(H_1)}{\Pr(H_2)}$$

We see that the PI relates the odds on paternity prior to considering the genetic evidence to those after considering that evidence. As with any Bayesian treatment the posterior probability of paternity can be calculated from the PI and the prior odds. The prior odds relate to the probability of paternity based on the non-genetic evidence. This could include statements of the mother as to with whom she had intercourse or evidence that may suggest that the alleged father was out of the country or in prison at the time of conception. Such evidence, if relevant and admissible, affects the prior odds.

However it has become customary to set the prior odds to 1:1, that is to assign prior probabilities of 50% to both H_1 and H_2 when calculating the probability of paternity. This assumption is hard to justify at the fundamental level[163,174] and must be seen simply as a pragmatic tool. It may be completely appropriate in many cases but equally may be totally inappropriate in others. It would seem wise, however, to make this assumption of equal prior odds explicit.

Utilizing this assumption we see that

$$\frac{\Pr(H_1 \mid E)}{\Pr(H_2 \mid E)} = \text{PI}$$

and hence that

$$\frac{\Pr(H_1 \mid E)}{1 - \Pr(H_2 \mid E)} = \text{PI}$$

yielding

$$\Pr(H_1 \mid E) = \frac{\text{PI}}{1 + \text{PI}}$$

Given the assumption of prior odds of 1:1, we can simply tabulate the posterior probability of paternity given the PI (Table 11.1).

A Discussion of the Methods

Strong support is given for the PI approach by many authorities, including Evett and Weir[257] and the Paternity Testing Commission of the International Society of Forensic Genetics (ISFG).[946,962] We agree. This is Recommendation R1 of the Paternity Testing Commission (PTC) of the ISFG.

All methods are in recent usage,[963,964] although the recommendations to use the PI alone or predominantly are clear. The number and type of statistics reported by the English-speaking working group of the ISFG is given in Table 11.2.[964]

All three methods use the frequency of certain alleles. These frequencies must be estimated from a relevant database as has been discussed in Chapter 5. A 'rare' allele could be an allele that has not previously been reported, or is not contained in the relevant database, or an allele with very few previous observations. Methods for dealing with rare alleles have been discussed in a general context in Chapter 6.

PTC Recommendation 2.1[946] suggests $\frac{x_i + 1}{N + 1}$ where there are x_i observations of allele i in a database of N alleles. This is perfectly reasonable in practice but cannot be obtained by any mathematical method of which we are aware. For example, we cannot obtain it from a beta-binomial. The NRC II* suggestion of replacing x_i with the $\max(x_i, 5)$ is equally pragmatic and *ad hoc*.

Table 11.1 The Posterior Probability of Paternity Given the Assumption of Equal Prior Odds	
Paternity Index	Probability of Paternity
10	0.9090909
100	0.9900990
1,000	0.9990010
10,000	0.9999000
100,000	0.9999900
1,000,000	0.9999990
10,000,000	0.9999999

Note: Probabilities are rounded to eight significant figures.

---

* *Second National Research Council report on forensic DNA evidence.*

Table 11.2 Statistics Reported in Paternity Testing							
Statistics Reported	2002 %	2003 %	2004 %	2005 %	2006 %	2007 %	2008 %
PI, paternity index	80	71	69	69	70	67	71
W, probability of paternity	70	61	78	79	86	86	85
Probability of exclusion	11	8	9	5	11	7	4
No statistic	2	10	5	2	–	–	–

Source: Thomsen, A.R., et al., *Forensic Science International: Genetics*, 3(4), 214–221, 2009.

Most laboratories have a requirement for issuing a report with a positive weight for paternity.[963–965] There is no theoretical requirement for a lower limit for reporting, and a decision to have such a limit is based on pragmatic reasons such as avoiding court cases where the biological evidence is evaluated as less than the limit.

Use of the Product Rule in the Evaluation of the Paternity Index

In the evaluation of the likelihood ratio in previous chapters we have discussed the small bias inherent in the use of the product rule when population substructure exists. The method of Balding and Nichols[358] can be used to evaluate likelihood ratios, or PIs, for paternity duos and trios when population substructure exists.

When the Balding and Nichols correction is applied to a whole race or when conservatively large values of θ are used, this is thought to be an overcorrection, which may err too much in one direction. This 'conservative' behaviour is considered desirable by some courts and scientists in criminal cases. However this property of the subpopulation correction does not have such an obvious justification in civil cases. Of course that is not to suggest that the population genetic fact of population subdivision has disappeared; however in civil proceedings the product rule may have more desirable properties. NRC II discusses this matter briefly in the US context in footnote 74.

Recommendation 2.4 of the PTC recommendations states, 'If a significant degree of substructuring is known to be present in a population, algorithms that take substructure into consideration shall be used'. In the guidance that follows there are comments that suggest the routine use of the product rule in many cases. We amplify these comments. The product rule probably has the lowest total bias and is most appropriate for civil casework irrespective of the existence of substructure. The subpopulation correction is most appropriate for criminal work.

Paternity Trios: Mother, Child and Alleged Father

We begin by considering at least two hypotheses. In the most common case these could be the following:

H_1: The alleged father is the true father (and the mother is the true mother).

H_2: A random person who is not related to the alleged father is the true father (and the mother is the true mother).

The assumption that the person labelled as the mother is the true mother of the child is usually unstated. Although these two hypotheses are the most commonly used, we note that they are not exhaustive, as the random person may be a relative of the alleged father. This again suggests an alternative approach based on the general form of Bayes' theorem. Such an approach is not in use in any laboratory of which we are aware.

Typically then we require

$$PI = \frac{\Pr(G_C, G_M, G_{AF} \mid H_1)}{\Pr(G_C, G_M, G_{AF} \mid H_2)}$$

It is customary to decompose these probabilities using the third law of probability. Usually to evaluate the probabilities of the observing genotypes of individuals they are conditioned on the genotypes of their ancestors. For example:

$$PI = \frac{\Pr(G_C, G_M, G_{AF} \mid H_1)}{\Pr(G_C, G_M, G_{AF} \mid H_2)} = \frac{\Pr(G_C \mid G_M, G_{AF}, H_1)\Pr(G_M, G_{AF} \mid H_1)}{\Pr(G_C \mid G_M, G_{AF}, H_2)\Pr(G_M, G_{AF} \mid H_2)}$$

where the genotype of the youngest person, the child, is conditioned on the parents, as opposed to

$$PI = \frac{\Pr(G_C, G_M, G_{AF} \mid H_1)}{\Pr(G_C, G_M, G_{AF} \mid H_2)} = \frac{\Pr(G_{AF} \mid G_M, G_C, H_1)\Pr(G_M, G_C \mid H_1)}{\Pr(G_{AF} \mid G_M, G_C, H_2)\Pr(G_M, G_C \mid H_2)}$$

Both decompositions are, of course, formally equivalent mathematically. However the former is easier to evaluate. Thus we will work with the former decomposition.

It is customary to assume that the joint probability of observing the genotypes of the putative parents does not depend on the particular hypothesis, i.e.

$$\Pr(G_M, G_{AF} \mid H_1) = \Pr(G_M, G_{AF} \mid H_2) = \Pr(G_M, G_{AF})$$

This assumption essentially states that the joint probability of observing the genotypes of the mother and alleged father is not conditioned on whether the alleged father is the true father or not. This is only true in the absence of any conditioning on the genotypes of any other children or descendants. Given this assumption the PI becomes:

$$PI = \frac{\Pr(G_C \mid G_M, G_{AF}, H_1)}{\Pr(G_C \mid G_M, G_{AF}, H_2)}$$

Evaluation of the PI can proceed directly from this equation. The numerator can be evaluated using a Punnett square at each locus where both parents are present in the conditioning.

Assuming that the mother is the true mother it is often possible to determine the maternal and paternal alleles, A_m, and A_p, unambiguously. This allows us to write

$$\Pr(G_C \mid G_M, G_{AF}, H_2) = \Pr(A_p, A_m \mid G_M, G_{AF}, H_2) = \Pr(A_m \mid G_M, G_{AF}, A_p, H_2)\,\Pr(A_p \mid G_M, G_{AF}, H_2)$$

Conventionally using the further assumption that

$$\Pr(A_m \mid G_M, G_{AF}, A_p, H_2) = \Pr(A_m \mid G_M)$$

allows the probability in the denominator of the PI to be written as

$$\Pr(G_C \mid G_M, G_{AF}, H_2) = \Pr(A_m \mid G_M)\,\Pr(A_p \mid G_M, G_{AF}, H_2)$$

Now $\Pr(A_m \mid G_M)$ is 1/2 or 1 depending on whether the genotype G_M containing the maternal allele is heterozygous or homozygous. We denote this probability as the maternal Mendelian factor M_M. Evaluation of $\Pr(A_p \mid G_M, G_{AF}, H_2)$ is slightly more problematic.

As with previous chapters we now turn to consideration of a series of examples and show in detail how to evaluate the PI for paternity trios.

Example 11.1: A Simple Paternity Trio: Mother Is a Heterozygote

	Genotype
Mother	cd
Child	ac
Alleged father	ab

Under H_1 we assume that the alleged father is the true father, and we may proceed by using a Punnett square:

		Genes from the Father	
		a	b
Genes from the Mother	c	ac	bc
	d	ad	bd

We see that the child's genotype is one of the four (equiprobable) outcomes and assign the probability $\Pr(G_C|G_M, G_{AF}, H_1) = 1/4$.

The mother is heterozygous for the maternal allele ($A_m = c$) and we can assign the value $M_M = 1/2$ to the maternal Mendelian factor. The paternal allele is $A_p = a$. Under the hypothesis H_2 we assign the probability $\Pr(A_p|G_M, G_{AF}, H_2) = p_a$, the allele probability of the a allele in this population. Hence the PI is

$$PI = \frac{\frac{1}{4}}{\frac{1}{2} \times p_a} = \frac{1}{2p_a}$$

Example 11.2: A Simple Paternity Trio: Mother is a Homozygote

	Genotype
Mother	cc
Child	ac
Alleged father	ab

Again under H_1 we assume that the alleged father is the true father, and the Punnett square becomes

		Genes from the Father	
		a	b
Genes from the Mother	c	ac	bc
	c	ac	bc

We see that the child's genotype occurs in two of the four (equiprobable) outcomes and assign the probability $\Pr(G_C|G_M, G_{AF}, H_1) = 1/2$.

The mother is homozygous for the maternal allele ($A_m = c$) and we can assign $M_M = 1$. The paternal allele $A_p = a$. As before we assign the probability $\Pr(A_p|G_M, G_{AF}, H_2) = p_a$ under the hypothesis H_2. Hence

$$PI = \frac{\frac{1}{2}}{1 \times p_a} = \frac{1}{2p_a}$$

Example 11.3: A Simple Paternity Trio: Paternal Allele Ambiguous

	Genotype
Mother	ab
Child	ab
Alleged father	bc

Under H_1 we assume that the alleged father is the true father, and we may proceed by a Punnett square:

		Genes from the Father	
		b	c
Genes from the Mother	a	ab	ac
	b	bb	bc

We see that the child's genotype occurs in one of the four (equiprobable) outcomes and assign the probability 1/4 to this genotype.

This example was introduced because of a small complexity that occurs under H_2. This arises because either of the mother's alleles may be the maternal allele, making attribution of both the maternal and the paternal allele ambiguous. Under H_2 we can see that the mother may contribute the a allele ($A_m = a$) with probability $M_M = 1/2$ or the b allele ($A_m = b$) with probability $M_M = 1/2$. If the maternal allele is $A_m = a$, then the paternal allele A_p must be b. If the maternal allele is $A_m = b$, then the paternal allele must be a. The denominator is therefore the sum of two terms. Hence

$$\text{PI} = \frac{\frac{1}{4}}{\frac{1}{2}p_a + \frac{1}{2}p_b} = \frac{1}{2(p_a + p_b)}$$

There are 15 distinct combinations of maternal and paternal genotypes possible, but if we use the product rule to evaluate the PI, we find that the PI takes only four possible forms, depending on whether the alleged father is a homozygote or a heterozygote and whether or not the child's paternal allele can be unambiguously identified.[966] In Table 11.3 we tabulate the possible combination of mother, child and alleged father along with the PI formulae utilizing the product rule.

Paternity Duos: Child and Alleged Father

As usual we begin by considering at least two hypotheses. In the most common case these could be the following:

H_1: The alleged father is the true father (and the true mother's genotype is unknown).

H_2: A random person who is not related to the alleged father is the true father (and the true mother's genotype is unknown).

We require

$$\text{PI} = \frac{\Pr\left(G_C, G_{AF} \mid H_1\right)}{\Pr\left(G_C, G_{AF} \mid H_2\right)} = \frac{\Pr\left(G_C \mid G_{AF}, H_1\right)\Pr\left(G_{AF} \mid H_1\right)}{\Pr\left(G_C \mid G_{AF}, H_2\right)\Pr\left(G_{AF} \mid H_2\right)}$$

Table 11.3 Form of PI for All Non-Excluded Combinations of Maternal and Paternal Genotypes

Genotype Mother	Genotype Child	Genotype Alleged Father	PI (Alleged Father Is True Father)
aa	aa	aa	$\dfrac{1}{p_a}$
ab			
bb	ab		
bc			
aa	aa	ab	$\dfrac{1}{2p_a}$
ab			
ac			
bb	ab		
bc			
bc	ac		
cc			
cd			
ab	ab	aa	$\dfrac{1}{p_a+p_b}$
		ab	
		ac	$\dfrac{1}{2(p_a+p_b)}$

Source: Lee, H-S., et al., *Forensic Science International*, 114, 57–65, 2000.

Next it is customary to assume $\Pr(G_{AF}|H_1) = \Pr(G_{AF}|H_2)$, hence

$$PI = \frac{\Pr\left(G_C|G_{AF},H_1\right)}{\Pr\left(G_C|G_{AF},H_2\right)}$$

This assumption is essentially stating that the genotype of the alleged father is unconditional on whether the alleged father is the true father or not. Evaluation of the PI proceeds directly from this equation.

If we assume allelic independence between people, we can write

$$PI = \frac{\Pr\left(G_C|G_{AF},H_1\right)}{\Pr\left(G_C|G_{AF},H_2\right)} = \frac{\Pr\left(G_C|G_{AF},H_1\right)}{\Pr\left(G_C|H_2\right)}$$

In Example 11.4 we give an example using the assumption of independence; a compilation of formulae appears in Table 11.4.

Table 11.4   Form of PI for All Non-Excluded Combinations of Paternal and Child Genotypes

Genotype of Child	Genotype of Alleged Father	PI (Alleged Father Is True Father)
aa	aa	$\dfrac{1}{p_a}$
aa	ab	$\dfrac{1}{2p_a}$
ab	aa	
ab	ab	$\dfrac{p_a + p_b}{4 p_a p_b}$
ab	ac	$\dfrac{1}{4 p_a}$

Note: We agree with Lee et al.[966]

Example 11.4: An Example of a Paternity Duo

	Genotype
Child	ab
Alleged father	ac

Under H_1 we assume that the alleged father is the true father. As the genotype of the true mother is unknown we cannot use a Punnett square to evaluate the numerator of the PI. It is easier to proceed by noting that the paternal allele under H_1 is a and this will be passed 1/2 of the time. Then the maternal allele (under H_1) must be b. We assign the probability $\Pr(b) = p_b$ to the event of this coming from a random person as before.

Under H_2 and the assumption of independence we see that we require the probability of the child's genotype but have neither the genotype of the true mother nor the true father to help us determine this. We assign the probability of this event as $\Pr(G_C = ab|H_2) = 2p_a p_b$, which is the product rule assignment for this genotype. Hence

$$\text{PI} = \frac{\frac{1}{2} p_b}{2 p_a p_b} = \frac{1}{4 p_a}$$

When the product rule is used to evaluate the case of a child/alleged father duo, the PI takes one of the four possible forms (set out in Table 11.4).

Linked Loci

Consider a paternity trio with a pair of linked loci (A and B). We consider the situation where these loci have recombination fractions R_F and R_M for the female and male, respectively. Label the parental alleles as shown in Figure 11.3.

We consider the phase of M and F to be unknown. In other words we do not know whether the A_3 and B_3 alleles in the mother are on the same chromosome or not. We assume that each phase is equiprobable. We ask the question, what is the chance that the mother will pass A_3, B_3? Label the two possible phases P_1 and P_2. In P_1 the A_3 and B_3 are on the same chromosome; in P_2 they are on different chromosomes.

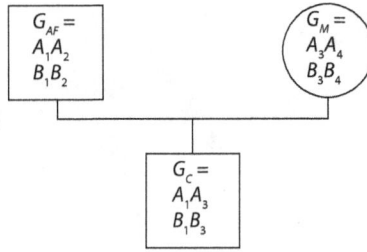

Figure 11.3   A paternity trio with two linked loci.

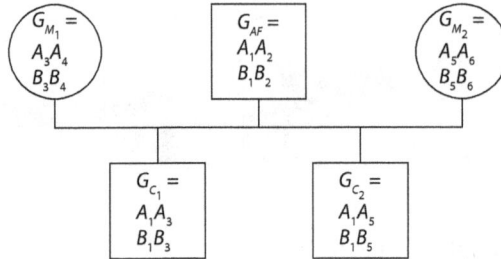

Figure 11.4   A pedigree involving multiple meioses of the same chromosome.

To pass the A_3,B_3 set we require that one of the following events occur:

P_1 *and* no recombination *and* this chromosome (of the two) chosen

P_2 *and* recombination *and* this chromosome (of the two post-recombination) chosen

This suggests that $\frac{1}{2}(1-R_F)\frac{1}{2}+\frac{1}{2}(R_F)\frac{1}{2}=\frac{1}{4}$, which is equal to the maternal Mendelian factor for two unlinked loci. The same result occurs for the male. This result holds true as long as each chromosome is only involved in one meiosis. The conclusion is that no correction for linked loci is necessary as long as we are only considering sets of single meioses (as in all trios and duos).[*]

For more complex pedigrees there is an effect, such as that shown in Figure 11.4. Consider the following hypotheses:

H_1: The alleged father (AF) is the father of C_2.

H_2: A random man is the father of C_2.

We again assume that the phases of the parents, M_1, M_2 and AF, are unknown. The two mothers are each involved in only one meiosis and hence we can use the result, given above, that their Mendelian factor for two loci will be the same as the unlinked factor. However the alleged father is involved in multiple meioses and hence there is an effect of linkage. Hence we will consider P_1^{AF} to be Phase 1 for AF and P_2^{AF} to be Phase 2 for AF. We arbitrarily assign P_1^{AF} to be the phase with A_1,B_1 on the same chromosome. Hence P_2^{AF} is the phase with A_1,B_2 on the same chromosome.

Consider

$$\Pr\left(C_1,C_2\mid M_1,M_2,AF,H_1\right)=\Pr\left(C_1,C_2\mid M_1,M_2,AF,P_1^{AF},H_1\right)\Pr\left(P_1^{AF}\right)$$
$$+\Pr\left(C_1,C_2\mid M_1,M_2,AF,P_2^{AF},H_1\right)\Pr\left(P_2^{AF}\right)$$

---

[*] Dr Charles Brenner made us aware of this fact.

Assuming, as before, that $P_1^{AF} = P_2^{AF} = 1/2$

$$\Pr(C_1,C_2 \mid M_1,M_2,AF,H_1) = \frac{\Pr(C_1,C_2 \mid M_1,M_2,AF,P_1^{AF},H_1) + \Pr(C_1,C_2 \mid M_1,M_2,AF,P_2^{AF},H_1)}{2}$$

Considering the recombination fraction we obtain

$$\Pr(C_1,C_2 \mid M_1,M_2,AF,H_1) = \frac{\dfrac{1}{4}\dfrac{(1-R_M)}{2}\dfrac{1}{4}\dfrac{(1-R_M)}{2} + \dfrac{1}{4}\dfrac{R_M}{2}\dfrac{1}{4}\dfrac{R_M}{2}}{2} = \frac{(1-R_M)^2 + R_M^2}{32}$$

For unlinked loci we have

$$\Pr(C_1,C_2 \mid M_1,M_2,AF,H_p) = \tfrac{1}{64}$$

which is equivalent to setting $R_M = \tfrac{1}{2}$ in the above equation.

As a numerical example consider the pair of linked CODIS loci CSF1PO and D5S818, which are reported to be separated by 25 centiMorgans (cM).[967] Using Haldane's distance this suggests a recombination fraction of 0.197.

$\Pr(C_1, C_2|M_1, M_2, AF, H_1) = 0.021$ as compared with 0.016 if we do not consider the linkage. We see that the effect of linkage at this distance (25 cM) is moderate.

Paternally Imprinted Alleles

Techniques are available that allow the identification of the paternal allele.[17] This requires no modification to our general approach but does cause some differences in detail. When the child's *maternal* allele can be determined unambiguously the PI in this situation is unchanged. When the child shares the same genotype as the mother the additional information provided by knowledge of the paternal allele leads to simpler formulae for the PI. We reproduce the table for the paternity trios using the product rule but accounting for knowledge of the paternal allele (Table 11.5).

Molar Paternity
Molar Paternity Complete*
A *complete mole* describes a clump of cells that grows in the uterus resulting from a fertilized egg that contained no maternal DNA. The sperm duplicates and forms the full complement of 46 chromosomes. The genotype at the gomosomes is usually XX but XY is also known.

The genotype of the tissue shows a simple peak at every locus.
Consider the following propositions:

H_1: The POI is the donor of the sperm that caused the mole.

H_2: An unknown man is the donor of the sperm that caused the mole.

Following Sliter the PI is assigned as shown in Table 11.6.

Molar Paternity Partial
A *partial mole* occurs when an egg carrying maternal DNA is fertilized by two sperm or by one sperm which reduplicates itself, yielding triploid or tetraploid genotypes.
Consider the following propositions:

H_1: The POI is the donor of the sperm that caused the mole.

H_2: An unknown man is the donor of the sperm that caused the mole.

---

* This subject and the mathematical solution were brought to our attention by Timothy J. Sliter, PhD, Section Chief – Physical Evidence, Dallas County Southwestern Institute of Forensic Sciences, Dallas, Texas, USA.

Table 11.5 Form of the PI for All Non-Excluded Trios Accounting for Knowledge of the Paternal Allele

Genotype Mother	Genotype Child	Genotype Alleged Father	PI (Alleged Father Is True Father)
aa	aa	aa	$\dfrac{1}{p_a}$
ab			
bb	ab		
bc			
aa	aa	ab	$\dfrac{1}{2p_a}$
ab			
ac			
bb	ab		
bc			
bc	ac		
cc			
cd			
ab	ab	aa	$\dfrac{1}{p_a}$
		ab	$\dfrac{1}{2p_a}$
		ac	

Note: The paternal allele is marked in bold.
PI, paternity index.

Table 11.6 Form of PI for All Non-Excluded Duos of Alleged Father and a Complete Molar Pregnancy

Genotype of AF	Genotype of Mole	PI
aa	aa	$\dfrac{1}{p_a}$
ab	aa	$\dfrac{1}{2p_a}$

PI, paternity index; AF, alleged father.

We assume that double-dose chromosomes can be detected from peak height. Following Sliter the PI is assigned as shown in Table 11.7.

Non-Autosomal DNA Markers
Y Chromosome Analysis
The Y chromosome is inherited patrilinearly and for most of its length does not recombine. Since there is no maternal allele, paternity duos and trios are treated in the same way. If the effect of mutation is ignored, even cases where the alleged father is untyped and a more distant paternal

Table 11.7   Form of PI for All Non-Excluded Duos of Alleged Father and a Complete Molar Pregnancy

Genotype of AF	Genotype of Mole	Genotype of Mother	PI
aa	aab	bb	$\dfrac{2}{p_a(1+p_a)}$
aa	aab	bc	$\dfrac{1}{p_a(1+p_a)}$
ab	aac	cc	$\dfrac{1}{2p_a(1+p_a)}$
ab	abc	cc	$\dfrac{1}{2p_ap_b}$

PI, paternity index; AF, alleged father.

relative is used as the reference sample lead to the same formula. The PI has a very simple form. Consider a mother/alleged father/child trio, an alleged father/child duo and an alleged paternal relative/child duo. In each case we assume an exact match of the haplotype of the Y chromosome between the alleged father or the paternal relative and the child under hypothesis H_1.

The exclusion probability is PE = $(1 - f)$, where f is the probability of observing the child's (and alleged father's) haplotype. For the PI we need to assess

$$PI = \frac{\Pr(G_C|G_{AF},H_1)}{\Pr(G_C|G_{AF},H_2)} = \frac{1}{f}$$

This formula does not account for mutation.[968]

X Chromosome Analysis

The X chromosome does not recombine in the father. Again paternity duos and trios and the use of more distant paternal relatives lead to the same formulae. Consider again a mother/alleged father/child trio, an alleged father/child duo and an alleged paternal relative/child duo. In each case we assume an exact match of the haplotype of the paternal X chromosome between the alleged father or the paternal relative and the child under the hypothesis H_1.

The exclusion probability is PE = $(1 - f)$, where f is the probability of observing the child's (and alleged father's) haplotype.

As usual we assess

$$PI = \frac{\Pr(G_C|G_{AF},H_1)}{\Pr(G_C|G_{AF},H_2)}$$

We use the same reasoning for the X and Y chromosomes so, ignoring the possibility of mutation, PI = $\frac{1}{f}$, where f is the probability of observing the child's multilocus X chromosomal type. We speculate that this frequency may be approximated as the product of single locus frequencies since recombination does occur in the female. Recall that linkage does not necessarily imply linkage disequilibrium (see Chapter 3). Szibor et al.[951] noted one instance in which they observed linkage disequilibrium among 16 loci in a set of 210 males. This result suggests that sufficient recombination occurs to bring the frequencies close to equilibrium expectations in this population. It is likely that the same modelling considerations given to autosomal DNA may apply to a large extent for the X chromosome. However more and larger studies would be welcome.

Maternity Analysis for X Chromosomes

In rare circumstances we may be required to consider a pedigree analysis where it is the mother whose parentage is under question. In such a case the linkage of the loci on the X chromosome will need to be considered. However since we cannot tell the phase of the mother the finding given above applies in the case of a single meiosis.

The exclusion probability calculation is analogous to autosomal DNA. The calculation of the PI makes use of the unknown phase of the mother and hence applies a factor of 1/2 per heterozygotic locus. Again ignoring the possibility of mutation $PI = \dfrac{1}{2^N f}$, where f is the multilocus genotype probability of the child's X chromosome and N is the number of heterozygotic X chromosome loci considered.

Mitochondrial DNA Analysis

For forensic purposes we typically assume that mitochondrial DNA is matrilineally inherited without recombination. Therefore it is of use in parentage testing only when the parentage of the mother is in question. The development and formulae are the same as for the Y chromosome and for paternity testing with the X chromosome. As in these cases each of child/father/alleged mother trios, alleged mother/child duos and duos incorporating a maternal relative yield the same result if mutation is ignored.

Following the Y chromosome analysis given above and assuming an exact match between the alleged mother and the child the exclusion probability is $PE = (1 - f)$ and the PI is $PI = \dfrac{1}{f}$, where f is the probability of observing the child's (and alleged mother's) mtDNA haplotype.

Use of the Subpopulation Model

Using the subpopulation model of Balding and Nichols[358,453,455,966,969] the evaluation of $\Pr(A_p|G_M, G_{AF}, H_1)$ for a paternity trio proceeds as we have outlined above. The probability of observing the paternal allele from an alternative donor in the same subpopulation may be affected by the genotypes of the mother and the alleged father. Hence in general $\Pr(A_p|G_M, G_{AF}, H_2) \neq \Pr(A_p|H_2)$.

A relatively easy way to evaluate the PI in this situation is to write the term containing the paternal allele $\Pr(A_p|G_M, G_{AF}, H_2)$ as the probability of the paternal allele conditioned on the correct selection of conditioning alleles. If we consider that both the mother and alleged father are not related and in the same subpopulation as the true father, then we condition on four alleles, those of the mother and alleged father. Equally if we consider the true father to belong to the same subpopulation as the alleged father but not that of the mother, then we condition on the two alleles of the alleged father. If we consider the true father to belong to the subpopulation of neither the mother nor the alleged father, then we condition on no alleles and the product rule is appropriate. Once again we will illustrate the implementation of this approach through a series of worked examples.

Example 11.5: A Paternity Trio Demonstrating Application of the Balding and Nichols Formulae

Consider the same trio of genotypes as in Example 11.1.

	Genotype
Mother	cd
Child	ac
Alleged father	ab

Under H_2 we can see that the mother is heterozygotic for the maternal allele ($A_m = c$) and we can assign the value $M_M = 1/2$ to the mother's Mendelian factor. The paternal allele is $A_p = a$. Assuming that we are going to condition on the genotypes of both the mother and the alleged father we write the probability $\Pr(A_p|G_M,G_{AF},H_2)$ as $\Pr(a|abcd)$. The procedure for evaluation of this term follows the same approach as described in Chapter 8 on mixtures. Here we reproduce some of the 'shortcut' rules for evaluating these terms.

SHORTCUT RULES

1. Replace each of the paternal allele frequencies with one of these terms.

1st allele a	$(1 - \theta)p_a$
2nd allele a	$\theta + (1 - \theta)p_a$
3rd allele a	$2\theta + (1 - \theta)p_a$
4th allele a	$3\theta + (1 - \theta)p_a$
.....	
nth allele	$(n - 1)\theta + (1 - \theta)p_a$

2. Divide by a correction term based on the number of alleles behind the conditioning bar.

2 behind	$(1 + \theta)$
4 behind	$(1 + 3\theta)$
6 behind	$(1 + 5\theta)$
...	
M behind	$(1 + (M - 1)\theta)$

In Example 11.5 we condition one copy of each of the four alleles, a, b, c and d. Thus PI becomes

$$\text{PI} = \frac{\frac{1}{4}}{\frac{1}{2} \times \Pr\left(a \,|\, abcd\right)}$$

$$= \frac{1}{2\Pr\left(a \,|\, abcd\right)}$$

$$= \frac{1+3\theta}{2\left(\theta + (1-\theta)p_a\right)}$$

Example 11.6: A Paternity Trio Demonstrating Application of the Balding and Nichols Formulae

Consider the following trio:

	Genotype
Mother	bc
Child	ab
Alleged father	aa

Under H_2 we can see that the mother is heterozygotic for the maternal allele ($A_m = b$) and we can assign the value $M_M = 1/2$ to the mother's Mendelian factor. The paternal allele is $A_p = a$ and under H_2 we condition on having observed two copies of the paternal allele from among the four alleles observed from this subpopulation. We write the conditional probability for this as $\Pr(a|aabc)$. Hence

$$PI = \frac{\frac{1}{2}}{\frac{1}{2} \times \Pr\left(a|aabc\right)}$$

$$= \frac{1}{\Pr\left(a|aabc\right)}$$

$$= \frac{1+3\theta}{2\theta+(1-\theta)p_a}$$

In Example 11.7 we consider the same set of trios as in Example 11.6, but in addition we assume that the mother comes from a different subpopulation than the alleged and true fathers.

Example 11.7: A Paternity Trio Demonstrating Application of the Balding and Nichols Formulae

Consider the following trio of genotypes:

	Genotype
Mother	bc
Child	ab
Alleged father	aa

The maternal and paternal alleles and their Mendelian factors are as described above. Under H_2 we condition on having observed two copies of the paternal allele from among a total of only two alleles from the same subpopulation as opposed to four. We write the conditional probability for this as $\Pr(a|aa)$. Hence

$$PI = \frac{\frac{1}{2}}{\frac{1}{2} \times \Pr\left(a|aa\right)}$$

$$= \frac{1}{\Pr\left(a|aa\right)}$$

$$= \frac{1+\theta}{2\theta+(1-\theta)p_a}$$

In Tables 11.8, 11.9 and 11.10 we give tables that allow the calculation of the PI for paternity trios and duos under situations where the mother is a member of the same subpopulation as the alleged and true fathers and also for situations when she is in a different subpopulation or race. We have considered whether we should change from mother and putative father to 'known parent' and 'putative parent' but have not adopted this change.

Drábek[970,971] reviews software that performs these and other calculations.

Table 11.8 *LR* for Calculation of the Paternity Index for Trios and Duos			
Genotype of Mother	**Genotype of Child**	**Genotype of Putative Father**	**LR**
aa	aa	aa	$\dfrac{1}{P_{a|X}}$
ab			
bb	ab		
bc			
aa	aa	ab	$\dfrac{1}{2P_{a|X}}$
ab			$\dfrac{1}{P_{a|X}}$
ac			
bb	ab		$\dfrac{1}{2P_{a|X}}$
bc			
bc	ac		
cc			
cd			
ab	ab	aa	$\dfrac{1}{P_{a|X}+P_{b|X}}$
		ab	
		ac	$\dfrac{1}{2\left(P_{a|X}+P_{b|X}\right)}$

LR, likelihood ratio.

Relatedness

We envisage three potential situations where relatedness must be considered in the course of a parentage testing case:

1. A person is alleged to be the father of a child but his genotype is not available (due to death for instance) and the paternity analysis proceeds using the genotypes of the mother, the child and the alleged father's relatives.

2. A plausible alternative father is a relative of the accused man.

3. The alleged father and mother are related (incest).

The structure for solving these problems is based on three-allele descent measures as demonstrated by Weir[257,424] (see also Berry and Geisser[972] or Brenner[484]). It is often possible to assume that neither the alleged father nor the mother are inbred and this reduces the complexity of the problem considerably. In such cases it is possible to deal with a single factor, θ', (θ_{AT} in Weir). This factor θ' is very similar to the factor θ discussed in Chapter 3 in that it is a two-allele measure giving the probability that the paternal allele and a random allele from the alleged father (or a genotyped person) are identical by descent (IBD).

Table 11.9 The Form of the Term X for Table 11.8

Genotype of Mother	Genotype of Putative Father	X of Mother and Putative Father	X of Putative Father
aa	aa	aaaa	aa
ab		aaab	
bb		aabb	
bc		aabc	
aa	ab	aaab	ab
ab		aabb	
ac		aabc	
bb		abbb	
bc		abbc	
cc		abcc	
cd		abcd	
ab	aa	aaab	aa
	ab	aabb	ab
	ac	aabc	ac

Table 11.10 The Conditional Probabilities for Table 11.8

X	$P_{a|X}$	
aaaa	$4\theta + (1 - \theta)P_a$	$\Big/(1+3\theta)$
aaab	$3\theta + (1 - \theta)P_a$	
aabb	$2\theta + (1 - \theta)P_a$	
aabc		
abbb	$\theta + (1 - \theta)P_a$	
abbc		
abcc		
abcd		
aa	$2\theta + (1 - \theta)P_a$	$\Big/(1+\theta)$
ab	$\theta + (1 - \theta)P_a$	
ac		
None	P_a	
	$P_{b|X}$	
aaab	$\theta + (1 - \theta)P_b$	$\Big/(1+3\theta)$
aabb	$2\theta + (1 - \theta)P_b$	
aabc	$\theta + (1 - \theta)P_b$	
aa	$(1 - \theta)P_b$	$\Big/(1+\theta)$
ab	$\theta + (1 - \theta)P_b$	
ac	$(1 - \theta)P_b$	
None	P_b	

Relationship	θ'
Siblings, parent/child	1/4
Uncle/nephew, grandparent/grandchild, half-siblings	1/8
Cousins	1/16

A Relative of the Accused Is Suggested as the Alleged Father

Consider a situation where the accused man (previously called the *alleged father*) puts forward the suggestion that his brother is the father of the child (hence, under H_2, the brother is the alleged father). Thus the pair of hypotheses being considered are as follows:

H_1: The accused man is the father of the child in question.

H_2: The brother of the accused man is the father of the child in question.

Let the genotype of the accused man be G_{AF} as before. Under H_2 we require the probability that the paternal allele A_p is a certain allele given the genotype, G_{AF}, of the brother of the donor of this allele. This requires us to consider IBD states between one allele from each of two brothers (or other relatives). Unlike the situation described in Chapter 4 the fact that two siblings may share two pairs of alleles does not cause extra complexity here.

Consider the situation where $G_M = cc$, $G_C = ac$ and $G_{AF} = ab$. We see that under both hypotheses, H_1 and H_2, the paternal allele can be unambiguously identified as $A_p = a$. We require the probability that $A_p = a$ given the fact that $G_{AF} = ab$ and given that the donor of the paternal allele is the brother (G_B) of the accused. There are four states that can occur:

1. G_B and G_{AF} possess two IBD alleles (with probability 1/4).

2. G_B and G_{AF} possess the first IBD allele, a (with probability 1/4).

3. G_B and G_{AF} possess the second IBD allele, b (with probability 1/4).

4. G_B and G_{AF} do not possess any IBD alleles (with probability 1/4).

Thus

In State 1, $\Pr(G_B = ab) = 1$ and G_B will pass along A_p with probability 1/2.

In State 2, $\Pr(G_B = ab) = p_b$ and G_B will pass along A_p with probability 1/2.
$\Pr(G_B = aa) = p_a$ and G_B will pass along A_p with probability 1.
$\Pr(G_B = aQ) = p_Q$ and G_B will pass along A_p with probability 1/2.

In State 3, $\Pr(G_B = ab) = p_a$ and G_B will pass along A_p with probability 1/2.

In State 4, $\Pr(G_B = ab) = 2p_a p_b$ and G_B will pass along A_p with probability 1/2.
$\Pr(G_B = aa) = p_a^2$ and G_B will pass along A_p with probability 1.
$\Pr(G_B = aQ) = 2p_a p_Q$ and G_B will pass along A_p with probability 1/2.

Hence $\Pr(A_p = a | G_{AF} = ab$ and $G_M = cc$ and $G_B = true\ father)$

$$= \frac{1}{4}\left[\frac{1}{2}\right] + \frac{1}{4}\left[\frac{p_b}{2} + p_a + \frac{p_Q}{2}\right] + \frac{1}{4}\left[\frac{p_a}{2}\right] + \frac{1}{4}\left[\frac{2p_a p_b}{2} + p_a^2 + \frac{2p_a p_Q}{2}\right]$$

$$= \frac{1}{8} + \frac{1}{8} + \frac{p_a}{8} + \frac{p_a}{8} + \frac{p_a}{4}$$

This is $\dfrac{1}{4}+\dfrac{p_a}{2}$ (or using the θ' values above $\theta'+(1-2\theta')P_{a|X}$), whereas under the assumption that the mother and the accused come from the same subpopulation

$$\Pr\left(A_p=a|G_{AF}=ab,G_M=cc\right)=\frac{1}{4}+\frac{\Pr\left(a|abcc\right)}{2}=\frac{1}{4}+\frac{1}{2}\frac{\theta+(1-\theta)p_a}{1+3\theta}*$$

We can calculate the probability in the numerator of the PI using Mendelian factors $\Pr\left(G_C|G_{AF},G_M,H_1\right)=\frac{1}{2}$. In all other relationship types considered (without inbreeding) there is no opportunity for both alleles to be IBD. Hence there is a possibility for an IBD allele with the relative to be the paternal allele in G_{AF}, a possibility for an IBD allele with the relative to be the non-paternal allele in G_{AF} and a possibility that neither allele in the relatives will be IBD (excluding parents/children who must possess at least one IBD allele). Hence a general formulation for the PI can be obtained as

$$PI=\frac{M_M}{(3-x)\left[x\theta'+(1-2\theta')P_{a|X}\right]}$$

where x is 1 or 2 depending on whether G_{AF} is heterozygous or homozygous for the paternal allele, respectively. The only exception to this is when the paternal allele is in question, i.e. in the case where $G_M=ab$, $G_C=ab$ and $G_{AF}=ab$, in which case the PI is obtained by the formula

$$PI=\frac{1}{2\theta'+(1-2\theta')\left(P_{a|X}+P_{b|X}\right)}$$

We provide a tabulated version of all formulae in Tables 11.11 and 11.12 for ease of reference.

Deficient Paternity Analysis (The Alleged Father Is Unavailable)
We envisage a situation where the alleged father is unavailable but where, for example, his brother is. In such a case the two hypotheses may be of the form

H_1: The person, X, is a sibling of the true father.

H_2: The person, X, is unrelated to the child.[†]

The evaluation of the probability in the denominator of the PI, $\Pr(G_C|G_X, G_M, H_2)$, is the same as for a paternity trio illustrated earlier since under H_2, person X is unrelated to the child.

In this case it is the numerator, $\Pr(G_C|G_X,G_M,H_1)$, that is not a product of simple Mendelian factors. Recall that the probability that a random allele from X will be IBD with an allele from AF is θ'. Under H_1, the paternal allele is a random choice from AF, and hence with probability θ' it will be IBD with a random allele from X. This gives a relatively straightforward structure for calculating the PI for any situation. Consider $G_M=cd$, $G_C=ac$ and $G_X=ab$. The maternal Mendelian factor $M_M=1/2$. Under H_1 the person X is a sibling of the father.

There are three cases to consider:

A_p is IBD with the a allele of X (with probability 1/4).

A_p is IBD with the b allele of X (probability 1/4).

A_p is not IBD with either allele of X (probability 1/2).

---

[*] Please note that we are conditioning on both the genotypes of the alleged father and the mother of the child. Other conditioning may be appropriate in certain cases.

[†] The conventional additional assumption is made that the genotype of the true mother is known and is common to both H_1 and H_2 but not explicitly stated.

Table 11.11   The *LR* for Trios when H_2 Is a Relative

Genotype of Mother	Genotype of Child	Genotype of Putative Father	LR
aa	aa	aa	$\dfrac{1}{2\theta' + (1-2\theta')P_{a|X}}$
ab bc	ab		$\dfrac{1}{2(2\theta' + (1-2\theta')P_{a|X})}$
ab	aa	ab	$\dfrac{1}{4(\theta' + (1-2\theta')P_{a|X})}$
ac			$\dfrac{1}{2(\theta' + (1-2\theta')P_{a|X})}$
aa bc	ab		
bc cd	ac		$\dfrac{1}{4(\theta' + (1-2\theta')P_{a|X})}$
cc			$\dfrac{1}{2(\theta' + (1-2\theta')P_{a|X})}$
ab	ab	aa	$\dfrac{1}{2(2\theta' + (1-2\theta')P_{a|X})}$
		ab	$\dfrac{1}{2\theta' + (1-2\theta')(P_{a|X} + P_{b|X})}$
		ac	$\dfrac{1}{4(\theta' + (1-2\theta')P_{a|X})}$

LR, likelihood ratio.

Table 11.12   The *LR* for Duos when H_2 Is a Relative

Genotype of Child	Genotype of Putative Father	LR[a]
aa	aa	$\dfrac{1}{2\theta' + (1-2\theta')P_{a|X}}$
ab		$\dfrac{P_b}{(2\theta' + (1-2\theta')P_{a|X})P_b + (1-2\theta')P_{b|X}P_a}$
aa	ab	$\dfrac{1}{\theta' + (1-2\theta')P_{a|X}}$
ab		$\dfrac{P_a + P_b}{2(\theta' + (1-2\theta')P_{a|X})P_b + 2(\theta' + (1-2\theta')P_{b|X})P_a}$
ac		$\dfrac{1}{\theta' + (1-2\theta')P_{a|X}}$

[a] Conditioning alleles for the father's side = *X*.

If

A_p is IBD with the a allele of AF, then it should always be type a: $\text{Pr}(A_p = a) = 1$.

A_p is IBD with the b allele of AF then it should never be type a: $\text{Pr}(A_p = a) = 0$.

A_p is not IBD with either allele of AF then it is a random allele: $\text{Pr}(A_p = a) = \text{Pr}(a|abcd)$.[*]

Hence

$$\text{Pr}\left(G_C \mid G_X, G_M, H_1\right) = M_M \times \left(\frac{1}{4} + \frac{\text{Pr}(a|abcd)}{2}\right)$$

and so

$$\text{PI} = \frac{M_M \times \left(\dfrac{1}{4} + \dfrac{\text{Pr}(a|abcd)}{2}\right)}{M_M \times \text{Pr}(a|abcd)} = \frac{1 + 2\text{Pr}(a|abcd)}{4\text{Pr}(a|abcd)}$$

Making the assumption of independence $\text{PI} = \dfrac{1 + 2p_a}{4p_a}$ and under the assumption that the mother and the alleged father are from the same subpopulation:

$$\text{PI} = \frac{1 + 5\theta + 2(1-\theta)p_a}{4\left[\theta + (1-\theta)p_a\right]}$$

The Alleged Father and Mother Are Related

We have come across cases of alleged incest where standard paternity trio propositions are used:

H_1: The alleged father (AF) is the father of the child (C).

H_2: A random man is the father of the child (C).

The added complexity is that the alleged father is a relative of the mother. In these instances a consideration of relatedness needs to be taken into account if the subpopulation model is being considered, as the information that is conditioned on will depend on which alleles in the mother and alleged father are IBD. For these calculations it is the posterior probability of alleles being IBD that is required, as the relationship between the mother and alleged father is accepted by both parties.

Consider an example where the alleged father is a sibling of the mother. In this calculation we will need the posterior probability of a number of alleles being IBD to give the genotypes of the two siblings, S_1 and S_2. For siblings the prior probability that zero, one or two alleles are IBD (written as Z_0, Z_1 and Z_2) is 1/4, 1/2 and 1/4 respectively. The single IBD allele scenario can then be split into the first and second alleles (Z_{1A} and Z_{1B}), which both have a prior probability of 1/4.

There are a number combinations of genotypes that the siblings can have in this scenario, for which the posterior probabilities of Z_0, Z_1 and Z_2 must be calculated. Consider the instance where the evidence (E) is $G_M = aa$ and $G_{AF} = aa$.

---

[*] Please note that we are only conditioning on the genotypes of the uncle and the mother. Other conditioning may be appropriate in certain cases.

For zero alleles IBD:

$$\Pr(Z_0|E) = \frac{\Pr(E|Z_0)\Pr(Z_0)}{\Pr(E)} = \frac{\Pr(E|Z_0)\Pr(Z_0)}{\sum_i \Pr(E|Z_i)\Pr(Z_i)}$$

$$= \frac{p_a^4 \times \frac{1}{4}}{\frac{1}{4} \times p_a^4 + \frac{1}{2} \times p_a^3 + \frac{1}{4} \times p_a^2} = \frac{p_a^2}{p_a^2 + 2p_a + 1} = \frac{p_a^2}{(p_a+1)^2}$$

Similarly for one-allele IBD:

$$\Pr(Z_1|E) = \frac{p_a^3 \times \frac{1}{4} + p_a^3 \times \frac{1}{4}}{\frac{1}{4} \times p_a^4 + \frac{1}{2} \times p_a^3 + \frac{1}{4} \times p_a^2} = \frac{2p_a}{p_a^2 + 2p_a + 1} = \frac{2p_a}{(p_a+1)^2}$$

And for two-allele IBD:

$$\Pr(Z_2|E) = \frac{p_a^2 \times \frac{1}{4}}{\frac{1}{4} \times p_a^4 + \frac{1}{2} \times p_a^3 + \frac{1}{4} \times p_a^2} = \frac{1}{p_a^2 + 2p_a + 1} = \frac{1}{(p_a+1)^2}$$

Table 11.13 shows the posterior probabilities for the IBD states of two individuals who are siblings.

Note that the posterior probabilities given in Table 11.13 have not incorporated a coancestry coefficient. Such an adjustment could be included in the posterior probabilities; however it would significantly increase complexity and is likely to have very little effect on the *LR* value that these probabilities are being applied to.

Table 11.13		Posterior Probability for IBD of Siblings		
G_{S_1}	G_{S_1}	$\Pr(Z_0|E)$	$\Pr(Z_1|E)$	$\Pr(Z_2|E)$
aa	aa	$\dfrac{p_a^2}{(p_a+1)^2}$	$\dfrac{2p_a}{(p_a+1)^2}$	$\dfrac{1}{(p_a+1)^2}$
aa	ab	$\dfrac{p_a}{p_a+1}$	$\dfrac{1}{p_a+1}$	0
aa	bb	1	0	0
aa	bc	1	0	0
ab	ab	$\dfrac{p_a p_b}{p_a p_b + p_a + p_b + 1}$	$\dfrac{p_a \text{ or } p_b}{p_a p_b + p_a + p_b + 1}$	$\dfrac{1}{p_a p_b + p_a + p_b + 1}$
ab	ac	$\dfrac{p_a}{p_a+1}$	$\dfrac{1}{p_a+1}$	0
ab	cc	1	0	0
ab	cd	1	0	0

IBD, identical by descent.

If we now consider the PI calculation for the scenario $G_M = aa$, $G_C = aa$ and $G_{AF} = aa$

$$Pr(G_C|G_{AF},G_M,H_1) = 1$$

$$Pr(G_C|G_M, G_{AF}, H_2) = Pr(Z_0|E)Pr(a|aaaa) + Pr(Z_1|E)Pr(a|aaa) + Pr(Z_2|E)\,Pr(a|aa)$$

$$= \left[\frac{p_a^2}{(p_a+1)^2}\right]\left(\frac{4\theta+(1-\theta)p_a}{1+3\theta}\right)$$

$$+ \left[\frac{2p_a}{(p_a+1)^2}\right]\left(\frac{3\theta+(1-\theta)p_a}{1+2\theta}\right) + \left[\frac{1}{(p_a+1)^2}\right]\left(\frac{2\theta+(1-\theta)p_a}{1+\theta}\right)$$

Putting these two together gives the PI:

$$PI = \frac{(1+3\theta)(1+2\theta)(1+\theta)(p_a+1)^2}{\begin{bmatrix}p_a^2\left[4\theta+(1-\theta)p_a\right](1+2\theta)(1+\theta)\\ +2p_a\left[3\theta+(1-\theta)p_a\right](1+3\theta)(1+\theta)\\ \left[+2\theta+(1-\theta)p_a\right](1+2\theta)(1+3\theta)\end{bmatrix}}$$

In Table 11.14 are the PI formulae for a paternity trio where the alleged father is a sibling of the mother.

G_M	G_C	G_{AF}	PI
aa		aa	$\dfrac{(1+3\theta)(1+2\theta)(1+\theta)(p_A+1)^2}{\begin{bmatrix}p_A^2\left[4\theta+(1-\theta)p_A\right](1+2\theta)(1+\theta)\\+2p_A\left[3\theta+(1-\theta)p_A\right](1+3\theta)(1+\theta)\\+\left[2\theta+(1-\theta)p_A\right](1+2\theta)(1+3\theta)\end{bmatrix}}$
ab	aa		$\dfrac{(1+2\theta)(1+3\theta)(p_A+1)}{\begin{bmatrix}p_A(1+2\theta)\left[3\theta+(1-\theta)p_A\right]\\+(1+3\theta)\left[2\theta+(1-\theta)p_A\right]\end{bmatrix}}$
ab			$\dfrac{(p_A+1)(1+2\theta)(1+3\theta)}{\begin{bmatrix}p_A(1+2\theta)\left[4\theta+(1-\theta)(p_A+p_B)\right]\\+(1+3\theta)\left[3\theta+(1-\theta)(p_A+p_B)\right]\end{bmatrix}}$
bb	ab		$\dfrac{1+3\theta}{2\theta+(1-\theta)p_A}$
bc			$\dfrac{1+3\theta}{2\left[2\theta+(1-\theta)p_A\right]}$

Table 11.14   PI Formulae for a Paternity Trio Where the Alleged Father Is a Sibling of the Mother

(Continued)

Table 11.14 *(Continued)* PI Formulae for a Paternity Trio Where the Alleged Father Is a Sibling of the Mother

G_M	G_C	G_{AF}	PI
aa		ab	$$\dfrac{(p_A+1)(1+2\theta)(1+3\theta)}{\left\{\begin{array}{l}2p_A\left[3\theta+(1-\theta)p_A\right](1+2\theta)\\ +2\left[2\theta+(1-\theta)p_A\right](1+3\theta)\end{array}\right\}}$$
ab	aa		$$\dfrac{\frac{1}{4}(p_Ap_B+p_A+p_B+1)(1+3\theta)(1+2\theta)(1+\theta)}{\left\{\begin{array}{l}p_Ap_B\left(2\theta+(1-\theta)p_A\right)(1+\theta)(1+2\theta)\\ +\left[\theta(2p_A+p_B)+(1-\theta)\left(p_A^2+p_Ap_B\right)\right](1+\theta)(1+3\theta)\\ +\left(\theta+(1-\theta)p_A\right)(1+2\theta)(1+3\theta)\end{array}\right\}}$$
ac			$$\dfrac{(p_A+1)(1+2\theta)(1+3\theta)}{\left\{\begin{array}{l}2p_A\left[2\theta+(1-\theta)p_A\right](1+2\theta)\\ +2\left[\theta+(1-\theta)p_A\right](1+3\theta)\end{array}\right\}}$$
ab	ab	ab	$$\dfrac{(p_Ap_B+p_A+p_B+1)(1+3\theta)(1+2\theta)(1+\theta)}{\left\{\begin{array}{l}p_Ap_B\left[4\theta+(1-\theta)(p_A+p_B)\right](1+2\theta)(1+\theta)\\ +(p_A+p_B)\left[3\theta+(1-\theta)(p_A+p_B)\right](1+3\theta)(1+\theta)\\ +\left[2\theta+(1-\theta)(p_A+p_B)\right](1+3\theta)(1+2\theta)\end{array}\right\}}$$
bb			$$\dfrac{(p_B+1)(1+2\theta)(1+3\theta)}{\left\{\begin{array}{l}2p_B\left[\theta+(1-\theta)p_A\right](1+2\theta)\\ +2\left[\theta+(1-\theta)p_A\right](1+3\theta)\end{array}\right\}}$$
bc			
ac			$$\dfrac{(p_A+1)(1+2\theta)(1+3\theta)}{\left\{\begin{array}{l}2p_A\left[3\theta+(1-\theta)(p_A+p_C)\right](1+2\theta)\\ +2\left[2\theta+(1-\theta)(p_A+p_C)\right](1+3\theta)\end{array}\right\}}$$
bc	ac		$$\dfrac{(p_B+1)(1+2\theta)(1+3\theta)}{\left\{\begin{array}{l}2p_B\left[\theta+(1-\theta)p_A\right](1+2\theta)\\ +2\left[\theta+(1-\theta)p_A\right](1+3\theta)\end{array}\right\}}$$
cc			$$\dfrac{1+3\theta}{2\left[\theta+(1-\theta)p_A\right]}$$
cd			

PI, paternity index.

Multiple Children

The approach outlined above does not work with more than one child if both children are to be considered together. This event rarely happens in criminal casework, but it does arise in immigration cases and provides an introduction to problems involving more complex pedigrees.

Consider a mother, M, alleged father, AF, N children $C_1 \ldots C_N$ and the following hypotheses:

H_1: The alleged father is the father of all the children (and the mother is the true mother).

H_2: The alleged father is the father of none of the children, but they all have the same father (and the mother is the true mother).

$$PI = \frac{\Pr(C_1 \ldots C_N, M, AF \mid H_1)}{\Pr(C_1 \ldots C_N, M, AF \mid H_2)}$$

For both hypotheses we require

$$= \frac{\Pr(C_1 \ldots C_N \mid M, AF, H_1)\Pr(M, AF \mid H_1)}{\Pr(C_1 \ldots C_N \mid M, AF, H_2)\Pr(M, AF \mid H_2)}$$

Assuming, as previously, that $\Pr(M, AF \mid H_1) = \Pr(M, AF \mid H_2)$ and after enumeration of all possible genotypes for the true father as $R_1 \ldots R_M$ we obtain the following:

$$PI = \frac{\Pr(C_1 \ldots C_N \mid M, AF, H_1)}{\displaystyle\sum_{i=1}^{M} \Pr(C_1 \ldots C_N \mid M, R_i, AF, H_2)\Pr(R_i \mid M, AF, H_2)} \tag{11.1}$$

If we make the assumption of independence between people

$$PI = \frac{\Pr(C_1 \ldots C_N \mid M, AF, H_1)}{\displaystyle\sum_{i=1}^{M} \Pr(C_1 \ldots C_N \mid M, R_i, H_2)\Pr(R_i \mid H_2)} \tag{11.2}$$

And with the assumption that given the genotypes of their parents the genotypes of the children are independent

$$PI = \frac{\displaystyle\prod_{j=1}^{N} \Pr(C_j \mid M, AF, H_1)}{\displaystyle\sum_{i=1}^{M} \Pr(R_i \mid H_2)\prod_{j=1}^{N} \Pr(C_j \mid M, R_i, H_2)}$$

In Example 11.8 we consider the situation with two children ($N = 2$).

Example 11.8: A Paternity Case with Two Children

	Genotype
Mother	cd
Child 1	ac
Child 2	ad
Alleged father	ab

$$\Pr(C_1, C_2 \mid M, AF, H_1) = \Pr(C_1 \mid M, AF, H_1) \times \Pr(C_2 \mid M, AF, H_1) = \tfrac{1}{4} \times \tfrac{1}{4} = \tfrac{1}{16}$$

This probability is the product of the Mendelian factors for each child. Under H_2 we see that the true father must have the a allele. Therefore we can restrict the possible candidates to those whose genotype, R_i, is either an aa homozygote or a heterozygote with a single copy of the a allele (aQ). Explicit use of this restriction is unnecessary but simplifies the calculation by suppressing many terms that ultimately turn out to be zero. We can set out the calculation for the denominator, $\Pr(C_1,C_2|M,AF,H_2)$, in a tabular form:

R_i	$\Pr(R_i|H_2)$	$\Pr(C_1,C_2|M,R_i,H_2)$	$\Pr(C_1,C_2|M,R_i,H_2) \times \Pr(R_i|H_2)$
aa	p_a^2	$\dfrac{1}{2}\times\dfrac{1}{2}=\dfrac{1}{4}$	$\dfrac{p_a^2}{4}$
aQ	$2p_a(1-p_a)$	$\dfrac{1}{4}\times\dfrac{1}{4}=\dfrac{1}{16}$	$\dfrac{p_a(1-p_a)}{8}$
		Sum	$\dfrac{p_a(1+p_a)}{8}$

In this table we make the assumption of independence (the product rule). The paternity index becomes $PI = \dfrac{1}{2p_a(1+p_a)}$. This expression may easily be extended to the subpopulation case by replacing the factors in the $\Pr(R_i|H_2)$ column with their subpopulation equivalents.

Mutation

A mutation is a change to the DNA sequence usually caused by an error during DNA replication at meiosis. Such a change will be transmitted to the next generation. Mutations can occur as either a single substitution in the nucleotide sequence (transition/transversion) or as deletions or insertions of tracts of DNA.

In 1912 Wilhelm Weinberg reported that children with short-limbed dwarfism were often the last-born children. Weinberg, correctly and with astonishing insight, suggested that this was due to a mutation. In 1955 Penrose showed that the effect observed by Weinberg was due to paternal age, not maternal age or birth order. These observations have led to the recognition of the phenomenon of the effect of paternal age on mutation rate. However this may not be as simple as initially envisaged. Direct examinations of sperm suggest only a small increase in the number of mutant sperm, many fewer than expected from clinical data. Crow[973] reviews the current knowledge and suggests that there are three classes of gene mutation:

- Nucleotide substitutions scattered along the gene, usually with substantial sex and age effects

- Small insertions and deletions, mainly deletions, with no age effect and a slight maternal excess

- Hotspots occurring almost exclusively in males and rising steeply with age

Crow also reviews the evidence for and against pre-mitotic selection (the preferential selection of mutant spermatogonia before the two cell divisions that give rise to sperm).

STR loci are particularly prone to mutation compared with coding sequences or non-coding and non-repetitive DNA sequences. This is one of the reasons that STR loci are often very polymorphic (along with supposed selective neutrality). In essence this is one of the properties that render such loci highly informative markers in forensic genetics. However substitutions cannot be detected by most imaging systems as they produce the same-sized allelic product as the unmutated sequence.

Observation of any putative paternal mutation will lower the value of the PI quite dramatically. Consequently it would seem sensible to avoid a locus with high mutation rates. However to be useful a locus should also be highly polymorphic. There is a general positive correlation between mutation rate and polymorphism, which makes the selection of microsatellite loci for investigating paternity difficult.

The relatively high mutation rates of STR loci stem from the tandem arrangement of their repeated sequences. STR loci are typically observed to mutate in a predictable and characteristic way by addition or loss of one or more units of the repeated sequence. At least two possible explanations have been advanced to account for this observation. By way of example consider an idealized structure of the hypothetical STR locus in Figure 11.5.

There are two theories as to how mutations at STR loci occur. The loop-out theory posits that during DNA replication *in vivo* the DNA polymerase enzyme must traverse a stretch of DNA containing a tandem array of a repeated sequence. If the repeats have the same sequence motif, then there exists the possibility that either the template strand or the replicating strand can 'loop out' one or more repeated units. The loop can be stabilized kinetically provided that it is in phase and that there is sufficient sequence homology at either side. The effect of this loop is that the copied DNA strand will either have increased or decreased in length by one or more full repeat units depending on which strand the loop-out occurred. It seems highly likely that stuttering is the result of a similar process occurring *in vitro* with Taq polymerase.[974]

The unequal crossover theory posits that during a recombination event, there is an unequal exchange of DNA between the chromatids, resulting in a reciprocal change to both alleles.

As the typing of STR alleles is based on length polymorphism, both types of event will spawn a new allele. The theory behind this process has become known as the *stepwise mutation model* and postulates that STR alleles mutate incrementally by integer expansions and contractions of the repeat motif.[975] A number of factors appear to affect the propensity for stepwise mutation (and stutter). A positive correlation between the mean number of uninterrupted repeats and mutation rate was reported by Brinkmann et al.[976] The longer the run of repeats and the greater the 'purity' of the repeat sequence, the greater is the propensity to mutate or stutter.

Although the large majority of mutational events occurring at STR loci appear to be changes to the number of repeated units, it is also possible for there to be other types of mutational events. The possible types of mutation that could theoretically occur at our hypothetical STR locus are shown in Figure 11.6.

Only events resulting in a change in the length of the DNA between the primer-binding sequences will be perceived as a mutation on typing with current capillary electrophoresis (CE) technology. Insertions or deletion events not involving whole repeated units may produce non-integer changes to the allele length. The commonly occurring HUMTH01 9.3 allele appears to be the result of an ancestral mutation deleting a single nucleotide from one of the repeated units in the repeat region. Other loci (e.g. D19S433, HUMD21S11 and HUMFIBRA/FGA) have a series of commonly encountered X.2 variants resulting from event(s) culminating in the loss or addition of two nucleotides in the flanking DNA. Changes to the nucleotide sequence of the flanking region and repeat region will result in sequence microheterogeneity but will not be perceived as affecting the Mendelian pattern. This is not, however, the case for mutational events occurring in the primer-binding sequences. Mutations in the primer-binding sequences can produce silent (or null) alleles depending on whether they occur towards the 5' or 3' ends of the primer-binding sequence, as shown in Figures 11.7 and 11.8.

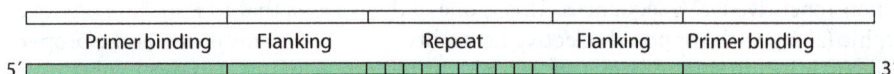

Figure 11.5   Idealized structure of a short tandem repeat locus.

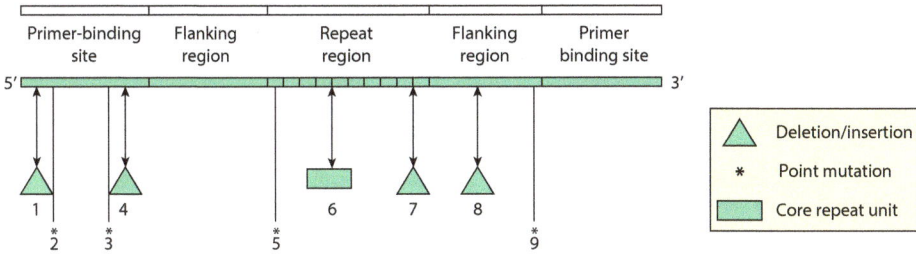

Figure 11.6 Possible mutations at a short tandem repeat locus.

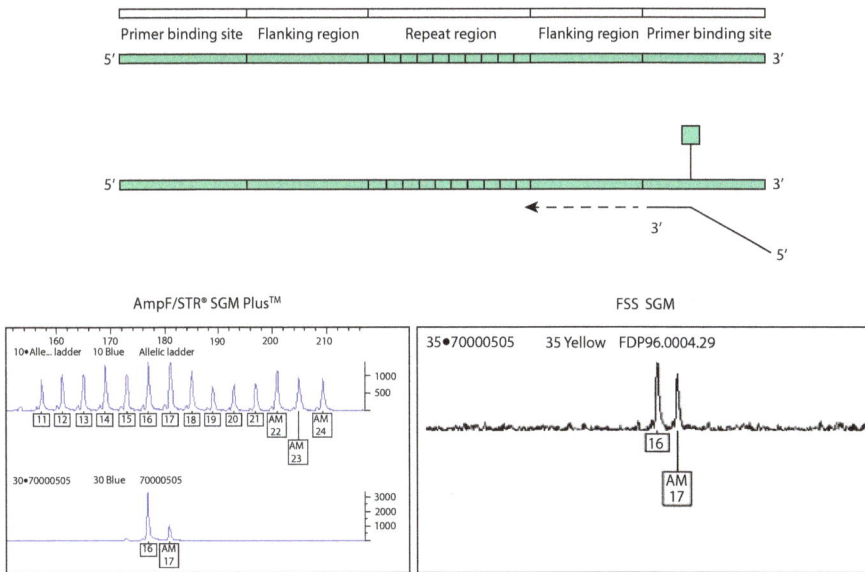

Figure 11.7 Primer binding site mutation affecting the amplification of the vWA 17 allele in the AmpF/STR® SGMPlus™ system (Applied Biosystems, Foster City, CA) whereas the allele has amplified efficiently using a different primer pair in the Forensic Science Service SGM Multiplex.

The existence of polar mutation at minisatellites has been reported.[976–985] The general conclusion is that most mutations involve the preferential gain of one or a few repeat units at one end of the tandem array (dissenting data is given in Refs. 986 and 987). However whether stepwise mutations have a propensity towards expansion is still the subject of debate.[985,987,988]

This discussion may be settled by the suggestion that longer alleles preferentially contract, whereas shorter alleles preferentially expand.[986,989–992] Huang et al. canvas the issue and provide

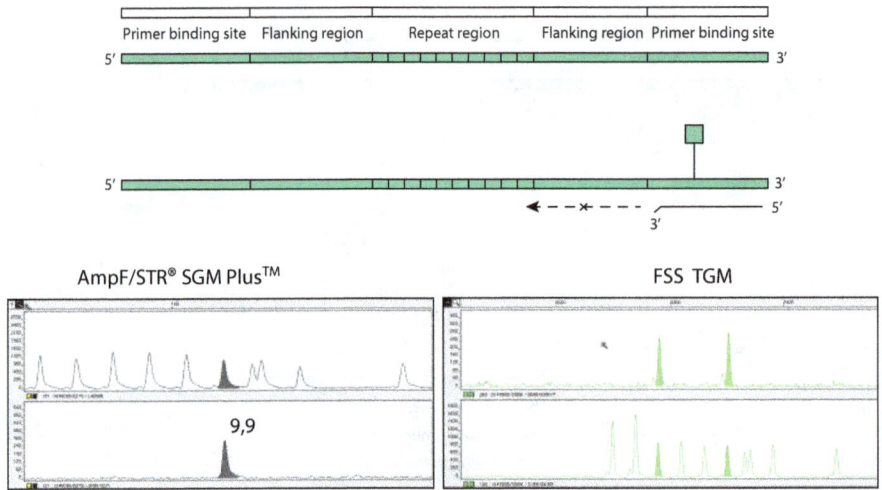

AmpF/STR® SGM Plus™

FSS TGM

9,9

Figure 11.8   Due to a primer binding site mutation the HUMTH01 locus amplified in the AmpF/STR SGMPlus appears as a 9,9 homozygote, whereas it is clearly a 6,9 heterozygote when analyzed under the FSS TGM (third generation multiplex). The primer binding site mutation has caused the 6 allele to be silent under the SGMPlus conditions.

further references to other papers discussing potential reasons why allele size does not increase endlessly, notably the absence of very large alleles. Note also the dissenting data regarding the prevalence of single step mutations in this paper.

There is a strong effect of sex, with paternal rates higher than maternal rates. The difference in mutation rates for male and female is plausibly explained by the observation that spermatozoa have undergone more cell divisions than ova during development. Crow discussed a dissenting report and gives an important overview.[993]

Some loci have higher mutation rates than others.

One accrediting body, NATA (National Association of Testing Authorities Australia),[994] states that loci with a mutation rate of greater than 0.25% cannot be used in parentage testing. This has caused some difficulty in court. This recommendation has been removed from the criminal testing guidelines but not the parentage testing guidelines.[995] We presume that the scientific motivation is to avoid apparent exclusions caused by mutation. However if a likelihood ratio approach utilizing a mutation model is employed, this type of recommendation is not required.

The simplest possible mutation model is based on two assumptions:

1. At any locus an allele has an equal probability of mutating to any other allele at that locus.

2. The rate of mutation from one allele to another is the same across all loci.

It is evident from empirical studies that such a model is a gross over-simplification. There is now compelling and cogent evidence that the probability of a mutation varies according to the sex of the individual and maybe the age, the locus being considered, which particular allele is being considered, the magnitude of change (number of steps) and the direction of that change.

A general mutation model relaxes these assumptions. At a given locus we denote allele-specific mutation probabilities where the probability that allele X mutates to allele Y denoted as $\mu_{X \to Y}$. Since paternal and maternal mutation rates differ, we will write these as $\mu^P_{X \to Y}, \mu^M_{X \to Y}$, respectively. Where we require the probability that allele X mutates to any other allele at the locus we will write this as $\mu_{X \to *}$. Currently the most prevalent data that exist are for locus mutation rates (μ).

Assume (probably falsely) that mutations occur independently from one another so that the probability of observing two mutations can be estimated by simple multiplication. Strictly, assuming the independence of mutational events may not be justified. For instance, a deficiency in a certain DNA repair enzyme may mean that multiple mutations occur in that individual with a greater frequency than might be expected. Or total mutation rates may be conditional on age, sex or another factor we have not yet discovered.

Dawid et al.[996] have recently developed a model based around these principles and comment, quite correctly, that 'the forensic treatment of sporadic parent/child inconsistency is sensitive to the mutation model assumed to underlie interallelic transitions'. They compare four possible models:

1. Uniform: Every interallelic transition is equiprobable.

2. Proportional: The probability of an interallelic transition is proportional to the frequency of the product allele.

3. Decreasing: This gives most probability to steps of ±1 repeat motif.

4. Stepwise stationary: Again this gives most probability to steps of ±1 repeat motif but it is modified by the frequency of the originating allele. This is the only model of the four that possesses stationarity, that is, the allele probabilities should not change over time for large populations.

Empirical data suggests that small alleles (those at the low molecular weight end of the allelic range) are most likely to mutate to increased motif number. The most likely transition is +1 motif. It appears, from limited data, that most multi-step transitions are equiprobable. The bias to positive change in motif number declines as the alleles become larger, until the bias is towards decrease in motif number for alleles at the high molecular weight end of the allelic range. It is conceivable that this model could also exhibit stationarity, although there is no absolutely compelling reason to expect stationarity in human populations.

Clayton et al. (unpublished results) suggest that mutations at differing loci may not be independent; this is to say that the rate of mutations at multiple loci may be in excess of the simple product of single locus mutation rates. Fortunately this effect is likely to lead to conservative *LRs* if ignored, for trios exhibiting apparent multiple mutations.

The work of Clayton et al. strongly suggests the need for specific locus *and* allelic mutation rates, preferably from empirical data or very robust models. One such potential source is the American Association of Blood Banks summary reports available online (http://www.aabb.org), which break down mutations by paternal/maternal status, locus, allele and step size.

Paternity Trios with 'Apparent Mutation'

The ISFG recommendations on biostatistics in paternity testing[946] state

> R1.3.1. Possible mutation PI shall be modified for possible mutation patterns between tested individuals when isolated mismatches among tested systems, which normally lead to an opinion of non-relationship, may be the result of mutant DNA causing false conclusions. The method for modifying PI shall be documented.*

We read this as stating the mutation should be considered if a Mendelian inconsistency is noted. Strictly mutation should be considered in all cases whether an inconsistency is noted or not. Doing so leads to a very large number of very small terms and the incorporation of many $(1 - \mu)$ factors. Collectively these add very little to accuracy and a lot to complexity; hence the usual and reasonable approach is to omit them unless a Mendelian inconsistency is noted.

---

* Reprinted from Gjertson, D.W., et al., *ISFG: Recommendations on biostatistics in paternity testing.* Forensic Science International: Genetics, 2007. **1**(3–4): 223–231, Copyright 2007, with permission from Elsevier.

Mother, Child and Alleged Father: Father Does Not Possess Paternal Allele

Hallenberg and Morling[965] report that the laboratories in their survey used four different formulae for calculating the PI when an apparent mutation had occurred. Unfortunately the formulae in use are not given.

Consider a situation where the alleged father does not possess the paternal allele, A_P, such as $G_M = A_M A_M$, $G_{AF} = A_1 A_2$, $G_C = A_M A_P$. Under H_1, we hypothesize that the alleged father, AF, is the true father; hence one of his alleles must have mutated. If we further add the possibility that the maternal alleles may have mutated, we end up with a complex sum of terms.

$$\Pr\left(G_C \mid G_M, G_{AF}, H_1\right) = \left(1 - \mu_{A_M \to *}^M\right) \frac{\mu_{A_1 \to A_p}^P + \mu_{A_2 \to A_p}^P}{2} + \mu_{A_M \to A_p}^M \frac{\mu_{A_1 \to A_M}^P + \mu_{A_2 \to A_M}^P}{2}$$

However the second term,

$$\mu_{A_M \to A_p}^M \frac{\mu_{A_1 \to A_M}^P + \mu_{A_2 \to A_M}^P}{2}$$

accounts for two mutational events and is expected to be small and may be ignored.

$\Pr\left(G_C \mid G_M, G_{AF}, H_d\right) = \left(1 - \mu_{A_M \to *}^M\right) p_{A_p} + \mu_{A_M \to A_p}^M p_{A_M}$, and the numerical value of the second term $\mu_{A_M \to A_p}^M p_{A_M}$ is small compared to the first term. Ignoring these terms of small order we have

$$\text{PI} \approx \frac{\mu_{A_1 \to A_p}^P + \mu_{A_2 \to A_p}^P}{2 p_{A_p}}$$

Dawid et al.[996] discuss a situation where it is unclear whether we have a maternal or a paternal mutation. We follow their treatment.

Consider $G_M = ab$, $G_C = ac$, $G_{AF} = aa$. It is unclear whether the paternal allele is a and has been passed unmutated (and hence that the maternal allele must have mutated) or whether the maternal allele is a (and hence that the paternal allele has mutated). Again ignoring those outcomes that posit simultaneous paternal and maternal mutations we have

$$\text{PI} \approx \frac{\dfrac{\mu_{a \to c}^M + \mu_{b \to c}^M}{2}\left(1 - \mu_{a \to *}^P\right) + \dfrac{\mu_{a \to c}^P}{2}\left(1 - \mu_{a \to *}^M + \mu_{b \to a}^M\right)}{p_c \dfrac{\left(1 - \mu_{a \to *}^M\right)}{2} + \dfrac{\mu_{a \to c}^M + \mu_{b \to c}^M}{2} p_a}$$

$$\approx \frac{\mu_{a \to c}^M + \mu_{b \to c}^M + \mu_{a \to c}^P}{p_c}$$

for small mutation rates. This result differs from Dawid in only minor detail. Ayres[997] discusses the addition of the subpopulation correction.

Mother, Child and AF: The Possibility of Silent (Null) Alleles

This issue arises when one alleged parent is an apparent homozygote, the child is an apparent homozygote for a different allele to the parent and we have a system that has silent alleles, collectively represented by the symbol ϕ. We present below expressions for the PI accounting for the uncertainty induced by silent alleles. Typically such silent alleles are caused by a primer-binding site mutation (see Chapter 1 for a brief discussion and some probabilities of observing silent alleles at different loci). However as Clayton[998] has suggested algebraic solutions are markedly inferior to a biological resolution of the uncertainty. The most obvious way to achieve this is to use a different primer to resolve the apparent silent allele.

Consider the situation $G_M = ab$, $G_C = b$, $G_{AF} = c$ and denote the allele probability of the silent allele as p_ϕ. Our treatment is completely general and could be applied to many other situations in this book where the use of a particular primer system suggests that a locus has silent alleles.

We have written the child's genotype as b rather than bb because in any system that has silent alleles it is difficult to be certain that the child has the homozygous genotype, bb, rather than the heterozygous $b\phi$ genotype. Similarly the alleged father may be either cc or $c\phi$.

Assuming Hardy–Weinberg equilibrium and in the absence of any other pedigree data, conditional probability arguments show that the apparent c homozygotes are composed of a fraction

$$\frac{p_c^2}{p_c^2 + 2p_c p_\phi} = \frac{p_c}{p_c + 2p_\phi}$$

who are actually cc homozygotes and a fraction

$$\frac{2p_c p_\phi}{p_c^2 + 2p_c p_\phi} = \frac{2p_\phi}{p_c + 2p_\phi}$$

who are $c\phi$ heterozygotes. Hence

$$\Pr\left(G_C \mid G_M, G_{AF}, H_1\right) = \frac{1}{2} \times \frac{1}{2} \times \frac{2p_c p_\phi}{p_c^2 + 2p_c p_\phi} = \frac{p_\phi}{2(p_c + 2p_\phi)}$$

if we consider a silent allele alone, and

$$\Pr\left(G_C \mid G_M, G_{AF}, H_1\right) \approx$$

$$\frac{1 - \mu_{b \to *}^{M} + \mu_{a \to b}^{M}}{2} \times \left(\begin{array}{l} \dfrac{p_\phi}{2(p_c + 2p_\phi)}\left(1 - \mu_{\phi \to *}^{P} + \mu_{\phi \to b}^{P} + \mu_{c \to b}^{P}\right) \\[2mm] + \dfrac{p_c}{p_c + 2p_\phi}\left(\mu_{c \to b}^{P} + \mu_{c \to *}^{P}\right) \end{array} \right)$$

$$+ \left(\frac{\mu_{a \to \phi}^{M} + \mu_{b \to \phi}^{M}}{2}\right)\left(\frac{p_\phi}{2(p_c + 2p_\phi)}\left(\mu_{\phi \to b}^{P} + \mu_{c \to b}^{P}\right) + \frac{p_c}{p_c + 2p_\phi}\mu_{c \to b}^{P}\right)$$

if we consider both silent alleles and mutation. Assuming small mutation rates:

$$\Pr\left(G_C \mid G_M, G_{AF}, H_1\right) \approx \frac{p_\phi + 2p_c\left(\mu_{c \to b}^{P} + \mu_{c \to *}^{P}\right)}{4(p_c + 2p_\phi)}$$

$$\Pr\left(G_C \mid G_M, G_{AF}, H_2\right) \approx \frac{1 - \mu_{b \to *}^{M} + \mu_{a \to b}^{M}}{2}\left(p_b + p_\phi\right) + \left(\frac{\mu_{a \to \phi}^{M} + \mu_{b \to \phi}^{M}}{2}\right)p_b$$

$$\approx \frac{\left(1 - \mu_{b \to *}^{M} + \mu_{a \to b}^{M}\right)p_\phi + \left(1 - \mu_{b \to *}^{M} + \mu_{a \to b}^{M} + \mu_{a \to \phi}^{M} + \mu_{b \to \phi}^{M}\right)p_b}{2}$$

$$\approx \frac{p_\phi + p_b}{2}$$

and hence

$$PI \approx \frac{p_\phi + 2p_c\left(\mu^P_{c \to b} + \mu^P_{c \to *}\right)}{2\left(p_c + 2p_\phi\right)\left(p_\phi + p_b\right)}$$

The important observation[999] has been made that silent alleles are usually ignored unless they are required under H_1. This leads to a non-negligible overestimation of paternity indices. This is a situation that requires action.

Brenner discusses the practice of declaring an exclusion if a certain number of Mendelian inconsistencies are observed. He concludes that this practice may have tended towards false exclusion in the past and in doing so affected mutation rate estimates.[1000]

Allele-Specific Mutation Rates or Silent Allele Probability Estimates Unavailable

At the time of writing data are scant for silent allele probabilities and the allele-specific mutation probabilities employed above. Butler[258, p. 370] gives an excellent review of emerging information. For mutation rates at STR loci we suggest using the average mutation rate at a locus modified for the step change. For example, if the mutation rate at a locus is μ and 90% of mutations are single step, assuming +1 and –1 are equally probable, then the +1 transition is assigned a probability $\frac{0.90 \times \mu}{2}$. This agrees with PTC Recommendation 1.3.[946] For silent alleles PTC suggests using a number of values in the plausible range. We can suggest nothing better. Again the American Association of Blood Banks summary reports provide a good source of mutation rate information.

Mutation and Non-Autosomal DNA
Y Chromosome

Consider a paternal relative/mother/child trio or paternal relative/child duo. We assume an exact match in haplotype of the Y chromosome between the paternal relative and the child. If we ignore mutation we obtain $PI \approx \frac{1}{f}$, where f is the frequency of the child's (and alleged father's) haplotype.

Assume a mutation rate μ_l at each locus, l, of the N loci typed on the Y chromosome. For the exact match described above

$$PI = \frac{\prod_{l=1}^{N}(1-\mu_l)}{f} \approx \frac{(1-\bar{\mu})^N}{f}$$

where $\bar{\mu}$ is the average mutation rate across loci. We can find a series of closer approximations to the actual value of the PI if we have an estimate of the variance of the mutation rates about their

mean, $s^2 = \dfrac{\displaystyle\sum_{i=1}^{N}(\bar{\mu}-\mu_i)^2}{N-1}$. The first approximation is given by

$$PI = \frac{\prod_{l=1}^{N}(1-\mu_l)}{f} \approx \frac{(1-\bar{\mu})^N}{f}\left(1 - \frac{N-1}{2}\frac{s^2}{(1-\bar{\mu})^2}\right)$$

Assume that the paternal relative and the child differ at locus k and that m meioses have occurred between the child's Y chromosome and that of the alleged paternal relative. At locus k the change is from allele x to y ($x{\to}y$).

$$PI \approx \frac{\prod_{l=1,l\neq k}^{N}(1-\mu_l)^m\, m\mu_k^{x\to y}(1-\mu_k)^{m-1}}{f}$$

Assuming that $\bar{\mu}$ is small we obtain

$$PI \approx \frac{m\mu_k^{x\to y}}{f}$$

Assuming further that the $x{\to}y$ transition is a single step and occurs in approximately 1/2 of all mutations at this locus, and also assuming a constant mutation rate across loci, leads to the approximation

$$PI \approx \frac{m\bar{\mu}}{2f}$$

as given by Rolf et al.,[968] where f is now the frequency of the child's (not the paternal relative's) haplotype.

Some data on Y chromosome mutation rates using deep-rooted pedigrees has been published and compare favourably with an average of 0.21% for Weber and Wong.[1001] Kayser et al.[981] note that their data show a mutational bias towards increased length. The ratio of increase to decrease was 10:4 for the 14 mutations observed. Thirteen of these mutations were a single repeat change and one was double repeat change.

X Chromosome Analysis

The interpretation of X chromosome evidence when used in paternity analysis follows the same principles as described for the Y chromosome. Assume a mutation rate μ_l at each locus, l of the N loci typed on the X chromosome. For the exact match

$$PI = \frac{\prod_{l=1}^{N}(1-\mu_l)}{f} \approx \frac{(1-\bar{\mu})^N}{f}$$

where $\bar{\mu}$ is the average mutation rate across loci. This may be approximated more closely as in the previous section (see Chapter 10 for mutation rates).

Assume that the paternal relative and the child differ at locus k and that m meioses have occurred between the child's X chromosome and that of the alleged paternal relative. At locus k the change is from allele x to y ($x{\to}y$).

$$PI \approx \frac{\prod_{l=1,l\neq k}^{N}(1-\mu_l)^m\, m\mu_k^{x\to y}(1-\mu_k)^{m-1}}{f}$$

Assuming $\bar{\mu}$ is small we obtain

$$PI \approx \frac{m\mu_k^{x\to y}}{f}$$

Further assuming that the $x \to y$ transition is a single step and occurs in approximately 1/2 of all mutations at this locus and a constant mutation rate across loci suggests the approximation

$$PI \approx \frac{m\bar{\mu}}{2f}$$

which is the X chromosome analogue to that given by Rolf et al.[968] for the Y chromosome. Now f is the frequency of the child's (not the paternal relative's) haplotype.

If the X chromosome is used in maternity analysis, the development is a composite of the recombination analysis given above and a mutation analysis. It requires no new principles. We make use of the result that linkage need not be considered if the phase of the mother is unknown and there is only one meiosis in the pedigree.

Assume that the mother and the child differ at locus k. At locus k the mother has alleles a and b. The child has a maternal allele y not possessed by the mother (and not from the father). Hence we have observed, under H_1, a mutation of $a \to y$ or $b \to y$. This leads to the expression

$$PI \approx \left(\frac{\mu_k^{a \to y} + \mu_k^{b \to y}}{2} \right) \frac{\prod_{l=1, l \neq k}^{N}(1-\mu_l)}{f}$$

Assuming constant μ and that $\bar{\mu}$ is small we obtain

$$PI \approx \left(\frac{\mu_k^{a \to y} + \mu_k^{b \to y}}{2} \right) \frac{1}{f}$$

Mitochondrial Maternity Analysis and Mutation

Consider a maternal relative/father[*]/child trio or a maternal relative/child duo. We assume an exact match in haplotype of the mtDNA between the maternal relative and the child. If we ignore mutation we obtain $PI \approx \frac{1}{f}$, where f is the frequency of the child's (and alleged maternal relative's) haplotype.

Assume a mutation rate μ_l at each nucleotide position, l, of the N positions typed on the mtDNA. For the exact match described above

$$PI = \frac{\prod_{l=1}^{N}(1-\mu_l)}{f} \approx \frac{(1-\bar{\mu})^N}{f}$$

where $\bar{\mu}$ is the average mutation rate across sites. This may also be approximated more closely as in the previous sections. Assume that the haplotypes differ at position k and that m meioses have occurred between the child's Y chromosome and that of the alleged maternal relative. At position k the change is from nucleotide x to y ($x \to y$).

$$PI \approx \frac{\prod_{l=1, l \neq k}^{N}(1-\mu_l)^m \, m\mu_k^{x \to y}(1-\mu_k)^{m-1}}{f}$$

---

[*] The father is irrelevant for mtDNA analysis.

Assuming $\bar{\mu}$ is very small we obtain

$$PI \approx \frac{m\mu_k^{x \to y}}{f}$$

Now f is the frequency of the child's (not the maternal relative's) haplotype.

Inconsistencies in the Mendelian Pattern

If the pattern of alleles at an STR locus is inconsistent with Mendelian principles, there can be several possible explanations, including the following:

- The pattern in an individual may contain three bands.
- The child may have a band not present in the genotype of either the mother of the alleged father or the child may not share an allele with either or both alleged parents.

In the latter situation either a mutation has occurred, a null allele is present or the individuals are not related as postulated. This situation is often referred to as an *exclusion*. Although we will continue to use this familiar terminology in subsequent sections, as we will illustrate, it is an inappropriate expression.

Three-Banded Patterns

There are at least three potential causes of three-banded patterns: somatic mutation, trisomy and translocation. These three phenomena affect familial testing in differing ways.

Somatic Mutation

Rolf et al.[1002] report a case of somatic mutation involving germline cells in which the alleles segregated separately. This is straightforward to interpret in the unlikely circumstance that the fraction of germ cells containing each allele is known. For sperm this should be estimable from relative peak areas of each allele in a sperm sample. Without such a sample, estimation of the fraction is difficult. There is also the possibility that an apparent heterozygote with genotype ab is, say, a mosaic of genotypes aa and ab.

Consider the trio of apparent genotypes:

	Genotype
Mother	dd
Child	ad
Alleged father	abc

Suppose that the fraction of sperm carrying allele a is q_a. Suppose further that the mother has genotype $G_M = dd$ (Mendelian factor $M_M = 1$) and the child has genotype $GC = ad$. Then the paternal Mendelian factor and numerator of the PI is q_a. The denominator of the PI is not affected by the mosaicism in any significant way (it is affected in a minor way when we assume correlation of genotypes such as implied by use of the subpopulation model). Using the product rule this is, as before, p_a. Thus if the alleged father is a mosaic for a standard paternity trio, the PI becomes $PI = \frac{q_a}{p_a}$.

If we assume that q_a cannot be estimated directly for this case, then it may be possible to infer its value from background studies on how often germline cells are affected by mosaicism when, say, buccal cells exhibits such mosaicism.

Trisomy and Translocation

Suppose that an alleged father shows the pattern abc with all alleles having same peak height, then trisomy or translocation may be suspected. These are difficult to differentiate from the electropherogram but trisomy can be determined by a number of other methods. Translocation can produce two copies of either the same or differing alleles on one chromosome. If the two copies are the same, they produce one band in the profile but of twice the expected area. When the translocated elements are strongly linked they will be inherited as one unit and can be treated as one rare allele (whether or not they are the same allele or they differ).

Suppose that we have the following trio of apparent genotypes:

	Genotype
Mother	*dd*
Child	*abd*
Alleged father	*abc*

where we believe that the alleged father has a translocation from his genotype *and* that trisomy has been excluded (this cannot be inferred from observation of the genotype of the child in question, although the genotype of other acknowledged children of the alleged father can provide information as to his genotype). Then we do not know whether the alleles *a,b* are a pair on the same chromosome or whether the alleged father has some other pairing of alleles. If we assume that alleles *a,b* are on the same chromosome, then $\Pr\left(G_C \mid G_{AF}, G_M, H_1\right) = \frac{1}{2} \times M_M$, where M_M is the mother's Mendelian factor. This assumption maximizes the numerator of the PI. This is not appropriate unless the alleged father has other children whose genotypes have been examined or if STR examination of a single sperm has been made. In the absence of such data it may be reasonable, *a priori*, to assume that each of the three possible pairs of the alleles *a*, *b* and *c* are equally likely. There are three combinations:

ab	*c*
ac	*b*
bc	*a*

and hence six possible sperm types. Accordingly we write

$$\Pr\left(G_C \mid G_{AF}, G_M, H_1\right) = \frac{M_M}{6}$$

Exclusions

For the purposes of illustration we consider the situation where STR tests have been employed at a number of loci to address the question of whether or not there is any evidence to support the proposition that the alleged father (*AF*) is the true biological father of a child (*C*). The alternative hypothesis is that some other unrelated man is *C*'s biological father. We could then pose the following question: 'If *AF* is not *C*'s father, how many inconsistent loci would be required for a declaration of non-paternity?'

Many laboratories use a system where, if a predetermined number of inconsistencies are present, 'exclusion' can be declared. Such a 'numerical standard' would be dependent on the number of loci tested. For example, consider the evidential weight of two inconsistencies in a panel of six loci compared to that from two inconsistencies in a panel of 66 loci. Accordingly for some laboratories this standard for exclusion is one, others two and some three out of a standard panel of anywhere between 10 and 20 loci. For example, Nutini et al.[1003] report a double inconsistency in what they conclude is a true trio.

Not all mutations should carry equivalent evidential weight. Certain types of mutations are inherently much less common than others.

We suggest that the most satisfactory approach is to use an *LR*, or PI, combined with a mutation model. There is no necessity for a laboratory standard stipulating the number of inconsistent loci that must be present in a panel of STR loci before an exclusion is declared. It is desirable that such a mutation model be able to weigh changes according to the particular type of mutation involved. Bayesian methods offer a simple and logically coherent method of incorporating the effects of a mutation into the overall calculation of the PI.

If the PI is greater than one, even though one or more exclusions have been observed there is still support for the proposition of parentage versus non-parentage, notwithstanding the observed inconsistencies.

Mutation and Exclusion Probabilities*

The paternity index, PI, is a far superior measure of evidential weight than an exclusion probability, PE. However it is possible to modify exclusion probabilities to account for mutations. There is an obvious interaction between what we define as an exclusion and the calculation of an exclusion probability. If we allow at most one apparent mutation in all L loci, then Chakraborty and Stivers[1004] give

$$1 - \prod_{l=1}^{L} (1 - PE_l) \left\{ 1 + \sum_{j=1}^{L} \frac{PE_j}{(1 - PE_j)} \right\}$$

(we can confirm their derivation of this formula). These authors also give a recursive equation that allows the calculation allowing any number of mutations.

Let $Q_l = \sum_i \Pr(A_i)$ where the index i enumerates all those alleles (at locus l) allowed to mutate to the paternal allele. Suppose that we only allow alleles to mutate by ± 1 repeat, then

$$Q_l = \Pr\left(A_{p-1}^l\right) + \Pr\left(A_{p+1}^l\right)$$

where A_{p+1}^l, and A_{p-1}^l are the alleles +1 and –1 repeats from the paternal allele $\left(A_p^l\right)$, respectively. Then

$$PE = 1 - \prod_{l=1}^{L} (1 - PE_l) \left\{ 1 + \sum_{l=1}^{L} \frac{Q_l\left(2 - Q_l - 2\Pr\left(A_p^l\right)\right)}{1 - PE_l} \right\}$$

If we allow the possibility that all alleles at a locus may mutate to the paternal allele, then $Q_l = 1 - \Pr\left(A_p^l\right)$ and we recover Chakraborty and Stivers' formula.

However we are concerned that under some circumstances the exclusion probability calculated in this way may be misleading. The PE may give an indication of some substantial evidential value, whereas the more reliable PI does not.

---

* This section was motivated by an inquiry by Tim Sliter.

12

Disaster Victim Identification, Identification of Missing Persons and Immigration Cases

John S. Buckleton, Jo-Anne Bright and Duncan Taylor*

Contents

---

* Based on earlier work by John Buckleton, Chris Triggs and Tim Clayton.

Introduction

In earlier chapters we considered the evaluation of evidence from single genetic profiles, from mixtures of profiles derived from two or more unrelated individuals and in Chapter 11 from three individuals, two of whom are the parents of the third. In this chapter we generalize the approach from a paternity trio to consider evidence from the profiles from a number of individuals who are members of a more complex pedigree. The methods discussed in this chapter will allow us to consider situations such as the identification of missing persons, the evaluation of the genetic closeness of relationships in immigration cases* and the identification of victims of disasters. In each of these cases we observe the profiles of several people and wish to use these to compare the likelihood of observing two or more postulated sets of relationships between the individuals.

The purpose of disaster victim identification may be to bring justice or closure to the families of the missing and also to show respect to the victims themselves by treating them with individual dignity.[1005] It is questionable whether scientific or historic curiosity is an adequate substitute for these motives and such endeavours must be dealt with very carefully. There are some mandated rights and responsibilities in this area. For example, the Geneva Convention defines the responsibility of states to help in the location of graves of persons who have died in their detention.[1006,1007]

The identification of human remains has been undertaken without the aid of DNA typing for many years, and a wide range of approaches are still appropriate for differing circumstances.[1008–1010] However in recent times DNA technology has been extensively and usefully applied to the identification problem. The identification of the remains may be only a part of the problem. It is important to remember that the position of the body or the burial may be a crime scene in itself and that much information may be obtained from a proper scene examination.[1011] However the identification of remains presents the forensic scientist with the dual problems of obtaining a profile from remains that are often in a state of advanced decomposition and obtaining a reference profile for the missing person† with which to compare. In this chapter we address these issues and discuss both the practical and interpretational difficulties surrounding them.

Mitochondrial or Nuclear DNA?

Before embarking on practical measures to identify human remains, it is usually necessary to consider several factors which will affect the decision as to whether to proceed with mitochondrial DNA (mtDNA) typing (see Chapter 10) or nuclear DNA profiling.[766]

Mitochondrial DNA

In certain circumstances mtDNA offers a number of advantages over nuclear DNA.[776,1012] The mtDNA molecule is present in high copy number; therefore there is greater chance of some template surviving degradation. It is relatively easy to extract typeable quantities of material from hair shafts and other skeletal structures where the amount of nuclear DNA may be very limited indeed. Last, in cases where reference samples from immediate genetic relatives are scant (so-called genetic deficiency cases) mtDNA is useful as it can bridge the gaps in the pedigree. Thus, any relative on the maternal lineage can be used for comparison even though they may be separated by more than one generation. In this way Gill et al.[785] were able to use surviving relatives of Tsar Nicholas II to identify his putative remains.

---

* We will often refer to the *body* in this chapter. For immigration cases this is inappropriate and a term such as *applicant* should be substituted. The mathematics, however, are identical.

† It is quite useful to use the term *missing person* to refer to the person from the pedigree. The body is not known to be from the pedigree; indeed that is the matter in question. Hence *missing person* can be used to refer to the identity of the body under H_1 but not under H_2.

However the relative lack of discriminating power associated with mtDNA typing needs to be balanced against these advantages. This may be a major factor if multiple sets of remains are present. Similarly, if those remains were from individuals who are matrilineally related, one would be unable to distinguish between them.

Nuclear DNA

Consideration should also be given to which nuclear DNA typing system to use. If patrilineal relatives are available in genetic deficiency cases, a panel of Y chromosome markers may be appropriate. Of course these markers do not have the advantage of multiple copy number. However, in the majority of cases, autosomal multiplex short tandem repeat (STR) profiling will be the method of choice. The very high discriminating power afforded by STR loci combined with gender information has proven to be an excellent tool especially when multiple sets of remains are present. In 1995 Clayton et al.[1013] applied such technology to identify multiple victims of the Waco incident. More recently we have seen this method used in a large number of incidents. This technology is now used routinely to identify human remains and has expanded into massive DNA programmes such as those to identify the victims of ethnic cleansing in the former Yugoslavia and the victims of the September 11th incident in New York. It has been used to successfully type the remains of a neonate who had been kept in a vinyl bag for 15 years.[1014] The value of a multidisciplinary approach is emphasized by an example from the World Trade Center Human Identification Project.[1015] Due to commingling of soft tissues, DNA testing alone would have led to problems and a partnership between forensic anthropologists and DNA specialists was advocated.

Human Remains: Obtaining a Profile from Bodily Remains

When human remains are found, they may be in a variety of conditions ranging from recently deceased to fully skeletonized. A body may be intact but, more often than not, the sorts of remains which are of forensic interest are fragmentary due to

- Physical forces (such as the violent impacts encountered in transport accidents, explosions or mechanical wave action)
- Scavenging and predation by land or marine organisms
- Dismemberment and/or disarticulation by an individual seeking to dispose of or conceal the body or its identity

Moreover, the remains may have been exposed to fire (thermal insult) or to aggressive compounds such as lime or acid (chemical insult). The level of decomposition of the tissues in human remains can vary dramatically according to the time since death and the prevailing environmental conditions. Extreme cold can preserve remains as though they had been deep frozen while hot dry conditions can lead to complete desiccation and mummification. Conversely warm damp conditions or water immersion can lead to rapid decomposition. By contrast, an aquatic but cold and/or anaerobic environment can sometimes serve to preserve tissue.

For the purposes of this discussion, it is useful to place remains into a categorization system based upon the extent of decomposition. The approach to obtaining DNA from the remains can differ depending on which category is being considered.

Category 1: Remains Displaying Relatively Few Signs of Decomposition

At the post-mortem examination it will generally be possible to obtain blood samples from some areas of the body and the internal organs and soft tissues will be largely unaffected. As the blood and soft tissues are rich sources of DNA, obtaining a DNA profile from remains in this category should present few, if any, technical difficulties.

Category 2: Remains Exhibiting Partial Decomposition

Generally, at the post-mortem examination no blood will be available and the superficial soft tissues may be exhibiting signs of putrefaction. Successful typing of the soft tissues and sera may still be possible depending on the temperature in the area of death and the pathological conditions that the victim experienced.[1016] Deep tissues such as psoas muscle or bone marrow will usually be in a reasonable condition. In this situation, targeting deeper tissues is often more successful than attempting to use more superficial tissues as a source of DNA. Contamination of the extract by decomposition products is known to inhibit subsequent polymerase chain reaction (PCR). Pusch et al.[766] review some potential inhibitors. These include Maillard reaction products, remains of porphyrines, degraded nucleic acids, soil components such as humic and fulvic acids, tannins and ferric ions but especially they mention degraded human collagen type I. Normally tissue samples will require additional treatment to release the DNA and purify it from the cell debris and other decomposition products. The most common protocol employed is to use a buffered solution containing Proteinase K, SDS and DTT followed by an organic clean-up using phenol or phenol/chloroform. Using ethanol precipitation or microfiltration further purifies the DNA. Other protocols have been published, all of which are designed to maximize recovery and minimize the presence of decomposition products.

DNA profiling may also reveal DNA degradation (exhibited as a gradual loss of signal from the high molecular weight loci first). This degradation may be extensive enough to prevent a full profile from being obtained.

Category 3: Remains in an Advanced State of Decomposition

Typically, in this situation, most of the soft tissues will have lost their integrity and some may have formed adipocere. If the remains are in such an advanced state of decay, obtaining a DNA profile from liquefied tissues or adipocere is seldom successful. The bone marrow can sometimes be better preserved and may provide sufficient DNA. However, if profiling from the putrefied soft tissues and marrow is unsuccessful, then recourse should be made to skeletal structures (see Category 4).

Category 4: Remains That Are Fully Skeletal (Including Mummified or Desiccated Remains)

At this stage of decomposition generally only hardy structures such as bone, hair, nails and teeth will be available. The skeletal structures, bone matrix and tooth pulp are rich in mtDNA. They also contain low, but typeable, quantities of nuclear DNA. As the DNA is 'encased' within a hardened calcified mass it requires special procedures to release and purify it (see section 'Extraction of DNA from Bone, Tooth, Hair and Nail'). Hair shafts are relatively rich sources of mtDNA (see Chapter 10) but contain only traces of highly fragmented nuclear DNA. Attempts have been made to prepare STR profiles from hair shafts or other sources using short amplicon strategies.[1017,1018] This is a very logical approach but has not yet been implemented widely.

Extraction of DNA from Bone, Tooth, Hair and Nail

Extraction of DNA from tooth,[1019,1020] hair,[650,651] nail[1021,1022] and bone[1023,1024] poses a significant technical challenge.[1025,1026] The preferred starting material is either a molar tooth (preferably free from an amalgam filing) or approximately 1 g of dense (non-cancellous) bone. First, the surface of the tooth or bone is cleaned to remove surface contamination. This is often done by sanding away the surface layer of bone or, in the case of a tooth, by transient acid immersion followed by washing. Next, the tooth or bone must be powdered. Two methods are generally employed. The first utilizes a specialized piece of 'bone-milling' equipment in which a bone chip is enclosed in a vial with a heavy metal bar. The vial is then submerged in liquid nitrogen to render the bone brittle. An oscillating magnetic field is then applied. This causes the metal bar to vibrate violently, pulverizing the bone chip into a fine powder. The same effect can be achieved by grinding using a drill bit but care must be taken to avoid generating high temperatures as a result of frictional forces. Once a fine powder has been produced the DNA is released by enzymatic digestion using a buffered solution of Proteinase K, DTT and Tween 60. The resulting extract is heavily contaminated with calcium salts leached from the bone that are then removed by mixing with a concentrated solution of EDTA. Finally, the extract is cleaned and concentrated by microfiltration. Nevertheless, the yields of nuclear DNA are typically low and, often, elevated cycle number PCR (>28 cycles) must be used to generate typing results.

Nakanishi et al. report the successful typing of nails after various environmental insults.[1027] Their findings confirm the usefulness of nail as a source of DNA.

Comparisons

Having successfully obtained a profile from the unidentified remains a comparison must then be carried out with the profile of the missing person. However it is often the case that the missing person's DNA profile is not available. Fortunately, there are a number of ways in which information can be obtained.

Surrogate Samples

Increasingly we are seeing the use of a 'surrogate' DNA sample, that is, a sample thought to be DNA from the missing person. All 155 victims of the Kaprun cable car disaster in 2000 were identified within 19 days based mainly on the use of surrogate samples.[1028] From an evidential perspective, perhaps the best type of surrogate sample one can obtain is an archival 'clinical' sample. Often clinics, hospitals and other medical institutions will retain labelled and indexed archival specimens that are traceable through patient records. The most common format is as a wax-embedded histology block. However microscope slides, deep frozen tissue specimens and neonatal blood cards have all been utilized in the past. Tissue 'well' preserved in formalin solution has proven to be highly refractory to PCR analysis.

In those cases with an active investigation, law enforcement agencies may obtain personal effects that may carry biological material. Generally, these are articles of a personal or individual nature such as a toothbrush, razor, underwear or hairbrush. However a variety of other samples have proven useful in the past, for example saliva beneath stamps, bedding, handkerchiefs and cigarette butts.

Many jurisdictions have now instituted National DNA Intelligence databases. These repositories often contain the DNA STR profiles from hundreds of thousands of individuals. The UK National DNA Database currently holds in excess of two million records. If a missing person is on record, then it may be possible to obtain a copy of that person's profile to assist in the identification of their remains.

Twins

If a sample from a surviving monozygotic twin is available, then the deceased should share the same DNA profile. However consideration should be given as to how the surviving individual knows that he or she is monozygotic. Similarity of appearance may provide strong evidence of monozygosity, but this is not in itself conclusive and generally genetic tests are required to establish that the individuals are monozygotic as opposed to dizygotic.

Pedigree Analysis

In the remainder of this chapter we will describe the last approach – use of pedigree (kinship) analysis. We will concentrate on the calculation of likelihood ratios (*LRs*) based on calculating the probability of the observed genotypes if the postulated relationship is true or false. This requires access to appropriate databases. Chakraborty and Jin[1029] and Ehm and Wagner[1030] have proposed summary measures based on the number of shared and non-shared alleles. This approach was tested on 315 mother/child and 91 full-sib pairs and by simulation.[1031] Such measures may be of some use as a screening tool or as a filter for computer software but are less powerful than

LR methods because they do not take account of the relative rareness of shared alleles. For example the evidence for a relationship is stronger if the shared alleles are rare than if they are common.

There are many possible variations in individual family trees. However general guidance on how to proceed has been published.[496] It is possible to formulate some simple guidelines in terms of the 'appropriateness' of obtaining samples from certain relatives. This stems from a consideration of the amount of genetic information they would contribute to the inference process. As a practical solution, investigators could be instructed to obtain samples from any or all first-degree relatives. In some cases this will lead to a redundancy of information. For instance, if both parents of the missing person are available, then the genotypes of his siblings are redundant (although those of his children are not). In certain instances there may be sufficient information from the children of missing persons to completely determine their genotype. In this case the information given by the genotypes of the missing person's parents is redundant. However obtaining samples from all available first degree relatives may be the most expedient course of action.

General Principles

A pedigree specifies the relationships between a set of individuals. Those individuals at the top of the pedigree whose parents are not specified are termed the *founders* of the pedigree. Those individuals at the base of the pedigree who have no offspring are termed the *final individuals*. Pictorially males are usually designated by squares, females by circles. In much of the work to come the sex of a member of a pedigree is not relevant. In such cases we may use a diamond as a general symbol.

We begin by considering unlinked loci. We imagine a situation where there is a body with genotype G_B. We have a pedigree of N people with genotypes $G_1 \dots G_N$. The pedigree information itself is I. Typically we seek to evaluate the evidence given two hypotheses:

H_1: The body is this person in this pedigree.

H_2: The body is not related to this pedigree.[*]

This suggests the evaluation of the *LR*

$$LR = \frac{\Pr\left(G_B, G_1 \dots G_N \mid H_1, I\right)}{\Pr\left(G_B, G_1 \dots G_N \mid H_2, I\right)}$$

The joint probabilities in the numerator and denominator of the *LR* are often evaluated by decomposition into a chain of conditional probabilities. For non-founders we condition on the genotypes of their parents. Sets of children can usefully be taken out together. Where the probability of a child is conditioned on both parents, conditioning on other members of the pedigree, either siblings or other ancestors, is not required. Where we have no genotype for a person in the pedigree we consider all possible genotypes for that person and sum over their mutually exclusive probabilities. For unlinked loci the equation

$$LR = \frac{\Pr\left(G_B, G_1 \dots G_N \mid H_1, I\right)}{\Pr\left(G_B, G_1 \dots G_N \mid H_2, I\right)}$$

can be approximated by

$$LR = \prod_{loci} LR_{locus}$$

These principles are difficult to follow in the abstract but become natural with practice.[487–490,495,1032–1034] We show an example of such a probabilistic decomposition in Box 12.1.

---

[*] Strictly speaking, the two hypotheses, H_1 and H_2, specify two different pedigrees. We illustrate the difference in the discussion of Example 12.1.

**BOX 12.1   EVALUATION OF THE PROBABILITY OF OBSERVING
A SET OF GENOTYPES CONDITIONAL ON A SPECIFIED PEDIGREE**

Suppose that we observe five genotypes, G_G, G_M, G_P, G_N and G_C. We further believe that individuals G and M are the parents of P, and that P and N are the parents of C, and denote this specification of relationships as H. We could also describe the relationships in a simple pedigree.

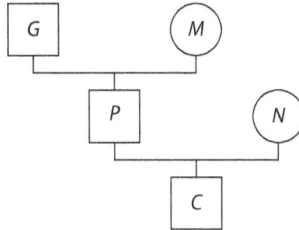

We now notice that the members of the pedigree fall into two classes: founders and non-founders. The founders, G, M and N, are defined as unrelated* and further we have not observed the genotypes of any of their parents. We can express the probability of observing the whole pedigree, $\Pr(G_P, G_G, G_M, G_N, G_C|H)$, as the product of the conditional probability of observing the non-founders given the genotypes of the founders and the unconditional probability of observing the founders.

$$\Pr(G_P, G_G, G_M, G_N, G_C \,|\, H) = \Pr(G_P, G_C \,|\, G_G, G_M, G_N, H) \times \Pr(G_G, G_M, G_N \,|\, H)$$

We can further simplify $\Pr(G_P, G_C|G_G, G_M, G_N, H)$ into a product of the conditional probabilities of observing the genotype of an individual given the genotypes of his parents. For the simple pedigree above,

$$\Pr(G_P, G_G \,|\, G_M, G_N, G_C, H) = \Pr(G_C \,|\, G_P, G_N, H) \times \Pr(G_P \,|\, G_G, G_M \,|\, H$$

If the genotypes of all of the founders of the pedigree are specified, evaluation of the probability of observing the pedigree is direct and follows Mendel's laws.

---

* Otherwise there would be more branches to the pedigree.

Parents

If samples are available from both of the deceased's parents, it enables strong inferences to be drawn regarding the profile of the deceased. Following the principles given in Chapter 11 it can be seen that depending on the pattern of parental alleles between one and four distinct combinations exist at each locus for their biological child.

We envisage a situation where we have a body with genotype G_B. We also assume that both the putative parents of the missing person are available, the mother (M) with genotype G_M and the father (F) with genotype G_F.

Evaluating the evidence in such a scenario requires hypotheses of the type:

H_1: The remains are from a biological child of M and F.

H_2: The remains are from an unknown person unrelated to M and F.

We evaluate the LR

$$LR = \frac{\Pr\left(G_B, G_F, G_M \,|\, H_1, I\right)}{\Pr\left(G_B, G_F, G_M \,|\, H_2, I\right)}$$

First, using the third law of probability, we take out the youngest person, which is the body.

$$LR = \frac{\Pr(G_B \mid G_F, G_M, H_1, I)\Pr(G_F, G_M \mid H_1, I)}{\Pr(G_B \mid G_F, G_M, H_2, I)\Pr(G_F, G_M \mid H_2, I)}$$

We assume that the joint probabilities of observing the genotypes of the founders of the pedigree, that is the mother and father, do not depend on the two hypotheses, H_1 and H_2, $\Pr(G_F, G_M \mid H_2, I) = \Pr(G_F, G_M \mid H_1, I)$, and hence

$$LR = \frac{\Pr(G_B \mid G_F, G_M, H_1, I)}{\Pr(G_B \mid G_F, G_M, H_2, I)}$$

The term $\Pr(G_B \mid G_F, G_M, H_1, I)$ can be assessed by applying Mendel's laws using a Punnett square. The term $\Pr(G_B \mid G_F, G_M, H_2, I)$ is the probability of observing the genotype of a person conditioned on those of two people to whom he or she is unrelated under H_2. This can be assessed either using the product rule or the subpopulation correction as desired.

It is worthwhile considering the usefulness of the subpopulation correction in this context. We believe that the product rule has a slight bias in favour of H_1, whereas the subpopulation correction has a strong bias in favour of H_2. This is especially so if a conservative value is assigned for θ. If the intent of the case is to identify bodies to return the remains to the correct relatives, then there seems to be little value to the subpopulation correction. If the case is criminal, then there may be some value in using the subpopulation correction in order to give a conservative LR to the court. If the subpopulation correction is applied, then we are assuming that the body is not part of this pedigree but is from the same subpopulation as the members of the pedigree. Birus et al.[470] give powerful evidence in support of this approach. Fung et al.[1035] outline the general approach to incorporating the subpopulation correction.

In Table 12.1 we give the formulae for the LR at a single locus. These formulae ignore mutation. For autosomal loci there is no need to differentiate the mother from the father, so that we can call these persons Parent 1 and 2. For the 10-locus SGMPlus system this typically leads to values of the LR of the order of 10^5 to 10^6.

If a sample from only one parent is available (because the identity of the other parent is unknown or because he or she is deceased), the LR can still be calculated. Although inferences can still be drawn regarding the profile of the deceased, the numerical value of the LR will be smaller and the 'power' of the analysis is dramatically reduced.

The hypotheses are likely to be of the following form:

H_1: The remains are from a biological child of the parent.

H_2: The remains are from an unknown individual unrelated to the parent.

Let G_B be the genotype of the body and G_P the genotype of the parent. We require

$$LR = \frac{\Pr(G_B \mid G_P, H_1, I)}{\Pr(G_B \mid G_P, H_2, I)}$$

The term $\Pr(G_B \mid G_P, H_1, I)$ can be assessed by simple Mendelian principles before considering a 'missing' parent. It is not necessary in this instance to enumerate all the possibilities for the missing parent as the expedient of a 'random allele' can be used, as described under 'Paternity Duos' in Chapter 11.*

---

* Recall that this expedient will not work if there are multiple children. In this formulation the body is the only typed child of the parent and the missing parent. If, for example, siblings of the missing person are available, then the possible genotypes of the missing parent must be enumerated.

Table 12.1   Formulae for the *LR* When Genotypes of Both Parents (But No Children) of a Missing Person Are Available as Reference Samples

Parent 1	Parent 2	Body	*LR* Assessed by the Product Rule	*LR* Assessed Using the Subpopulation Correction
aa	aa	aa	$\dfrac{1}{p_a^2}$	$\dfrac{(1+3\theta)(1+4\theta)}{(4\theta+(1-\theta)p_a)(5\theta+(1-\theta)p_a)}$
	ab	aa	$\dfrac{1}{2p_a^2}$	$\dfrac{(1+3\theta)(1+4\theta)}{2(3\theta+(1-\theta)p_a)(4\theta+(1-\theta)p_a)}$
		ab	$\dfrac{1}{4p_ap_b}$	$\dfrac{(1+3\theta)(1+4\theta)}{4(3\theta+(1-\theta)p_a)(\theta+(1-\theta)p_b)}$
	bb	ab	$\dfrac{1}{2p_ap_b}$	$\dfrac{(1+3\theta)(1+4\theta)}{2(2\theta+(1-\theta)p_a)(2\theta+(1-\theta)p_b)}$
	bc	ab	$\dfrac{1}{4p_ap_b}$	$\dfrac{(1+3\theta)(1+4\theta)}{4(2\theta+(1-\theta)p_a)(\theta+(1-\theta)p_b)}$
ab	ab	aa	$\dfrac{1}{4p_a^2}$	$\dfrac{(1+3\theta)(1+4\theta)}{4(2\theta+(1-\theta)p_a)(3\theta+(1-\theta)p_a)}$
		ab	$\dfrac{1}{4p_ap_b}$	$\dfrac{(1+3\theta)(1+4\theta)}{4(2\theta+(1-\theta)p_a)(2\theta+(1-\theta)p_b)}$
	ac	ab	$\dfrac{1}{4p_ap_b}$	$\dfrac{(1+3\theta)(1+4\theta)}{8(2\theta+(1-\theta)p_a)(\theta+(1-\theta)p_b)}$
		aa	$\dfrac{1}{4p_a^2}$	$\dfrac{(1+3\theta)(1+4\theta)}{4(2\theta+(1-\theta)p_a)(3\theta+(1-\theta)p_a)}$
	cd	ac	$\dfrac{1}{8p_ap_b}$	$\dfrac{(1+3\theta)(1+4\theta)}{8(\theta+(1-\theta)p_a)(\theta+(1-\theta)p_c)}$

Note: Recall we advocate no subpopulation correction in non-criminal work; hence θ may be set to 0 to return the product rule.

LR, likelihood ratio.

The term $\Pr(G_B \mid G_P, H_2, I)$ is the probability of observing the genotype of a person conditioned on the genotype of another person to whom he or she is unrelated. This probability can be assessed using the product rule or the subpopulation correction as desired. Table 12.2 gives some *LR*s which can be applied to a single parent situation ignoring mutation.

The values of the *LR* obtained using the 10 loci from the SGMPlus system are typically reduced to the order of 10^2 to 10^3.

If only a single parent is available, then the paucity of genetic information can often be supplemented by reference to other members of the pedigree if they are available.

Children

A sample from a child provides information regarding its biological parent. If the deceased had a number of children, then testing all of them will provide the most information regarding his

Table 12.2   Formulae for the *LR* When the Genotype of One Relative of the Missing Person Is Available as a Reference Sample

Genotype of Comparison Relative	Genotype of the Missing Person	*LR* Assessed by the Product Rule	*LR* Asessed Using the Subpopulation Correction
aa	aa	$\dfrac{Z_2}{p_a^2}+\dfrac{Z_1}{p_a}+Z_0$	$\dfrac{Z_2(1+\theta)(1+2\theta)}{\big(2\theta+(1-\theta)p_a\big)\big(3\theta+(1-\theta)p_a\big)}$ $+\dfrac{Z_1(1+2\theta)}{\big(3\theta+(1-\theta)p_a\big)}+Z_0$
	bb	Z_0	Z_0
	ab	$\dfrac{Z_1}{2p_a}+Z_0$	$Z_1\dfrac{(1+2\theta)}{2\big(2\theta+(1-\theta)p_a\big)}+Z_0$
	bc	Z_0	Z_0
ab	aa	$\dfrac{Z_1}{2p_a}+Z_0$	$\dfrac{Z_1(1+2\theta)}{2\big(2\theta+(1-\theta)p_a\big)}+Z_0$
	ab	$\dfrac{2Z_2+Z_1(p_a+p_b)}{4p_ap_b}$ $+Z_0$	$\dfrac{\big[2Z_2(1+\theta)+Z_1\big(2\theta+(1-\theta)(p_a+p_b)\big)\big](1+2\theta)}{4\big(\theta+(1-\theta)p_a\big)\big(\theta+(1-\theta)p_b\big)}$ $+Z_0$
	ac	$\dfrac{Z_1}{4p_a}+Z_0$	$\dfrac{Z_1(1+2\theta)}{4\big(\theta+(1-\theta)p_a\big)}+Z_0$
	cc	Z_0	Z_0
	cd		

LR, likelihood ratio. *Z* values for common relatives are given in Table 4.1.

or her genotype. Moreover, if a sample is available from the children's other parent, the process is aided as this often allows the determination of which allele was contributed by the deceased.

Consider a situation where the male deceased has a wife (genotype *ab*) and two children (genotypes *aa* and *bc*). From this it can be deduced that at this locus the deceased's genotype is *ac*. Without the sample from the deceased's wife, there would have been two possible genotypes (*ab* or *ac*).

The magnitude of the *LR* obtained from the analysis of children will be governed by the availability of a sample from the other parent and also the number of children available for testing.

We consider a situation where there is one child and the partner of the missing person is available. The hypotheses are likely to be of the following form:

H_1: The remains are from the biological parent of the child.

H_2: The remains are from an unknown individual unrelated to the child.

Let G_B be the genotype of the body, G_C the genotype of the child and G_P the genotype of the partner of the missing person. We require

$$LR=\dfrac{\Pr\big(G_B,G_P,G_C\,|\,H_1,I\big)}{\Pr\big(G_B,G_P,G_C\,|\,H_2,I\big)}$$

As usual first we condition the genotype of the youngest person in the pedigree on the genotypes in the rest of the pedigree. In this example the youngest person is the child.

$$LR = \frac{\Pr\left(G_B, G_P, G_C \mid H_1, I\right)}{\Pr\left(G_B, G_P, G_C \mid H_2, I\right)} = \frac{\Pr\left(G_C \mid G_B, G_P, H_1, I\right)\Pr\left(G_B, G_P \mid H_1, I\right)}{\Pr\left(G_C \mid G_B, G_P, H_2, I\right)\Pr\left(G_B, G_P \mid H_2, I\right)}$$

Again assuming that $\Pr(G_B, G_P \mid H_1, I) = \Pr(G_B, G_P \mid H_2, I)$ we see that

$$LR = \frac{\Pr\left(G_C \mid G_B, G_P, H_1, I\right)}{\Pr\left(G_C \mid G_B, G_P, H_2, I\right)}$$

The term $\Pr(G_C \mid G_B, G_P, H_1, I)$ can be assessed by simple Mendelian principles as before.

When we turn to the consideration of the pedigree under H_2, the term $\Pr(G_C \mid G_B, G_P, H_2, I)$ is the probability of observing the genotype of a child given that of one parent (recall that B is not related to C and P under H_2) and should be assessed as previously for paternity duos. As usual this can be assessed using the product rule or the subpopulation correction as desired. Some formulae for typical situations are given in Table 12.3. Table 12.2 can be used to give the *LRs* when the partner of the deceased is not available.

Table 12.3   Formulae for the *LR* for Situations Where the Genotypes of the Partner and One Child of the Missing Person Are Available as Reference Samples

Body	Child	Partner of the Missing Person	LR Assessed by the Product Rule	LR Assessed Using the Subpopulation Correction
aa	aa	aa	$\dfrac{1}{p_a}$	$\dfrac{1+3\theta}{4\theta+(1-\theta)p_a}$
		ab	$\dfrac{1}{p_a}$	$\dfrac{1+3\theta}{3\theta+(1-\theta)p_a}$
	ab	ab	$\dfrac{1}{p_a+p_b}$	$\dfrac{1+3\theta}{4\theta+(1-\theta)\left[p_a+p_b\right]}$
		bb or bc	$\dfrac{1}{p_a}$	$\dfrac{1+3\theta}{2\theta+(1-\theta)p_a}$
ab	aa	aa	$\dfrac{1}{2p_a}$	$\dfrac{1+3\theta}{2\left[3\theta+(1-\theta)p_a\right]}$
		ab or ac	$\dfrac{1}{2p_a}$	$\dfrac{1+3\theta}{2\left[2\theta+(1-\theta)p_a\right]}$
	ab	ab	$\dfrac{1}{p_a+p_b}$	$\dfrac{1+3\theta}{4\theta+(1-\theta)\left[p_a+p_b\right]}$
		bb or bc	$\dfrac{1}{2p_a}$	$\dfrac{1+3\theta}{2\left[\theta+(1-\theta)p_a\right]}$
	ac	cc or cd	$\dfrac{1}{2p_a}$	$\dfrac{1+3\theta}{2\left[\theta+(1-\theta)p_a\right]}$

LR, likelihood ratio.

It is worth noting a further feature of an analysis using children. Suppose that the genotype of the deceased's wife was pr and the four children at a locus were pq, pq, qr and qr. On this occasion the deceased can be inferred to carry the q allele. There are at least two possible explanations for this observation:

- The deceased has genotype qq at this locus.

- The deceased has genotype qx at the locus (where x is any allele other than q).

From this finding it can be seen that the first explanation, that the deceased is a qq homozygote, becomes more probable and the second explanation, that he is a heterozygote, less probable. If the deceased was in fact qx, then the probability of transmitting only allele q to each of his four children is $(\frac{1}{2})^4$, i.e. 1 in 16. We see that one will never be certain that the deceased is a qq homozygote at this locus although this may be overwhelmingly the most supported genotype.

Siblings

It is possible for two full siblings to have no alleles in common at a locus. If two or more siblings are available, the information increases concomitantly. Only when all four distinct alleles are represented among the surviving siblings, will it be possible to deduce the four parental alleles at a locus. It will still be impossible to determine which genotype is paternal. When multiple loci have all four alleles present, there will be ambiguity about the multilocus paternal and maternal genotypes. The ambiguity in the deceased is influenced by the ambiguity in the parental profiles and by Mendelian factors.

The magnitude of the LR obtained from the analysis of siblings will depend upon the number of siblings available for testing and on the rarity of shared alleles. In addition it is possible that a match may exist between the deceased and, for example, two putative siblings, but that the calculated LR value across multiple loci is less than 1. In other words, there is support for the alternative proposition (that these individuals are not siblings of the body) despite the apparent match. This tends to happen when the profile from the body has several loci where it shares no alleles in common with either of the putative siblings. At such a locus the value of the LR is 1/4. As a very rough rule of thumb, where the body shares one allele at a locus the LR is generally close to 1 and when both alleles are shared it will be greater than 1, although its magnitude depends on the rarity of the alleles concerned.

Table 12.2 can be used to give the LRs when one sibling of the missing person is available.

Other Combinations of First Degree Relatives

On many occasions, the pedigree contains combinations of relatives, e.g. a child and sib. In these instances the formulae for the LR must be derived on a case-by-case and locus-by-locus basis depending on the specific pattern of alleles.[496] Software programmes such as Charles Brenner's symbolic kinship programme[484,485] have excellent algorithms and offer considerable savings of labour in this regard. Dawid et al.[1036] describe the adaptation of general-purpose computer software such as Hugin,[1037] GeNIe[1038] or XBAIES[1039] to the problem by reformulating the pedigree as a probabilistic expert system. We give a few examples of this derivation below.

Example 12.1: Missing Body Given Putative Parent and Child

Suppose that we have a simple three-generation pedigree as depicted below. The person labelled D is missing and a body, B, has been found which may belong to this person.

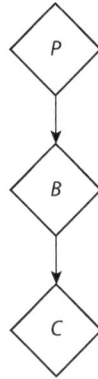

We take the following hypotheses:

H_1: The body is the missing person.

H_2: The body is unrelated to this pedigree.

For these hypotheses, we require

$$LR = \frac{\Pr(G_C, G_B, G_P \mid H_1, I)}{\Pr(G_C, G_B, G_P \mid H_2, I)}$$

Using the third law we decompose this to arrange for children to be conditioned on parents (if any are present in the pedigree).

$$LR = \frac{\Pr(G_C \mid G_B, G_P, H_1, I)\Pr(G_B \mid G_P, H_1, I)\Pr(G_P \mid H_1, I)}{\Pr(G_C \mid G_B, G_P, H_2, I)\Pr(G_B \mid G_P, H_2, I)\Pr(G_P \mid H_2, I)}$$

Next we can simplify this if we make a series of assumptions. The assumptions are of two types. The first type is an assumption that the joint probabilities of observing the genotypes of the founders of the pedigree under the two hypotheses are the same.

1. The probability of observing the genotypes of the founder(s) of the pedigree does not depend on the specific hypothesis being considered, $\Pr(G_P \mid H_1, I) = \Pr(G_P \mid H_2, I)$. The genotype of P does not depend on whether B is in the pedigree or not (recall that we do not know G_B at this point).

   The second type of assumption follows from the application of Mendel's laws to the pedigree.

2. $\Pr(G_C \mid G_B, G_P, H_1, I) = \Pr(G_C \mid G_B, H_1, I)$, since the conditioning on P is redundant, under the assumptions of H_1.
3. $\Pr(G_B \mid G_P, H_2, I) = \Pr(G_B \mid H_2, I)$, since under H_2, B and P are unrelated.
4. $\Pr(G_C \mid G_B, G_P, H_2, I) = \Pr(G_C \mid G_P, H_2, I)$, since under H_2, C and B are unrelated.

Note that if we use the subpopulation correction we leave the general conditioning in place in Steps 2 and 3 but treat the genotypes as coming from unrelated individuals.

Hence

$$LR = \frac{\Pr(G_C \mid G_B, H_1, I)\Pr(G_B \mid G_P, H_1, I)}{\Pr(G_C \mid G_P, H_2, I)\Pr(G_B \mid H_2, I)}$$

Let $G_P = ab$, $G_B = bc$ and $G_C = cd$. Now $\Pr(G_C \mid G_B, H_1, I) = \dfrac{p_d}{2}$, $\Pr(G_B \mid G_P, H_1, I) = \dfrac{p_c}{2}$ and $\Pr(G_B \mid H_2, I) = 2p_b p_c$.

To assess the term $\Pr(G_C|G_P, H_2, I)$ in general[*] it is necessary to consider the genotype of the missing person, D. This genotype is unknown so we denote by G_{Di}, $i = 1 \ldots n$, the range of possible genotypes for this person. Suppose that the locus that is being considered has m alleles; there are then m possible homozygous genotypes and $\frac{1}{2}m(m-1)$ possible heterozygous genotypes to consider. However unless the genotype G_{Di} has (at least) one allele in common with that of P, then $\Pr(G_{Di}|G_P, H_2, I) = 0$. Similarly $\Pr(G_C|G_{Di}, H_2, I) = 0$ unless the genotype, G_{Di}, has (at least) one allele in common with that of C. Hence once the genotypes of P and C are known the length, n, of the list of genotypes, G_{Di}, that needs to be considered is greatly reduced. Thus

$$\Pr(G_C|G_P, H_2, I) = \sum_{i=1}^{n} \Pr(G_C|G_{Di}, G_P, H_2, I)\Pr(G_{Di}|G_P, H_2, I)$$

Note that $\Pr(G_C|G_{Di}, G_P, H_2, I) = \Pr(G_C|G_{Di}, H_2, I)$ since the genotype of G_C is independent of the genotype G_P conditional on H_2 if the genotype of D, the child of P and parent of C, is specified.

This term is amenable to evaluation using a tabular approach, with one row of the table below for each possible genotype G_{Di}. Any possible genotype must contain one allele in common with G_P and one in common with G_C.

$$G_P = ab, \ G_B = bc \text{ and } G_C = cd$$

G_{Di}	$\Pr(G_{Di}|G_P, H_2, I)$	$\Pr(G_C|G_{Di}, H_2, I)$	$\Pr(G_C|G_{Di}, G_P, H_2, I)$ $\times \Pr(G_{Di}|G_P, H_2, I)$
ac	$\dfrac{p_c}{2}$	$\dfrac{p_d}{2}$	$\dfrac{p_c p_d}{4}$
ad	$\dfrac{p_d}{2}$	$\dfrac{p_c}{2}$	$\dfrac{p_c p_d}{4}$
bc	$\dfrac{p_c}{2}$	$\dfrac{p_d}{2}$	$\dfrac{p_c p_d}{4}$
bd	$\dfrac{p_d}{2}$	$\dfrac{p_c}{2}$	$\dfrac{p_c p_d}{4}$

$$\sum_{i=1}^{n} \Pr(G_C|G_{Di}, H_d, I)\Pr(G_{Di}|G_P, H_d, I) = p_c p_d$$

Assembling the above terms we find that $LR = \dfrac{1}{8 p_b p_c}$.

We can write the LR as the product of two terms

$$LR = \frac{1}{\Pr(G_B|H_2, I)} \times \frac{\Pr(G_C|G_B, H_1, I)\Pr(G_B|G_P, H_1, I)}{\Pr(G_C|G_P, H_2, I)}$$

The first,

$$\frac{1}{\Pr(G_B|H_2, I)} = \frac{1}{2 p_b p_c},$$

---

[*] There are shortcuts at this point that work well for one child but are more difficult for multiple children. By using identical by descent (IBD) states we see that there is a 1/2 chance that neither of the alleles in P is IBD with the alleles in C. If neither are IBD, then a cd child will result with probability $2p_c p_d$. This directly yields $\frac{1}{2} \times 2 p_c p_d = p_c p_d$.

is the *LR* that would be obtained if we knew the genotype of person *D*. The second can be expressed as a fraction, since

$$\frac{\Pr\left(G_C\,|\,G_B,H_p,I\right)\Pr\left(G_B\,|\,G_P,H_1,I\right)}{\Pr\left(G_C\,|\,G_P,H_2,I\right)} = \frac{\Pr\left(G_C\,|\,G_B,H_p,I\right)\Pr\left(G_B\,|\,G_P,H_1,I\right)}{\sum\limits_{i=1}^{n}\Pr\left(G_C\,|\,G_{D_i},H_2,I\right)\Pr\left(G_{D_i}\,|\,G_P,H_2,I\right)}$$

After we have enumerated the genotypes $D_1, \ldots, D_n$ we can drop the conditioning on the hypotheses H_1 and H_2. The genotype of the (non-excluded) body *B* must be one of the genotypes in the list, D_k, say, $G_B = G_{Dk}$. We thus have

$$\frac{\Pr\left(G_C\,|\,G_B,H_1,I\right)\Pr\left(G_B\,|\,G_P,H_1,I\right)}{\Pr\left(G_C\,|\,G_P,H_2,I\right)} = \frac{\Pr\left(G_C\,|\,G_B,I\right)\Pr\left(G_B\,|\,G_P,I\right)}{\sum\limits_{i=1}^{n}\Pr\left(G_C\,|\,G_{D_i},I\right)\Pr\left(G_{D_i}\,|\,G_P,I\right)}$$

Hence the fraction is always less than 1 in value if there is more than one possible genotype for the missing body which is consistent with the pedigree. In this example there are four possible genotypes and, coincidentally, the *LR* is 1/4 of that for a simple identification.

Example 12.2: Missing Body Given Putative Parent, Partner and Child

We have the simple three-generation pedigree as depicted below. The person labelled *D* is missing and a body, *B*, has been found which may belong to this person.

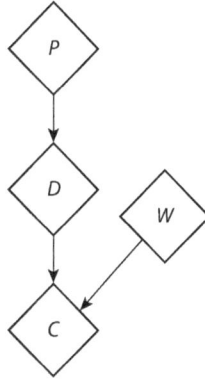

Consider the following hypotheses:

H_1: The body is the missing person.

H_2: The body is unrelated to *P*, *W* and *C*.

For these hypotheses we require

$$LR = \frac{\Pr\left(G_C,G_B,G_W,G_P\,|\,H_1,I\right)}{\Pr\left(G_C,G_B,G_W,G_P\,|\,H_2,I\right)}$$

Using the third law we decompose this to arrange for genotypes of children to be conditioned on the genotypes of their parents (if any are present in the pedigree), hence

$$LR = \frac{\Pr\left(G_C\,|\,G_B,G_W,G_P,H_1,I\right)\Pr\left(G_B\,|\,G_W,G_P,H_1,I\right)\Pr\left(G_W,G_P\,|\,H_1,I\right)}{\Pr\left(G_C\,|\,G_B,G_W,G_P,H_2,I\right)\Pr\left(G_B\,|\,G_W,G_P,H_2,I\right)\Pr\left(G_W,G_P\,|\,H_2,I\right)}$$

As in the previous example we can simplify this by making the same four assumptions plus one further assumption:

1. The joint probability of observing the genotypes of the founders of the pedigree P and W is the same for both hypotheses.

   The remaining assumptions are the implications of Mendel's laws for the probabilities of observing the genotypes G_P, G_B, G_W and G_C under the two hypotheses, H_1 and H_2.

2. Under H_1 the genotype of C is determined by those of B and W, so $\Pr(G_C|G_B,G_W,G_P,H_1,I) = \Pr(G_C|G_B,G_W,H_1,I)$.

3. Under H_2 the genotype of B is independent of those of P and W.

4. Under H_2 the genotypes of B and C are unrelated and hence the probability of observing the genotype of B is determined by the genotypes of P and W.

5. In addition we further assume that W and B are unrelated and so $\Pr(G_B|G_W,G_P,H_1,I) = \Pr(G_B|G_P,H_1,I)$.

Note that if we use the subpopulation correction we leave the general conditioning in place in Steps 2, 3 and 4 but treat the genotypes as coming from unrelated individuals.

Hence

$$LR = \frac{\Pr(G_C|G_B,G_W,H_1,I)\Pr(G_B|G_P,H_1,I)}{\Pr(G_C|G_W,G_P,H_2,I)\Pr(G_B|H_2,I)}$$

Let $G_P = ab$, $G_B = bc$, $G_W = de$ and $G_C = cd$. Now $\Pr(G_C|G_B,G_W,H_1,I) = \frac{1}{4}$, $\Pr(G_B|G_P,H_1,I) = \frac{p_c}{2}$ and $\Pr(G_B|H_2,I) = 2p_bp_c$.

The term $\Pr(G_C|G_W,G_P,H_2,I)$ is assessed as before by considering the range of possible genotypes, G_{Di}, for the missing person, D.

$$\Pr(G_C|G_W,G_P,H_2,I) = \sum_{i=1}^{n} \Pr(G_C|G_{Di},G_W,G_P,H_2,I)\Pr(G_{Di}|G_W,G_P,H_2,I)$$

$\Pr(G_{Di}|G_W,G_P,H_2,I) = \Pr(G_{Di}|G_P,H_2,I)$ since D and W are unrelated and $\Pr(G_C|G_{Di},G_W,G_P,H_2,I) = \Pr(G_C|G_{Di},G_W,H_2,I)$ since the genotype of the child is independent of that of P under H_1 if the genotypes of the child's parents are specified.

Hence we can write

$$\Pr(G_C|G_W,G_P,H_2,I) = \sum_{i=1}^{n} \Pr(G_C|G_{Di},G_W,H_2,I)\Pr(G_{Di}|G_P,H_2,I)$$

The LR can be written as

$$LR = \frac{1}{\Pr(G_B|H_2,I)} \times \frac{\Pr(G_C|G_B,G_W,H_1,I)\Pr(G_B|G_P,H_1,I)}{\Pr(G_C|G_P,G_W,H_2,I)}$$

$$= \frac{1}{\Pr(G_B|H_2,I)} \times \frac{\Pr(G_C|G_{D_k},G_W,I)\Pr(G_{D_k}|G_P,G_W,I)}{\sum_{i=1}^{n}\Pr(G_C|G_{D_i},G_W,I)\Pr(G_{D_i}|G_P,G_W,I)}$$

As in the previous example we can enumerate the list of possible genotypes, D_i, and evaluate the sum in the denominator using the table below. The table includes rows for each of the same set of genotypes as in Example 11.1 but for two genotypes the term $\Pr(G_C|G_{Di},G_W,H_2,I) = 0$.

$$G_P = ab, \; G_B = bc, \; G_W = de \text{ and } G_C = cd$$

G_{Di}	$\Pr(G_{Di}\mid G_P,H_2,I)$	$\Pr(G_C\mid G_{Di},G_W,H_2,I)$	$\Pr(G_C\mid G_{Di},G_W,H_2,I)$ $\times \Pr(G_{Di}\mid G_P,H_2,I)$
ac	$\dfrac{p_c}{2}$	$\dfrac{1}{4}$	$\dfrac{p_c}{8}$
ad	$\dfrac{p_d}{2}$	0	0
bc	$\dfrac{p_c}{2}$	$\dfrac{1}{4}$	$\dfrac{p_c}{8}$
bd	$\dfrac{p_d}{2}$	0	0
	$\displaystyle\sum_{i=1}^{n}\Pr(G_C\mid G_{Di},G_W,H_2,I)\Pr(G_{Di}\mid G_P,H_2,I)=\dfrac{p_c}{4}$		

Assembling the above terms we find that $LR=\dfrac{1}{4\,p_b\,p_c}$. Reducing the list of possible genotypes for the missing person, D, from four to two has coincidently increased the LR by a factor of 2.

Example 12.3: Missing Body Given Putative Parent, Partner and Two Children

We consider a simple three-generation pedigree as depicted below. The person labelled D is missing and a body, B, has been found that may belong to this person.

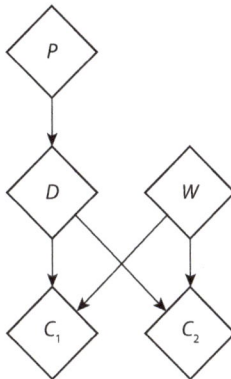

Consider the following pair of hypotheses:

H_1: The body is the missing person.

H_2: The body is unrelated to this pedigree.

For these hypotheses, we require

$$LR=\frac{\Pr\big(G_{C1},G_{C2},G_B,G_W,G_P\mid H_1,I\big)}{\Pr\big(G_{C1},G_{C2},G_B,G_W,G_P\mid H_2,I\big)}$$

$$=\frac{\Pr\big(G_{C1},G_{C2}\mid G_B,G_W,G_P,H_1,I\big)\Pr\big(G_B\mid G_W,G_P,H_1,I\big)\Pr\big(G_W,G_P\mid H_1,I\big)}{\Pr\big(G_{C1},G_{C2}\mid G_B,G_W,G_P,H_2,I\big)\Pr\big(G_B\mid G_W,G_P,H_2,I\big)\Pr\big(G_W,G_P\mid H_2,I\big)}$$

If we make the same five assumptions as in the previous example, we can write the LR as

$$LR = \frac{1}{\Pr(G_B \mid H_2, I)} \times \frac{\Pr(G_{C1}, G_{C2} \mid G_B, G_W, H_1, I)\Pr(G_B \mid G_P, H_1, I)}{\Pr(G_{C1}, G_{C2} \mid G_W, G_P, H_2, I)}$$

Let $G_P = ab$, $G_B = bc$, $G_W = de$, $G_{C1} = bd$ and $G_{C2} = ce$. Now $\Pr(G_{C1}, G_{C2} \mid G_B, G_W, H_1, I) = \frac{1}{16}$, $\Pr(G_B \mid G_P, H_1, I) = \frac{p_c}{2}$ and $\Pr(G_B \mid H_2, I) = 2p_b p_c$.

The term $\Pr(G_{C1}, G_{C2} \mid G_W, G_P, H_2, I)$ is assessed as before by considering the range of possible genotypes, G_{Di}, for the missing person, D, which are consistent with the genotypes of W, P, C_1 and C_2 and then evaluating the sum

$$\Pr(G_{C1}, G_{C2} \mid G_W, G_P, H_2, I) = \sum_{i=1}^{n} \Pr(G_{C1}, G_{C2} \mid G_{Di}, G_W, I)\Pr(G_{Di} \mid G_P, I)$$

This pedigree differs from that in Example 11.2 because under H_2 the genotypes of the two children, C_1 and C_2, together with the genotype of the partner suffice to determine the genotype of the missing person. Our table now only has a single row. Three of the previously considered genotypes lead to a value of 0 for $\Pr(G_{C1}, G_{C2} \mid G_{Di}, G_W, I)$.

G_{Di}	$\Pr(G_{Di} \mid G_P, I)$	$\Pr(G_{C1}, G_{C2} \mid G_{Di}, G_W, I)$	$\Pr(G_{C1}, G_{C2} \mid G_{Di}, G_W, I) \times \Pr(G_{Di} \mid G_P, I)$
bc	$\frac{p_c}{2}$	$\frac{1}{16}$	$\frac{p_c}{32}$

$$\sum_{i=1}^{n} \Pr(G_{C1}, G_{C2} \mid G_{Di}, G_W, I)\Pr(G_{Di} \mid G_P, I) = \frac{p_c}{32}$$

The numerator and denominator of the second term in the expression for the LR are the same and hence we find that $LR = \frac{1}{2p_b p_c}$. Its value is now the same as that for a simple identification.

Example 12.4: Missing Body Given Putative Parent, Partner and Two Children

We consider the same pedigree as in the previous three examples when the genotype of the recovered body, B, is homozygous.

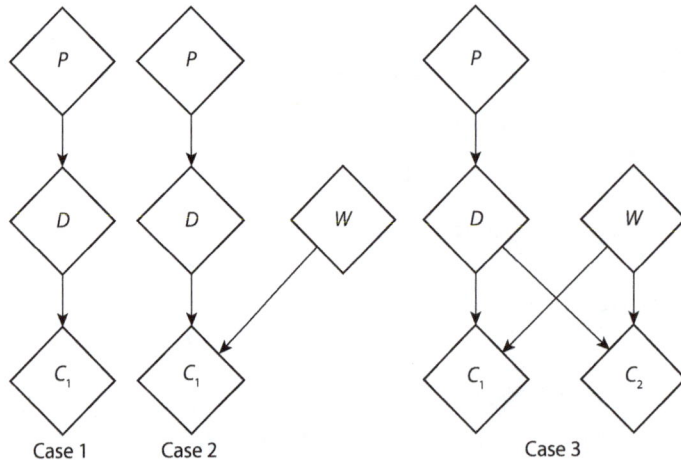

Case 1   Case 2   Case 3

414

Person	Case 1	Case 2	Case 3
P	ab	ab	ab
W	–	cd	cd
B	aa	aa	aa
C_1	ac	ac	ac
C_2	–	–	ad

Taking the same pair of hypotheses and making the same assumptions as in the three previous examples we use the same method to evaluate the LR. Under H_1 we can enumerate the lists of possible genotypes D_i which lead to non-zero probabilities in each of the three cases.

D_i	Case 1	Case 2	Case 3
D_1	aa	aa	aa
D_2	ab	ab	ab
D_3	ac	ac	ac
D_4	bc	–	–
D_5	ax	ax	ax

The allele x is taken to be any allele other than a, b or c. In each case $\Pr(G_B \mid H_2, I) = p_a^2$. We consider the tables for each case in turn.

Case 1. $P = ab$, $B = aa$, $C_1 = ac$

G_{Di}	$\Pr(G_{Di} \mid G_P, I)$	$\Pr(G_{C_1} \mid G_{Di}, I)$	$\Pr(G_{C_1} \mid G_{Di}, I) \times \Pr(G_{Di} \mid G_P, I)$
$G_B = aa$	$\dfrac{p_a}{2}$	p_c	$\dfrac{p_a p_c}{2}$
ab	$\dfrac{p_a + p_b}{2}$	$\dfrac{p_c}{2}$	$\dfrac{(p_a + p_b) p_c}{4}$
ac	$\dfrac{p_c}{2}$	$\dfrac{p_a + p_c}{2}$	$\dfrac{(p_a + p_c) p_c}{4}$
bc	$\dfrac{p_c}{2}$	$\dfrac{p_a}{2}$	$\dfrac{p_a p_c}{4}$
ax	$\dfrac{1 - p_a - p_b - p_c}{2}$	$\dfrac{p_c}{2}$	$\dfrac{(1 - p_a - p_b - p_c) p_c}{4}$
	$\displaystyle\sum_{i=1}^{n} \Pr(G_{C_1} \mid G_{Di}, I)\Pr(G_{Di} \mid G_P, I) = $		$\dfrac{(1 + 4p_a) p_c}{4}$

We find that

$$LR = \frac{2}{p_a(1 + 4p_a)} = \frac{1}{p_a^2} \times \frac{2p_a}{1 + 4p_a}$$

Its value is very much less than that for a simple identification if the a allele is rare.

415

Case 2. Inclusion of other parent of the child of the missing person. $P = ab$, $B = aa$, $W = cd$, $C_1 = ac$

G_{Di}	$\Pr(G_{Di} \mid G_P, I)$	$\Pr(G_{C1} \mid G_{Di}, I)$	$\Pr(G_{C1} \mid G_{Di}, I) \times \Pr(G_{Di} \mid G_P, I)$
$G_B = aa$	$\dfrac{p_a}{2}$	$\frac{1}{2}$	$\dfrac{p_a}{4}$
ab	$\dfrac{p_a + p_b}{2}$	$\frac{1}{4}$	$\dfrac{(p_a + p_b)}{8}$
ac	$\dfrac{p_c}{2}$	$\frac{1}{4}$	$\dfrac{p_c}{8}$
ax	$\dfrac{1 - p_a - p_b - p_c}{2}$	$\frac{1}{4}$	$\dfrac{(1 - p_a - p_b - p_c)}{8}$

$$\sum_{i=1}^{n} \Pr(G_{C1} \mid G_{Di}, I)\Pr(G_{Di} \mid G_P, I) = \frac{(1 + 2p_a)}{8}$$

We find that

$$LR = \frac{2}{p_a(1 + 2p_a)} = \frac{1}{p_a^2} \times \frac{2p_a}{1 + 2p_a}$$

Its value is a little greater than that for Case 1 but is still less than that for a simple identification.

Case 3. Inclusion of a second child. $P = ab$, $B = aa$, $W = cd$, $C_1 = ac$, $C_2 = ad$

G_{Di}	$\Pr(G_{Di} \mid G_P, I)$	$\Pr(G_{C1} \mid G_{Di}, I)$	$\Pr(G_{C1} \mid G_{Di}, I) \times \Pr(G_{Di} \mid G_P, I)$
$G_B = aa$	$\dfrac{p_a}{2}$	$\frac{1}{4}$	$\dfrac{p_a}{8}$
ab	$\dfrac{p_a + p_b}{2}$	$\frac{1}{16}$	$\dfrac{(p_a + p_b)}{32}$
ac	$\dfrac{p_c}{2}$	$\frac{1}{16}$	$\dfrac{p_c}{32}$
ax	$\dfrac{1 - p_a - p_b - p_c}{2}$	$\frac{1}{16}$	$\dfrac{(1 - p_a - p_b - p_c)}{32}$

$$\sum_{i=1}^{n} \Pr(G_{C1} \mid G_{Di}, I)\Pr(G_{Di} \mid G_P, I) = \frac{(1 + 4p_a)}{32}$$

We find that $LR = \dfrac{4}{p_a(1 + 4p_a)} = \dfrac{1}{p_a^2} \times \dfrac{4p_a}{1 + 4p_a}$. In the following table we compare the numerical value for the LR in each of the four cases for a range of allele frequencies for the a allele.

Allele Frequency, p_a	Simple Identification	Case 1	Case 2	Case 3
0.005	40,000	390	400	780
0.010	10,000	190	200	380
0.025	1,600	73	76	150
0.050	400	33	36	67

Continued

Allele Frequency, p_a	Simple Identification	Case 1	Case 2	Case 3
0.100	100	14	17	29
0.250	16	4.0	5.3	8.0
0.350	8.2	2.4	3.4	4.8

Example 12.5: Missing Body Given Two Siblings

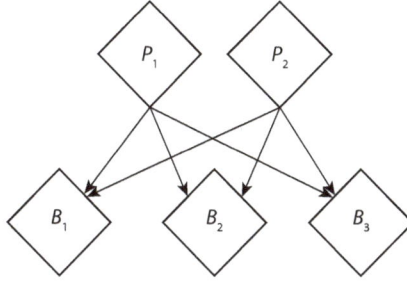

In this instance we consider three siblings whose parents have not been typed. The parents are drawn in the pedigree but recall that their genotypes are not available. Sibling B_3 is missing and a body, B, has been found that may belong to this person.

Consider the following hypotheses:

H_1: The body is the missing person.

H_2: The body is unrelated to this pedigree.

For these hypotheses we require

$$LR = \frac{\Pr\left(G_{B1}, G_{B2}, G_{B3} \mid H_1, I\right)}{\Pr\left(G_{B1}, G_{B2}, G_{B3} \mid H_2, I\right)}$$

Assuming that B_1 and B_2, B_3 are independent if unrelated this yields

$$LR = \frac{\Pr\left(G_{B1}, G_{B2}, G_{B3} \mid H_1, I\right)}{\Pr\left(G_{B1} \mid H_2, I\right)\Pr\left(G_{B2}, G_{B3} \mid H_2, I\right)}$$

Evaluation of the denominator is relatively straightforward. $\Pr(G_{B1} \mid H_2, I)$ can be assessed by the product rule; $\Pr(G_{B2}, G_{B3} \mid H_2, I)$ is the joint probability for two siblings and is tabulated in Chapter 4. This leaves $\Pr(G_{B1}, G_{B2}, G_{B3} \mid H_1, I)$. This is the joint probability for the genotypes of three siblings. Two approaches are available.

1. Complete enumeration of the possible genotypes for the parents. This approach is consistent with the approach used in Examples 12.1 through 12.4. If there are $1 \ldots n$ possibilities for the parents, P_1 and P_2, then

$$\Pr\left(G_{B1}, G_{B2}, G_{B3} \mid H_1, I\right) = \sum_{i=1}^{n} \left(\begin{array}{c} \Pr\left(G_{B1}, G_{B2}, G_{B3} \mid G_{P1}, G_{P2}, H_1, I\right) \\ \times \Pr\left(G_{P1}, G_{P2} \mid H_1, I\right) \end{array} \right)$$

2. The use of six-allele descent measures, which are the logical extension of Weir's four-allele measures presented in Chapter 4.

Six-allele descent measures were discussed by Thompson[496] in the context of two siblings and an aunt or a niece or half-sib. We illustrate their use in this case. Let $G_{B1} = ab$, $G_{B2} = ab$ and $G_{B3} = cd$ (this is the easiest three-sibling calculation since all four distinct alleles are present).

417

Enumeration of the possibilities for the genotypes of parents leads to a calculation which can be set out in a table as in the examples above.

P_1	P_2	$\Pr(G_{P1}, G_{P2}|H_1, I)$	$\Pr(G_{B1}, G_{B2}, G_{B3}|G_{P1}, G_{P2}, H_1, I)$
ac	bd	$4p_a p_b p_c p_d$	$\dfrac{1}{64}$
ad	bc	$4p_a p_b p_c p_d$	$\dfrac{1}{64}$
bd	ac	$4p_a p_b p_c p_d$	$\dfrac{1}{64}$
bc	ad	$4p_a p_b p_c p_d$	$\dfrac{1}{64}$

$$\sum_{i=1}^{n}\Pr(G_{B1}, G_{B2}, G_{B3}|G_{P1}, G_{P2}, H_1, I)\Pr(G_{P1}, G_{P2}|H_1, I) = \frac{p_a p_b p_c p_d}{4}$$

Now $\Pr(G_{B1}|H_2, I) = 2p_a p_b$, and from Chapter 4 we see that

$$\Pr(G_{B2}, G_{B3}|H_2, I) = p_a p_b p_c p_d$$

Hence

$$LR = \frac{1}{8p_a p_b}$$

In order to apply the six-allele* descent measures we label the alleles from the parents a to f. We consider that the alleles a and c could be identical by descent (IBD) since they have come from the same parent. This will occur 1/2 of the time. Hence the alleles a, c and e will be IBD ($a \equiv b \equiv c$) 1/4 of the time. The alleles b, d and f will be IBD 1/4 of the time. Hence the event $a \equiv b \equiv c$ and $b \equiv d \equiv f$ will occur 1/16 of the time.

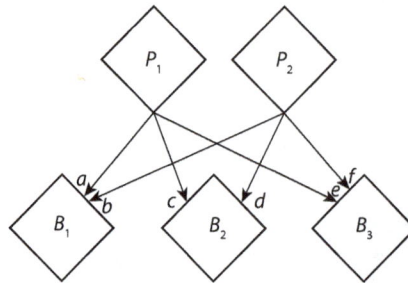

IBD State		Pr(IBD State)	$\Pr(G_{B1}, G_{B2}, G_{B3}|$IBD State$)$
$a \equiv b \equiv c$	$b \equiv d \equiv f$	$\frac{1}{16}$	0
	$b \equiv d$	$\frac{1}{16}$	0
	$b \equiv f$	$\frac{1}{16}$	0
	$d \equiv f$	$\frac{1}{16}$	0

Continued

---

* The extension to N alleles is discussed by Thompson.[495,496]

IBD State		Pr(IBD State)	Pr(G_{B1}, G_{B2}, G_{B3} | IBD State)
a≡c	b≡d≡f	$\frac{1}{16}$	0
	b≡d	$\frac{1}{16}$	$4p_a p_b p_c p_d$
	b≡f	$\frac{1}{16}$	0
	d≡f	$\frac{1}{16}$	0
a≡e	b≡d≡f	$\frac{1}{16}$	0
	b≡d	$\frac{1}{16}$	0
	b≡f	$\frac{1}{16}$	0
	d≡f	$\frac{1}{16}$	0
c≡e	b≡d≡f	$\frac{1}{16}$	0
	b≡d	$\frac{1}{16}$	0
	b≡f	$\frac{1}{16}$	0
	d≡f	$\frac{1}{16}$	0
Taking the product across the rows and the sum down yields→			$\dfrac{p_a p_b p_c p_d}{4}$

The result yielded in the last row of the table is the same result as that achieved by enumerating the parental possibilities.

Example 12.6: Missing Body Given Two Siblings

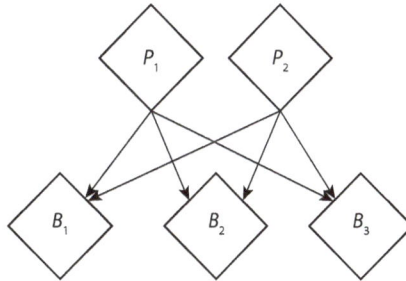

In this instance we consider the same pedigree of three siblings whose parents have not been typed, as given in Example 11.5. Consider the following hypotheses:

H_1: The body is the missing person.

H_2: The body is unrelated to this pedigree.

We evaluate

$$LR = \frac{\Pr\left(G_{B1}, G_{B2}, G_{B3} \mid H_1, I\right)}{\Pr\left(G_{B1} \mid H_2, I\right)\Pr\left(G_{B2}, G_{B3} \mid H_2, I\right)}$$

as usual; however in this example we consider a more difficult arrangement of genotypes. Let $G_{B1} = ab$, $G_{B2} = ab$ and $G_{B3} = ac$.

Enumeration of the possibilities for the parents can be attempted by the tabular approach again. The asterisk (*) is used to mean 'not a'.

P_1	P_2	$\Pr(G_{P1}, G_{P2} \mid H_1, I)$	$\Pr(G_{B1}, G_{B2}, G_{B3} \mid G_{P1}, G_{P2}, H_1, I)$
aa	bc	$2p_a^2 p_b p_c$	$\frac{1}{8}$
ac	ab	$4p_a^2 p_b p_c$	$\frac{1}{64}$
a*	bc	$4p_a p_b p_c (1-p_a)$	$\frac{1}{64}$
bc	aa	$2p_a^2 p_b p_c$	$\frac{1}{8}$
ab	ac	$4p_a^2 p_b p_c$	$\frac{1}{64}$
bc	a*	$4p_a p_b p_c (1-p_a)$	$\frac{1}{64}$

$$\sum_{i=1}^{n} \frac{\Pr(G_{B1}, G_{B2}, G_{B3} \mid G_{P1}, G_{P2}, H_1, I)}{\times \Pr(G_{P1}, G_{P2} \mid H_1, I)} = \frac{p_a p_b p_c}{8}(1+4p_a)$$

$$\Pr(G_{B1} \mid H_2, I) = 2p_a p_b \; \Pr(G_{B2}, G_{B3} \mid H_2, I) = \Pr(G_{B3} \mid G_{B2}, H_2, I) \Pr(G_{B2} \mid H_2, I)$$

$$\Pr(G_{B2} \mid H_2, I) = 2p_a p_b \text{ and } \Pr(G_{B3} \mid G_{B2}, H_2, I) = \frac{p_c}{4}(1+2p_a)$$

This last equation could be obtained from Table 4.4 using Row 7 and setting $\theta = 0$, $Z_1 = 1/2$ and $Z_0 = 1/4$ so

$$LR = \frac{1+4p_a}{8 p_a p_b (1+2p_a)}$$

Use of the descent measures leads to the table below.

IBD State		Pr(IBD State)	$\Pr(G_{B1}, G_{B2}, G_{B3} \mid \text{IBD State})$
a≡b≡c	b≡d≡f	$\frac{1}{16}$	0
	b≡d	$\frac{1}{16}$	$p_a p_b p_c$
	b≡f	$\frac{1}{16}$	0
	d≡f	$\frac{1}{16}$	0
a≡c	b≡d≡f	$\frac{1}{16}$	$p_a p_b p_c$
	b≡d	$\frac{1}{16}$	$4p_a^2 p_b p_c$
	b≡f	$\frac{1}{16}$	$p_a^2 p_b p_c$
	d≡f	$\frac{1}{16}$	$p_a^2 p_b p_c$

Continued

420

IBD State		Pr(IBD State)	Pr(G_{B1}, G_{B2}, G_{B3} | IBD State)
a≡e	b≡d≡f	$\frac{1}{16}$	0
	b≡d	$\frac{1}{16}$	$p_a^2 p_b p_c$
	b≡f	$\frac{1}{16}$	0
	d≡f	$\frac{1}{16}$	0
c≡e	b≡d≡f	$\frac{1}{16}$	0
	b≡d	$\frac{1}{16}$	$p_a^2 p_b p_c$
	b≡f	$\frac{1}{16}$	0
	d≡f	$\frac{1}{16}$	0
Taking the product across the rows and the sum down yields		$\rightarrow$	$\dfrac{p_a p_b p_c}{8}(1+4p_a)$

The value

$$LR = \frac{p_a p_b p_c \left(1 + 4 p_a\right)}{8}$$

is the same result as that achieved by enumerating the possible parental genotypes.

Example 12.7: Missing Body Given Two Siblings

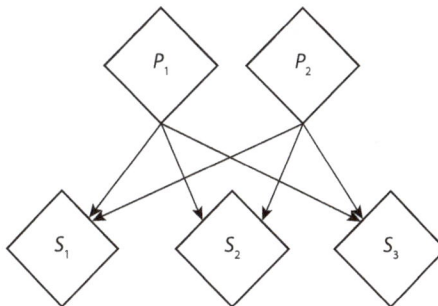

In this instance we consider the same pedigree of three siblings. No parents have been typed but two siblings have, S_1 and S_2. Consider the following hypotheses:

H_1: S_3 is a sibling of S_1 and S_2.

H_2: S_3 is unrelated to S_1 and S_2.

			$\Pr(S_1, S_2 \mid P_1, P_2)$		$\Pr(S_3 = aa \mid P_1, P_2)$	$\Pr(S_3 = ab \mid P_1, P_2)$	$\Pr(S_3 = bb \mid P_1, P_2)$	$\Pr(S_3 = bc \mid P_1, P_2)$
P_1	P_2			$\Pr(P_1, P_2)$				
Column j		Row i	1	2	3			
aa	aa	1	1	p_a^4	1	0	0	0
aa	ab	2	¼	$4p_a^3 p_b$	½	½	0	0
ab	ab	3	¹⁄₁₆	$4p_a^2 p_b^2$	¼	½	¼	0
ab	ac	4	¹⁄₁₆	$8p_a^2 p_b p_c$	¼	¼	0	¼
aa	aQ	5	¼	$4p_a^3(1 - p_a - p_b - p_c)$	½	0	0	0
aQ	aQ	6	¹⁄₁₆	$4p_a^2(1 - p_a - p_b - p_c)^2$	¼	0	0	0

$S_1 = S_2 = aa$

$$LR = \frac{\displaystyle\sum_{i=1\ldots6} \prod_{j=1\ldots3} x_{ij}}{\Pr(S_3) \displaystyle\sum_{i=1\ldots6} \prod_{j=1,2} x_{ij}}$$

			$\Pr(S_1, S_2 \mid P_1, P_2)$		$\Pr(S_3 = aa \mid P_1, P_2)$	$\Pr(S_3 = ab \mid P_1, P_2)$	$\Pr(S_3 = ac \mid P_1, P_2)$	$\Pr(S_3 = bb \mid P_1, P_2)$	$\Pr(S_3 = bc \mid P_1, P_2)$
P_1	P_2			$\Pr(P_1, P_2)$					
Column j		Row i	1	2	3				
aa	ab	1	¼	$4p_a^3 p_b$	½	½	0	0	0
ab	ab	2	⅛	$4p_a^2 p_b^2$	¼	½	0	¼	0
ab	ac	3	¹⁄₁₆	$8p_a^2 p_b p_c$	¼	¼	¼	0	¼
ab	aQ	4	¹⁄₁₆	$8p_a^2 p_b(1 - p_a - p_b - p_c)$	¼	¼	0	0	0

$S_1 = aa\ S_2 = ab$

$$LR = \frac{\displaystyle\sum_{i=1\ldots4} \prod_{j=1\ldots3} x_{ij}}{\Pr(S_3) \displaystyle\sum_{i=1\ldots4} \prod_{j=1,2} x_{ij}}$$

$S_1 = aa\ S_2 = bb$, $S_1 = aa\ S_2 = bc$, $S_1 = ab\ S_2 = cc$, $S_1 = ab\ S_2 = cd$

These are easy since the parents are certain but we will carry out the same process.

P₁	P₂	Column j / Row i	Pr(S₁,S₂|P₁,P₂)	Pr(P₁,P₂)	Pr(S₃=aa|P₁,P₂)	Pr(S₃=ab|P₁,P₂)	Pr(S₃=bb|P₁,P₂)
		Column j	1	2	3		
ab	ab	Row i : 1	$\frac{1}{16}$	$4p_a^2 p_b^2$	¼	½	¼

$$LR = \frac{\sum\limits_{i=1}\prod\limits_{j=1\ldots 3} x_{ij}}{Pr(S_3)\sum\limits_{i=1}\prod\limits_{j=1,2} x_{ij}} = \frac{x_{13}}{Pr(S_3)}$$

$S_1 = ab \; S_2 = bc \; p_Q = 1 - p_a - p_b - p_c - p_d$

P₁	P₂	Column j / Row i	Pr(S₁|P₁,P₂)	Pr(S₂|P₁,P₂)	Pr(P₁)	Pr(P₂)	Reversible	Pr(S₃=aa|P₁,P₂)	Pr(S₃=ab|P₁,P₂)	Pr(S₃=ac|P₁,P₂)	Pr(S₃=bb|P₁,P₂)	Pr(S₃=bc|P₁,P₂)	Pr(S₃=cc|P₁,P₂)	Pr(S₃=cd|P₁,P₂)
		Column j	1	2	3	4	5	6						
ab	ac	1	¼	¼	$2p_a p_b$	$2p_a p_c$	2	¼	¼	¼	0	¼	0	0
ab	bc	2	¼	¼		$2p_b p_c$	2	0	¼	¼	¼	¼	0	0
ac	bb	3	½	½	$2p_a p_c$	p_b^2	2	0	½	0	0	½	0	0
ac	bc	4	¼	¼		$2p_b p_c$	2	0	¼	¼	0	¼	¼	0
ac	bd	5	¼	¼		$2p_b p_d$	2	0	¼	0	0	¼	0	¼
ac	bQ	6	¼	¼		$2p_b p_Q$	2	0	¼	0	0	¼	0	0

$$LR = \frac{\sum\limits_{i=1\ldots 6}\prod\limits_{j=1\ldots 6} x_{ij}}{Pr(S_3)\sum\limits_{i=1\ldots 6}\prod\limits_{j=1\ldots 5} x_{ij}}$$

			$S_1 = ab$ $S_2 = ab$ $p_Q = 1 - p_a - p_b - p_c - p_d$										
P_1	P_2		$\Pr(S_1 \mid P_1, P_2)$	$\Pr(S_2 \mid P_1, P_2)$	$\Pr(P_1)$	$\Pr(P_2)$	Reversible	$\Pr(S_3 = aa \mid P_1, P_2)$	$\Pr(S_3 = ab \mid P_1, P_2)$	$\Pr(S_3 = ac \mid P_1, P_2)$	$\Pr(S_3 = bb \mid P_1, P_2)$	$\Pr(S_3 = bc \mid P_1, P_2)$	$\Pr(S_3 = cc \mid P_1, P_2)$	$\Pr(S_3 = cd \mid P_1, P_2)$
Column j		Row i	1	2	3	4	5	6						
aa	ab	1	½	½	p_a^2	$2p_ap_b$	2	½	½	0	0	0	0	0
aa	bb	2	1	1		p_b^2	2	0	1	0	0	0	0	0
aa	bc	3	½	½		$2p_bp_c$	2	0	½	½	0	0	0	0
aa	bd	4	½	½		$2p_bp_d$	2	0	½	0	0	0	0	0
aa	bQ	5	½	½		$2p_bp_Q$	2	0	½	0	0	0	0	0
ab	ab	6	½	½	$2p_ap_b$	$2p_ap_b$	1	¼	½	0	¼	0	0	0
ab	ac	7	¼	¼		$2p_ap_c$	2	¼	¼	¼	0	¼	0	0
ab	ad	8	¼	¼		$2p_ap_d$	2	¼	¼	0	0	0	0	0
ab	aQ	9	¼	¼		$2p_ap_Q$	2	¼	¼	0	0	0	0	0
ab	bb	10	½	½		p_b^2	2	0	½	0	½	0	0	0
ab	bc	11	¼	¼		$2p_bp_c$	2	0	¼	¼	¼	¼	0	0
ab	bd	12	¼	¼		$2p_bp_d$	2	0	¼	0	¼	0	0	0
ab	bQ	13	¼	¼		$2p_bp_Q$	2	0	¼	0	¼	0	0	0
ac	bb	14	½	½	$2p_ap_c$	p_b^2	2	0	½	0	0	½	0	0
ac	bc	15	¼	¼		$2p_bp_c$	2	0	¼	¼	0	¼	¼	0
ac	bd	16	¼	¼		$2p_bp_d$	2	0	¼	0	0	¼	0	¼
ac	bQ	17	¼	¼		$2p_bp_Q$	2	0	¼	0	0	¼	0	0
ad	bb	18	½	½	$2p_ap_d$	p_b^2	2	0	½	0	0	0	0	0
ad	bc	19	¼	¼		$2p_bp_c$	2	0	¼	¼	0	0	0	¼
ad	bd	20	¼	¼		$2p_bp_d$	2	0	¼	0	0	0	0	0
ad	bQ	21	¼	¼		$2p_bp_Q$	2	0	¼	0	0	0	0	0
aQ	bb	22	½	½	$2p_ap_Q$	p_b^2	2	0	½	0	0	0	0	0
aQ	bc	23	¼	¼		$2p_bp_c$	2	0	¼	¼	0	0	0	0
aQ	bd	24	¼	¼		$2p_bp_d$	2	0	¼	0	0	0	0	0
aQ	bQ	25	¼	¼		$2p_bp_Q$	2	0	¼	0	0	0	0	0

$$LR = \frac{\displaystyle\sum_{i=1\ldots25} \prod_{j=1\ldots6} x_{ij}}{\Pr(S_3) \displaystyle\sum_{i=1\ldots25} \prod_{j=1\ldots5} x_{ij}}$$

Complicating Factors

There are some factors that are liable to complicate a pedigree analysis. These include the following:

- Biological non-paternity of one (or more) of the individuals in the pedigree
- Germline mutation
- Linkage

Unfortunately, human relationships are such that biological non-paternity is a real possibility, however 'convinced' a party may be that a man is the true father of a certain child. For this reason any assumptions made during analysis regarding paternity should be explicitly stated. In some situations, it may be possible to carry out comparisons first based on maternal profiles.

The issue of germline mutation has been discussed previously in Chapter 11. The possibility of germline mutation must be borne in mind, especially when a large number of parent/child transmissions have been studied. It is likely that such an effect will be restricted to a single locus. The effects on the analysis may be negligible if the mutation occurs in a 'known' sample.

The analysis given above was for unlinked loci. In such cases the LR may be calculated on a locus-by-locus basis and the results multiplied across all the loci considered,

$$LR = \prod_{loci} LR_{locus}$$

For linked loci, such as the pair D5S818 and CSF1PO in the CODIS set, this equation applies only when there is no information about the phase of the people in dispute. Information about phase is present whenever a relevant individual in the supposed pedigree is involved in two or more meioses.[1040]

Consider the following pedigree:

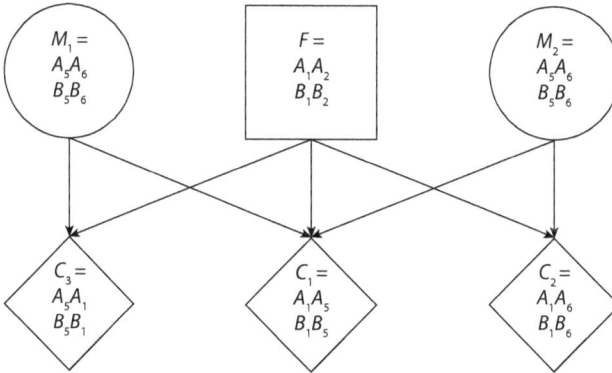

Let us take the following hypotheses:

H_1: C_3 is the person indicated in this pedigree.

H_2: C_3 is unrelated to this pedigree.

For these hypotheses, the LR is

$$LR = \frac{\left(1 - R_M\right)^3 + R_M^3}{8\left\{\left(1 - R_M\right)^2 + R_M^2\right\} p_{A1} p_{A5} p_{B1} p_{B5}}$$

where the male and female recombination fractions are R_M and R_F, respectively. This compares with

$$LR = \frac{1}{16 p_{A1} p_{A5} p_{B1} p_{B5}}$$

if the loci were unlinked. This is because the genotypes of the children C_1 and C_2 either singly or together give information about the phase of F.

An approach to incorporating linkage was given in Chapter 4. The practical implications are likely to be confined to only a fraction of the pedigrees, and unless there are multiple linked loci the implications will be small. Linkage tends to improve the power of relationship testing.

Mass Disasters

In a mass disaster situation some of the difficulties of body identification by genetic means are compounded.

First, in many cases a cataclysmic physical event such as an impact or explosion will have caused severe fragmentation of the bodies. In such a situation simply locating and recovering the post-mortem remains is a major organizational and technical challenge. A key part of the identification process will be to reunify fragmentary remains as well as to identify the deceased.

Second, the remains may have been subjected to extreme thermal, chemical or microbial insult due to the environmental conditions. In turn this will increase the difficulty of obtaining DNA in satisfactory concentrations and of sufficient quality.

Third, it may be the case that a number of individuals from the same family are thought to be victims. This creates the twofold problem of coping with the inter-relatedness of some of the remains and obtaining sufficient genetic information via surviving relatives (see Clayton[1041]).

Lastly, the sheer scale of the exercise may present difficulties. For instance, tracking and collating results from tens of thousands of samples, actioning rework and comparing a large number of ante-mortem samples with a large number of post-mortem samples may be too great an endeavour for a single individual or group of individuals. Ballantyne[1042] reports that Olaisen's group operated around the clock for three weeks on the 1996 Spitsbergen crash, which involved 141 victims. The situation following the terrorist attacks on the Work Trade Center Towers on September 11, 2001 precipitated the development of a specialist software package (MFISys, Mass Fatality Identification System) by a bioinformatics company (Genecode Forensics, Ann Arbor, MI) to handle the vast quantities of data and information generated.

Brenner and Weir[1043,1044] identify three steps in the identification process.

Collapsing. This refers to the association of like profiles to condense the amount of data. These authors describe an approximate probabilistic approach to dealing with the 'collapse' of partial profiles. Olaisen et al.[1045] and Ballantyne[1042] report DNA typing of the 141 victims of the crash of a Tupolev 154 aircraft into Operafjellet mountain on the island of Spitsbergen, Norway, in 1996. The DNA results from 257 fragmented remains could be collapsed to 141 different genotypes equating to the number of victims. The 1277 tested remains from the crash of Swissair Flight 111 could be collapsed to the 228 genotypes expected from the 229 victims, which contained one pair of identical twins.[1046] Goodwin et al.[776] describe the analysis of 187 tissue samples from 104 victims of Cebu Pacific Flight 387 in 1998. The tissue samples could be collapsed into 55 groups by mtDNA, subdivided into 80 groups when STR results were added and further into 95 groups when post-mortem results were considered. The 14,249 typing results from the World Trade Center tragedy were collapsed to at least 1487 distinct profiles. There are 2792 missing persons in this set.[1043]

Screening. This refers to the comparison of every victim profile in the collapsed list with every missing person profile. Brenner and Weir point out that screening of direct comparisons between a victim and a sample from the missing person, from a toothbrush for example, is straightforward, whereas screening against relatives is more difficult. The problem of false positives was highlighted since the number of pairings will give a number of false indications of membership of a given pedigree.

Testing. This is the confirming calculation of *LR*s and was undertaken as described in the equations and tables above and in Brenner.[484]

Closed Set Matching

Consider a situation where there are N persons associated with a mass disaster. We denote the missing people $M_1 \ldots M_N$. The bodies are denoted $B_1 \ldots B_N$ with genotypes $G_1 \ldots G_N$. We have the records of the people who are missing. In addition a sample known to be from each person is available from, say, a toothbrush, hair or database sample or some pedigree information. We denote the known sample or pedigree information as $P_1 \ldots P_N$. This is termed *closed set* matching because the issue is to match a finite number of bodies or body parts to a finite set of missing people.[1043,1047,1048] It uses the information more effectively than open set matching since both the consistency with a pedigree and the dissimilarity to other pedigrees are used.

The direct match comparisons between bodies, body parts and complete profiles of missing people presents few statistical problems. However Leclair et al.[1046] reported that in 5 of 47 instances in the Swissair Flight 111 crash investigation the reference sample was incorrect, being that of another family member. This does suggest the use of confirmatory pedigree analysis. Let us assume that L bodies can be assigned without error to missing people in this way. There are $N–L$ bodies unassigned and hence there are $(N–L)!$ possible assignments of the remaining bodies to pedigrees. To keep the subscripting simple we arrange to label the 'directly assigned' bodies and missing people as $B_1 \ldots B_L$ and $M_1 \ldots M_L$. In principle for small sets of missing people and bodies the remaining assignments can be assessed by direct enumeration. We label each of the possible sets of assignments of the unassigned bodies to missing people as $A_{L+1} \ldots A_{(N-L)!}$ and evaluate the equation

$$\Pr\left(A_j \mid G_{L+1}...G_N, P_{L+1}...P_N\right) = \frac{\Pr\left(G_{L+1}...G_N \mid P_{L+1}...P_N, A_j\right)\Pr\left(A_j\right)}{\displaystyle\sum_{i=L+1}^{(N-L)!} \Pr\left(G_{L+1}...G_N \mid P_{L+1}...P_N, A_i\right)\Pr\left(A_i\right)}$$

for each possible assignment, j, in this set. The prior probabilities $\Pr(A_j)$ can be assigned from physical examination of the bodies, location or other information or may be set to a flat prior for the remaining assignments (after the direct comparisons have been removed). Egeland et al.[1048,1049] give advice on how this may be undertaken in an elegant manner. They also suggest giving low priors to highly incestuous pedigrees, those involving what they term *promiscuity* and to pedigrees that extend over multiple generations.

This process yields the posterior probability for each member of the possible set of assignments. However we will probably be interested, not in the posterior probability for the entire set, which may be quite small, but the posterior probability for each assignment of a certain body to a certain missing person. This is obtained by summing the terms $\Pr(A_j \mid G_{L+1}...G_N, P_{L+1}...P_N)$ for those assignments A_j which contain this pairing.

The term $\Pr(G_{L+1} \ldots G_N \mid P_{L+1} \ldots P_N, A_j)$ may be approximated by assuming no interpersonal correlations within the set of missing people by

$$\prod_{i=L+1}^{N} \Pr\left(G_i \mid P_{L+1}...P_N, A_j\right)$$

This is clearly incorrect, especially for related persons, but may be an adequate approximation. Any assignment A_j which produces $\Pr(G_i \mid P_{M+1}...P_N, A_j) = 0$ for any genotype G_i can be tentatively eliminated.[485] Such an elimination is tentative as mutation or a pedigree error, for example a person thinks he or she is a parent but is in fact not, will produce a false exclusion. This provides a quick screen to eliminate potential assignments. However it may be appropriate to 'keep this combination alive' by assigning it a small number in case a mutation or a pedigree error may have occurred. Olaisen et al.[1045] reported four mutations in their analysis while Leclair et al. reported one.[1046] A superior approach[1048] would include a full mutation model but would be computationally expensive.

Egeland et al. demonstrated this approach on the nine bodies found in the grave in Ekaterinburg and thought to include most of the Russian royal family. In this set there are 4536 possible family relationships. The number of permutations may be reduced by dividing the bodies into children (who cannot themselves have children in this example) and adults on an age determination.[1049] However the full-scale closed set approach given above may be impractical in many cases due to the size of the problem. A more typical approach is to eliminate possible assignments, for instance body j cannot be from pedigrees x.... In addition it may be possible to break the remaining assignments into male and female using amelogenin[1049] or other methods. This may leave two smaller sets of missing persons, one of female and one of male, to be assigned to bodies also divided by sex. Brenner also describes an elegant 'lattice' approach to reducing the number of permutations that need be considered. The use of mitochondrial DNA and Y chromosome typing to simplify the number of comparisons has great promise. Cowell and Mostad[1050] suggested a method for identifying small clusters of closely related people based on a LR-based measure of distance. They demonstrated the effectiveness of their approach using real examples and simulations.

Next we assume that pedigree information is not available for some missing persons. For such persons the term $\Pr(G_i \mid P_{L+1} \dots P_N, A_j)$ can be set to the product rule estimate $\Pr(G_i)$ since it is an unconditional probability. Under such situations there will be some sets of assignments with equivalent posteriors. These will be those A_j with alternate arrangements of the people with no pedigree information.

In many circumstances there will be fewer recovered bodies or parts than missing persons. After collapsing of the DNA profiles down to the subset of unique profiles, there will be even fewer profiles to assign to pedigrees. Hence, in a practical example, we may have fewer pedigrees than required and fewer unique DNA profiles than we have missing persons.

Let the number of unique DNA profiles be X, which will be less than N. Of these unique profiles, L are assigned by direct comparison to samples from the missing person (toothbrushes etc.). This leaves X–L unassigned bodies to assign to N–L missing persons of which Q do not have pedigree information.* In such cases X–L < N–L. Again all that is required is to assess the equation

$$\Pr\left(A_j \mid G_{X-L+1} \dots G_X, P_{L+1} \dots P_{N-L-Q}\right) = \frac{\Pr\left(G_{X-L+1} \dots G_X \mid P_{L+1} \dots P_{N-L-Q}, A_j\right)\Pr\left(A_j\right)}{\displaystyle\sum_{i=L+1}^{N} \Pr\left(G_{X-L+1} \dots G_X \mid P_{L+1} \dots P_{N-L-Q}, A_i\right)\Pr\left(A_i\right)}$$

$$= \frac{\displaystyle\prod_{k=X-L+1}^{X} \Pr\left(G_k \mid P_{L+1} \dots P_{N-L-Q}, A_j\right)\Pr\left(A_j\right)}{\dfrac{1}{(N-L)!}\displaystyle\sum_{i=L+1}^{X}\prod_{k=X-L+1}^{X} \Pr\left(G_k \mid P_{L+1} \dots P_{N-L-Q}, A_i\right)\Pr\left(A_i\right)}$$

Even with these expedients this may be an insurmountable computational problem. The larger the number of bodies unrecovered and the larger the number of missing persons without pedigree or direct comparison information, the less the advantage to closed set matching. There will come a point where this approach is not worthwhile. Brenner and Weir discuss a number of shortcuts.[1043]

---

* For example, no reference samples were available for 2 of the 141 victims in the 1996 Tupolev 154 crash.[1042]

13

DNA Intelligence Databases

*Simon J. Walsh, Jo-Anne Bright and John S. Buckleton**

Contents

The growth of DNA intelligence databases has increased the involvement of forensic science in law enforcement. Having succeeded at their primary function of linking crimes and suspects, DNA intelligence databases have continued to expand, including expansion into transnational systems. DNA intelligence databases frequently produce links in a wide range of crime types, which, when analyzed, provide a repository of information on crimes and criminals. In addition, DNA databases require us to consider interpretation issues specific to their utilization.

A Brief History

The ability of DNA to incriminate or exonerate was extended during the 1990s by the advent of DNA intelligence databases. The first jurisdiction to pass legislation allowing the collection and storage of DNA samples from convicted offenders was the Commonwealth of Virginia, USA, in 1989.[1051] During these early years the databases often comprised VNTR profiles and were sometimes constructed on an *ad hoc* basis.[1052,1053]

* We warmly acknowledge valuable comments from Dr Kees van der Beek.

In 1994 the Netherlands[1054] and in 1995 the United Kingdom established national DNA profile databases based on a platform of short tandem repeat (STR) technology.[43,1055,1056] This model was followed shortly afterwards by many other countries. Currently, over 50 countries operate a national DNA database (INTERPOL Global Survey, 2011).

Virginia was also the first state to execute a person convicted on the basis of DNA evidence when Timothy W. Spencer was sent to the electric chair in 1993.[1057] The first execution of an individual identified through a DNA database search occurred in Virginia in April 2002 when James Earl Patterson was put to death by lethal injection.[1058] While imprisoned for another matter, Patterson's DNA sample 'hit' samples associated with the 1987 rape and murder of 56-year-old Joyce Alridge in 1999. Following the DNA match, Patterson confessed and pled guilty to the allegations.

Since the completion of the first edition of this book, China has established a national DNA database programme that grew from 28,000 in 2005 to over 1,500,000 by 2008 and over 13,500,000 in 2012. Profiles are contributed by over 380 laboratories at a rate approaching 5 million profiles per year. A national DNA database has been created in India and despite slow progress towards wide-scale implementation, mechanisms are being put in place to allow this to happen.

While widespread international exchange has yet to be achieved, heightened awareness around the threat of transnational crime and terrorism and the increased frequency and ease of international travel has precipitated significant early steps towards the formation of international DNA database capabilities. The outputs observed to date from existing state or national databases lead to a low expectation that networking national systems will improve domestic crime clearance rates. The primary return from DNA databases is in the area of high-volume property crime, rather than serious, violent or organized crime. Forerunner international systems have generally reflected an awareness of these issues. Rather than placing an emphasis on generating a single multi-national system, the preference has been to encourage the concept of developing a strong national database programme while reinforcing a commitment to share and exchange information when needed. The Prüm network in Europe is the best example of such a framework.

An example of *bona fide* international databasing is the Interpol DNA Database, set up by the Interpol General Secretariat in 2003.[1059] The database (or Gateway) provides a resource through which Interpol's member countries can exchange and compare DNA profile data. Access to the Interpol database (by what are termed *beneficiaries* or *users*) is allowable only following a written undertaking. Existing users can also object to any new beneficiary being granted access. The submitting countries retain ownership of the profiles and have direct control of submission, access and deletion, in accordance with (their own) national legislation. Once a match occurs and the submitting country has been notified, then that country can communicate or request additional material to or from another country, subject to restrictions imposed by that country. The notified countries can determine what information can be released once a match with one of their profiles occurs and whether, after a match occurs, they will release further information pertaining to the specific DNA profile.

From the above summary it can be seen that while there has been an increased focus on the development of national DNA database operations in over 50 countries, the approaches that have been taken vary widely and there is considerable development yet to occur. Notably, the world's two most populous nations (China and India) have commenced activities that will lead to enormous national holdings. Expansion of DNA databases has been brought about by gradual broadening of the legislative regimes that expand the categories of entrants. That progress is now leading to the consideration and implementation of global exchange instruments. This is one of the new frontiers for DNA database applications. In general, some level of international exchange is necessary and inevitable and is mostly occurring either through *ad hoc* bilateral instruments, through existing regional or strategic political groupings or via global networks administered by agencies such as Interpol, for example.

Functional Aspects

Typically DNA intelligence databases consist of two separate collections of profiles: a database of the profiles of individuals who have either volunteered or been compelled to submit samples and a database of profiles obtained from samples from crime scenes or exhibits associated with an alleged offence (Figure 13.1).[1060] Often the operator of a database has a programme that can compare the following:

- Crime samples to other crime samples
- Crime samples to individuals
- Individuals to individuals

Corresponding profiles revealed through the above comparisons could each be termed a *hit*, but each hit has a very different meaning. Obviously, crime-to-crime hits may suggest that the same person was at both scenes. Crime-to-individual hits may suggest that a particular individual was at a particular scene and may lead investigators to others who were involved. Blakey[*,1061,1062] observed the following:

- On average every identification[†] leads to 1.4 detections.
- Over 61% of all identifications contribute some form of intelligence.

Individual-to-individual hits may contain information regarding the discriminating power of our systems and have implications for the reliability of our estimation procedure. In many cases databases are not 'clean'. By this we mean that the same individual may be in the database more than once either under the same name or under aliases. This makes aspects of individual-to-individual comparisons difficult, particularly as the database grows.

Blakey noted an issue with multiple false identities appearing in the UK National DNA Database (NDNAD).[1061] The same issue occurred in New Zealand and we abandoned attempts to remove all duplicates from the database.

Administration and Legislation

As the technology that forms the basis for DNA intelligence databases is specialized, the operational components (producing the profile) have remained the responsibility of forensic biology laboratories. In general, the database and its products are the property of law enforcement

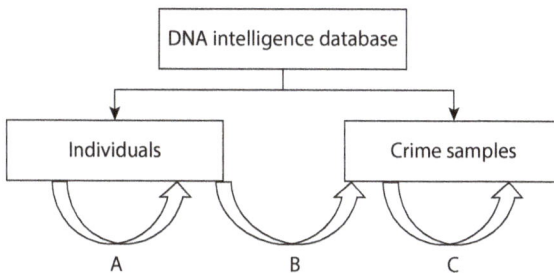

Figure 13.1   A diagrammatic representation of DNA database structure and match process, where A = individual to individual, B = crime to individual and C = crime to crime. (Reproduced from Walsh, S.J., et al., *Science & Justice*, 42(4), 205–214, 2002, with the kind permission of the editor.)

---

* The Blakey quotations are reproduced with the kind permission of Her Majesty's Stationary Office.
† Blakey uses the term *identification* synonymously with *hit*. *Detection* is used to mean that a person is charged.

agencies with the analytical and matching processes administered on their behalf by forensic institutions. All aspects of the process whether handled by police or scientists are subject to governing legislation, as summarized further below. The United Kingdom is an example where the custodial and contributor functions of the database are separated. The UK National DNA Database does no profiling itself but sets standards and administers the matching functions of the database. Contributors include other government and private laboratories, all of whom may contribute to the national database.

Prior to the establishment of DNA databases, the mainstream introduction of forensic DNA evidence into criminal courts had already brought challenges regarding the legality of samples taken from suspects, particularly surrounding the issue of informed consent. One example was the New Zealand matter of *R v Montella*.[1063] In *Montella* the Crown sought to adduce evidence of the results of DNA analysis which indicated a 'match' between samples from the complainant's underwear and a blood sample provided by the accused. There was a dispute as to whether the accused had consented to the taking of a blood sample for DNA analysis, or, as attested by the defence, to allow for HIV testing in order to placate fears held by the complainant's father. A secondary issue to be considered was whether the court exercised its discretion to allow 'evidence improperly obtained' to be admitted on the basis of its relevance. Justice Williamson stated that the onus of establishing free and informed consent was clearly on the Crown and that in this case it had not been so established. In his ruling on this discretionary issue in the absence of clear statutory guidance Justice Williamson made a specific plea for 'legislators to give urgent consideration to providing a statute which sets out the position both of the police and of an accused when DNA testing is a possibility' [at 68].

At the same time that these consent issues were arising from the routine use of forensic DNA evidence, there were growing desires to begin development of forensic DNA databases. To achieve this it was necessary to obtain large numbers of DNA samples for database inclusion, a process which in almost all circumstances required the alteration of existing legislation or the creation of entirely new laws. These laws sought to address the needs expressed by Justice Williamson (above) by codifying the rights of the police to obtain and store DNA samples as well as the rights of those approached.

In general DNA sampling laws cover the grounds under which DNA samples can be obtained from suspects and convicted offenders; they provide the legal framework for the creation and administration of a DNA database. Many differences exist between different jurisdictional legal regimes, although the intent is consistent.

For example, the United Kingdom has an aggressive version of DNA laws in comparison with other international jurisdictions. Any person convicted of, charged with or suspected to have had involvement in the pursuance of a 'recordable offence' may be required to provide a DNA sample.[1064,1065] The right to order a sample rests with a police officer with a minimal rank of superintendent. The 2001 UK act (*Criminal Justice and Police Act 2001* (UK)) has been referred to as a 'compendious "catch-all" criminal justice package'.[1066] In a highly significant case[1067] a suspect was identified following a DNA database match to a reference profile that should have been destroyed several months earlier (according to the legislative model of the time, the *Police and Criminal Evidence Act 1984* or PACE Act).* The House of Lords overruled the trial judge's decision to exclude the evidence. The legislative response was to remove the requirement to destroy samples following acquittal and in its place insert a rule that allows samples retained in such circumstances to be used for 'purposes related to the prevention and detection of crime, the investigation of any offence or the conduct of any prosecution' (s.82). This amendment allows any sample that should have been destroyed, but has not been, to be used in the investigation of subsequent crimes. Wasik expresses alarm not only at the legal decision to allow evidence that appeared to have been improperly obtained but also at the willingness of governments to extend

---

* In particular s.64, which stated that 'any sample (intimate or non-intimate) must be destroyed if a suspect is cleared of an offence or not prosecuted'.

police powers, despite obvious breaches of legally enshrined individual liberties. 'In the case where the police have acted in breach of PACE by retaining DNA evidence which quite clearly should have been destroyed, the legislative response has been to change the law with retrospective effect so as to legitimize what was improperly done.'[1066]

In 2003 the law was extended again to allow police to take DNA samples, fingerprints and other personal information without consent from anyone arrested or suspected of any recordable offence (which is most offences). This information can be retained indefinitely even if the person is never charged.[1068] The retention of samples from those charged but never convicted was challenged in the cases of *Marper and S*, which went through the Court of Appeal to the House of Lords. The House of Lords upheld the judgment that the retention was 'proportionate and justified'. At the time of sampling 'S' was a 12-year-old boy. The rulings were recently overturned in the European Court of Human Rights,[1069] who found the retention of profiles of innocent persons was unlawful. This ruling imposed corrective action on the UK Government, which has subsequently altered the legislative basis of the NDNAD, removing some of the powers previously available to police.

In 2013–14, 1,384,905 DNA profiles from individuals were deleted from the NDNAD. Of these 1,352,356 were deleted under the provisions of the Protection of Freedoms Act*; 31,690 profiles taken by Scottish forces were deleted under Scottish law. A further 6837 crime scene profiles were deleted because the crimes had been solved.[1070]

The United States provides another interesting example of the willingness to clear a legislative path for the use of DNA evidence and the construction of DNA databases. As discussed earlier in this chapter, US states began to consider laws covering the compulsory acquisition of DNA samples from convicted offenders (usually sex offenders) as early as 1988. By 1994, 29 states had passed some form of DNA legislation and by 1998 all states had done so, the last being Rhode Island.[1071] In 1994 Congress introduced the DNA Identification Act, specifically authorizing the FBI to create an index of DNA profiles collected from all persons convicted of crimes, evidence recovered from crime scenes and missing persons. In *Maryland v King*,[1072] the US Supreme Court majority opinion stated that 'when officers make an arrest supported by probable cause … taking and analyzing a cheek swab of the arrestee's DNA is, like fingerprinting and photographing, a legitimate police booking procedure that is reasonable under the Fourth Amendment'.

From a forensic scientist's perspective, the legal basis for the administration of DNA databases represents an additional level of legislative governance over their work. Almost ubiquitously, DNA laws contain sections that prescribe the appropriate conditions under which a DNA sample can be collected, analyzed, stored, compared and disclosed, as well as the criminal sanctions that are enforceable for individuals in breach of these provisions. Although it is not possible to itemize all the various offence categories here, they generally include intentionally or recklessly supplying forensic material for analysis, improperly accessing or disseminating information stored on the DNA database and matching profiles on the database unlawfully. Penalties can include fines and/or prison sentences. Some legal commentators feel that the sanctions are too lenient and do not provide sufficient deterrence to prevent a rogue scientist acting to pervert the course of justice through inappropriate use of a DNA database.[1073] We differ. Often this legislation contains clauses that facilitate external review of operations by delegated parliamentary authorities. This is highly desirable.

The recent issues surrounding the UK NDNAD illustrate some important points. First, when establishing a DNA database three policy approaches to sampling from citizens can be followed: (1) a population-wide biometric surveillance database, (2) a broad sampling regime aiming to input as many profiles as possible onto the system or (3) a strategic sampling regime

---

* The Protection of Freedoms Act 2012 (https://www.gov.uk/government/publications/protection-of-freedoms-act-2012-dna-and-fingerprint-provisions/protection-of-freedoms-act-2012-how-dna-and-fingerprint-evidence-is-protected-in-law).

that targets individuals selectively due to an increased likelihood they are an active offender. While following Approach 3 is obviously more palatable and cost-effective to the community, it will bring fewer actual results than following Approaches 1 and 2. Approach 1 is virtually never recommended on the basis of extreme cost and controversy, but Approach 2 is widespread – and is symbolic of the approach undertaken in the United Kingdom. Approach 2 results in a higher probability that the person of interest (POI) is among those on the database and will generate more database links than Approach 3 and for this reason it is often favoured. However, the obvious tradeoff is that there is much greater redundancy in Approach 2, and while there are more links (overall) there are also a great many more people sampled and profiled who will never be associated with any crime or indeed any database link. This creates a risk that the model is seen as over-reaching and unnecessarily imposing itself on otherwise innocent people.

Performance Management

Forensic DNA databases have altered the landscape of the criminal justice system and reshaped the field of forensic science. They have provided new challenges to the mechanisms by which forensic evidence can be utilized and have brought pressures and increased responsibility upon those who administer their use. At the time of their inception there was widespread review and commentary regarding the legal and socio-political basis of DNA databases. Most debate in this area has emanated from the legal community.[1074] Now that DNA intelligence databases are more well established, current complexities are more operationally focussed and encompass DNA database performance and effectiveness. It is important that the forensic community acknowledge this shift, reflect effectively on the lessons of our experiences and represent the impact of forensic DNA databases in the criminal justice context.

To date, there has been little attention given to the assessment of database performance – due mainly to the fact that through their history there has been minimal demand for such evaluation. Forensic DNA databases have always provided results, many of which involve spectacular and unprecedented contributions to the most serious of cases. These results have taken little strategic thought to achieve, and to some degree this will always be the case. However an era is arriving where more profound performance management and consideration of database effectiveness will be essential to ensure an ongoing contribution and to manage future challenges.

In order to assess database performance we need to define and decide how we might measure the success of forensic DNA databases. This is a complex undertaking that requires the coalescence of a range of experimental methodologies across numerous domains of society. Mostly this does not occur and instead jurisdictions monitor the performance of their databases by reporting a one-dimensional index of output relating to the number or proportion of hits.

As a database ages, a number of changes occur, some of which are detrimental. Consider the crime sample database. These are samples from crime scenes and may be from the true offender or may be from an irrelevant source – such as the owner of a house that has been burgled. Scenes of crime officers seek to keep the fraction of relevant samples high. However certain types of samples, such as cigarette butts and surprisingly blood, have a risk of irrelevancy. As time passes crimes are solved, which sometimes results in the removal of relevant samples from the database. However, case resolution does nothing for irrelevant samples, and so those samples largely remain on the database. Therefore the fraction of irrelevant samples on the unsolved part of the crime database may slowly rise.

Even relevant samples that generate hits also gradually diminish in their overall value over time. This is because resolving old crimes is of less value and often harder than resolving recent crimes. While this is a general statement, it is certainly true of property crimes, which make up the vast bulk of database cases and hits.

The database which is composed of samples from people also ages. In a very coarse model this database is composed of active offenders and non-offenders. In general there is a movement of some active offenders towards non-offending. This occurs as active offenders retire from crime, die or become imprisoned. The fraction of active offenders on the person database has a tendency to decline over time. This decline can be exaggerated if selection criteria for inclusion on the database decrease the fraction of offenders sampled.

While the fraction of active offenders may decline, it is possible that the absolute number may be stable or increase if new additions to the database add new active offenders. Hence the match rate may plateau and then remain stable. This may be visible in the UK NDNAD data (see Figure 13.2, generated from data in Ref. 1070).

We acknowledge that this description is very simplistic and that the division of people into active offenders and non-offenders overlooks the large range of behaviours exhibited by people. However we have found this thinking very useful when considering the value of database sampling strategies and how they interrelate with performance.

An additional factor that further compromises the efficacy of the person database is that there is a small but almost unavoidable accrual of duplicate samples as people are sampled twice due, for example, to subterfuge, sampling under aliases or the existence of numerous legislative models feeding into the one national database (each requiring samples to be collected from locally apprehended suspects or offenders). This latter example exists in Australia.

Presently, assessment of the effectiveness of forensic DNA databases is almost exclusively limited to primary indexes such as profile inclusions, 'match rates' or 'hit rates'. Generally these are calculated by the total number of hits (or matches) divided by the total number of crime samples loaded to the crime sample (or forensic) database. Crime samples may come into the forensic laboratory from no-suspect cases or from cases where the police already have a suspect. There is logic to putting those cases where the police already have a suspect onto the database. This may be to see if that crime links to any others or it may simply be that the police already know that the suspect is on the database and are conserving resources. The hits in the no-suspect type case are termed 'cold' hits but in those cases where there is a suspect this term is not appropriate. Such hits are sometimes referred to as 'warm' hits. Different organizations have different reporting policies for these cold and warm hits, and this leads to difficulties in comparison. This is just one factor that makes comparison difficult.

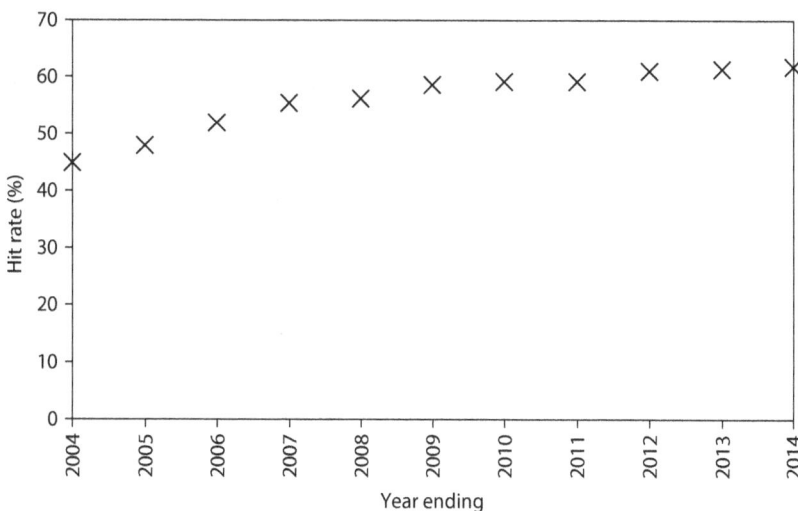

Figure 13.2   Hit rates over time for the UK National DNA Database.

These indices are one-dimensional and limited in their informativeness, particularly in relation to using them to determine optimal strategies for database operation. They measure output (hits) rather than outcomes (verdicts) and are not corrected for influencing factors such as cost. More recently the Dutch DNA database has been considering factoring in costs.[*]

Walsh et al.[1075] suggest some statistics that could be used to measure the effectiveness of databases (as defined largely by hits). From this modelling it is possible to construct hypotheses regarding the factors that drive or limit DNA database effectiveness. They suggest that the number of relevant crime-to-person hits is determined in the early stages of database development predominantly by the product of the number of people in the person and crime databases times two quality factors:

α_t: the fraction of active offenders on the database at time t.

ω_t: the fraction of the crime sample database at time t that is relevant.

This modelling suggests that views such as those of political proponents of sampling on arrest or sampling everyone focus on increasing the number of people on the person database but not on increasing the crime databases, thereby constraining a crucial determinant of success. They suggest that the notion of quality factors will be highly instructive and correlate ultimately to database performance.

To balance the ongoing and increasing use of such technology, with its associated cost and privacy, rights and misuse concerns, the benefits must be clear and must substantially outweigh the risks.

Familial Searching (John Buckleton and Steven Myers)

The fact that close relatives of an offender may share genetic material has led to a search strategy known as *familial searching*.[1076] The profile associated with a crime is often termed the *target profile*. This is searched against a database using a different search strategy to that employed for standard searches. Two strategies are in use:

1. Allele counting

2. Likelihood ratio (*LR*)

For allele counting a count is kept of matching alleles and mismatching alleles. For example, the SGMPlus multiplex has 10 loci and hence a full profile has 20 alleles. A search may return the results 14,6 meaning 14 matching alleles and 6 mismatching. For partial profiles the total does not need to add to 20. For example, a partial profile may return the numbers 10,4. Profiles are ranked in descending order of matching alleles but some mental allowance needs to be made for the partial profiles with high matching allele counts that will appear further down the list.

For the *LR* approach, an *LR* is usually calculated for two relationships, siblings and parent/child. The formulae from Table 12.2 may be used and there is no need for a θ correction. The *LR*s produced are ranked in descending order.

The *LR* approach has better power to find relatives and cannot be improved using a composite of the *LR* and any other statistic.[1077] However there are a number of complicating factors, few of which have been resolved. The assignment of an *LR* requires allele probabilities. If there are N ethnic databases in use, then there will be $2N$ *LR*s produced for each profile, one for siblings and one for parent/child for every set of allele probabilities. The set of allele probabilities producing the lowest *LR* is the one more likely to be applicable. Older databases often contain profiles typed with multiplexes now retired. They are likely to have fewer loci typed. It is the issue of balancing the multiple lists and the varying number of typed loci that requires solution.

---

[*] There is currently no English language reference for this. The Dutch language report can be accessed at http://dnadatabank.forensischinstituut.nl/dna_dossier/jaarverslagen_dna_databank/index.aspx

> ## BOX 13.1 FAMILIAL SEARCHING HINTS
>
> ### Adam Shariff
>
> *UK National DNA Database*
>
> 1. Everyone on the list did not commit the crime.
> 2. You cannot be the same age as your parents or your children.
> 3. Criminals do not travel too far – using a likelihood ratio (*LR*) for DNA, coupled with an *LR* for age and an *LR* for geography has proven useful.
> 4. You may not need to look too far – the vast majority of UK cases had the person of interest (i.e. the familial match) which led to the offender in the top 30 of the names on the list.

However once the lists are produced they are then examined. Often the top, say, 10 are examined first. The entries are investigated as to whether the person has a relative of appropriate age with opportunity. This is termed *metadata* and includes a consideration of geography and age.

Simulation experiments suggest a remarkable power for the technique.[1078] Linked loci will improve the power of familial searching.

With familial searching it is important that expectations are managed carefully. The Forensic Science Service was the first to begin familial searching and reported success in 41 of 188 investigations. This is higher than the success rate in New Zealand (2 of 42). In order to have a successful familial search the true offender must have a relative on the database, Mendel must be kind and there must be suitable metadata to help identify the correct person from the list. In Box 13.1 we give some insightful comments from Adam Shariff of the NDNAD.

Searching Mixed DNA Profiles Directly against DNA Databases

The database matching strategies discussed above assume the crime profile has originated from a single contributor (single source) or those where a contributor could unambiguously be determined from a mixed DNA profile. Under these conditions a significant number of profiles are unsuitable for database searching.

The advent of continuous methods for the interpretation of DNA profiles offers a way to circumvent this restriction. Using these methods, each profile on the database may be considered a possible contributor to a mixture and an *LR* can be formed. Those profiles which produce a sufficiently large *LR* can serve as an investigative lead. Typically, database search algorithms do not calculate an *LR* but simply report the number of concordant and non-concordant alleles. However for unresolvable or low level mixtures the use of an *LR* confers considerable advantages. The hypotheses being considered in the *LR* calculation are as follows:

H_p: Database individual and $N - 1$ unknown contributors

H_d: N unknown contributors

where N is the number of contributors under consideration.

One such method has been described by Bright et al.[757] In this work a number of mixed DNA profiles were compared against the New Zealand DNA Profile Database and the number and magnitude of adventitious matches observed. Direct searching of unresolved mixtures against databases of known individuals was shown to be feasible as an investigative technique with the use of a suitable *LR* threshold to filter out low grade adventitious links. A 'list management' threshold of *LR* = 1,000,000 was recommended to mitigate the risk of reporting an adventitious match when interpreting extreme low level profiles. The choice of a threshold is undertaken as part of a risk assessment. Setting the threshold too low risks increasing the chance of obtaining an adventitious match, whereas setting the threshold too high risks missing true, legitimate matches.

It is acknowledged that the adoption of an *LR* matching strategy may be dependent on individual jurisdiction legislation and is restricted by the availability of software. This type of database matching was introduced in New Zealand in March 2013 where over 120 profiles have been searched (to June 2015) with a success rate greater than 70%.

Social and Ethical Considerations

The success of DNA databasing occurs because individuals included on the database may commit or are likely to commit further crimes. Initially the selection of persons for inclusion on a database tended to start with people convicted of serious crimes.[1079] There was little objection from the public and much support for the inclusion of these individuals. Some felt that any rights that an individual may have to object to inclusion were forfeit by the commission of a serious crime. Initially in DNA database development a situation existed where the law enforcement community targeted a group of individuals that had few social or legal rights to object to mandatory sampling of their DNA and for whom it was thought the high recidivist tendencies would prevent and resolve future heinous crimes. Kaye and Smith refer to these twin justifications as the *forfeiture* and *predictivist* theories.[1080]

An exception to this pattern occurred in the Netherlands. At commencement of databasing in 1994, DNA testing of persons was initially permitted only to aid investigations. Hence only suspects were tested and subsequently included in the Dutch DNA database, from which they had to be (and still have to be) removed if they are not convicted. It took until 2005 before all convicted persons (of certain types of crime) had to provide a DNA sample for the Dutch DNA database. This was reflected in the growth of the number of persons in the Dutch DNA database, which was slow until 2005 but then exploded.*

Most jurisdictions started slowly with databasing. Inexperience and available resource limited the number of samples that could be profiled. At one time in an unnamed laboratory there were people urgently finding freezer space to store unprofiled samples. Time rapidly fixed inexperience and there was often political and public support to extend the mandate, that is extend the range of persons who could be compelled to submit a sample. The widest inclusionary rule for mandatory sampling of which we are aware is inclusion upon arrest regardless of later conviction or acquittal.

Such a scheme has considerable ramifications. Kaye and Smith[1080, p. 456] comment that an arrest-only database 'would have the look and feel of a universal DNA database for black males, whose already jaundiced view of law enforcement's legitimacy is itself a threat to public safety'.

One way to avoid this potential for racial discrimination is a very broad mandatory scheme, in the extreme a 'sample everyone at birth' scheme.[1080] Universal sampling actually reduces any stigma associated with inclusion on a database. Goode argues, on the one hand, that the latter approach of 'having a huge national DNA offenders databank including every common or garden assault in or near a drinking establishment uses a sledge hammer to crack a nut and is an invasion of privacy quite out of proportion to the offence committed'.[1081, p. 70] We could add that this would be beyond the current resource of most jurisdictions and would load databases with non-offenders. The loading of databases with non-offenders may seem an innocuous event, other than being wasteful of resources. However there is some evidence that a fraction, potentially as much as one-half, of samples submitted to the crime sample database from volume crime is not from the offender. Presumably it is from the homeowner or repairman or is simply irrelevant for some other reason. These samples will hit an 'all persons at birth' database. The effect of this will require some thought but it might lead to a reversal of the onus of proof. Innocent people may be asked to prove that they are innocent instead of the prosecution proving that they are guilty.

---

* See http://dnadatabank.forensischinstituut.nl/resultaten/groei_dna_databank_strafzaken/

Criminology had a lot to offer this undertaking, but there is scant evidence that it was used by the political policy makers. The observations that individuals convicted of certain types of crime are more likely to reoffend could have informed decision making. The observation of the youthfulness of many offenders was more problematic. If offending is likely to peak in frequency in late teen males, then it is desirable to have them on the database early in their criminal careers, which is in their early teens. Public acceptance of databasing children is limited. However a considered strategy that incorporates forensic DNA databases as part of crime reduction initiatives provides a justification to counteract the ethical imposition of mandatory sampling upon an individual or a community.

While some of these issues may seem non-forensic in origin, it is impossible for us to isolate discussion that is relevant only to a single discipline and/or irrelevant to another. Forensic scientists must now be aware of their legislative obligations under DNA laws and the socio-legal and ethical controversy associated with the regime under which they work. The forensic community must continue to refine not only the technology but, most crucially, the manner in which it is applied, so that the most effective and judicious use of DNA databases is ensured. We must be receptive, rather than reactionary, to social, ethical and cultural concerns.

Interpretation Issues Associated with DNA Databases

The advent of DNA intelligence databases has not only altered operational features of the role of forensic DNA evidence, but also the context within which this evidence is interpreted. Interpretation models for forensic DNA evidence have evolved considerably. As a recent adaptation, it is understandable that testimony relating to DNA databases is now being scrutinized. Issues associated with this area are discussed here.

Adventitious Matches

In this section we attempt to show how to estimate the chance of adventitious matches in a database of size N. This is a very difficult task, largely because of the following:

1. The structure of databases.

2. The fact that the match probabilities between two people, or between people and crime samples, are not constant.

3. Databases have different matching strategies, allowing for example zero, one or rarely two mismatching alleles.*

4. The presence of profiles with alleles recorded as 'rare'.

5. The presence, most often in the crime database, of alleles recorded as potentially dropped. For example 7,F means the 7 allele is recorded but there may or may not be another allele.†

The simplest model, and the one most often employed, assumes that databases have no structure. In other words they have no pairs of brothers or other relatives and no ethnic structure, and the match probability for any two people taken from the database or from the contributors

---

* The reason for allowing mismatches is to detect false negative matches (matches between profiles, one of which contains a mistake).

† CODIS does not allow the use of wild cards. However homozygote loci are registered with only one allele value and will match a corresponding heterozygote locus if the search stringency 'moderate' is used. In this way allelic dropouts in low template DNA profiles can be detected.

to the crime database is the same (p). If the person database is of size N and the crime database of size C, then the number of adventitious matches is approximately pNC. The match probability p may incorporate any matching strategy that allows zero, one or two mismatching alleles. Weir[431] gave efficient formulae for this calculation.

One terminology system in use is to term a match with all alleles matching and no mismatching alleles an 'N – 0 match'. This could also be termed a 'full stringency match'. One mismatching allele is termed N – 1 and so on. This same terminology uses the allele designation R for any rare allele but may differentiate, for example, 10,R from R,10. In the former the rare allele is larger than the 10 and in the latter it is smaller. As mentioned above the code 10,F stands for the 10 allele and potentially any other allele.

To make full use of the available information databases have evolved some quite complex matching strategies. For example, using an N – 0 strategy an 8,10 may match an 8,10; 8,R; 8,F; R,10 or 10,F but not R,8; 10,R; 10,10 or 8,8. When checked by human hand or repeat analysis the 8,10 match to 8,R and R,10 will be eliminated. Hence true adventitious hits after checking are only affected by the F designation, not the R. Most databases require that the person profiles be complete. This means that the F designation appears only in the crime sample database.

Following Weir,[1082] modelling the behaviour of the F designation is not too difficult. However we have struggled to model the behaviour of the R designation in an easily implementable way. In Table 13.1 we give the average probability of a match between two genotypes. We assume that all matches involving R designations have been investigated.

Table 13.1 Average Probability of Two Genotypes, G_1 and G_2

G_1	G_2	Number of Matching Alleles	Joint Probability
A_iA_i	A_iA_i	2	S_4
A_iA_i	A_jA_j	0	$S_2^2 - S_4$
A_iA_i	A_iA_j	1	$4(S_3 - S_4)$
A_iA_i	A_jA_k	0	$2(S_2 - 2S_3 - S_2^2 + 2S_4)$
A_iA_j	A_iA_j	2	$2(S_2^2 - S_4)$
A_iA_j	A_iA_k	1	$4(S_2 - 2S_3 - S_2^2 + 2S_4)$
A_iA_j	A_kA_l	0	$1 - 6S_2 + 8S_3 + 3S_2^2 - 6S_4$

Note: The probability of the ith allele is p_i, $\sum_i p_i^2 = S_2$,

$$\sum_i p_i^3 = S_3 \text{ and } \sum_i p_i^4 = S_4.$$

Number of Matching Alleles	Joint Probability
2	$2S_2^2 - S_4$
1	$4(S_2 - S_3 - S_2^2 + S_4)$
0	$1 - 4S_2 + 4S_3 + 2S_2^2 - 3S_4$

Table 13.2 Average Probability of Two Genotypes, G_1 and G_2, for Crime Profiles with an F Designation

G_1	G_2	Number of Matching	Alleles-Joint Probability
A_iA_i	A_iF	2	S_3
A_iA_i	A_jF	1	$S_2 - S_3$
A_iA_j	A_iF	2	$2S_2 - 2S_3$
A_iA_j	A_kF	1	$1 - 3S_2 + 2S_3$

Number of Matching Alleles	Joint Probability
2	$2S_2 - S_3$
1	$1 - 2S_2 + S_3$

If we allow the crime database but not the person database to have an F designation, we may adjust Table 13.1 to give the joint probabilities for an F designation (Table 13.2).

It would be wise to curtail this process at some sensible point. The modelling above is an attempt, albeit only partially successful, to incorporate the effect of the F allelic designation into assessing the risk of adventitious hits. However these equations do not account for relatedness and substructure. At multiple loci relatedness is likely to be the larger effect.

Again the only scientific safeguard is confirmation at additional loci. We must recommend continued scientific investigation to foster an understanding and assessment of these risks. It seems likely that the public is not fully informed of these risks nor has informed public debate occurred.

While it is the vanishingly small random match probabilities (RMPs) that are derived from direct matches between 13-locus STR profiles that have encouraged approaches such as the assignment of source attribution[1083] or the abandonment of reporting actual figures in favour of capped values,[1084] the collation of large-scale DNA databases has refocused this issue somewhat. If a database of individuals is of size N, with C entries on the crime stain database, this means there are $N(N - 1)/2$ pairs of individual profiles, $C(C - 1)/2$ pairs of crime profiles (involved in the crime-to-crime matching process) and NC person-to-crime comparisons during the matching of the two databases to each other. These numbers are not always at the front of people's minds and it is interesting to see how quickly they become large. With their increasing size comes the increasing likelihood of adventitious database matches.[1074,*] This effect will be offset by the increased use of highly discriminating 15-, 21- or 24-locus multiplexes.

The likely event of adventitious matches seems counter-intuitive for those unaccustomed to the mathematics, and we imagine it could confuse or alarm the general public. Perhaps for this reason, the issue has recently emerged in court as part of evidence questioning the validity of DNA match statistics (for example, in Australia see Ref. 1085). On occasions these issues have been raised on the basis of observed results from databases of forensic DNA profiles. For example, reports exist in the literature relating to parentage[1086] and kinship[1087,1088] testing experiences that

---

* *Adventitious matches* refer to genuine links provided through the DNA database where an individual was not the donor of the crime scene DNA.

describe observed levels of matching or allele sharing that appear contradictory in the context of associated DNA match statistics. There have also been occasional instances reported of coincidental matches at nine or more STR loci (Carmen Eckhoff, Australia, Northern Territory Police, Fire and Emergency Services, personal communication). All of these observations have involved comparisons with a database of some kind.

One of the limitations of forensic statistical approaches, and one for which they are often criticized,[1089] is the inability to validate empirically the estimates produced and, thereby, the models that underpin them. This is compounded by the fact that the numbers themselves are so large (or small) that they raise justifiable concerns about their level of accuracy. As the examples above have shown, large DNA databases have recently emerged as attractive pools of empirical data that, despite the earlier mentioned limitations, may provide some realistic basis by which theoretical estimates could in certain circumstances be evaluated.

Weir[1082] first addressed this issue using combined Australian profile data (~15,000 nine-locus profiles) and focussing not only on the fully matching profiles but also on those that partially match (for example, a profile where eight loci fully match and one allele or no alleles of the last locus match). The breakthrough made by Weir was to observe that the partially matching profiles do not suffer from the disadvantage that they may be the same person. Curran et al.[371,1090,1091] have recently extended this approach to include corrections in expected estimates for the common relationships (siblings, cousins and parent/child) as well as unrelated persons. A variety of large datasets were utilized, comprised of diverse population groups: Caucasian, New Zealand Maori, Australian Aborigine and even the Croatian populations where elevated allele sharing had been previously identified.[1087,1088] The comparison of observed and expected numbers of partially matching profiles shows that when subpopulation effects and relatedness are taken into consideration, the existing models can give an excellent fit to empirical observations.

From this period of development some interesting ironies have emerged. The assembly of large databases of DNA profiles has brought the issue of adventitious sharing of DNA into sharp focus. In turn this has brought into question policies such as source attribution. Associated with DNA there remains a significant issue around the expectation of the uninitiated. The majority of the general public see DNA as a unique identifier and they are befuddled when adventitious matches occur. These misappropriated expectations are easily exploitable (and are exploited) by anyone wishing to denigrate the basis of the DNA match statistics, as at first blush the facts appear contradictory. Yet where the DNA databases themselves have facilitated this confusion, they also provide a resource for resolving long-held ambiguity about the validity of statistical estimates. In fact the scientific analysis of these data that has so far been undertaken[371,1082,1090,1091] provides the strongest direct evidence yet as to the robustness of DNA interpretation models.

Assessing the Strength of the Evidence from a Match Derived from the Intelligence Database

The strength of the DNA evidence resulting from an intelligence database match is often presented without any mention that the hit was obtained from a database. It is usually not in the suspect's interest to let a jury know that he or she has a sample on the DNA database. The question of whether searching an intelligence database for a match affects the strength of the evidence has been discussed extensively and forcefully in the literature. The issue also affects any search among suspects, whether they are on a database or not. Unfortunately there is much confused writing and it would be very difficult for a court to make a reasoned decision based on a simple assessment of literature recommendations.

The first National Research Council (NRC) report[473] suggested that those loci used in the matching process should not be used in assessing the weight of evidence. The second NRC report[176, pp. 133–135] recommended that an adjustment be applied by multiplying the match probability (Pm) by the number of people on the database. Using an example of an intelligence database of 1000 and a multiplex with a Pm of 10^{-6} this would result in a Pm of 0.001. To date Weir, Evett, Gittelson, Foreman, Balding, Nichols, Donnelly, Friedman, Dawid, Mortera, Aitken, Berry, Finklestein and Levin[219,236,258,270,275,310,1092–1098] have all suggested that the evidence is slightly stronger after a database search and hence no correction is required. Meester and Sjerps[241] suggest that a flat prior be assumed and that the posterior probability be reported, but they essentially support the 'unadjusted' LR. Taroni et al.[346], Biedermann et al.[1099] and Gittelson et al.[1098] take a Bayes network approach and reach the same conclusion, 'the result of the database search has the character of an *additional* piece of information'.

The two NRC reports, Devlin and Stockmarr[176,473,506,1100–1103] have suggested that the match probability be multiplied by the number of people on the database (termed the *NP approach*). Lempert[506] suggests multiplying by the size of the suspect population not the database. Morton[1104] suggests confirmatory markers or the use of the NP approach. The National Commission on the Future of DNA Evidence appears undecided.[1105] It is unclear what Goldman and Long[1106] desired but they did suggest that 'the estimated match probability must be adjusted to take into account multiple testing'.

Here is one of our favourite pieces: 'Because the probative effect of a match does not depend on what occasioned the testing, we conclude that the adjustment recommended by the committee (NRC II) should not be made. The use of Bonferroni's adjustment (multiplying by the size of the database) may be seen as a frequentist attempt to give a result consistent with Bayesian analysis without a clear-cut Bayesian formulation,' Finklestein and Levin.[219]

What would a biologist or court make of this? The mathematical arguments given by either side appear impressive; however we believe that the weight of logical argument is on the 'no correction' side.

We attempt here to formulate a summary of the most well-supported approach based on quality of the mathematical argument. We use terms familiar from Chapters 3 through 5 and follow Berger et al.[1107] Rearranging Bayes' rule

$$LR = \frac{\text{posterior odds}}{\text{prior odds}}$$

Let the population size be N, n of which are on the database, and a match probability to the profile of interest, f. Let us have one match in the database search.

Assuming that the POI is as likely as the average of all other $N - 1$ individuals, the prior odds are $\dfrac{1}{N-1}$. The expected number of matching individuals outside the database is $f(N - n)$. Assuming that the POI is as likely as the average of these $f(N - n)$ people to be the true donor, then the posterior odds are $\dfrac{1}{f(N-n)}$. This gives $LR = \dfrac{N-1}{f(N-n)} \geq \dfrac{1}{f}$.

We supplement these mathematical arguments with some fables given by Buckleton and Curran[1108] that may be more use in court than reasoned mathematical arguments.

Fable 13.1 Three people enter an empty train carriage, which is then locked. When the carriage is unlocked by the police, it is discovered that one of these passengers has been stabbed to death. The remaining two passengers immediately become suspects. Not surprisingly, each states that the other did it. What are the police to do? On examining the suspects they find that one is a tetraplegic and could never hold a knife, let alone stab a person with it. Therefore the police charge the other passenger.

Moral: Excluding alternative suspects increases the probability of guilt for those suspects remaining.

Fable 13.2 Consider a case where we have typed many loci of a stain at the scene of a crime. The estimated match probability is one in four billion. We search a database of every person in the world and find that one (and only one) person matches. Clearly we believe that this is the true perpetrator. Why? Because he matches the crime stain *and* because no one else does (remember there could have been two or more matches, as the match probability is not a count in the population).

Moral: Excluding other persons increases our belief that the profile is rare.

Fable 13.3 Consider a case where we have investigated two crimes that are identical. A stain has been left at the scene and a partial driver's license giving an address and surname has also been left behind. In the one case we type brother A (of five from this address with this surname) first. He matches. We stop. In the second case we find a stain at the scene and type brothers B–E first. They are excluded. Then we type brother A. He matches. Stockmarr's analysis would have us down-weight the evidence in this second scenario since we have searched among five persons. However, we have eliminated the persons most likely to also match (his brothers) who are also the other primary suspects due to the partial driver's licence evidence. Surely this does not down-weight the evidence but increases it?

Moral: Eliminating genetically close relatives is sound practice and increases the weight of evidence.

It seems plausible that, if the suspect has been identified by a database search, the prior odds are lower than if he has been identified by some other means (such as an eyewitness identification). We see therefore that the possible effect on the posterior odds of a database search is not via a lowering of the *LR* but by plausibly lower prior odds (although this is not necessarily always the case).

It is important that we continue to encourage the following:

• The development of evidence that a certain profile is, indeed rare

• Continuing to eliminate other likely suspects

• The investigation either genetically or otherwise of brothers who may be potential alternative suspects

For an elegant analysis of the same issue in fingerprints see Champod and Ribaux.[1109] We would like to draw attention to their illuminating scenarios on pages 475 and 476.

It is important that an incorrect analysis of database searches not be allowed to damage interpretation in this area. In Box 13.2 we give insightful comments from van der Beek.

BOX 13.2   COMMENTS ON ADVENTITIOUS MATCHES IN DATABASES

Dr. ir. C.P. (Kees) van der Beek, MBA

Custodian Dutch DNA-database, Netherlands Forensic Institute, Netherlands Ministry of Security and Justice, The Hague, The Netherlands

The expected number of adventitious matches (of a single search) is dependent on the random match probabilities (RMPs) and the size of the searched DNA-database. Missing person profiles usually have a very low RMP (full profiles) and missing person DNA databases are usually much smaller than criminal DNA databases, so the expected number of adventitious matches can usually be ignored in missing person situations. The problem of adventitious matches becomes real with partial profiles and big DNA databases. In Europe this is a real problem. All European Union countries are required to make their DNA databases available for automated searches from other countries. Until a few years ago only the seven old European standard set (ESS) loci were used by all countries (now there are 12 ESS loci). Hence six- and seven-locus matches may be found in the DNA database of another country. I have studied this problem both theoretically and empirically and talked about it at the Promega meeting in San Antonio, TX, in 2010 (see http://www.promega.com/resources/articles/profiles-in-dna/2011/forensic-dna-profiles-crossing-borders-in-europe/). In the meantime we have 'upgraded' over 500 six- and seven-locus matches and have found that in the present European situation about 6% of all seven-locus matches and over 60% of all six-locus matches are false positives (adventitious matches). We have now also calculated all the RMPs of the original six- and seven-locus matches and have seen that even an RMP of less than one in one billion is no guarantee that a seven-locus match is a reliable match.

I prefer the expression 'expected number of adventitious matches' over 'DMP' (database match probability) because the expression DMP suggests that the RMP is modified in some way by the size of the DNA database, which is not true. The RMP is the RMP and remains the RMP even after a DNA database search. What is actually happening can easily be explained by Bayes statistics. Prior probability $\times LR$ = posterior probability. If somebody becomes a suspect through a DNA database match, this means that apparently there was no pre-existing evidence pointing at this person. Hence the prior probability was close to zero, resulting in a posterior probability which is much lower (weaker evidence) than the LR.

Summary

Undeniably the introduction and expansion of DNA intelligence databases has modified the landscape of forensic science significantly. Through the use of DNA intelligence databases forensic science has become

- More important as a potential source of law enforcement intelligence
- More widely applied in crime investigation
- More able to contribute proactively to strategies of crime reduction and prevention

When coupled with developments such as portable, miniaturized, diagnostic laboratory tools, this impact is destined to increase even further. As the focus of law enforcement becomes increasingly transnational, there is the potential for DNA intelligence databases to contribute to criminal investigation at a global level.

As with all areas of forensic science we must continue to challenge and refine our understanding of this technology.

References

1. Weir, B.S. Court experiences in the USA: *People v. Simpson*. In *First International Conference on Human Identification*, London, 1999.
2. Rudin, N. and K. Inman. *An Introduction to Forensic DNA Analysis*. 2nd ed. Boca Raton, FL: CRC Press; 2002.
3. Rudin, N. and K. Inman. *An Introduction to Forensic DNA Analysis*. Boca Raton, FL: CRC Press; 1997.
4. Butler, J.M. *Fundamentals of Forensic DNA Typing*. Academic Press; 2009.
5. Wambaugh, J. *The Blooding*. New York: William Morrow; 1989.
6. Seton, C. Life for sex killer who sent decoy to take genetic test. *The Times*, London, 1988.
7. Jeffreys, A.J., V. Wilson, and S.L. Thein. Hypervariable minisatellite regions in human DNA. *Nature*, 1985; 314: 67–72.
8. Jeffreys, A.J., A.C. Wilson, and S.L. Thein. Individual specific "fingerprints" of human DNA. *Nature*, 1985; 316: 75–79.
9. Gill, P., A. Jeffreys, and D. Werrett. Forensic application of DNA 'fingerprints'. *Nature*, 1985; 318(12 December): 577–579.
10. Weir, B.S. The status of DNA fingerprinting. *The World and I*, 1993, pp. 214–219.
11. Ago, K., et al. Polymerase chain reaction amplification of samples from Japanese monkeys using primers for human short tandem repeat loci. *Legal Medicine*, 2003; 5: 204–206.
12. Capelli, C., F. Tschentscher, and V.L. Pascali. "Ancient" protocols for the crime scene? Similarities and differences between forensic genetics and ancient DNA analysis. *Forensic Science International*, 2003; 131(1): 59–64.
13. Sykes, B.C. *Adam's Curse*. London: Bantham Press; 2003.
14. Huang, D., et al. Parentally imprinted allele (PIA) typing in the differentially methylated region upstream of the human H19 gene. *Forensic Science International: Genetics*, 2008; 2(4): 286–291.
15. Xu, H.D., et al. Parentally imprinted allele typing at a short tandem repeat locus in intron 1a of imprinted gene KCNQ1. *Legal Medicine*, 2006; 8(3): 139–143.
16. Naito, E., et al. Novel paternity testing by distinguishing parental alleles at a VNTR locus in the differentially methylated region upstream of the human H19 gene. *Journal of Forensic Science*, 2003; 48(6): 1275–1279.
17. Jirtle, R.L. *Imprinted genes: By Species*. Available at: http://www.geneimprint.com/site/genes-by-species.Homo+sapiens.imprinted-All
18. Miozzo, C., et al. A case of chimerism in a paternity study. *Forensic Science International: Genetics Supplement Series*, 2009; 2(1): 228–229.
19. Li, C., et al. Identical but not the same: The value of DNA methylation profiling in forensic discrimination within monozygotic twins. *Forensic Science International: Genetics Supplement Series*, 2011; 3(1): e337–e338.
20. Johnston, M. and G.D. Stormo. Heirlooms in the attic. *Science*, 2003; 302: 997–999.
21. Mattick, J.S. Introns: Evolution and function. *Current Opinions in Genetics and Development*, 1994; 4: 823–831.
22. Mattick, J.S. Non-coding RNA's: The architects of eukaryotic complexity. *European Molecular Biology Organisation Reports*, 2001; 2(11): 986–991.
23. Pai, C.-Y., et al. Allelic alterations at the STR markers in the buccal tissue cells of oral cancer patients and the oral epithelial cells of healthy betel quid chewers: An evaluation of forensic applicability. *Forensic Science International*, 2002; 129: 158–167.
24. Liu, B., et al. Mismatch repair gene defects in sporadic colorectal cancers with microsatellite instability. *Nature Genetics*, 1995; 9: 48–53.
25. Jiricny, J. Colon cancer and DNA repair: Have mismatches met their match? *Trends in Genetics*, 1994; 10(5): 164–168.
26. Budowle, B., et al. *DNA Typing Protocols: Molecular Biology and Forensic Analysis*. BioTechniques. Natick, MA: Eaton; 2000.

References

27. Edwards, A., et al. DNA typing and genetic mapping at five trimeric and tetrameric tandem repeats. *American Journal of Human Genetics*, 1991; 49: 746–756.

28. Findlay, I., A. Taylor, and P. Quirke. DNA fingerprinting from single cells. *Nature*, 1997; 389: 555–556.

29. Budowle, B., R. Chakraborty, and A. van Daal. Response to commentary by Gill and Buckleton and concerns about practices of bias. *Journal of Forensic Sciences*, 2010; 55: 269–272.

30. Budowle, B., A.J. Eisenberg, and A. van Daal. Validity of low copy number typing and applications to forensic science. *Croatian Medical Journal*, 2009; 50: 207–217.

31. Budowle, B., R. Chakraborty, and A. van Daal. Author's response to Gill P, Buckleton J. Commentary on: Budowle B, Onorato AJ, Callaghan TF, Della Manna A, Gross AM, Guerrieri RA, Luttman JC, McClure DL. Mixture interpretation: Defining the relevant features for guidelines for the assessment of mixed DNA profiles in forensic casework. J Forensic Sci 2010;55:265–268. *Journal of Forensic Sciences*, 2010; 55(1).

32. Budowle, B. and A. van Daal. Reply to comments by Buckleton and Gill on "Low copy number typing has yet to achieve 'general acceptance'" by Budowle, B., et al., 2009. *Forensic Science International: Genetics: Supplement Series 2*, 551–552. *Forensic Science International: Genetics*, 2011; 5(1): 12–14.

33. Buckleton, J. and P. Gill. Further comment on "Low copy number typing has yet to achieve 'general acceptance'" by Budowle, B., et al., 2009. *Forensic Science International: Genetics: Supplement Series 2*, 551–552. *Forensic Science International: Genetics*, 2011; 5(1): 7–11.

34. Budowle, B., A.J. Eisenberg, and A. van Daal. Low copy number typing has yet to achieve "general acceptance." *Forensic Science International: Genetics Supplement Series*, 2009; 2(1): 551–552.

35. Caddy, B., G. Taylor, and A. Linacre. A review of the science of low template DNA analysis. 2008. Available at: http://police.homeoffice.gov.uk/news-and-publications/publication/operational-policing/Review_of_Low_Template_DNA_1.pdf?view=Binary

36. The Forensic Science Regulator. Response to Professor Brian Caddy's review of the science of low template DNA analysis. 2008. Available at: http://police.homeoffice.gov.uk/news-and-publications/publication/operational-policing/Review_of_Low_Template_DNA_1.pdf?view=Binary

37. Kimpton, C.P., et al. Automated DNA profiling employing multiplex amplification of short tandem repeat loci. *PCR Methods and Applications*, 1993; 3: 13–22.

38. Sullivan, K.M., et al. A rapid and quantitative DNA sex test fluorescence-based PCR analysis of X-Y homologous gene amelogenin. *Biotechniques*, 1994; 15: 636–641.

39. Sparkes, R., et al. The validation of a 7-locus multiplex STR test for use in forensic casework (II) mixtures, ageing, degradation and species studies. *International Journal of Legal Medicine*, 1996; 109(4): 195–204.

40. Sparkes, R., et al. The validation of a 7-locus multiplex STR test for use in forensic casework (I) mixtures, ageing, degradation and species studies. *International Journal of Legal Medicine*, 1996; 109(4): 186–194.

41. Mills, K.A., D. Even, and J.C. Murray. Tetranucleotide repeat polymorphism at the human alpha fibrinogen locus (FGA). *Human Molecular Genetics*, 1992; 1: 779.

42. Werrett, D.J. The national DNA database. *Forensic Science International*, 1997; 88: 33–42.

43. Harbison, S.A., J.F. Hamilton, and S.J. Walsh. The New Zealand DNA databank: Its development and significance as a crime solving tool. *Science & Justice*, 2001; 41: 33–37.

44. FBI. Available at: http://www.fbi.gov/about-us/lab/codis/ndis-statistics

45. Ruitberg, C.M., D.J. Reeder, and J.M. Butler. STRBase: A short tandem repeat DNA database for the human identity testing community. *Nucleic Acids Research*, 2001; 29(1): 320–322.

46. Gill, P., et al. The evolution of DNA databases—Recommendations for new European STR loci. *Forensic Science International*, 2006; 156(2–3): 242–244.

47. Schneider, P.M. Expansion of the European standard set of DNA database loci—The current situation. *Profiles in DNA*, 2009; 12(1): 6–7.

48. Hares, D.R. Expanding the CODIS core loci in the United States. *Forensic Science International: Genetics*, 2012; 6(1): e52–e54.

49. Butler, J.M. and C.R. Hill. Biology and genetics of new autosomal STR loci useful for forensic DNA analysis. *Forensic Science Review*, 2012; 24(1): 15–26.

50. Butler, J.M. Genetics and genomics of core short tandem repeat loci used in human identity testing. *Journal of Forensic Sciences*, 2006; 51(2): 253–265.

51. Haldane, J.B.S. A combination of linkage values, and the calculation of distances between loci of linked factors. *Journal of Genetics*, 1919; 8: 299–309.

52. Kosambi, D.D. The estimation of map distances from recombination values. *Annals of Eugenics*, 1943; 12: 172–175.

53. Bright, J.A., et al. A Guide to forensic DNA interpretation and linkage. Promega Corporation. Available at: https://www.promega.in/resources/profiles-in-dna/2014/a-guide-to-forensic-dna-interpretation-and-linkage/

54. Gill, P., et al. An evaluation of potential allelic association between the STRs vWA and D12S391: Implications in criminal casework and applications to short pedigrees. *Forensic Science International: Genetics*, 2012; 6(4): 477–486.

55. Bright, J.-A., J.M. Curran, and J.S. Buckleton. Relatedness calculations for linked loci incorporating subpopulation effects. *Forensic Science International: Genetics*, 2013; 7(3): 380–383.

56. Gill, P., et al. An evaluation of potential allelic association between the STRs vWA and D12S391: Implications in criminal casework and applications to short pedigrees. *Forensic Science International: Genetics*, 2012; 6(4): 477–486.

57. Wu, W., et al. Analysis of linkage and linkage disequilibrium for syntenic STRs on 12 chromosomes. *International Journal of Legal Medicine*, 2014; 128: 735–739.

58. O'Connor, K.L., et al. Linkage disequilibrium analysis of D12S391 and vWA in U.S. population and paternity samples. *Forensic Science International: Genetics*, 2011; 5(5): 538–540.

59. The Forensic Science Regulator. Codes of practice and conduct. In *Allele Frequency Databases and Reporting Guidance for the DNA* (Short Tandem Repeat) profiling FSR-G-213 ISSUE 1. 2014.

60. Budowle, B., et al. Population genetic analyses of the NGM STR loci. *International Journal of Legal Medicine*, 2011; 125: 101–109.

61. Urquhart, A., et al. Variation in short tandem repeat sequences—A survey of twelve microsatellite loci for use as forensic identification markers. *International Journal of Legal Medicine*, 1994; 107: 13–20.

62. Polymeropolous, M.H., et al. Tetranucleotide repeat polymorphism at the human tyrosine hydrolase gene (TH). *Nucleic Acids Research*, 1991; 19: 3753.

63. Puers, C., et al. Identification of repeat sequence heterogeneity at the polymorphic short tandem repeat locus HUMTH01 [AATG]n and reassignment of alleles on population analysis by using a locus specific ladder. *American Journal of Human Genetics*, 1993; 53: 953–958.

64. Kimpton, C.P., A. Walton, and P. Gill. A further tetranucleotide repeat polymorphism in the vWF gene. *Human Molecular Genetics*, 1992; 1: 287.

65. Sharma, V. and M. Litt. Tetranucleotide repeat polymorphism at the D21S11 locus. *Human Molecular Genetics*, 1992; 1(1): 67.

66. Butler, J.M. and D.J. Reeder. Short Tandem Repeat DNA Internet DataBase. Available at: www. cstl.nist.gov/biotech/strbase

67. Walsh, S.J., et al. Characterisation of variant alleles at the HumD21S11 locus implies unique Australasian genotypes and re-classification of nomenclature guidelines. *Forensic Science International*, 2003; 135: 35–41.

68. Warne, D.C., et al. Tetranucleotide repeat polymorphism at the human beta actin related pseudogene 2 (ACTBP2) detected using the polymerase chain reaction. *Nucleic Acids Research*, 1991; 19: 6980.

69. Urquhart, A.J., C.P. Kimpton, and P. Gill. Sequence variability of the tetranucleotide repeat of the human beta-actin related pseudogene H-beta-Ac-psi-2 (ACTBP2) locus. *Human Genetics*, 1993; 92: 637–638.

70. Gill, P., et al. A new method of STR interpretation using inferential logic—Development of a criminal intelligence database. *International Journal of Legal Medicine*, 1996; 109: 14–22.

71. Elder, J.K. and E.M. Southern. Measurement of DNA length by gel electrophoresis II: Comparison of methods for relating mobility to fragment length. *Analytical Biochemistry*, 1983; 128(1): 227–231.

72. Elder, J.K., et al. Measurement of DNA length by gel electrophoresis. I. Improved accuracy of mobility measurements using a digital microdensitometer and computer processing. *Analytical Biochemistry*, 1983; 128(1): 223–226.

73. Gill, P., R.L. Sparkes, and C.P. Kimpton. Development of guidelines to designate alleles using a STR multiplex system. *Forensic Science International*, 1997; 89: 185–197.

74. Bar, W., et al. DNA recommendations. Further report of the DNA Commission of the ISFH regarding the use of short tandem repeat systems. International Society for Forensic Haemogenetics. *International Journal of Legal Medicine*, 1997; 110: 175–176.

References

75. Olaisen, B., et al. DNA recommendations 1997 of the International Society for Forensic Genetics. *Vox Sanguinis*, 1998; 74: 61–63.
76. Gill, P., et al. Considerations from the European DNA profiling group (EDNAP) concerning STR nomenclature. *Forensic Science International*, 1997; 87(3): 185–192.
77. Caliebe, A., et al. No shortcut solution to the problem of Y-STR match probability calculation. *Forensic Science International: Genetics*, 2015; 15: 69–75.
78. Overballe-Petersen, S., L. Orlando, and E. Willerslev. Next-generation sequencing offers new insights into DNA degradation. *Trends in Biotechnology*, 2012; 30(7): 364–368.
79. Scheible, M., et al. Short tandem repeat sequencing on the 454 platform. *Forensic Science International: Genetics Supplement Series*, 2011; 3(1): e357–e358.
80. Van Neste, C., et al. Forensic STR analysis using massive parallel sequencing. *Forensic Science International: Genetics*, 2012; 6(6): 810–818.
81. Loreille, O., et al. Application of next generation sequencing technologies to the identification of highly degraded unknown soldiers' remains. *Forensic Science International: Genetics Supplement Series*, 2011; 3(1): e540–e541.
82. Irwin, J., et al. Assessing the potential of next generation sequencing technologies for missing persons identification efforts. *Forensic Science International: Genetics Supplement Series*, 2011; 3(1): e447–e448.
83. Rockenbauer, E., et al. Characterization of mutations and sequence variants in the D21S11 locus by next generation sequencing. *Forensic Science International: Genetics*, 2014; 8(1): 68–72.
84. Bandelt, H.-J. and A. Salas. Current next generation sequencing technology may not meet forensic standards. *Forensic Science International: Genetics*, 2012; 6(1): 143–145.
85. Lejeune, J., M. Gauthier, and R. Turpin. Les chromosomes humains en culture de tissus. *Comptes Rendus de l' Académie des Sciences*, 1959; 248: 602–603.
86. Johnson, C.L., et al. Validation and uses of a Y-Chromosome STR 10-plex for forensic and paternity laboratories. *Journal of Forensic Science*, 2003; 48(6): 1260–1268.
87. Crouse, C.A., et al. Analysis and interpretation of short tandem repeat microvariants and three-banded allele patterns using multiple detection systems [published erratum appears in *J Forensic Sci* 1999 May;44(3)]. *Journal of Forensic Sciences*, 1999; 44(1): 87–94.
88. Picanço, J.B., et al. Tri-allelic pattern at the TPOX locus: A familial study. *Gene*, 2014; 535(2): 353–358.
89. Díaz, V., P. Rivas, and A. Carracedo. The presence of tri-allelic TPOX genotypes in Dominican Population. *Forensic Science International: Genetics Supplement Series*, 2009; 2(1): 371–372.
90. Lane, A.B. The nature of tri-allelic TPOX genotypes in African populations. *Forensic Science International: Genetics*, 2008; 2(2): 134–137.
91. Picanço, J.B., et al. Identification of the third/extra allele for forensic application in cases with TPOX tri-allelic pattern. *Forensic Science International: Genetics*, 2015; 16: 88–93.
92. Picanço, J.B., et al. Tri-allelic pattern at the TPOX locus: A familial study. *Gene*, 2014; 535(2): 353–358.
93. Lukka, M., et al. Triallelic patterns in STR loci used for paternity analysis: Evidence for a duplication in chromosome 2 containing the TPOX STR locus. *Forensic Science International*, 2006; 164(1): 3–9.
94. Mertens, G., et al. Observation of tri-allelic patterns in autosomal STRs during routine casework. *Forensic Science International: Genetics Supplement Series*, 2009; 2(1): 38–40.
95. Alves, C., et al. Contribution for an African autosomic STR database (AmpFlSTR Identifiler and Powerplex 16 system) and a report on genotypic variations. *Forensic Science International*, 2004; 139: 201–205.
96. Whittle, M.R., N.L. Romano, and V.A.C. Negreiros. Updated Brazilian genetic data, together with mutation rates, on 19 STR loci, including D10S1237. *Forensic Science International*, 2004; 139: 207–210.
97. Gill, P., J. Curran, and K. Elliot. A graphical simulation model of the entire DNA process associated with the analysis of short tandem repeat loci. *Nucleic Acids Research*, 2005; 33(2): 632–643.
98. Buckleton, J.S., C.M. Triggs, and S.J. Walsh. *DNA Evidence*. Boca Raton, FL: CRC Press; 2004.
99. Parys-Proszek, A. Application of STR analysis to the profiling of biological traces containing low DNA mounts. *Problems of Forensic Sciences*, 2004; LIX: 100–114.
100. Budowle, B., et al. Low copy number—Consideration and caution. In *Twelfth International Symposium on Human Identification*, Biloxi, MS, 2001.

101. Gill, P. Application of low copy number DNA profiling. *Croatian Medical Journal*, 2001; 42(3): 229–232.

102. Budowle, B., et al. Mixture interpretation: Defining the relevant features for guidelines for the assessment of mixed DNA profiles in forensic casework. *Journal of Forensic Sciences*, 2009; 54(3): 810–821.

103. Gill, P., et al. An investigation of the rigor of interpretation rules for STRs derived from less than 100 pg of DNA. *Forensic Science International*, 2000; 112: 17–40.

104. Petricevic, S., et al. Low copy number DNA profiling a valid forensic technique? *Forensic Science International: Genetics*, 2010; 4(5): 305–310.

105. Butler, J.M., SWGDAM autosomal STR interpretation guidelines, Scientific Working Group on DNA Analysis Methods (SWGDAM). *SWGDAM* Interpretation Guidelines for Autosomal STR Typing by Forensic DNA Testing Laboratories. 2010. Available at: https://www.fbi.gov/about-us/lab/biometric-analysis/codis/swgdam-interpretation-guidelines

106. Gill, P. and H. Haned. A new methodological framework to interpret complex DNA profiles using likelihood ratios. *Forensic Science International: Genetics*, 2013; 7(2): 251–263.

107. Lohmueller, K. and N. Rudin. Calculating the weight of evidence in low-template forensic DNA casework. *Journal of Forensic Sciences*, 2013; 58(1): 234–259.

108. Steele, C.D., M. Greenhalgh, and D.J. Balding. Verifying likelihoods for low template DNA profiles using multiple replicates. *Forensic Science International: Genetics*, 2014; 13: 82–89.

109. Taylor, D., J.-A. Bright, and J. Buckleton. The interpretation of single source and mixed DNA profiles. *Forensic Science International: Genetics*, 2013; 7(5): 516–528.

110. Perlin, M.W., et al. Validating TrueAllele® DNA mixture interpretation. *Journal of Forensic Sciences*, 2011; 56: 1430–1447.

111. Gilder, J.R., et al. Magnitude-dependent variation in peak height balance at heterozygous STR loci. *International Journal of Legal Medicine*, 2011; 125(10): 87–94.

112. Bregu, J. *Investigation of Baseline Noise: Establishing an RFU Threshold for Forensic DNA analysis.* B.S., Biomedical Forensic Sciences, Boston University, 2009.

113. Balding, D.J. and J. Buckleton. Interpreting low template DNA profiles. *Forensic Science International: Genetics*, 2009; 4(1): 1–10.

114. Buckleton, J. and C.M. Triggs. Is the 2p rule always conservative? *Forensic Science International*, 2006; 159: 206–209.

115. Perlin, M.W., et al. Validating TrueAllele® DNA mixture interpretation. *Journal of Forensic Sciences*, 2011; 56: 1430–1447.

116. Gill, P., et al. An investigation of the rigor of interpretation rules for STRs derived from less than 100 pg of DNA. *Forensic Science International*, 2000; 112: 17–40.

117. Bright, J.-A., J. Turkington, and J. Buckleton. Examination of the variability in mixed DNA profile parameters for the Identifiler(TM) multiplex. *Forensic Science International: Genetics*, 2009; 4(2): 111–114.

118. Bright, J.-A., et al. Determination of the variables affecting mixed MiniFiler™ DNA profiles. *Forensic Science International: Genetics*, 2011; 5(5): 381–385.

119. Bright, J.-A., et al. Developing allelic and stutter peak height models for a continuous method of DNA interpretation. *Forensic Science International: Genetics*, 2013; 7(2): 296–304.

120. Weusten, J. and J. Herbergs. A stochastic model of the processes in PCR based amplification of STR DNA in forensic applications. *Forensic Science International: Genetics*, 2012; 6: 17–25.

121. Haned, H. Forensim: An open-source initiative for the evaluation of statistical methods in forensic genetics. *Forensic Science International: Genetics*, 2011; 5(4): 265–268.

122. Gill, P., J. Curran, and K. Elliot. A graphical simulation model of the entire DNA process associated with the analysis of short tandem repeat loci. *Nucleic Acids Research*, 2005; 33(2): 632–643.

123. Haned, H., et al. Estimating drop-out probabilities in forensic DNA samples: A simulation approach to evaluate different models. *Forensic Science International: Genetics*, 2011; 5(5): 525–531.

124. Bright, J.-A., et al. A comparison of stochastic variation in mixed and unmixed casework and synthetic samples. *Forensic Science International: Genetics*, 2012; 6(2): 180–184.

125. Findlay, I., et al. High throughput genetic diagnosis of single and small numbers of cells. *Today's Life Science*, 2001; 13: 40–46.

126. Findlay, I., et al. Allelic dropout and preferential amplification in single cells and human blastomeres: Implications for preimplantation diagnosis of sex and cystic fibrosis. *Molecular Human Reproduction*, 1995; 10(6): 1609–1618.

References

127. Bright, J.-A., et al. Degradation of forensic DNA profiles. *Australian Journal of Forensic Sciences*, 2013; 45(4): 445–449.

128. Shinde, D., et al. Taq DNA polymerase slippage mutation rates measured by PCR and quasi-likelihood analysis: (CA/GT)n and (A/T)n microsatellites. *Nucleic Acids Research*, 2003; 31(3): 974–980.

129. Fazekas, A.J., R. Steeves, and S.G. Newmaster. Improving sequencing quality from PCR products containing long mononucleotide repeats. *BioTechniques*, 2010; 48(4): 277–283.

130. Forster, L., J. Thomson, and S. Kutranov. Direct comparison of post-28-cycle PCR purification and modified capillary electrophoresis methods with the 34-cycle "low copy number" (LCN) method for analysis of trace forensic DNA samples. *Forensic Science International: Genetics*, 2008; 2(4): 318–328.

131. Hill, C.R., et al. Concordance and population studies along with stutter and peak height ratio analysis for the PowerPlex® ESX 17 and ESI 17 Systems. *Forensic Science International: Genetics*, 2011; 5(4): 269–275.

132. Westen, A.A., et al. Assessment of the stochastic threshold, back- and forward stutter filters and low template techniques for NGM. *Forensic Science International: Genetics*, 2012; 6(6): 708–715.

133. Brookes, C., et al. Characterising stutter in forensic STR multiplexes. *Forensic Science International: Genetics*, 2012; 6(1): 58–63.

134. Walsh, P.S., N.J. Fildes, and R. Reynolds. Sequence analysis and characterization of stutter products at the tetranucleotide repeat locus vWA. *Nucleic Acids Research*, 1996; 24: 2807–2812.

135. Weusten, J. and J. Herbergs. A stochastic model of the processes in PCR based amplification of STR DNA in forensic applications. *Forensic Science International: Genetics*, 2012; 6: 17–25.

136. Gibb, A.J., et al. Characterisation of forward stutter in the AmpFlSTR® SGM Plus® PCR. *Science & Justice*, 2009; 49(1): 24–31.

137. Gill, P., et al. New multiplexes for Europe—Amendments and clarification of strategic development. *Forensic Science International*, 2006; 163(1–2): 155–157.

138. Sailus, J., et al. Considerations for the evaluation of Plus Stutter for AmpFℓSTR® PCR Amplification Kits in human identification laboratories. *Forensic News*, 2012. Available at: http://www3.appliedbiosystems.com/cms/groups/applied_markets_marketing/documents/generaldocuments/cms_102368.pdf

139. Bright, J.-A., et al. Modelling forward stutter: Towards increased objectivity in forensic DNA interpretation. *Electrophoresis*, 2014; 35(21–22): 3152–3157.

140. Buckleton, J. Validation issues around DNA typing of low level DNA. *Forensic Science International: Genetics*, 2009; 3(4): 225–260.

141. Gill, P. and A. Kirkham. Development of a simulation model to assess the impact of contamination in casework using STRs. *Journal of Forensic Sciences*, 2004; 49(3): 485–491.

142. Vincent, F.H.R. Inquiry into the circumstances that led to the conviction of Mr Farah Abdulkadir Jama. 2010. Available at: http://assets.justice.vic.gov.au/justice/resources/4cd228fd-f61d-4449-b655-ad98323c4ccc/vincentreportfinal6may2010.pdf

143. Willis, S. ENFSI Guideline for evaluative reporting in forensic science. 2015. Available at: http://www.enfsi.eu/news/enfsi-guideline-evaluative-reporting-forensic-science

144. Gross, T., J. Thomson, and S. Kutranov. A review of low template STR analysis in casework using the DNA SenCE post-PCR purification technique. *Forensic Science International: Genetics Supplement Series*, 2009; 2: 5–7.

145. Forster, L., J. Thomson, and S. Kutranov. Direct comparison of post-28-cycle PCR purification and modified capillary electrophoresis methods with the 34-cycle "low copy number" (LCN) method for analysis of trace forensic DNA samples. *Forensic Science International: Genetics*, 2008; 2(4): 318–328.

146. Buckleton, J.S. and P.D. Gill, Personal Communication.

147. Puch-Solis, R. A dropin peak height model. *Forensic Science International: Genetics*, 2014; 11: 80–84.

148. Butler, J.M. DNA mixture statistics. In *Advanced Topics in Forensic DNA Typing: Interpretation*, J.M. Butler, Ed. San Diego, CA: Academic Press; 2015, pp. 309–332.

149. Life Technologies Corporation. *Considerations for Evaluating Carryover on Applied Biosystems Capillary Electrophoresis Platforms in a HID Laboratory.* 2012.

150. Gusamo, L., et al. Point mutations in the flanking regions of the Y-chromosome specific STR's DYS391, DYS437, and DYS438. *International Journal of Legal Medicine*, 2002; 116: 322–326.

151. Alves, C., et al. VWA STR genotyping: Further inconsistencies between Perkin-Elmer and Promega kits. *International Journal of Legal Medicine*, 2001; 115: 97–99.

152. Budowle, B. STR allele concordance between different primer sets—A brief summary. *Profiles DNA*, 2000; 3: 10.

153. Walsh, S. Commentary on: Kline MC, Jenkins B, Rogers, S. *Journal of Forensic Science*, 1998; 43: 1103.

154. Chang, Y.M., L.A. Burgoyne, and K. Both. Higher failures of Amelogenin sex test in an Indian population group. *Journal of Forensic Science*, 2003; 48(6): 1309–1313.

155. Clayton, T.M., et al. Primer binding site mutations affecting the typing of STR loci contained within the AMPFlSTR® SGM Plus™ kit. *Forensic Science International*, 2004; 139: 255–259.

156. Clayton, T.M., et al. Primer binding site mutations affecting the typing of STR loci contained within the AMPFlSTR® SGM Plus™ kit. *Forensic Science International*, 2004; 139: 255–259.

157. Grgicak, C.M., S. Rogers, and C. Mauterer. Discovery and identification of new D13S317 primer binding site mutations. *Forensic Science International*, 2006; 157(1): 36–39.

158. Kline, M.C., et al. STR sequence analysis for characterizing normal, variant, and null alleles. *Forensic Science International: Genetics*, 2011; 5(4): 329–332.

159. Tsuji, A., et al. A silent allele in the locus D19S433 contained within the AmpFℓSTR® Identifiler™ PCR Amplification Kit. *Legal Medicine*, 2010; 12(2): 94–96.

160. Chambers, G.K., et al. Forensic DNA profiling: The importance of giving accurate answers to the right questions. *Criminal Law Forum*, 1997; 8(3): 445–459.

161. Robertson, B. and G.A. Vignaux. Explaining evidence logically. *New Law Journal*, 1998; 148(6826): 159–162.

162. *R v T*, in *EWCA Crim 2439*, C.o.A.C. Division, Editor. 2010.

163. Robertson, B. and G.A. Vignaux. *Interpreting Evidence—Evaluating Forensic Science in the Courtroom*. Chichester: Wiley; 1995.

164. Triggs, C.M. and J.S. Buckleton. Comment on "Why the effect of prior odds should accompany the likelihood ratio when reporting DNA evidence" Meester, R. and Sjerps, M. Law, Probability and Risk 2004; 3(1). *Law, Probability & Risk*, 2004; 3(1): 73–82.

165. Henderson, J.P. The use of DNA statistics in criminal trials. *Forensic Science International*, 2002; 128: 183–186.

166. Freckleton, I. Expert evidence. In *Expert Evidence*, I. Freckleton and H. Selby, Eds. Sydney: Law Book Company; 2001, pp. 3600–3864.

167. Gans, J. and G. Urbas. *DNA Identification in the Criminal Justice System*. Canberra: Australian Institute of Criminology; 2002, pp. 1–6.

168. Robertson, B. and G.A. Vignaux. DNA on appeal—II. *New Zealand Law Journal*, 1997, pp. 247–250.

169. Robertson, B. and G.A. Vignaux. DNA on appeal. *New Zealand Law Journal*, 1997, pp. 210–212.

170. Robertson, B. and G.A. Vignaux. Bayes' theorem in the court of appeal. *The Criminal Lawyer*, January, 1998, pp. 4–5.

171. Roberts, H. Interpretation of DNA evidence in courts of law—A survey of the issues. *Australian Journal of Forensic Sciences*, 1998; 30: 29–40.

172. Court of Appeal. Regina v Doheny and Adams, Royal Courts of Justice—The Strand—London WC2, 1996.

173. Robertson, B. and G.A. Vignaux. DNA evidence: Wrong answers or wrong questions? In *Human Identification: The Use of DNA Markers*, B.S. Weir, Ed. Dordrecht: Kluwer Academic Publishers; 1995, pp. 145–152.

174. Good, P.I. *Applying Statistics in the Courtroom*. London: Chapman & Hall/CRC; 2001.

175. Inman, K. and N. Rudin. *Principles and Practice of Criminalistics. The Profession of Forensic Science*. Boca Raton, FL: CRC Press; 2001.

176. NRC II. *National Research Council Committee on DNA Forensic Science, The Evaluation of Forensic DNA Evidence*. Washington, DC: National Academy Press; 1996.

177. Lempert, R.O. Some caveats concerning DNA as criminal identification evidence: With thanks to the Reverend Bayes. *Cardozo Law Review*, 1991; 13(3): 303–341.

178. Robertson, B. and G.A. Vignaux. Don't teach statistics to lawyers! In *Fifth International Conference on Teaching of Statistics*. Singapore, 1998.

179. Koehler, J.J. Error and exaggeration in the presentation of DNA evidence at trial. *Jurimetrics Journal*, 1993; 34(1): 21–39.

180. Koehler, J.J. DNA matches and statistics: Important questions, surprising answers. *Judicature*, 1993; 76(5): 222–229.

References

181. Koehler, J.J., A. Chia, and S. Lindsey. The random match probability in DNA evidence: Irrelevant and prejudicial? *Jurimetrics Journal*, 1995; 35(2): 201–219.
182. Koehler, J.J. The base rate fallacy reconsidered: Descriptive, normative, and methodological challenges. *Behavioral and Brain Sciences*, 1996; 19: 1–53.
183. Koehler, J.J. On conveying the probative value of DNA evidence: Frequencies, likelihood ratios and error rates. *University of Colorado Law Review*, 1996; 67(4): 859–886.
184. Koehler, J.J. When are people persuaded by DNA match statistics? *Law and Human Behavior*, 2001; 25(5): 493–513.
185. Thompson, W.C. Are juries competent to evaluate statistical evidence? *Law and Contemporary Problems*, 1989; 52(4): 9–41.
186. Thompson, W.C. Subjective interpretation, laboratory error and the value of forensic DNA evidence: Three case studies. In *Human Identification: The Use of DNA Markers*, B.S. Weir, Ed. Dordrecht: Kluwer Academic Publishers; 1995, pp. 153–168.
187. Balding, D.J. and P. Donnelly. The prosecutor's fallacy and DNA evidence. *Criminal Law Review*, October, 1994, pp. 711–721.
188. Buckleton, J., B. Robertson, and G.A. Vignaux. Interpreting evidence—Evaluating forensic-science in the courtroom. *Nature*, 1995; 377(6547): 300.
189. Lawton, M.E., J.S. Buckleton, and K.A.J. Walsh. An international survey of the reporting of hypothetical cases. *Journal of the Forensic Science Society*, 1988; 28: 243–252.
190. Monahan, S.L., S.J. Cordiner, and J.S. Buckleton. The use of likelihood ratios in reporting difficult forensic cases. In *Advances in Forensic Haemogenetics*, A. Carracedo, B. Brinkmann, and W. Bär, Eds. Berlin: Springer Verlag; 1996, pp. 87–89.
191. Thompson, W.C. and E.L. Schumann. Interpretation of statistical evidence in criminal trials— The prosecutors fallacy and the defense attorneys fallacy. *Law and Human Behavior*, 1987; 11: 167–187.
192. Fairley, W.B. and F. Mosteller. A conversation about Collins. *University of Chicago Law Review*, 1974; 41: 242–253.
193. Panckhurst, P. All Swahili to court. *NZ Herald*, 1994, p. 2.
194. Goos, L.M., et al. The influence of probabilistic statements on the evaluation of a DNA match. *Canadian Society of Forensic Science*, 2002; 35(2): 77–90.
195. Taroni, F. and C.G.G. Aitken. Probabilistic reasoning and the law. Part 1: Assessment of probabilities and explanation of the value of DNA evidence. *Science & Justice*, 1998; 38(3): 165–177.
196. Taroni, F. and C.G.G. Aitken. Probabilistic reasoning and the law. Part 2: Assessment of probabilities and explanation of the value of trace evidence other than DNA. *Science & Justice*, 1998; 38(3): 179–188.
197. Findlay, M. and J. Grix. Challenging forensic evidence? Observations on the use of DNA in certain criminal trials. *Current Issues in Criminal Justice*, 2003; 14(3): 269–282.
198. Berger, C.E.H., et al. Evidence evaluation: A response to the court of appeal judgment in R v T. *Science & Justice*, 2011; 51(2): 43–49.
199. De Kinder, J. and T. Olsson. Expressing evaluative opinions: A position statement. *Science & Justice*, 2011; 51(1): 1–2.
200. Found, B. and J. Ganas. The management of domain irrelevant context information in forensic handwriting examination casework. *Science & Justice*, 2013; 53(2): 154–158.
201. Lindley, D.V. Probability. In *The Use of Statistics in Forensic Science*, C.G.G. Aitken and D.A. Stoney, Eds. New York; Ellis Horwood; 1991, pp. 27–50.
202. Robertson, B. and G.A. Vignaux. Extending the conversation About Bayes. *Cardozo Law Review*, 1991; 13(2–3): 629–645.
203. Geigerenzer, G. *Reckoning with Risk*. London: Penguin Books; 2002.
204. Neyman, J. and E. Pearson. On the problem of the most efficient tests of statistical hypotheses. *Philosophical Transactions of the Royal Society, Series A*, 1933; 231: 289–337.
205. Fisher, R.A. On a significance test in Pearson's biometrika tables (no. 11). *Journal of the Royal Statistical Society, Series B*, 1956; 18: 56–60.
206. Pearson, K. *The History of Statistics in the 17th and 18th Centuries against the Changing Background of Intellectual, Scientific and Religious Thought*, E.S. Pearson, Ed. London: Charles Griffin, 1978.
207. Berger, C.E.H., et al. Evidence evaluation: A response to the court of appeal judgment in R v T. *Science & Justice*, 2011; 51(2): 43–49.
208. Lindley, D.V. *Understanding Uncertainty*. Wiley; 2006.

209. Taroni, F., C.G.G. Aitken, and P. Garbolino. De Finetti's subjectivism, the assessment of probabilities and the evaluation of evidence: A commentary for forensic scientists. *Science & Justice*, 2001; 3: 145–150.

210. Thompson, W.C. DNA evidence in the O.J. Simpson trial. *University of Colorado Law Review*, 1996; 67(4): 827–857.

211. Lord Justice Phillips, Mr Justice Jowitt, and Mr Justice Keene, *R. v. Adams and R. v. Doheny*, 1996.

212. Cook, R., et al. A hierarchy of propositions: Deciding which level to address in casework. *Science & Justice*, 1998; 38(4): 231–240.

213. Cook, R., et al. A model for case assessment and interpretation. *Science & Justice*, 1998; 38(3): 151–156.

214. Evett, I.W., G. Jackson, and J.A. Lambert. More in the hierarchy of propositions: Exploring the distinction between explanations and propositions. *Science & Justice*, 2000; 40(1): 3–10.

215. Jackson, G., et al. The nature of forensic science opinion—A possible framework to guide thinking and practice in investigation and in court proceedings. *Science & Justice*, 2006; 46(1): 33–44.

216. *R v Weller*. Royal Courts of Justice, Strand, London, WC2A 2LL; 2010.

217. Vuille, J., A. Biedermann, and F. Taroni. The importance of having a logical framework for expert conclusions in forensic DNA profiling: Illustrations from the Amanda Knox case. In *Wrongful Convictions and Miscarriages of Justice: Causes and Remedies in North-American and European Criminal Justice Systems*, C.R. Huff and M. Killias, Eds. New York: Routledge/Chapman & Hall; 2013, pp. 137–159.

218. Langley, W. The case against DNA. *The Telegraph*, 2012.

219. Finkelstein, M.O. and B. Levin. *Statistics for Lawyers*. New York: Springer-Verlag; 2001.

220. Buckleton, J.S. Bayes beats frequentist. *The Forensic Panel Letter*, 1999; 3(11): 5.

221. Evett, I.W. A discussion of the deficiencies of the coincidence method for evaluating evidential value and a look towards the future. In *The 10th IAFS Triennial Meeting*, Oxford, UK, 1984.

222. Robertson, B. and G.A. Vignaux. Taking fact analysis seriously. *Michigan Law Review*, 1993; 91: 1442–1464.

223. Lindley, D.V. Probabilities and the Law. In *Utility, Probability and Human Decision Making*, D. Wendt and C. Vlek, Eds. D. Dordrecht: Reidel; 1975, pp. 223–232.

224. Lindley, D.V. A problem in forensic science. *Biometrika*, 1977; 64(2): 207–213.

225. Lindley, D.V. Probability and the law. *The Statistician*, 1977; 26(3): 203–220.

226. Evett, I.W. What is the probability that this blood came from that person? A meaningful question. *Journal of the Forensic Science Society*, 1983; 23: 35–39.

227. Lavine, M. and M.J. Schervish. Bayes factors: What they are and what they are not. *The American Statistician*, 1999; 53(2): 119–122.

228. Lee, P.M. *Bayesian Statistics—An Introduction*. 2nd ed. New York: Wiley; 1997.

229. Essen-Moller, E. Die Beweiskraft der Ahnlichkeit im Vatershaftsnachweis. Theoretische Grundlagen. *Mitteilungen der Anthropologischen Gesellschaft*, 1938; 68: 9–53.

230. Taroni, F., C. Champod, and P. Margot. Forerunners of Bayesianism in early forensic science. *Jurimetrics*, 1998; 38: 183–200.

231. Aitken, C.G.G. The use of statistics in forensic science. *Journal of the Forensic Science Society*, 1987; 27: 113–115.

232. Curran, J.M., T.N. Hicks, and J.S. Buckleton. *Forensic Interpretation of Glass Evidence*. Boca Raton, FL: CRC Press; 2000.

233. Champod, C. and F. Taroni. Interpretation of fibres evidence—The Bayesian approach. In *Forensic Examination of Fibres*, M. Grieve and J. Robertson, Eds. London: Taylor & Francis; 1999, pp. 379–398.

234. Champod, C. and F. Taroni. Bayesian framework for the evaluation of fibre transfer evidence. *Science & Justice*, 1997; 37(2): 75–83.

235. Champod, C. and I.W. Evett. A probabilistic approach to fingerprint evidence. *Journal of Forensic Identification*, 2001; 51(2): 101–122.

236. Aitken, C.G.G. *Statistics and the Evaluation of Evidence for Forensic Scientists*. Statistics in Practice, V. Barnett, Ed. Chichester: Wiley; 1995.

237. George, K.H. DNA profiling: What should the jury be told? *The Journal of NIH Research*, 1996; 8: 24–26.

238. Bar, W. DNA profiling: Evaluation of the evidentiary value. *Legal Medicine*, 2003; 5: 41–44.

239. Bayes, T. An essay towards solving a problem in the doctrine of chances. *The Philosophical Transactions*, 1763; 53: 370–418.

References

240. Evett, I.W., et al. The impact of the principles of evidence interpretation on the structure and content of statements. *Science & Justice*, 2000; 40(4): 233–239.

241. Meester, R. and M. Sjerps. The evidential value in the DNA database search controversy and the two-stain problem. *Biometrics*, 2003; 59(3): 727–732.

242. Dawid, A.P. Which likelihood ratio? *Law, Probability & Risk*, 2004; 3(1): 65–71.

243. Walsh, K.A.J., J. Buckleton, and C.M. Triggs. Assessing prior probabilities considering geography. *Journal of the Forensic Science Society*, 1994; 34: 47–51.

244. Triggs, C., K.A.J. Walsh, and J. Buckleton. Assessing probabilities considering eyewitness evidence. *Science & Justice*, 1995; 35(4): 263–266.

245. Bodziak, W.B. Traditional conclusions in footwear examinations versus the use of the Bayesian approach and likelihood ratio: A review of a recent UK appellate court decision. *Law, Probability and Risk*, 2012; 11(4): 279–287.

246. Champod, C., I.W. Evett, and G. Jackson. Establishing the most appropriate databases for addressing source level propositions. *Science & Justice*, 2004; 44(3): 153–164.

247. Pfannkuch, M., G.A.F. Seber, and C.J. Wild. Probability with less pain. *Teaching Statistics*, 2002; 24: 24–30.

248. Fenton, N.E. and M. Neil. The jury observation fallacy and the use of Bayesian networks to present probabilistic legal arguments, mathematics today. *Bulletin of the IMA*, 2000; 36: 180–187.

249. Biedermann, A., et al. E-learning initiatives in forensic interpretation: Report on experiences from current projects and outlook. *Forensic Science International*, 2013; 230: 2–7.

250. Good, I.J. *Probability and the Weighing of Evidence.* London: Charles Griffin; 1950.

251. Riancho, J.A. and M.T. Zarrabeitia. The prosecutor's and defendants's Bayesian nomograms. *International Journal of Legal Medicine*, 2002; 116: 312–313.

252. Champod, C., et al. Comments on the scale of conclusions proposed by the ad hoc committee of the ENFSI Marks Working Group. *Information Bulletin for Shoeprint/Toolmark Examiners*, 2000; 6(3): 11–18.

253. Evett, I.W. and J.S. Buckleton. Some aspects of the Bayesian approach to evidence evaluation. *Journal of the Forensic Science Society*, 1989; 29(5): 317–324.

254. Evett, I.W. Verbal conventions for handwriting opinions. *Journal of Forensic Sciences*, 2000; 45(2): 508–509.

255. Aitken, C.G.G. and F. Taroni. A verbal scale for the interpretation of evidence. *Science & Justice*, 1998; 38(4): 279–281.

256. Broeders, A.P.A. Some observations on the use of probability scales in forensic identification. *Forensic Linguistics*, 1999; 6(2): 228–241.

257. Evett, I.W. and B.S. Weir. *Interpreting DNA Evidence—Statistical Genetics for Forensic Scientists.* Sunderland, MA: Sinauer Associates; 1998.

258. Butler, J.M. *Advanced Topics in Forensic DNA Typing: Interpretation.* Elsevier; 2014.

259. Aitken, C. and F. Taroni. *Statistics and the Evaluation of Evidence for Forensic Sciences.* 2nd ed. Wiley; 2012.

260. Association of Forensic Science Providers. Standards for the formulation of evaluative forensic science expert opinion. *Science & Justice*, 2009; 49(3): 161–164.

261. Martire, K.A. and I. Watkins. Perception problems of the verbal scale: A reanalysis and application of a membership function approach. *Science & Justice*, 2015; 55(4): 264–274.

262. Champod, C. Identification/individualization—Overview and meaning. In *Encyclopedia of Forensic Sciences*, S.P. Siegel and J.A. Siegel, Eds. London: Elsevier; 2013, pp. 303–309.

263. *R v Nealon* in *EWCA Crim 574.* 2014.

264. Steele, C.D. and D.J. Balding. Choice of population database for forensic DNA profile analysis. *Science & Justice*, 2014; 54(6): 487–493.

265. Nordgaard, A., et al. Scale of conclusions for the value of evidence. *Law, Probability and Risk*, 2012; 11: 1–24.

266. Volckeryck, G. Fifth meeting of the committee on the harmonisation of conclusion scales in footwear casework. *Information Bulletin for Shoeprint/Toolmark Examiners*, 2002; 8(1): 17–32.

267. Conclusion Scale Committee. Conclusion scale for interpreting findings in proficiency tests and collaborative exercises within the WG marks. *The Information Bulletin for Shoeprint/Toolmark Examiners*, 2005; 11(2): 15–18.

268. Bodziak, W.J. Footwear impression evidence—Detection, recovery and examination. In *Practical Aspects of Criminal and Forensic Investigations*, 2nd ed., V.J. Geberth, Ed. Boca Raton, FL: CRC Press; 2000.

269. *R v Craig Paul Meyboom*, in *ACTSC 13* 2011, Supreme Court of the Australian Capital Territories.

270. Balding, D.J., P. Donnelly, and R.A. Nichols. Some causes for concern about DNA profiles—Comment. *Statistical Science*, 1994; 9(2): 248–251.

271. Aitken, C.G.G. and A.J. Gammerman. Probabilistic reasoning in evidential assessment. *Journal of the Forensic Science Society*, 1989; 29: 303–316.

272. Aitken, C.G.G. and D.A. Stoney, Eds. *The Use of Statistics in Forensic Science*. Ellis Horwood Series in Forensic Science, J. Robertson, Ed. Chichester: Ellis Horwood; 1991, p. 242.

273. Aitken, C. and F. Taroni. Interpretation of scientific evidence. *Science & Justice*, 1996; 36(4): 290–292.

274. Aitken, C.G.G. and F. Taroni. Interpretation of scientific evidence (Part II). *Science & Justice*, 1997; 37(1): 65.

275. Balding, D.J. and P. Donnelly. Inference in forensic identification. *Journal of the Royal Statistical Society: Series A*, 1995; 158(1): 21–53.

276. Balding, D.J. and P. Donnelly. Inferring identity from DNA profile evidence. *Proceedings of the National Academy of Sciences of the United States America*, 1995; 92: 11741–11745.

277. Balding, D.J. *Weight-of-Evidence for Forensic DNA Profiles*. Chichester: Wiley; 2005.

278. Budowle, B., et al. Reply to weir. *Forensic Science Communications*, 2001; 3(1).

279. Taroni, F., et al. *Bayesian Networks for Probabilistic Inference and Decision Analysis in Forensic Science*. 2nd ed. Chichester: Wiley; 2014.

280. Buckleton, J., C. Triggs, and C. Champod. An extended likelihood ratio framework for interpreting evidence. *Science & Justice*, 2006; 46: 69–78.

281. Champod, C., Personal Communication. 2003.

282. Wiersema, S. Is the Bayesian approach for you? *Presented at the European Meeting for Shoeprint/Toolmark Examiners*, 2001.

283. Robertson, B. and G.A. Vignaux. Crime investigation and the criminal trial. *Journal of the Forensic Science Society*, 1994; 34(4): 270.

284. Bille, T., J.-A. Bright, and J. Buckleton. Application of random match probability calculations to mixed STR profiles. *Journal of Forensic Sciences*, 2013; 58(2): 474–485.

285. Taroni, F., et al. *Bayesian Networks and Probabilistic Inference in Forensic Science*. Chichester: Wiley; 2006.

286. Evett, I.W. Avoiding the transposed conditional. *Science & Justice*, 1995; 35(2): 127–131.

287. Weir, B.S. Interpreting DNA course notes. In *NCSU Summer School in Statistical Genetics*, Raleigh, NC; 2001.

288. Aitken, C.G.G. Statements of probability. *Journal of the Forensic Science Society*, 1988; 28: 329–330.

289. Leung, W.-C. The prosecutor's fallacy—A pitfall in interpreting probabilities in forensic evidence. *Medicine, Science and the Law*, 2002; 42(1): 44–50.

290. Carracedo, A., et al. Focusing the debate on forensic genetics. *Science & Justice*, 1996; 36(3): 204–206.

291. Robertson, B. and G.A. Vignaux. Probability—The logic of the law. *Oxford Journal of Legal Studies*, 1993; 13(4): 457–478.

292. Fienberg, S.E., S.H. Krislov, and M.L. Straf. Understanding and evaluating statistical evidence in litigation. *Jurimetrics Journal*, 1995; 36(1): 1–32.

293. Salmon, C. Commentary—DNA evidence. *Criminal Law Review*, 1997, pp. 669–673.

294. Eddy, S.R. and D.J.C. MacKay. Is the Pope the Pope? *Nature*, 1996; 382: 490.

295. Brownlie, A.R. Does justice require less precision than chemistry? *Science & Justice*, 1997; 37(2): 73–74.

296. *Regina v Galli*, 2001.

297. *Regina v GK*, 2001.

298. Robertson, B. and G.A. Vignaux. Expert evidence: Law, practice and probability. *Oxford Journal of Legal Studies*, 1992; 12: 392–403.

299. Berry, D.A. DNA, statistics, and the Simpson case. *Chance: New Directions for Statistics and Computing*, 1994; 7(4): 9–12.

References

300. Hazlitt, G. DNA statistical evidence: Unravelling the strands. *Judicial Officers' Bulletin*, 2002; 14(9): 66–69.
301. Robertson, B., G.A. Vignaux, and C.E.H. Berger. Extending the confusion about Bayes. *The Modern Law Review*, 2011; 74(3): 444–455.
302. Evett, I.W., Personal communication, 2001.
303. Weir, B.S. DNA statistics in the Simpson matter. *Nature Genetics*, 1995; 11: 365–368.
304. Horgan, J. High profile. *Scientific American*, October, 1994, pp. 18–19.
305. Holder, E.H., M.L. Leary, and J.H. Laub. *DNA for the Defense Bar*. 2012. Available at: https://www.ncjrs.gov/pdffiles1/nij/237975.pdf
306. Sandiford, A. *Expert Witness*. Auckland: Harper Collins; 2010.
307. Brookfield, J. DNA profiling on trial—Correspondence. *Nature*, 1994; 369: 351.
308. Weir, B.S. DNA profiling on trial—Correspondence. *Nature*, 1994; 369: 351.
309. Brenner, C.H. Understanding Y haplotype matching probability. *Forensic Science International: Genetics*, 2014; 8(1): 233–243.
310. Berry, D.A. Comment in Roeder, K (1994). DNA fingerprinting: A review of the controversy. *Statistical Science*, 1994; 9(2): 252–255.
311. Lempert, R. Comment: Theory and practice in DNA fingerprinting. *Statistical Science*, 1994; 9(2): 255–258.
312. Roeder, K. DNA fingerprinting: A review of the controversy. *Statistical Science*, 1994; 9(2): 222–278.
313. Lewontin, R. Forensic DNA typing dispute. *Nature*, 1994; 372: 398.
314. Thompson, W.C. Comment in Roeder, K (1994). DNA fingerprinting: A review of the controversy. *Statistical Science*, 1994; 9(2): 263–266.
315. Nowak, R. Forensic DNA goes to court with O.J. *Science*, 1994; 265: 1352–1354.
316. Thompson, W.C., F. Taroni, and C.G.G. Aitken. How the probability of a false positive affects the value of DNA evidence. *Journal of Forensic Science*, 2003; 48(1): 1–8.
317. Clarke, G.W. Commentary on: "How the probability of a false positive affects the value of DNA evidence." *Journal of Forensic Science*, 2003; 48(5).
318. Cotton, R.W. and C.J. Word. Commentary on: "How the probability of a false positive affects the value of DNA evidence." *Journal of Forensic Science*, 2003; 48(5).
319. Thompson, W.C., F. Taroni, and C.G.G. Aitken. Authors' response. *Journal of Forensic Science*, 2003; 48(5).
320. Koehler, J.J. Proficiency tests to estimate error rates in the forensic sciences. *Law, Probability and Risk*, 2012, pp. 1–10.
321. Kloosterman, A., M. Sjerps, and A. Quak. Error rates in forensic DNA analysis: Definition, numbers, impact and communication. *Forensic Science International: Genetics*, 2014; 12: 77–85.
322. Chakraborty, R. DNA profiling on trial—Correspondence. *Nature*, 1994; 369: 351.
323. Committee on Identifying the Needs of the Forensic Sciences Community, National Research Council. *Strengthening Forensic Science in the United States: A Path Forward*. Washington, DC: National Academy Press; 2009.
324. Parson, W., et al. The EDNAP mitochondrial DNA population database (EMPOP) collaborative exercises: Organisation, results and perspectives. *Forensic Science International*, 2004; 139: 215–226.
325. van Oorschot, R.A.H., K.N. Ballantyne, and R.J. Mitchell. Forensic trace DNA: A review. *Investigative Genetics*, 2010; 1: 14.
326. Rutty, G.N., S. Watson, and J. Davison. DNA contamination of mortuary instruments and work surfaces: A significant problem in forensic practice? *International Journal of Legal Medicine*, 2000; 114: 56–60.
327. Krone, T. Raising the alarm? Role definition for prosecutors in criminal cases. *Australian Journal of Forensic Sciences*, 2012; 44(1): 15–29.
328. Daniel, R. and R.A.H. van Oorschot. An investigation of the presence of DNA on unused laboratory gloves. *Forensic Science International: Genetics Supplement Series*, 2011; 3(1): e45–e46.
329. Himmelreich, C. Germany's Phantom serial killer: A DNA blunder. *Time Magazine*, 2009.
330. Rutty, G.N., A. Hopwood, and A. Tucker. The effectiveness of protective clothing in the reduction of potential DNA contamination of the scene of crime. *International Journal of Legal Medicine*, 2003; 117: 170–174.
331. MI6 death: Gareth Williams's family in 'dark arts' fear. *BBC News*, 2012. Available at: http://www.bbc.com/news/uk-england-london-17562112

332. Rutty, G.N. An investigation into the transference and survivability of human DNA following simulated manual strangulation with consideration of the problem of third party contamination. *International Journal of Legal Medicine*, 2002; 116: 170–173.

333. Thompson, W.C. Painting the target around the matching profile: The Texas sharpshooter fallacy in forensic DNA interpretation. *Law, Probability and Risk*, 2009; 8: 257–276.

334. Risinger, D.M., et al. The Daubert/Kuhmo implications of observer effects in forensic science: Hidden problems of expectation and suggestion. *California Law Review*, 2002; 90(1): 1–56.

335. Saks, M.J., et al. Context effects in forensic science: A review and application of the science of science to crime laboratory practice in the United States. *Science & Justice*, 2003; 43(2): 77–90.

336. Dror, I.E. and G. Hampikian. Subjectivity and bias in forensic DNA mixture interpretation. *Science & Justice*, 2011; 51(4): 204–208.

337. Baker, H. *The Microscope Made Easy Ch 15: Cautions in Viewing Objects*. Lincolnwood, IL: Science Heritage; 1742.

338. Caesar, C.J. *Commentaries on the Gallic War*. F.H. Dewey, Ed. New York: Translation Publishing; 1918.

339. Dror, I.E., D. Charlton, and A.E. Peron. Contextual information renders experts vulnerable to making erroneous identifications. *Forensic Science International*, 2006; 156: 74–78.

340. Associated Press. U.S. widens probe of FBI's DNA analysis. *USA Today*, 2003.

341. King, J. *DOJ Aware of Problems in FBI's DNA Lab*. 2003. Available at: www/nacdl.org/MEDIA/proooo96.htm

342. ASCLD/LAB. *Guiding principles of professional responsibility for crime laboratories and forensic scientists*. 2009. Available at: http://www.ascld-lab.org/about_us/guidingprinciples.html#iii

343. Bourn, J. *Improving service delivery. The Forensic Science Service*. Report of the Comptroller and Auditor General. HC 523 session 2002–2003. 2003.

344. Hagerman, P.J. DNA typing in the forensic arena. *American Journal of Human Genetics*, 1990; 47(5): 876–877.

345. Weir, B.S. Population genetics in the forensic DNA debate. *Proceedings of the National Academy of Sciences of the United States of America*, 1992; 89: 11654–11659.

346. Taroni, F., et al. A general approach to Bayesian networks for the interpretation of evidence. *Forensic Science International*, 2004; 139: 5–16.

347. Evett, I.W. Establishing the evidential value of a small quantity of material found at a crime scene. *Journal of the Forensic Science Society*, 1993; 33(2): 83–86.

348. Lynch, M. God's signature: DNA profiling, the new gold standard in forensic science. *Endeavour*, 2003; 27(2): 93–97.

349. Goodman-Delahunty, J., T. Gumbert-Jourjon, and S. Hale. The biasing influence of linguistic variations in DNA profiling evidence. *Australian Journal of Forensic Sciences*, 2014; 46: 348–360.

350. McKie, I.A.J. There's nane ever fear'd that the truth should be heard but they whom the truth would indite. *Science & Justice*, 2003; 43(3): 161–165.

351. Forrest, A.R.W. Sally Clark—A lesson for us all. *Science & Justice*, 2003; 43(2): 63–64.

352. Dingley, J. The Bombing of Omagh, 15 August 1998: The bombers, their tactics, strategy, and purpose behind the incident. *Studies in Conflict & Terrorism*, 2001; 24: 451–465.

353. Potter, S.J.O. and G.E. Carter. The Omagh Bombing—A medical perspective. *Journal of the Royal Army Medical Corps*, 2000; 146: 18–21.

354. McDonald, H. Omagh bomb police witnesses cleared of lying. *The Guardian*, 2009.

355. Evett, I.W., G. Jackson, and J.A. Lambert. More in the hierarchy of propositions: Exploring the distinction between explanations and propositions. *Science & Justice*, 2000; 40(1): 3–10.

356. Evett, I.W. A quantitative theory for interpreting transfer evidence in criminal cases. *Applied Statistics*, 1984; 33(1): 25–32.

357. Taroni, F., et al. Whose DNA is this? How relevant a question? (a note for forensic scientists). *Forensic Science International: Genetics*, 2013; 7(4): 467–470.

358. Balding, D.J. and R.A. Nichols. DNA profile match probability calculation: How to allow for population stratification, relatedness, database selection and single bands. *Forensic Science International*, 1994; 64: 125–140.

359. Robertson, B. and G.A. Vignaux. Inferring beyond reasonable doubt. *Oxford Journal of Legal Studies*, 1991; 11: 431–438.

360. Zaykin, D., L.A. Zhivotovsky, and B.S. Weir. Exact tests for association between alleles at arbitrary numbers of loci. *Genetica*, 1995; 96: 169–178.

References

361. Zaykin, D., et al. Truncated product method for combining p-values. *Genetic Epidemiology*, 2002; 22(2): 170–185.
362. Evett, I.W. and J.S. Buckleton. Statistical analysis of STR Data. In *Advances in Forensic Haemogenetics*, A. Carracedo, B. Brinkmann, and W. Bär, Eds. Berlin: Springer Verlag; 1996, pp. 79–86.
363. Law, B., et al. Effects of population structure and admixture on exact tests for association between loci. *Genetics*, 2003; 164: 361–387.
364. Triggs, C.M. and J.S. Buckleton. Logical implications of applying the principles of population genetics to the interpretation of DNA profiling evidence. *Forensic Science International*, 2002; 128: 108–114.
365. Curran, J.M., J.S. Buckleton, and C.M. Triggs. What is the magnitude of the subpopulation effect? *Forensic Science International*, 2003; 135(1): 1–8.
366. Buckleton, J., J. Curran, and S. Walsh. How reliable is the sub-population model in DNA testimony? *Forensic Science International*, 2006; 157(1–2): 144–148.
367. Weir, B.S. Matching and partially-matching DNA profiles. *Journal of the Forensic Sciences*, 2004; 49(5): 1009–1014.
368. Tvedebrink, T., et al. Analysis of matches and partial-matches in a Danish STR data set. *Forensic Science International: Genetics*, 2012; 6(3): 387–392.
369. Lauc, G., et al. Empirical support for the reliability of DNA interpretation in Croatia. *Forensic Science International: Genetics*, 2008; 3(1): 50–53.
370. Curran, J., S.J. Walsh, and J.S. Buckleton. Empirical support for the reliability of DNA evidence interpretation in Australia and New Zealand. *Australian Journal of Forensic Sciences*, 2008; 40(2): 99–108.
371. Curran, J.M., S.J. Walsh, and J.S. Buckleton. Empirical testing of estimated DNA frequencies. *Forensic Science International: Genetics*, 2007; 1(3–4): 267–272.
372. Mueller, L. Can simple population genetic models reconcile partial match frequencies observed in large forensic databases? *Journal of Genetics*, 2008; 87(2): 101–108.
373. Buckleton, J. and C. Triggs. Relatedness and DNA: Are we taking it seriously enough? *Forensic Science International*, 2005; 152: 115–119.
374. Crow, J.F. and M. Kimura. *An Introduction to Population Genetics Theory*. London: Harper & Row; 1970.
375. Walsh, K. and J.S. Buckleton. A discussion of the law of mutual independence and its application to blood-group frequency data. *Journal of the Forensic Science Society*, 1988; 28(2): 95–98.
376. Walsh, K.A.J. and J.S. Buckleton. Calculating the frequency of occurrence of a blood type for a 'random man'. *Journal of the Forensic Science Society*, 1991; 31: 49–58.
377. Hardy, G.H. Mendelian proportions in a mixed population. *Science*, 1908; 28: 49–50.
378. Weinberg, W. Uber den Nackweis der Vererbung beim Menschen. *Jahresh. Verein f. Varerl Naturk. Wurtemb*, 1908; 64: 368–382.
379. Yule, G.U. Mendel's laws and their probable relation to inter-racial heredity. *New Phytologist*, 1902; 1: 192–207, 222–238.
380. Pearson, K. On a generalized theory of alternative inheritance, with special references to Mendel's laws. *Philosophical Transactions of the Royal Society of London. Series A*, 1904; 203: 53–86.
381. Castle, W.E. The law of heredity of Galton and Mendel and some laws governing race improvement by selection. *Proceedings of the American Academy of Science*, 1903; 39: 233–242.
382. Mendel, G. Experiments in plant hybridisation. In *English Translation and Commentary by R.A. Fisher.*, J.H. Bennett, Ed., Edinburgh: Oliver & Boyd; 1866 (1965).
383. Geiringer, H. Further remarks on linkage theory in Mendelian heredity. *The Annals of Mathematical Statistics*, 1945; 16: 390–393.
384. Bennett, J.H. On the theory of random mating. *Annals of Eugenics*, 1954; 18: 311–317.
385. Hudson, R.R. Linkage disequilibrium and recombination. In *Handbook of Statistical Genetics*, D.J. Balding, M. Bishop, and C. Cannings, Eds. Chichester: Wiley; 2001.
386. Morgan, T.H. *The Theory of Genes*. New Haven: Yale University Press; 1928.
387. Morgan, T.H. Random segregation versus coupling in Mendelian inheritance. *Science*, 1911; 34: 384.
388. Sturtevant, A.H. The linear arrangement of six sex-linked factors in Drosophila as shown by their mode of association. *Journal of Experimental Zoology*, 1913; 14: 43–59.
389. Ott, J. *Analysis of Human Genetic Linkage*. 3rd ed. London: The Johns Hopkins University Press; 1985.

390. Ardlie, K.G., L. Kruglyak, and M. Seielstad. Patterns of linkage disequilibrium in the human genome. *Nature Reviews Genetics*, 2002; 3: 299–309.

391. Cerda-Flores, R.M., et al. Maximum likelihood estimates of admixture in Northeastern Mexico using 13 short tandem repeat loci. *American Journal of Human Biology*, 2002; 14: 429–439.

392. Kimura, M. and T. Ohta. Mutation and evolution at the molecular level. *Genetics*, 1973; 73(Suppl): 19–35.

393. Kimura, M. and J. Crow. The number of alleles that can be maintained in a finite population. *Genetics*, 1964; 49: 725–738.

394. DiRienzo, A., et al. Mutational processes of simple-sequence repeat loci in human populations. *Proceedings of the National Academy of Sciences of the United States of America*, 1994; 91: 3166–3170.

395. Estoup, A. and J.-M. Cornuet. Microsatellite evolution: Inferences from population data. In *Microsatellites Evolution and Applications*, D.B. Goldstein and C. Schlötterer, Eds. Oxford University Press; 1999.

396. Rosenberg, N.A., et al. Genetic structure of human populations. *Science*, 2002; 298: 2381–2385.

397. Excoffier, L. and G. Hamilton. Comment on "Genetic structure of human populations." *Science*, 2003; 300: 1877b.

398. Rosenberg, N.A., et al. Response to comment on "Genetic structure of human populations." *Science*, 2003; 300: 1877.

399. Neuhauser, C. Mathematical models in population genetics. In *Handbook of Statistical Genetics*, D.J. Balding, M. Bishop, and C. Cannings, Eds. Chichester: Wiley; 2001.

400. Jorde, L.B., et al. Microsatellite diversity and the demographic history of modern humans. *Proceedings of the National Academy of Sciences of the United States of America*, 1997; 94: 3100–3103.

401. Ohno, S. So much 'junk' DNA in our genome. *Brookhaven Symposia in Biology*, 1972; 23: 366–370.

402. Makalowski, W. Not junk after all. *Science*, 2003; 300: 1246–1247.

403. Laird, R., P.M. Schneider, and S. Gaudieri. Forensic STRs as potential disease markers: A study of VWA and von Willebrand's disease. *Forensic Science International: Genetics*, 2007; 1(3–4): 253–261.

404. ENCODE Consortium. Available at: www.encodeproject.org

405. Electronic Frontier Foundation. Available at: https://www.eff.org/document/haskell-v-harris%E2%80%94eff-letter-ninth-circuit-re-junk-dna

406. Carroll, S.B. Genetics and the making of *Homo sapiens. Nature*, 2003; 422: 849–857.

407. Wagner, J.K. Out with the "Junk DNA" phrase. *Journal of Forensic Sciences*, 2013; 58(1): 292–294.

408. Cavalli-Sforza, L.L., P. Menozzi, and A. Piazza. *The History and Geography of Human Genes*. Princeton: Princeton University Press; 1994.

409. Mourant, A.E. Blood groups and diseases. *Haematologia*, 1974; 8(1–4): 183–194.

410. Orkin, S.T., et al. Linkage of β-thalassaemia mutations and β-globin gene polymorphisms with DNA polymorphisms in human β-globin gene cluster. *Nature*, 1982; 296: 627–631.

411. Katsanis, S.H. and J.K. Wagner. Characterization of the standard and recommended CODIS markers. *Journal of Forensic Sciences*, 2013; 58(Suppl 1): S169–S172.

412. Thibaut, F., et al. Association of DNA polymorphism in the first intron of the tyrosine hydroxylase gene with disturbances of the catecholaminergic system in schizophrenia. *Schizophrenia Research*, 1997; 23(3): 259–264.

413. Burgert, E., et al. No association between the tyrosine hydroxylase microsatellite marker HUMTH01 and schizophrenia or bipolar I disorder. *Psychiatric Genetics*, 1998; 8(2): 45–48.

414. Sharma, P., et al. Positive association of tyrosine hydroxylase microsatellite marker to essential hypertension. *Hypertension*, 1998; 32: 676–682.

415. Klintschar, M., et al. HumTH01 and blood pressure. An obstacle for forensic applications? *International Congress Series*, 2004; 1261: 589–591.

416. Klintschar, M., et al. DNA polymorphisms in the tyrosin hydroxylase and GNB3 genes: Association with unexpected death from acute myocardial infarction and increased heart weight. *Forensic Science International*, 2005; 153(2–3): 142–146.

417. Phillips, C., et al. The recombination landscape around forensic STRs: Accurate measurement of genetic distances between syntenic STR pairs using HapMap high density SNP data. *Forensic Science International: Genetics*, 2012; 6(3): 354–365.

418. Chakraborty, R., et al. Relative mutation rates at di-, tri-, and tetranucleotide microsatellite loci. *Proceedings of the National Academy of Sciences of the United States of America*, 1997; 94: 1041–1046.

419. Diamond, J. *The Rise and Fall of the Third Chimpanzee*. London: Vintage; 1991.

References

420. Lewontin, R.C. Comment: The use of DNA profiles in forensic contexts. *Statistical Science*, 1994; 9(2): 259–262.
421. Lewontin, R.C. and D.L. Hartl. Population genetics in forensic DNA typing. *Science*, 1991; 254: 1745–1750.
422. Excoffier, L. Analysis of population subdivision. In *Handbook of Statistical Genetics*, D.J. Balding, M. Bishop, and C. Cannings, Eds. Chichester: Wiley; 2001.
423. Wahlund, S. Zuzammensetzung von populationen und korrelationserscheinungen vom standpunkt der vererbungslehre aus betrechtet. *Hereditas*, 1928; 11: 65–106.
424. Weir, B.S. *Genetic Data Analysis II*. Sunderland, MA: Sinauer; 1996.
425. Ohta, T. and M. Kimura. Linkage disequilibrium due to random genetic drift. *Genetical Research*, 1969; 13: 47–55.
426. Nei, M. and W.H. Li. Linkage disequilibrium in subdivided populations. *Genetics*, 1973; 75: 213–219.
427. Li, W.H. and M. Nei. Stable linkage disequilibrium without epistasis in subdivided populations. *Theoretical Population Biology*, 1974; 6: 173–183.
428. Ohta, T. Linkage disequilibrium due to random genetic drift in finite subdivided populations. *Proceedings of the National Academy of Sciences of the United States of America*, 1982; 79: 1940–1944.
429. Lander, E. DNA fingerprinting on trial. *Nature*, 1989; 339: 501–505.
430. Lander, E. Invited editorial: Research on DNA typing catches up with courtroom application. *American Journal of Human Genetics*, 1991; 48: 819–823.
431. Weir, B.S. Matching and partially-matching DNA profiles. *Journal of Forensic Sciences*, 2004; 49: 1009–1014.
432. Laurie, C. and B.S. Weir. Dependency effects in multi-locus match probabilities. *Theoretical Population Biology*, 2003; 63(3): 207–219.
433. Zhang, K., et al. Randomly distributed crossovers may generate block-like patterns of linkage disequilibrium: An act of genetic drift. *Human Genetics*, 2003; 113: 51–59.
434. Mourant, A. *Blood Relations: Blood groups and anthropology*. New York: Oxford University Press; 1983.
435. Bowcock, A.M., et al. High resolution of human evolutionary trees with polymorphic microsatellites. *Nature*, 1994; 368: 455–457.
436. Bright, J.-A., J.S. Buckleton, and C.E. McGovern. Allele frequencies for the four major subpopulations of New Zealand for the 15 Identifiler loci. *Forensic Science International: Genetics*, 2010; 4(2): e65–e66.
437. Goetz, R., et al. Population data from the New South Wales Aboriginal Australian sub-population for the profiler plus autosomal short tandem repeat (STR) loci. *Forensic Science International*, 2008; 175(2–3): 235–237.
438. Buckleton, J., S. Walsh, and J. Mitchell. *Autosomal Microsatellite Diversity within the Australian Population*. Report of the National Institute of Forensic Sciences Standing Committee on Sub-Population Data, 2007.
439. Walsh, S.J. and J. Buckleton. Autosomal microsatellite allele frequencies for 15 regionally defined Aboriginal Australian population datasets. *Forensic Science International*, 2007; 168: e29–e42.
440. Walsh, S.J. and J.S. Buckleton. Autosomal microsatellite allele frequencies for a nationwide dataset from the Australian Caucasian sub-population. *Forensic Science International*, 2007; 168(2–3): e47–e50.
441. Walsh, S.J., et al. A comprehensive analysis of microsatellite diversity in Aboriginal Australia. *Journal of Human Genetics*, 2007; 52(2): 712–728.
442. Eckhoff, C., S.J. Walsh, and J.S. Buckleton. Population data from sub-populations of the Northern Territory of Australia for 15 autosomal short tandem repeat (STR) loci. *Forensic Science International*, 2007; 171(2–3): 237–249.
443. Walsh, S.J., et al. Examining genetic diversity among the people of Aotearoa, New Zealand. *Journal of Forensic Science*, 2003; 48(5): 1091–1093.
444. Bagdonavicius, A., et al. Western Australian sub-population data for the thirteen AMPFlSTR Profiler Plus™ and COfiler™ STR loci. *Journal of Forensic Sciences*, 2002; 47(5): 1–5.
445. Wild, C.J. and G.A.F. Seber. *Chance Encounters*. New York: Wiley; 2000.
446. Budowle, B., et al. The assessment of frequency estimates of Hae III-generated VNTR profiles in various reference databases. *Journal of Forensic Sciences*, 1994; 39: 319–352.

447. Budowle, B., et al. The assessment of frequency estimates of Hinf I-generated VNTR profiles in various ethnic databases. *Journal of Forensic Sciences*, 1994; 39(4): 988–1008.

448. Hartmann, J.M., et al. The effect of ethnic and racial population substructuring on the estimation of multi-locus fixed-bin VNTR RFLP genotype probabilities. *Journal of Forensic Sciences*, 1997; 42(2): 232–240.

449. Sawyer, S., et al. Fingerprinting Loci do show population differences: Comments on Budowle et al. *American Journal of Human Genetics*, 1996; 59: 272–274.

450. Gill, P.D., et al. A comparison of adjustment methods to test the robustness of an STR DNA database comprised of 24 European populations. *Forensic Science International*, 2003; 131: 184–196.

451. Regina v Karger, 2001.

452. Ayres, K.L., J. Chaseling, and D.J. Balding. Implications for DNA identification arising from an analysis of Australian forensic databases. *Forensic Science International*, 2002; 129(1): 90–98.

453. Balding, D.J. and R.A. Nichols. Significant genetic correlations among Caucasians at forensic DNA loci. *Heredity*, 1997; 78: 583–589.

454. Wright, S. The genetical structure of populations. *Annals of Eugenics*, 1951; 15: 323–354.

455. Balding, D.J. and R.A. Nichols. A method for quantifying differentiation between populations at multi-allelic loci and its implications for investigating identity and paternity. *Genetica*, 1995; 96: 3–12.

456. Weir, B.S. Forensics. In *Handbook of Statistical Genetics*, D.J. Balding, M. Bishop, and C. Cannings, Eds. Chichester: Wiley; 2001.

457. Evett, I.W., et al. DNA profiling: A discussion of issues relating to the reporting of very small match probabilities. *Criminal Law Review*, May, 2000, pp. 341–355.

458. Foreman, L.A. and I.W. Evett. Statistical analysis to support forensic interpretation of a new ten-locus STR profiling system. *International Journal of Legal Medicine*, 2001; 114: 147–155.

459. Buckleton, J. Lecture notes DNA workshop. Subsequently subsumed into FSS training material. In *Millennium Conference*, London, 1999.

460. Lander, E. and B. Budowle. DNA fingerprinting dispute laid to rest. *Nature*, 1994; 371: 735–738.

461. Hartl, D., Forensic DNA typing dispute. *Nature*, 1994; 372: 398–399.

462. Steele, C.D. and D.J. Balding. Statistical evaluation of forensic DNA profile evidence. *Annual Review of Statistics and Its Application*, 2014; 1: 361–384.

463. Tippett, C.F., et al. Paint flakes from sources other than vehicles. *Journal of the Forensic Science Society*, 1965; 8(2): 61–65.

464. Evett, I.W., et al. Statistical analysis of a large file of STR profiles of British Caucasians to support forensic casework. *International Journal of Legal Medicine*, 1996; 109: 173–177.

465. Foreman, L.A., A.F.M. Smith, and I.W. Evett. Bayesian Validation of a Quadruplex STR Profiling System for Identification Purposes. *Journal of Forensic Science*, 1999; 44(3): 478–486.

466. Weir, B.S., Personal Communication.

467. Weir, B.S. The rarity of DNA profiles. *Annals of Applied Statistics*, 2007; 1: 358–370.

468. Hopwood, A.J., et al. Consideration of the probative value of single donor 15-plex STR profiles in UK populations and its presentation in UK courts. *Science & Justice*, 2012; 52(3): 185–190.

469. Overall, A.D.J., L.A. Foreman, and J.A. Lambert. Genetic differentiation within and between four UK ethnic groups. *Forensic Science International*, 2000; 114: 7–20.

470. Birus, I., et al. How high should paternity index be for reliable identification of war victims by DNA typing? *Croatian Medical Journal*, 2003; 44(3): 322–326.

471. Lempert, R.O. DNA, science and the law: Two cheers for the ceiling principle. *Jurimetrics Journal*, 1993; 34(1): 41–57.

472. Devlin, B., N. Risch, and K. Roeder. NRC report on DNA typing. *Science*, 1993; 260: 1057–1058.

473. Committee on DNA Technology in Forensic Science, Board on Biology, Commission on Life Sciences, National Research Council. *DNA Technology in Forensic Science*. Washington, DC: National Academy Press; 1992.

474. Foreman, L.A., J.A. Lambert, and I.W. Evett. *Rationale Behind QMS Guidelines (FSS-TS-404) for Match Probability Calculations*. FSS Report No. TN 823, 1997.

475. Weir, B.S. DNA match and profile probabilities: Comment on Budowle et al. (2000) and Fung and Hu (2000). *Forensic Science Communications*, 2001; 3(1).

476. Sun, G., et al. Global genetic variation at nine short tandem repeat loci and implications on (sic) forensic genetics. *European Journal of Human Genetics*, 2003; 11: 39–49.

References

477. Budowle, B., et al. Population studies on three Native Alaska population groups using STR loci. *Forensic Science International*, 2002; 129(1): 51–57.

478. Budowle, B. and R. Chakraborty. Author's response to Buckleton et al. Detection of deviations from genetic equilibrium—A commentary on Budowle B. et al. Population data on the thirteen CODIS core short tandem repeat loci in African Americans, US Caucasians, Hispanics, Bahamians, Jamaicans, and Trinidadians. *Journal of Forensic Sciences*, 2001; 46: 201–202.

479. Bertoni, B., et al. Admixture in Hispanics: Distribution of ancestral population contributions in the continental United States. *Human Biology*, 2003; 75(1): 1–11.

480. Budowle, B. Population studies on 17 STR loci routinely used in forensic cases. *International Congress Series*, 2003; 1239: 71–74.

481. Beyleveld, D. Ethics in the use of statistics in genetics. In *Handbook in Statistical Genetics*, D.J. Balding, M. Bishop, and C. Cannings, Eds. Chichester: Wiley; 2001.

482. Graham, J., J. Curran, and B.S. Weir. Conditional genotypic probabilities for microsatellite loci. *Genetics*, 2000; 155: 1973–1980.

483. Thompson, E.A. Two-locus and three-locus gene identity by descent in pedigrees. *IMA Journal of Mathematics Applied in Medicine and Biology*, 1988; 5: 261–279.

484. Brenner, C.H. Symbolic kinship program. *Genetics*, 1997; 145: 535–542.

485. Brenner, C.H. Kinship analysis when there are many possibilities. In *Progress in Forensic Genetics 8*, G.F. Sensabaugh, P.J. Lincoln, and B. Olaisen, Eds. Elsevier Science; 1999, pp. 94–96.

486. Evett, I.W. Evaluating DNA profiles in a case where the defence is "it was my brother." *Journal of the Forensic Science Society*, 1992; 32(1): 5–14.

487. Cotterman, C.W. *A Calculus for Statistical Genetics*. Columbus, OH: Ohio State University; 1940.

488. Malecot, G. *Les mathematigues de l'heredite*. Paris: Masson et Cie; 1948.

489. Li, C.C. and L. Sacks. The derivation of joint distribution and correlation between relatives by the use of stochastic measures. *Biometrics*, 1954; 10: 347–360.

490. Jacquard, A. Genetics information given by a relative. *Biometrics*, 1972; 28: 1101–1114.

491. Wright, S. Systems of mating II. *Genetics*, 1921; 6: 124–143.

492. Haldane, J.B.S. Some theoretical results of continued brother-sister mating. *Journal of Genetics*, 1937; 34: 265–274.

493. Fisher, R.A. *Theory of Inbreeding*. Edinburg: Oliver & Boyd; 1949.

494. Cockerham, C.C. and B.S. Weir. Sib mating with two linked loci. *Genetics*, 1968; 60: 629–640.

495. Thompson, E.A. Gene identities and multiple relationships. *Biometrics*, 1974; 30: 667–680.

496. Thompson, E.A. *Statistical Inference from Genetic Data on Pedigrees*. Beachwood, OH: Institute of Mathematical Statistics; 2000.

497. Weir, B.S. *Summer School in Statistical Genetics Course Notes*. 2003.

498. Li, C.C., D.E. Weeks, and A. Chakravarti. Similarity of DNA fingerprints due to chance and relatedness. *Human Heredity*, 1993; 43: 45–52.

499. Buckleton, J.S. and C.M. Triggs. The effective of linkage on the calculation of DNA match probabilities for siblings and half siblings. *Forensic Science International*, 2006; 160: 193–199.

500. Kling, D., T. Egeland, and A.O. Tillmar. FamLink—A user friendly software for linkage calculations in family genetics. *Forensic Science International: Genetics*, 2012; 6(5): 616–620.

501. Strom, C.M. More on DNA typing dispute. Correspondence. *Nature*, 1995; 373: 98–99.

502. Budowle, B., et al. Population data on the thirteen CODIS core short tandem repeat loci in African Americans, US Caucasians, Hispanics, Bahamanians, Jamaicans and Trinidadians. *Journal of Forensic Science*, 1999; 44: 1277–1286.

503. Lewontin, R. Which population? *American Journal of Human Genetics*, 1993; 52: 205.

504. Lempert, R.O. The suspect population and DNA identification. *Jurimetrics Journal*, 1993; 34(1): 1–7.

505. Evett, I.W. and B.S. Weir. Flawed Reasoning in Court. *Chance: New Directions for Statistics and Computing*, 1991; 4(4): 19–21.

506. Lempert, R. After the DNA wars: Skirmishing with NRC II. *Jurimetrics Journal*, 1997; 37: 439–468.

507. Weir, B.S. and I.W. Evett. Whose DNA? *American Journal of Human Genetics*, 1992; 50: 869.

508. Robertson, B., T. Vignaux, and J. Buckleton. R v Meyboom (2011) 28 A Crim R 551, "Flawed reasoning about DNA." *Criminal Law Journal*, 2013; 37: 137–143.

509. Buckleton, J.S., K.A.J. Walsh, and I.W. Evett. Who is "Random Man"? *Journal of the Forensic Science Society*, 1991; 31(4): 463–468.

510. Triggs, C.M., S.A. Harbison, and J.S. Buckleton. The calculation of DNA match probabilities in mixed race populations. *Science & Justice*, 2000; 40: 33–38.

511. Brinkmann, B. Overview of PCR-based systems in identity testing. *Methods in Molecular Biology*, 1998; 98: 105–119.

512. Romualdi, C., et al. Patterns of human diversity, within and among continents, inferred from biallelic DNA polymorphisms. *Genome Research*, 2002; 12: 602–612.

513. Buckleton, J.S., et al. A stratified approach to the compilation of blood group frequency surveys. *Journal of the Forensic Science Society*, 1987; 27: 103–122.

514. Fung, W.K. Are convenience DNA samples significantly different? *Forensic Science International*, 1996; 82: 233–241.

515. Walsh, S.J., et al. Evidence in support of self-declaration as a sampling method for the formation of sub-population databases. *Journal of Forensic Sciences*, 2003; 48(5): 1091–1093.

516. Walsh, S.J., et al. *Genetic Diversity among the People of Aotearoa, New Zealand.* 2002.

517. Law, B. *Statistical Interpretation of DNA Evidence.* PhD Thesis, Department of Statistics, University of Auckland, New Zealand, 2002.

518. Guo, S.W. and E.A. Thompson. Performing the exact test of Hardy-Weinberg proportion for multiple alleles. *Biometrics*, 1992; 48: 361–372.

519. Maiste, P.J. and B.S. Weir. A comparison of tests for independence in the FBI RFLP databases. *Genetica*, 1995; 96: 125–138.

520. Brown, A.H.D. and M.W. Feldman. Multilocus structure of natural populations of Hordeum spontaneum. *Genetics*, 1980; 96: 523–536.

521. Chakraborty, R. Detection of nonrandom association of alleles from the distribution of the number of heterozygous loci in a sample. *Genetics*, 1984; 108: 719–731.

522. Buckleton, J.S., C.M. Triggs, and J.M. Curran. Detection of deviations from genetic equilibrium— A commentary on Budowle B, Moretti TR, Baumstark AL, Defenbaugh DA, Keys KM. Population data on the thirteen CODIS core short tandem repeat loci in African Americans, Caucasians, Hispanics, Bahamians, Jamaicans and Trinidadians. *J Forensic Sci* 1999;44:1277–86. *Journal of Forensic Sciences*, 2001; 46(1): 198–202.

523. Triggs, C.M., Personal communication: unpublished results. 2002.

524. Buckleton, J.S., J.M. Curran, and S.J. Walsh. R v Bropho: Careful interpretation of DNA evidence required for courtroom decision making. *Australian Law Journal*, 2005; 79: 709–721.

525. Nuzzo, R. Scientific method: Statistical errors. *Nature News Feature*, 2014.

526. Budowle, B., et al. STR primer concordance study. *Forensic Science International*, 2001; 124: 47–54.

527. O'Connor, K.L., et al. Linkage disequilibrium analysis of D12S391 and vWA in U.S. population and paternity samples. *Forensic Science International: Genetics*, 2011; 5(5): 538–540.

528. O'Connor, K.L., et al. Corrigendum to "linkage disequilibrium analysis of D12S391 and vWA in U.S. population and paternity samples." *Forensic Science International: Genetics*, 2011; 5(5): 541–542.

529. Budowle, B., et al. Population genetic analyses of the NGM STR loci. *International Journal of Legal Medicine*, 2011; 125: 101–109.

530. Gill, P., et al. An evaluation of potential allelic association between the STRs vWA and D12S391: Implications in criminal casework and applications to short pedigrees. *Forensic Science International: Genetics*, 2012; 6(4): 477–486.

531. Bittles, A.H. and J.V. Neel. The costs of human inbreeding and their implications for variations at the DNA level. *Nature Genetics*, 1994; 8: 117–121.

532. Bittles, A.H. The role and significance of consanguinity as a demographic variable. *Population and Development Review*, 1994; 20(3): 561–584.

533. Ottenheiner, M. Lewis Henry Morgan and the prohibition of cousin marriage in the United States. *Journal of Family History*, 1990; 15: 325–334.

534. Coleman, D. A note on the frequency of consanguineous marriages in Reading, England in 1972/1973. *Human Heredity*, 1980; 30: 278–285.

535. Lebel, R.R. Consanguinity studies in Wisconsin. I: Secular trends in consanguineous marriages, 1843–1981. *American Journal of Medical Genetics*, 1983; 15: 543–560.

536. Imaizumi, Y. A recent survey of consanguineous marriages in Japan. *Clinical Genetics*, 1986; 30: 230–233.

537. Shinozaki, N. and H. Aoki. Inbreeding in Japan: Results of a nationwide study. *Japanese Journal of Human Genetics*, 1975; 20: 91–107.

References

538. Bittles, A.H., et al. Reproductive behavior and health in consanguineous marriages. *Science*, 1991; 252: 789–794.

539. Bhatia, G., et al. Estimating and interpreting Fst: The impact of rate variants. *Genome Research*, 2013; 23: 1514–1521.

540. Rębała, K., et al. Northern Slavs from Serbia do not show a founder effect at autosomal and Y-chromosomal STRs and retain their paternal genetic heritage. *Forensic Science International: Genetics*, 2014; 8(1): 126–131.

541. Perez-Lezaun, A., et al. Allele frequencies of 13 short tandem repeats in population samples from the Iberian Peninsula and Northern Africa. *International Journal of Legal Medicine*, 2000; 113: 208–214.

542. Zhivotovsky, L.A., et al. A comprehensive population survey on the distribution of STR frequencies in Belarus. *Forensic Science International*, 2007; 172(2–3): 156–160.

543. Rocchi, A., et al. Italian data of 23 STR loci amplified in a single multiplex reaction. *Forensic Science International: Genetics*, 2012; 6(6): e157–e158.

544. Novokmet, N. and Z. Pavcec. Genetic polymorphisms of 15 AmpFlSTR identifiler loci in Romani population from Northwestern Croatia. *Forensic Science International*, 2007; 168(2–3): e43–e46.

545. Ross, J., et al. Multiplex PCR amplification of eight STR loci in Austrian and Croatian populations. *International Journal of Legal Medicine*, 2001; 115: 57–60.

546. Walsh, S.J. and J. Buckleton. Autosomal microsatellite allele frequencies for 15 regionally defined Aboriginal Australian population datasets. *Forensic Science International*, 2007; 168: e29–e42.

547. Gorostiza, A., et al. Allele frequencies of the 15 AmpF/Str Identifiler loci in the population of Metztitlán (Estado de Hidalgo), México. *Forensic Science International*, 2007; 166(2–3): 230–232.

548. Muñoz, A., et al. Allele frequencies of 15 STRs in the Calchaqui Valleys population (North-Western Argentina). *Forensic Science International: Genetics*, 2012; 6(1): e58–e60.

549. Mohammed, A.A.A., et al. STR data for the GenePrint(TM) PowerPlex(TM) 1.2 system loci from three United Arab Emirates populations. *Forensic Science International*, 2001; 119(3): 328–329.

550. Rangel-Villalobos, H., et al. Forensic evaluation of the AmpFℓSTR identifiler kit in nine Mexican native populations from the pre-Columbian Mesoamerican region. *International Journal of Legal Medicine*, 2014; 128(3): 467–468.

551. Paredes, M., et al. Analysis of the CODIS autosomal STR loci in four main Colombian regions. *Forensic Science International*, 2003; 137(1): 67–73.

552. Schlebusch, C.M., H. Soodyall, and M. Jakobsson. Genetic variation of 15 autosomal STR loci in various populations from southern Africa. *Forensic Science International: Genetics*, 2012; 6(1): e20–e21.

553. Chen, T., et al. Population genetics of nine STR loci from Baoan population in NW China. *Forensic Science International*, 2006; 157(2–3): 218–220.

554. Kraaijenbrink, T., et al. Allele frequency distribution of 21 forensic autosomal STRs in 7 populations from Yunnan, China. *Forensic Science International: Genetics*, 2014; 3(1): e11–e12.

555. Tong, D., et al. Polymorphism analysis of 15 STR loci in a large sample of the Han population in southern China. *Forensic Science International: Genetics*, 2009; 4(1): e27–e29.

556. Zhai, D., et al. The allele frequency of 15 STRs among three Tibeto-Burman-speaking populations from the southwest region of mainland China. *Forensic Science International: Genetics*, 2014; 13: e22–e24.

557. Tereba, A. Tools for analysis of population statistics. *Promega Corporation Profiles in DNA*, 1999; 2: 14–16.

558. Chakraborty, R., P.E. Smouse, and J.V. Neel. Population amalgamation and genetic variation: Observations on artificially agglomerated tribal populations of central and South America. *American Journal of Human Genetics*, 1988; 43: 709–725.

559. Nei, M. *Molecular Evolutionary Genetics*. New York: Columbia University Press; 1987.

560. Fisher, R.A. Standard calculations for evaluating a blood-group system. *Heredity*, 1951; 5(8): 95–102.

561. Jones, D.A. Blood samples: Probability of discrimination. *Journal of Forensic Science Society*, 1972; 12: 355–359.

562. Botstein, D., et al. Construction of a genetic linkage map in man using restriction fragment length polymorphisms. *American Journal of Human Genetics*, 1980; 32: 314–331.

563. Ohno, Y., I.M. Sebetan, and S. Akaishi. A simple method for calculating the probability of excluding paternity with any number of codominant alleles. *Forensic Science International*, 1982; 19: 93–98.

564. Brenner, C. and J.W. Morris. Paternity index calculations in single locus hypervariable DNA probes: Validation and other studies. In *International Symposium on Human Identification*, Promega Corporation, 1989.

565. Nijenhuis, L.E. *Inclusion Probabilities in Parentage Testing*, R. Walker, Ed. Arlington, VA: AABB; 1983.

566. Schneider, S., et al. *Arlequin: A Software for Population Genetic Data Analysis*. Geneva, Switzerland: Genetics and Biometry Laboratory; 1997.

567. Brenner, C.H. *DNA Frequency Uncertainty—Why Bother*. 1997. Available at: www.dna-view.com/noconfid.htm

568. Chakraborty, R., M.R. Srinivasan, and S.F. Daiger. Evaluation of standard errors and confidence intervals of estimated multilocus genotype probabilities and their implications in DNA. *American Journal of Human Genetics*, 1993; 52: 60–70.

569. Eriksen, B. and O. Svensmark. The effect of sample size on the estimation of the frequency of DNA-profiles in RFLP-analysis. *Forensic Science International*, 1994; 65: 195–205.

570. Balding, D.J. Estimating products in forensic identification using DNA profiles. *Journal of American Statistical Association*, 1995; 90(431): 839–844.

571. Curran, J.M., et al. Assessing uncertainty in DNA evidence caused by sampling effects. *Science & Justice*, 2002; 42(1): 29–37.

572. Chakraborty, R. Sample size requirements for addressing the population genetic issues of forensic use of DNA typing. *Human Biology*, 1992; 64: 141–160.

573. Budowle, B., K.L. Monson, and R. Chakraborty. Estimating minimum allele frequencies for DNA profile frequency estimates for PCR-based loci. *International Journal of Legal Medicine*, 1996; 108: 173–176.

574. Weir, B.S., et al., Personal communication: Assessing sampling error in DNA evidence. 2000.

575. Weir, B.S. Forensic population genetics and the National Research Council (NRC). *American Journal of Human Genetics*, 1993; 52: 437.

576. Beecham, G.W. and B.S. Weir. Confidence interval of the likelihood ratio associated with mixed stain DNA evidence. *Journal of Forensic Sciences*, 2011; 56: S166–S171.

577. NRC II. *National Research Council Committee on DNA Forensic Science, The Evaluation of Forensic DNA Evidence*. Washington, DC: National Academy Press; 1996.

578. Curran, J.M., SPURS II (Statistical Probability Using Re-Sampling), software.

579. Parson, W., et al. DNA Commission of the International Society for Forensic Genetics: Revised and extended guidelines for mitochondrial DNA typing. *Forensic Science International: Genetics*, 2014; 13: 134–142.

580. Triggs, C.M. and J.M. Curran. The sensitivity of the Bayesian HPD method to the choice of prior. *Science & Justice*, 2006; 46(3): 169–178.

581. Curran, J.M. and J.S. Buckleton. An investigation into the performance of methods for adjusting for sampling uncertainty in DNA likelihood ratio calculations. *Forensic Science International: Genetics*, 2011; 5(5): 512–516.

582. Scranage, J. and R.A. Pinchin. The Forensic Science Service. *DNASYS*. Birmingham; 1995.

583. Ahrens, J.H. and U. Dieter. Generating gamma variates by a modified rejection technique. *Communications of the Austrian Research Council*, 1982; 25: 47–54.

584. Ahrens, J.H. and U. Dieter. Computer methods for sampling from gamma, beta, Poisson and binomial distributions. *Computing*, 1974; 12: 223–246.

585. Weir, B.S. Independence tests for VNTR alleles defined as fixed bins. *Genetics*, 1992; 130: 873–878.

586. *R v T*, in *Neutral Citation Number: [2010] EWCA Crim 2439*. 2010, Court of Appeal.

587. Taylor, D., et al. An illustration of the effect of various sources of uncertainty on DNA likelihood ratio calculations. *Forensic Science International: Genetics*, 2014; 11: 56–63.

588. Bright, J.-A., et al. Consideration of the probative value of single donor 15-plex STR profiles in UK populations and its presentation in UK courts II. *Science & Justice*, 2013; 53(3): 371.

589. Budowle, B., et al. *DNA Typing Protocols: Molecular Biology and Forensic Analysis*. BioTechniques. Natick, MA: Eaton; 2000.

590. Holden, C. DNA fingerprinting comes of age. *Science*, 1997; 278: 1407.

591. Budowle, B., et al. Source attribution of a forensic DNA profile. *Forensic Science Communications*, 2000; 2(3). Available at: www.fbi.gov/programs/lab/fsc/backissu/july2000/source.html

592. McKasson, S. I think therefore I probably am. *Journal of Forensic Identification*, 2001; 51(3): 217–221.

593. Crispino, F. Comment on JFI 51(3). *Journal of Forensic Identification*, 2001; 51(5): 449–456.

594. Stoney, D.A. Letters to the editor—Source individuality versus expressed individuality—Discussion of "Probability analysis and the evidential value of bolt arrangements." *Journal of Forensic Sciences*, 1989; 34: 1295–1296.

References

595. Stoney, D.A. What made us ever think we could individualize using statistics. *Journal of the Forensic Science Society*, 1991; 31(2): 197–199.
596. Champod, C. Identification/individualisation. In *Encyclopedia of Forensic Sciences*, J. Seigel, Ed. New York: Academic Press; 2000, pp. 1077–1084.
597. Galton, F. Personal identification and description I. *Nature*, 1888; 21: 173–177.
598. Galton, F. Personal identification and description II. *Nature*, 1888; 38: 201–202.
599. Galton, F. Identification of finger tips. *Nineteenth Century*, 1891; 30: 303.
600. Galton, F. The pattern in thumb and finger—On their arrangement into naturally distinct classes, the permanence of the papillary ridges that make them, and the resemblance of their class to ordinary Genera. *Philosophical Transactions of the Royal Society of London*, 1891; 182: 1–23.
601. Galton, F. *Finger Prints*. London: Macmillan; 1892.
602. Galton, F. *Fingerprint Directories*. London: Macmillan; 1895.
603. Stoney, D.A. Fingerprint identification, §21–2. In *Modern Scientific Evidence: The Law and Science of Expert Testimony*, D.L. Faigman, et al., Eds. St. Paul, MN: West Publishing; 1997, pp. 55–78.
604. Stoney, D.A. and J.I. Thornton. A critical analysis of quantitative fingerprint individuality models. *Journal of Forensic Sciences*, 1986; 31(4): 1187–1216.
605. Stoney, D.A. and J.I. Thornton. A Systematic Study of Epidermal Ridge Minutiæ. *Journal of Forensic Sciences*, 1987; 32: 1182–1203.
606. Stoney, D.A. and J.I. Thornton. Author's response for discussion of "a critical analysis of quantitative fingerprint individuality models." *Journal of Forensic Sciences*, 1988; 33(1): 11–12.
607. Stoney, D.A. and J.I. Thorton. A method for the description of minutiæ pairs in epidermal ridge patterns. *Journal of Forensic Sciences*, 1986; 31: 1217–1234.
608. Champod, C. Reconnaissance automatique et analyse statistique des minuties sur les empreintes digitales. In *Institut de Police Scientifique et de Criminologie*. Lausanne: Université de Lausanne; 1996, p. 384.
609. Champod, C. Fingerprints (dactyloscopy): Standard of proof. In *Encyclopedia of Forensic Science*, J. Siegel, P. Saukko, and G. Knupfer, Eds. London: Academic Press; 2000, pp. 884–890.
610. Champod, C., C. Lennard, and P.A. Margot. Alphonse Bertillon and dactyloscopy. *Journal of Forensic Identification*, 1993; 43: 604–625.
611. Champod, C. and P. Margot. Analysis of minutiæ occurrences in fingerprints—The search for non-combined minutiæ. In *14th Meeting of the International Association of Forensic Sciences*, Tokyo, Japan, 1996.
612. Champod, C. and P.A. Margot. Computer assisted analysis of minutiæ occurrences on fingerprints. In *International Symposium on Fingerprint Detection and Identification*, J. Almog and E. Springer, Eds. Israel National Police, Ne'urim, Israel, June 26–30, 1995, 1995, pp. 305–318.
613. Champod, C. and P.A. Margot. Fingermarks, shoesole impressions, ear impressions and toolmarks: A review (Sept. 1995—Aug. 1998). In *12th Interpol Forensic Science Symposium*, Forensic Sciences Foundation Press, Lyon, France, 1998.
614. LaBonne, S. Source attribution. *Discussion on Forensic DNA*, April 2nd, 2010, 2010.
615. Aaronson, J.H. Ballistics, *Like Fingerprint, Evidence — Non-Scientific but Nonetheless Admissible under Daubert*. Available at: http://www.jha.com/us/blog/?blogID=713. Accessed 18 November 2015.
616. Kaye, D.H. Probability, individualization and uniqueness in forensic science evidence: Listening to the academies. *Brooklyn Law Review*, 2010; 75(4): 1163–1185.
617. National Commission on Forensic Science. *Testimony Using the Term "Reasonable Scientific Certainty."* 2015. Available at: http://www.regulations.gov/#!documentDetail;D=DOJ-LA-2015-0004-0008
618. Balding, D.J. When can a DNA profile be regarded as unique? *Science & Justice*, 1999; 39(4): 257–260.
619. Stoney, D.A., What Made Us Ever Think We Could Individualize Using Statistics. *Journal of The Forensic Science Society*, 1991; 31(2): 197–199.
620. New Zealand Legislation. 2009. Judicature Act 1908. Schedule 4 Code of conduct for expert witnesses. Available at: http://www.legislation.govt.nz/act/public/1908/0089/latest/DLM1817947.html
621. Kaye, D.H. Identification, individualisation and uniqueness: What's the difference? *Law, Probability and Risk*, 2009; 8: 85–94.
622. Foreman, L.A., et al. Interpreting DNA evidence: A review. *International Statistical Review*, 2003; 71(3): 473–495.
623. Cole, S.A. Where the rubber meets the road: Thinking about expert evidence as expert testimony. *Villanova Law Review*, 2008; 52: 101–115.

624. Roth, A. Safety in Numbers?: Deciding when DNA Evidence Alone is Enough to Convict. *New York University Law Review, Vol. 85*, 2010.

625. Zaken, N., et al. Can brothers share the same STR profile? *Forensic Science International: Genetics*, 2013; 7(5): 494–498.

626. Pontikinas, E., M. Attwell, and C. Nicholls. Allele sharing at 12/15 STR loci between full siblings. *Forensic Science International: Genetics*, 2015; 16: 163–164.

627. Strom, C.M., et al. Reliability of polymerase chain reaction (PCR) analysis of single cells for preimplantation genetic analysis. *Journal of Assisted Reproduction and Genetics*, 1994; 11: 55–62.

628. Taberlet, P., et al. Reliable genotyping of samples with very low DNA quantities using PCR. *Nucleic Acids Research*, 1996; 24(16): 3189–3194.

629. Strom, C.M. and S. Rechitsky. Use of nested PCR to identify charred human remains and minute amounts of blood. *Journal of Forensic Science*, 1998; 43(3): 696–700.

630. Leclair, B., et al. STR DNA Typing: Increased sensitivity and efficient sample consumption using reduced PCR reaction volumes. *Journal of Forensic Science*, 2003; 48(5): 1001–1013.

631. Frégeau, C.J., et al. AmpflSTR profiler plus short tandem repeat analysis of casework samples, mixture samples, and nonhuman DNA samples amplified under reduced PCR volume conditions (25μl). *Journal of Forensic Science*, 2003; 48(5): 1014–1034.

632. Petricevic, S., et al. Validation and development of interpretation guidelines for low copy number (LCN) DNA profiling in New Zealand using the AmpFlSTR® SGM Plus(TM) multiplex. *Forensic Science International: Genetics*, 2010; 4(5): 305–310.

633. Lagoa, A.M., T. Magalhães, and M.F. Pinheiro. Genetic analysis of fingerprints—Could WGA or nested-PCR be alternatives to the increase of PCR cycles number? *Forensic Science International: Genetics Supplement Series*, 2008; 1(1): 48–49.

634. Jeffreys, A.J., et al. Amplification of human minisatellites by polymerase chain reaction: Towards DNA fingerprinting of single cells. *Nucleic Acids Research*, 1988; 10(23): 10953–10971.

635. Snabes, M.C., et al. Preimplantation single-cell analysis of multiple genetic loci by whole genome amplification. *Proceedings of the National Academy of Sciences of the United States of America*, 1994; 91: 6181–6185.

636. Findlay, I. and P. Quirke. Fluorescent polymerase chain reaction: Part 1. A new method allowing genetic diagnosis and DNA fingerprinting of single cells. *Human Reproduction Update*, 1996; 2(2): 137–152.

637. Findlay, I., et al. Simultaneous DNA 'fingerprinting', diagnosis of sex and single-gene defect status from single cells. *Molecular Human Reproduction*, 1995; 10(4): 1005–1013.

638. Findlay, I., et al. Genetic diagnosis of single cells: Multiplex PCR using seven fluorescent primers to diagnose sex and DNA fingerprint. In *Biotechnology European Symposium*, Miami, 1994.

639. Findlay, I. Single cell PCR. In *Methods in Molecular Medicine*, Y.M.D. Lo, Ed. Totowa, NJ: Humana Press; 1998, pp. 233–263.

640. Van Oorschot, R.A. and M. Jones. DNA fingerprints from fingerprints. *Nature*, 1997; 387(6635): 767.

641. van Hoofstst, D.E.O., et al. DNA typing of fingerprints and skin debris: Sensitivity of capillary electrophoresis in forensic applications using multiplex PCR. In *2nd European Symposium of Human Identification, Promega Corporation*, Innsbruck, Austria, 1998.

642. van Rentergeum, P., D. Leonard, and C. de Greef. Use of latent fingerprints as a source of DNA for genetic identification. In *Progress in Forensic Genetics*, G.F. Sensabaugh, P. Lincoln, and B. Olaisen, Eds. Amsterdam: Elsevier; 2000, pp. 501–503.

643. Van Oorschot, R.A. and M. Jones. Retrieval of DNA from touched objects. In *The 14th International Australia and New Zealand Forensic Science Society Symposium for Forensic Sciences*, Adelaide, Australia, 1998.

644. Balogh, M.K., et al. STR genotyping and mtDNA sequencing of latent fingerprint on paper. *Forensic Science International*, 2003; 137: 188–195.

645. Pizzamiglio, M., et al. DNA typing on latex gloves. In *Progress in Forensic Genetics*, G.F. Sensabaugh, P. Lincoln, and B. Olaisen, Eds. Amsterdam: Elsevier; 2000, pp. 504–507.

646. Wiegand, T., T. Bajanowski, and B. Brinkmann. DNA typing of debris from fingernails. *International Journal of Legal Medicine*, 1993; 106: 81–83.

647. Harbison, S.A., S.F. Petricevic, and S.K. Vintiner. The persistence of DNA under fingernails following submersion in water. *International Congress Series, Elsevier Science*, 2003; 1239: 809–813.

648. Wiegand, P. and M. Kleiber. DNA typing of epithelial cells after strangulation. *International Journal of Legal Medicine*, 1997; 110: 181–183.

References

649. Wiegand, P. and M. Kleiber. DNA typing of epithelial cells. In *Progress in Genetics*, B. Olaisen, B. Brinkmann, and P. Lincoln, Eds. Amsterdam: Elsevier; 1998. pp. 165–167.
650. Uchihi, R., et al. Deoxyribonucleic acid (DNA) typing of human leukocyte antigen (HLA)-DQA1 from single hairs in Japanese. *Journal of Forensic Sciences*, 1992; 37(3): 853–859.
651. Higuchi, R., et al. DNA typing from single hairs. *Nature*, 1988; 332(7): 543–546.
652. Schultz, M.M. and W. Reichert. A strategy for STR-analysis of cryptic epithelial cells on several textiles in practical casework. In *Progress in Forensic Genetics*, G.F. Sensabaugh, P. Lincoln, and B. Olaisen, Eds. Amsterdam: Elsevier; 2000, pp. 514–516.
653. Bright, J. and S.F. Petricevic. Recovery of trace DNA and its application to DNA profiling of shoe insoles. *Forensic Science International*, 2004; 145(1): 7–12.
654. Watanabe, Y., et al. DNA typing from cigarette butts. *Legal Medicine*, 2003; 5: 177–179.
655. Nascimento, E., et al. Genotyping of DNA samples under adverse conditions of low copy number—LCN (formolisados tissue samples and embedded in parraffin). *Forensic Science International: Genetics Supplement Series*, 2009; 2(1): 155–156.
656. Wiegand, P., K. Trubner, and M. Kleiber. STR typing of biological stains on strangulation tools. In *Progress in Forensic Genetics*, G.F. Sensabaugh, P. Lincoln, and B. Olaisen, Eds. Amsterdam: Elsevier; 2000, pp. 508–510.
657. Sutherland, B., J.-A. Bright, and S.J. Walsh. Commentary on: Wickenheiser RA. Trace DNA: A review, discussion of theory, and application of the transfer of trace quantities of DNA through skin contact. *Journal of Forensic Sciences*, 2002; 47(3): 442–450. *Journal of Forensic Sciences*, 2003; 48(2): 467.
658. Hedman, J. Extended survey on LCN analysis in DNA WG laboratories. In *22nd Meeting of the ENFSI DNA Working Group*, 2005.
659. Raymond, J.J., et al. Trace DNA: An underutilized resource or Pandora's box? A review of the use of trace DNA analysis in the investigation of volume crime. *Journal of Forensic Identification*, 2004; 54(6): 668–686.
660. Gill, P., et al. National recommendations of the technical UK DNA working group on mixture interpretation for the NDNAD and for court going purposes. *Forensic Science International: Genetics*, 2008; 2(1): 76–82.
661. Gill, P., et al. Report of the European Network of Forensic Science Institutes (ENSFI): Formulation and testing of principles to evaluate STR multiplexes. *Forensic Science International*, 2000; 108: 1–29.
662. Gill, P., R. Puch-Solis, and J. Curran. The low-template DNA (stochastic) threshold—Its determination relative to risk analysis for national DNA databases. *Forensic Science International: Genetics*, 2009; 3(2): 104–111.
663. Whitaker, J.P., E.A. Cotton, and P. Gill. A comparison of the characteristics of profiles produced with the AMPFlSTR®SGM Plus™ multiplex system for both standard and low copy number (LCN) STR DNA analysis. *Forensic Science International*, 2001; 123: 215–223.
664. Abaz, J., et al. Comparison of variables affecting the recovery of DNA from common drinking containers. *Forensic Science International*, 2002; 126(3): 233–240.
665. Lowe, A., et al. The propensity of individuals to deposit DNA and secondary transfer of low level DNA from individuals to inert surfaces. *Forensic Science International*, 2002; 129: 25–34.
666. Ladd, C., et al. A systematic analysis of secondary DNA transfer. *Journal of Forensic Sciences*, 1999; 44(6): 1270–1272.
667. Dominick, A.J., et al. Is there a relationship between fingerprint donation and DNA shedding? *Journal of Forensic Identification*, 2009; 59(2): 133–143.
668. Quinones, I. and B. Daniel. Cell free DNA as a component of forensic evidence recovered from touched surfaces. *Forensic Science International: Genetics*, 2012; 6(1): 26–30.
669. Kamphausen, T., et al. Good shedder or bad shedder—The influence of skin diseases on forensic DNA analysis from epithelial abrasions. *International Journal of Legal Medicine*, 2012; 126(1): 179–183.
670. Lowe, A., et al. Use of low copy number DNA in forensic inference. *International Congress Series*, 2003; 1239: 799–801.
671. van Oorschot, R.A.H., et al. Impact of relevant variables on the transfer of biological substances. *Forensic Science International: Genetics Supplement Series*, 2009; 2(1): 547–548.
672. Sullivan, K., et al. New developments and challenges in the use of the UK DNA database: Addressing the issue of contaminated consumables. *Forensic Science International*, 2004; 146(Suppl): S175–S176.

673. Schwark, T., et al. Phantoms in the mortuary-DNA transfer during autopsies. *Forensic Science International*, 2012; 216(1–3): 121–126.

674. Rutty, G.N., S. Watson, and J. Davison. DNA contamination of mortuary instruments and work surfaces: A significant problem in forensic practice? *International Journal of Legal Medicine*, 2000; 114: 56–60.

675. van Oorschot, R.A.H., K.N. Ballantyne, and R.J. Mitchell. Forensic trace DNA: A review. *Investigative Genetics*, 2010; 1: 14.

676. Preuße-Prange, A., et al. The problem of DNA contamination in forensic case work—How to get rid of unwanted DNA? *Forensic Science International: Genetics Supplement Series*, 2009; 2(1): 185–186.

677. Wickenhieser, R.A. Trace DNA: A review, discussion of theory, and application of the transfer of trace quantities of DNA through skin contact. *Journal Forensic Science*, 2002; 47(3): 442–450.

678. *R v Wallace*, in *CA590/2007 [2010] NZCA 46*. 2010, Court of Appeal of New Zealand.

679. Benschop, C.C.G., et al. Low template STR typing: Effect of replicate number and consensus method on genotyping reliability and DNA database search results. *Forensic Science International: Genetics*, 2011; 5(4): 316–328.

680. Bright, J.-A., P. Gill, and J. Buckleton. Composite profiles in DNA analysis. *Forensic Science International: Genetics*, 2012; 6(3): 317–321.

681. Buckleton, J.S., J.M. Curran, and P. Gill. Towards understanding the effect of uncertainty in the number of contributors to DNA stains. *Forensic Science International: Genetics*, 2007; 1(1): 20–28.

682. Paoletti, D.R., et al. Empirical analysis of the STR profiles resulting from conceptual mixtures. *Journal of Forensic Sciences*, 2005; 50: 1361–1366.

683. Anon. Low copy number DNA analysis (LCN)—Prosecutors' checklist of questions. 2008.

684. Balding, D. *likeLTD*. Available at: https://sites.google.com/site/baldingstatisticalgenetics/

685. Gill, P., et al. DNA commission of the International Society of Forensic Genetics: Recommendations on the evaluation of STR typing results that may include drop-out and/or drop-in using probabilistic methods. *Forensic Science International: Genetics*, 2012; 6(6): 678–688.

686. Mitchell, A.A., et al. Validation of a DNA mixture statistics tool incorporating allelic drop-out and drop-in. *Forensic Science International: Genetics*, 2012; 6(6): 749–761.

687. Perlin, M.W. and A. Sinelnikov. An information gap in DNA evidence interpretation. *PLoS One*, 2009; 4(12): e8327.

688. Gill, P., A. Kirkham, and J. Curran. LoComatioN: A software tool for the analysis of low copy number DNA profiles. *Forensic Science International*, 2007; 166(2–3): 128–138.

689. Gill, P., et al. DNA commission of the International Society of Forensic Genetics: Recommendations on the interpretation of mixtures. *Forensic Science International*, 2006; 160: 90–101.

690. Morling, N., et al. Interpretation of DNA mixtures—European consensus on principles. *Forensic Science International: Genetics*, 2007; 1(3–4): 291–292.

691. Stringer, P., et al. Interpretation of DNA mixtures—Australian and New Zealand consensus on principles. *Forensic Science International: Genetics*, 2009; 3(2): 144–145.

692. Budowle, B., Personal Communication: *Presentation to the National Academy of Sciences*. 2009.

693. Puch-Solis, R. and T. Clayton. Evidential evaluation of DNA profiles using a discrete statistical model implemented in the DNA LiRa software. *Forensic Science International: Genetics*, 2014; 11: 220–228.

694. Ge, J. and B. Budowle. Modeling one complete versus triplicate analyses in low template DNA typing. *International Journal of Legal Medicine*, 2014; 128: 259–267.

695. Cerri, N., et al. Mixed stains from sexual assault cases: Autosomal or Y-chromosome short tandem repeats? *Croatian Medical Journal*, 2003; 44(3): 289–292.

696. Budowle, B., A.J. Eisenberg, and A. van Daal. Response to comment on "Low copy number typing has yet to achieve 'general acceptance'" (Budowle et al., 2009. *Forensic Sci. Int. Genetics: Supplement Series 2*, 551–552) by Theresa Caragine, Mechthild Prinz. *Forensic Science International: Genetics*, 2011; 5(1): 5–7.

697. Budowle, B. and A. van Daal. Comment on "A universal strategy to interpret DNA profiles that does not require a definition of low copy number" by Peter Gill and John Buckleton, 2010, *Forensic Sci. Int. Genetics 4*, 221–227. *Forensic Science International: Genetics*, 2011; 5(1): 15.

698. Budowle, B. Statistics and mixture interpretation workshop. In *12th International Symposium on Human Identification*, Bioloxi, MS, 2001.

699. Bille, T.W., et al. Comparison of the performance of different models for the interpretation of low level mixed DNA profiles. *Electrophoresis*, 2014; 35(21–22): 3125–3133.

References

700. Harbison, S.A. and J. Buckleton. Applications and extensions of sub-population theory: A case-workers guide. *Science & Justice*, 1998; 38: 249–254.
701. Buckleton, J., Personal communication. 1996.
702. Paoletti, D.R., et al. Empirical analysis of the STR profiles resulting from conceptual mixtures. *Journal of Forensic Sciences*, 2005; 50: 1361–1366.
703. Gill, P., et al. The evolution of DNA databases—Recommendations for new European STR loci. *Forensic Science International*, 2006; 156(2–3): 242–244.
704. Egeland, T., I. Dalen, and P.F. Mostad. Estimating the number of contributors to a DNA profile. *International Journal of Legal Medicine*, 2003; 117: 271–275.
705. Haned, H., et al. The predictive value of the maximum likelihood estimator of the number of contributors to a DNA mixture. *Forensic Science International: Genetics*, 2011; 5(4): 281–284.
706. Haned, H., et al. Estimating the number of contributors to forensic DNA mixtures: Does maximum likelihood perform better than maximum allele count? *Journal of Forensic Sciences*, 2011; 56(1): 23–28.
707. Swaminathan, H., et al. NOCIt: A computational method to infer the number of contributors to DNA samples analyzed by STR genotyping. *Forensic Science International: Genetics*, 2015; 16: 172–180.
708. Biedermann, A., et al. Inference about the number of contributors to a DNA mixture: Comparative analyses of a Bayesian network approach and the maximum allele count method. *Forensic Science International: Genetics*, 2012; 6(6): 689–696.
709. *R v Donnelly*. New Zealand Courts. 2010.
710. Brenner, C. What's wrong with the "exclusion probability." 1997. Available at: www.dna-view.com/exclusn.htm
711. Buckleton, J. and J. Curran. A discussion of the merits of random man not excluded and likelihood ratios. *Forensic Science International: Genetics*, 2008; 2(4): 343–348.
712. Van Nieuwerburgh, F., et al. Impact of allelic drop-out on evidential value of forensic DNA profiles using RMNE. *Bioinformatics*, 2009; 25(2): 225–229.
713. Milot, E., et al. Inclusion probability with dropout: An operational formula. *Forensic Science International: Genetics*, 2015; 16: 71–76.
714. Evett, I.W. Letter to the DNA commission of the ISFG entitled: "Some comments on the draft ISFG recommendations on DNA mixtures." 2006.
715. Evett, I.W., et al. A guide to interpreting single locus profiles of DNA mixtures in forensic cases. *Journal of the Forensic Science Society*, 1991; 31(1): 41–47.
716. Weir, B.S., et al. Interpreting DNA mixtures. *Journal of Forensic Sciences*, 1997; 42(2): 213–222.
717. Mortera, J., A.P. Dawid, and S.L. Lauritzen. Probabilistic expert system for DNA mixture profiling. *Theoretical Population Biology*, 2003; 63: 191–205.
718. Curran, J.M., et al. Interpreting DNA mixtures in structured populations. *Journal of Forensic Sciences*, 1999; 44(5): 987–995.
719. Evett, I.W., P.D. Gill, and J.A. Lambert. Taking account of peak areas when interpreting mixed DNA profiles. *Journal of Forensic Sciences*, 1998; 43(1): 62–69.
720. Clayton, T., et al. Analysis and interpretation of mixed forensic stains using DNA STR profiling. *Forensic Science International*, 1998; 91: 55–70.
721. Gill, P., et al. Interpreting simple STR mixtures using allele peak areas. *Forensic Science International*, 1998; 91(1): 41–53.
722. Kirkham, A., Personal communication. 2002.
723. Gill, P., B. Sparkes, and J.S. Buckleton. Interpretation of simple mixtures when artefacts such as stutters are present—With special reference to multiplex STRs used by the Forensic Science Service. *Forensic Science International*, 1998; 95(3): 213–224.
724. Kelly, H., et al. The interpretation of low level DNA mixtures. *Forensic Science International: Genetics*, 2012; 6(2): 191–197.
725. Prieto, L., et al. Euroforgen-NoE collaborative exercise on LRmix to demonstrate standardization of the interpretation of complex DNA profiles. *Forensic Science International: Genetics*, 2014; 9: 47–54.
726. Tvedebrink, T., et al. Estimating the probability of allelic drop-out of STR alleles in forensic genetics. *Forensic Science International: Genetics*, 2009; 3(4): 222–226.
727. Tvedebrink, T., et al. Allelic drop-out probabilities estimated by logistic regression—Further considerations and practical implementation. *Forensic Science International: Genetics*, 2012; 6(2): 263–267.

728. Tvedebrink, T., et al. Statistical model for degraded DNA samples and adjusted probabilities for allelic drop-out. *Forensic Science International: Genetics*, 2012; 6(1): 97–101.

729. Nicklas, J.A., T. Noreault-Conti, and E. Buel. Development of a real-time method to detect DNA degradation in forensic samples. *Journal of Forensic Sciences*, 2012; 57(2): 466–471.

730. Chung, D.T., et al. A study of the effects of degradation and template concentration on the amplification efficiency of the STR miniplex primer sets. *Journal of Forensic Sciences*, 2004; 49(4): 733–740.

731. Bright, J.-A., et al. The effect of cleaning agents on the ability to obtain DNA profiles using the Identifiler (TM) and PowerPlex (R) Y multiplex kits. *Journal of Forensic Sciences*, 2011; 56(1): 181–185.

732. Taylor, D., J.-A. Bright, and J. Buckleton. Considering relatives when assessing the evidential strength of mixed DNA profiles. *Forensic Science International: Genetics*, 2014; 13: 259–263.

733. Taylor, D., J.A. Bright, and J. Buckleton. The 'factor of two' issue in mixed DNA profiles. *Journal of Theoretical Biology*, 2014; 363: 300–306.

734. Whittaker, R., Personal Communication.

735. Evett, I.W. On meaningful questions: A two-trace transfer problem. *Journal of the Forensic Science Society*, 1987; 27: 375–381.

736. Aitken, C.G.G. *Statistics and the Evaluation of Evidence for Forensic Scientists*. Statistics in Practice, V. Barnett, Ed. Chichester: Wiley; 1995.

737. Chapman, R., Personal communication. 2001.

738. Triggs, C.M. and J. Buckleton. The two trace transfer problem revisited. *Science & Justice*, 2003; 43(3): 127–134.

739. Gittelson, S., et al. Bayesian networks and the value of the evidence for the forensic two-trace transfer problem. *Journal of Forensic Sciences*, 2012; 57(5): 1199–1216.

740. Gittelson, S., et al. Modeling the forensic two-trace problem with Bayesian networks. *Artificial Intelligence and the Law*, 2013; 21(2): 221–252.

741. Perlin, M.W. and B. Szabady. Linear mixture analysis: A mathematical approach to resolving mixed DNA samples. *Journal of Forensic Sciences*, 2001; 46(6): 1372–1377.

742. Cowell, R.G., S.L. Lauritzen, and J. Mortera. Probabilistic modelling for DNA mixture analysis. *Forensic Science International: Genetics Supplement Series*, 2008; 1(1): 640–642.

743. Cowell, R.G., S.L. Lauritzen, and J. Mortera. Probabilistic expert systems for handling artifacts in complex DNA mixtures. *Forensic Science International: Genetics*, 2011; 5(3): 202–209.

744. Robert G.C. Validation of an STR peak area model. *Forensic Science International: Genetics*, 2009; 3(3): 193–199.

745. Bright, J.-A., et al. Determination of the variables affecting mixed MiniFiler™ DNA profiles. *Forensic Science International: Genetics*, 2011; 5(5): 381–385.

746. Taylor, D. Using continuous DNA interpretation methods to revisit likelihood ratio behaviour. *Forensic Science International: Genetics*, 2014; 11: 144–153.

747. Puch-Solis, R., et al. Evaluating forensic DNA profiles using peak heights, allowing for multiple donors, allelic dropout and stutters. *Forensic Science International: Genetics*, 2013; 7(5): 555–563.

748. Edwards, A., et al. DNA typing and genetic mapping at five trimeric and tetrameric tandem repeats. *American Journal of Human Genetics*, 1991; 49: 746–756.

749. Ballantyne, J., E.K. Hanson, and M.W. Perlin. DNA mixture genotyping by probabilistic computer interpretation of binomially-sampled laser captured cell populations: Combining quantitative data for greater identification information. *Science & Justice*, 2012; 53(2): 103–114.

750. Bill, M., et al. PENDULUM—A guideline-based approach to the interpretation of STR mixtures. *Forensic Science International*, 2005; 148(2–3): 181–189.

751. Kelly, H., et al. Modelling heterozygote balance in forensic DNA profiles. *Forensic Science International: Genetics*, 2012; 6(6): 729–734.

752. Chung, D.T., et al. A study of the effects of degradation and template concentration on the amplification efficiency of the STR miniplex primer sets. *Journal of Forensic Sciences*, 2004; 49(4): 733–740.

753. McCord, B., et al. *An Investigation of the Effect of DNA Degradation and Inhibition on PCR Amplification of Single Source and Mixed Forensic Samples*. 2011.

754. Cotton, E.A., et al. Validation of the AMPFlSTR® SGM Plus™ system for use in forensic casework. *Forensic Science International*, 2000; 112(2–3): 151–161.

755. Diegoli, T.M., et al. An optimized protocol for forensic application of the PreCR™ repair mix to multiplex STR amplification of UV-damaged DNA. *Forensic Science International: Genetics*, 2012; 6(4): 498–503.

References

756. Taylor, D. and J.S. Buckleton. Do low template DNA profiles have useful quantitative data? *Forensic Science International: Genetics*, 2015; 16: 13–16.

757. Bright, J.-A., et al. Searching mixed DNA profiles directly against profile databases. *Forensic Science International: Genetics*, 2014; 9: 102–110.

758. Bright, J.-A., J.M. Curran, and J.S. Buckleton. The effect of the uncertainty in the number of contributors to mixed DNA profiles on profile interpretation. *Forensic Science International: Genetics*, 2014; 12: 208–214.

759. Taylor, D., J. Buckleton, and I. Evett. Testing likelihood ratios produced from complex DNA profiles. *Forensic Science International: Genetics*, 2015; 16: 165–171.

760. Coble, M.D. MIX13: An interlaboratory study on the present state of DNA mixture interpretation in the U.S. In *5th Annual Prescription for Criminal Justice Forensics*, Fordham University School of Law, 2014.

761. *Frye v The United States of America, 54 AppDC 46, 293Fed 1013 (1923)*. 1923.

762. Bright, J.-A. and J.M. Curran. Investigation into stutter ratio variability between different laboratories. *Forensic Science International: Genetics*, 2014; 13: 79–81.

763. Bright, J.-A., J.M. Curran, and J.S. Buckleton. Investigation into the performance of different models for predicting stutter. *Forensic Science International: Genetics*, 2013; 7(4): 422–427.

764. Manabe, S., et al. Mixture interpretation: Experimental and simulated reevaluation of qualitative analysis. *Legal Medicine*, 2013; 15: 66–71.

765. Clisson, I., et al. Genetic analysis of human remains from a double inhumation in a frozen kurgan in Kazakhstan (Berel site, early 3rd Century BC). *International Journal of Legal Medicine*, 2002; 116: 304–308.

766. Pusch, C.M., M. Broghammer, and N. Blin. Molecular phylogenetics employing modern and ancient DNA. *Journal of Applied Genetics*, 2003; 44(3): 269–290.

767. Sykes, B. *The Seven Daughters of Eve*. London: Norton; 2001.

768. Sykes, B., et al. The origins of the polynesians: An interpretation from mitochondrial lineage analysis. *American Journal of Human Genetics*, 1995; 57: 1463–1475.

769. Mesa, N.R., et al. Autosomal, mtDNA, and Y chromosome diversity in Amerinds: Pre and post-Columbian patterns of gene flow in South America. *American Journal of Human Genetics*, 2000; 67: 1277–1286.

770. Richards, M.B., et al. Tracing European founder lineages in the near eastern mtDNA pool. *American Journal of Human Genetics*, 2000; 67: 1251–1276.

771. Carvajal-Carmona, L.G., et al. Strong Amerind/white sex bias and a possible Shepardic contribution among the founders of a population in Northwest Colombia. *American Journal of Human Genetics*, 2000; 67: 1287–1295.

772. Macauley, V., et al. The emerging tree of West Eurasian mtDNAs: A synthesis of control-region sequences and RFLPs. *American Journal of Human Genetics*, 1999; 64: 232–249.

773. Bobrowski, A., et al. Non-homogeneous infinite sites model under demographic change: Mathematical description and asymptotic behavior of pairwise distributions. *Mathematical Biosciences*, 2002; 175: 83–115.

774. Adcock, G.J., et al. Mitochondrial DNA sequences in ancient Australians: Implications for modern human origins. *Proceedings of the National Academy of Science of the United States of America*, 2001; 98(2): 537–542.

775. Horstman, M. Maori men and women from different homelands. *News in Science*, 2003.

776. Goodwin, W., A. Linacre, and P. Vanevis. The use of mitochondrial DNA and short tandem repeat typing in the identification of air crash victims. *Electrophoresis*, 1999; 20: 1707–1711.

777. Goodwin, W., G. Curry, and P. Vanezis. Mitochondrial DNA analysis of individuals from a mass grave. *Progress in Forensic Genetics*, 1998; 7: 80–83.

778. Sanger, F., S. Nicklen, and A.R. Coulson. DNA sequencing with chain terminating inhibitors. *Proceedings of the National Academy of Sciences of the United States of America*, 1977; 74: 5463–5467.

779. LaBerge, G.S., R.J. Shelton, and P.B. Danielson. Forensic utility of mitochondrial DNA analysis based on denaturing high-performance liquid chromatography. *Croatian Medical Journal*, 2003; 44(3): 281–288.

780. Bar, W., et al. Guidelines for mitochondrial DNA typing. *Vox Sanguinis*, 2000; 79: 121–125.

781. Warshauer, D.H., et al. Validation of the PLEX-ID™ mass spectrometry mitochondrial DNA assay. *International Journal of Legal Medicine*, 2013; 127(2): 277–286.

782. Eduardoff, M., et al. Mass spectrometric base composition profiling: Implications for forensic mtDNA databasing. *Forensic Science International: Genetics*, 2013; 7(6): 587–592.

783. Holland, M.M. Second generation sequencing allows for mtDNA mixture deconvolution and high resolution detection of heteroplasmy. *Croatian Medical Journal*, 2011; 52(3): 299–313.

784. Parson, W., et al. Evaluation of next generation mtGenome sequencing using the Ion Torrent Personal Genome Machine (PGM). *Forensic Science International: Genetics*, 2013; 7(5): 543–549.

785. Gill, P., et al. Identification of the remains of the Romanov family by DNA analysis. *Nature Genetics*, 1994; 6: 130–135.

786. Ivanov, P.L. Mitochondrial DNA sequence heteroplasmy in the Grand Duke of Russia Georgij Romanov establishes the authenticity of the remains of Tsar Nicholas II. *Nature Genetics*, 1996; 12(4): 417–420.

787. Coble, M.D. Mystery solved: The identification of the two missing Romanov children using DNA analysis. *PLoS One*, 2009; 4(3): e4838.

788. Stoneking, M., et al. Establishing the identity of Anna Anderson Manahan. *Nature Genetics*, 1995; 9: 9–10.

789. Anon. Anastasia and the tools of justice. *Nature Genetics*, 1994; 8(3): 205–206.

790. Lidor, D. *Be All that DNA Can Be*. 2002. Available at: www.wired.com/news/print/0,1294,54631,00.html

791. Stone, A.C., J.E. Starrs, and M. Stoneking. Mitochondrial DNA analysis of the presumptive remains of Jesse James. *Journal of Forensic Sciences*, 2001; 46(1): 173–176.

792. Anslinger, K., et al. Identification of the skeletal remains of Martin Bormann by mtDNA analysis. *International Journal of Legal Medicine*, 2001; 114: 194–196.

793. Holland, M.M. and T.J. Parsons. Mitochondrial DNA sequence analysis—Validation and use for forensic casework. *Forensic Science Review*, 1999; 11(1): 21–50.

794. Aloni, Y. and G. Attardi. Symmetrical in vivo transcription of mitochondrial DNA in HeLa cells. *Proceedings of the National Academy of Science of the United States of America*, 1971; 68: 1757–1761.

795. Murphy, W., et al. Evidence for complete symmetrical transcription in vivo of mitochondrial DNA in HeLa cells. *Journal of Molecular Biology*, 1975; 99: 809–814.

796. Cantatore, P. and G. Attardi. Mapping of nascent light and heavy strand transcripts on the physical map of HeLa cell mitochondrial DNA. *Nucleic Acids Research*, 1980; 8: 2605–2625.

797. Ojala, D., J. Montoya, and G. Attardi. tRNA punctuation model of RNA processing in human mitochondrial DNA. *Nature*, 1981; 99: 470–474.

798. Chang, D.D. and D.A. Clayton. Precise identification of individual promoters for transcription of each strand of human mitochondrial DNA. *Cell*, 1984; 36: 635–643.

799. Hixson, J.E. and D.A. Clayton. Initiation of transcription from each of the two human mitochondrial promoters requires unique nucleotides at the transcriptional start sites. *Proceedings of the National Academy of Sciences of the United States of America*, 1985; 82: 2660–2664.

800. Suzuki, H., et al. Common protein-binding sites in the 5′-flanking regions of human genes for cytochrome c1 and ubiquinone-binding protein. *The Journal of Biological Chemistry*, 1990; 265: 8159–8163.

801. Suzuki, H., et al. Existence of common homologous elements in the transcriptional regulatory regions of human nuclear genes and mitochondrial gene for the oxidative phosphorylation system. *The Journal of Biological Chemistry*, 1991; 266: 2333–2338.

802. Ohno, K., et al. Identification of a possible control element, Mt5, in the major noncoding region of mitochondrial DNA by intraspecific nucleotide conservation. *Biochemistry International*, 1991; 24: 263–272.

803. Fisher, R.P. and D.A. Clayton. A transcription factor required for promoter recognition by human mitochondrial RNA polymerase. *The Journal of Biological Chemistry*, 1985; 260: 11330–11338.

804. Fisher, R.P., J.N. Topper, and J.A. Clayton. Promoter selection in human mitochondria involves binding of a transcription factor to orientation-dependent upstream regulatory elements. *Cell*, 1987; 50: 247–258.

805. Crews, S., et al. Nucleotide sequence of a region of human mitochondrial DNA containing the precisely identified origin of replication. *Nature*, 1979; 277: 192–198.

806. Doda, J.N., C.T. Wright, and D.A. Clayton. Elongation of displacement-loop strands in human and mouse mitochondrial DNA is arrested near specific template sequences. *Proceedings of the National Academy of Sciences of the United States of America*, 1981; 78: 6116–6120.

References

807. Lutz, S., et al. Location and frequency of polymorphic positions in the mtDNA control region of individuals from Germany. *International Journal of Legal Medicine*, 1998; 111: 67–77.
808. Erratum, *International Journal of Legal Medicine*, 1999; 112: 145–150.
809. Bini, C., et al. Different informativeness of the three hypervariable mitochondrial DNA regions in the population of Bologna (Italy). *Forensic Science International*, 2003; 135: 48–52.
810. Tully, G., et al. Considerations of the European DNA Profiling (EDNAP) group on the working practices, nomenclature and interpretation of mitochondrial DNA profiles. *Forensic Science International*, 2001; 124(1): 83–91.
811. Birky, W.C.J. Uniparental inheritance of mitochondrial and chloroplast genes: Mechanisms and evolution. *Proceedings of the American Academy of Sciences of the United States of America*, 1995; 92: 11331–11338.
812. Ankel-Simons, F. and J.M. Cummins. Misconceptions about mitochondria and mammalian fertilization: Implications for theories on human evolution. *Proceedings of the National Academy of Sciences of the United States of America*, 1996; 93: 13859–13863.
813. Shitara, H., et al. Maternal inheritance of mouse mtDNA in interspecific hybrids: Segregation of the leaked paternal mtDNA followed by prevention of subsequent paternal leakage. *Genetics*, 1998; 148: 851–857.
814. Shitara, H., et al. Selective and continuous elimination of mitochondria microinjected into mouse eggs from spermatids, but not from liver cells, occurs throughout embryogenesis. *Genetics*, 2000; 156: 1277–1284.
815. Cummins, J.M., T. Wakayama, and R. Yanagimachi. Fate of microinjected spermatid mitochondria in mouse oocyte and embryo. *Zygote*, 1998; 6: 213–222.
816. Birky, W.C.J. The inheritance of genes in mitochondria and chloroplasts: Laws, mechanisms, and models. *Annual Review of Genetics*, 2001; 35: 125–148.
817. St John, J., et al. Failure of elimination of paternal mitochondrial DNA in abnormal embryos. *The Lancet*, 2000; 355: 200.
818. Houshmand, M., et al. Is paternal mitochondrial DNA transferred to the offspring following intracytoplasmic sperm injection? *Journal of Assisted Reproduction and Genetics*, 1997; 14(4): 223–227.
819. Yoneda, M., et al. Marked replicative advantage of human mtDNA carrying a point mutation that causes the MELAS encephalomyopathy. *Proceedings of the National Academy of Sciences of the United States of America*, 1992; 89: 11164–11168.
820. Schwartz, M. and J. Vissing. Paternal inheritance of mitochondrial DNA. *The New England Journal of Medicine*, 2002; 347(8): 576–580.
821. Bandelt, H.-J., et al. More evidence of non-maternal inheritance of mitochondrial DNA? *Journal of Medical Genetics*, 2005; 42: 957–960.
822. Birky, C.W., Jr. *Annual Review of Genetics*, 1978; 12: 471–512.
823. Birky, C.W., Jr., et al. Mitochondrial transmission genetics: replication, recombination, and segregation of mitochondrial DNA and its inheritance in crosses. In *Mitochondrial Genes*, P. Slonimski, P. Borst, and G. Attardi, Eds. Plainview, NY: Cold Spring Harbor Laboratory Press; 1982; 333–348.
824. Wolfe, K. In *Gene Structure in Eukaryotic Microbes*, J.R. Kinghorn, Ed. Oxford: IRL; 1987; 69–91.
825. Rowlands, R.T. and G. Turner. *Molecular and General Genetics*, 1974; 133: 151–161.
826. Kawano, S., et al. A genetic system controlling mitochondrial fusion in the slime mould, Physarum polycephalum. *Genetics*, 1993; 133(2): 213–224.
827. Awadalla, P., A. Eyre-Walker, and J. Maynard Smith. Linkage disequilibrium and recombination in hominoid mitochondrial DNA. *Science*, 1999; 286: 2524–2525.
828. Parsons, T.J., et al. A high observed substitution rate in the human mitochondrial DNA control region. *Nature Genetics*, 1997; 15: 363–368.
829. Giles, R.E., et al. Maternal inheritance of human mitochondrial DNA. *Proceedings of the National Academy of Sciences of the United States of America*, 1980; 77(11): 6715–6719.
830. Eyre-Walker, A., N.H. Smith, and J.M. Smith. How clonal are human mitochondria? *Proceedings of the Royal Society, London, B*, 1999; 266: 477–483.
831. Parsons, T.J. and J.A. Irwin. Questioning evidence for recombination in human mitochondrial DNA. *Science*, 2000; 288: 1931.
832. Gibbons, A. Calibrating the mitochondrial clock. *Science*, 1998; 279: 28–29.
833. Soares, P., et al. Correcting for purifying selection: An improved human mitochondrial molecular clock. *American Journal of Human Genetics*, 2009; 84: 740–759.

834. von Wurmb-Schwark, N., et al. Mitochondrial mutagenesis in the brain in forensic and pathological research. *Legal Medicine*, 2003; 5: 1–6.

835. Golding, G.B. Estimates of DNA and protein sequence divergence: An examination of some assumptions. *Molecular Biology and Evolution*, 1983; 1: 125–142.

836. Kocher, T.D. and A.C. Wilson. Sequence evolution of mitochondrial DNA in humans and chimpanzees: Control region and protein coding region. In *Evolution of Life: Fossils, Molecules and Culture*, S. Osawa and T. Honjo, Eds. Tokyo: Springer-Verlag; 1991, pp. 391–413.

837. Hasegawa, M., H. Kishino, and T. Yano. Dating of the human-ape splitting by a molecular clock of mitochondrial DNA. *Journal of Molecular Evolution*, 1985; 32: 37–42.

838. Hasegawa, M. and S. Horai. Time of the deepest root for polymorphism in human mitochondrial DNA. *Journal of Molecular Evolution*, 1991; 32: 37–42.

839. Wakeley, J. Substitution rate variation among sites in hypervariable region 1 of human mitochondrial DNA. *Journal of Molecular Evolution*, 1993; 37: 613–623.

840. Wilkinson-Herbots, H.M., et al. Site 73 in hypervariable region II of the human mitochondrial genome and the origin of European populations. *Annuals of Human Genetics*, 1996; 60: 499–508.

841. Excoffier, L. and Z. Yang. Substitution rate variation among sites in the mitochondrial DNA hypervariable region I of humans and chimpanzees. *Molecular Biology and Evolution*, 1999; 16: 1357–1368.

842. Meyer, S., G. Weiss, and A. von Haeseler. Pattern of nucleotide substitution and rate heterogeneity in the hypervariable regions I and II of human mtDNA. *Genetics*, 1999; 152: 1103–1110.

843. Wilson, M.R., et al. A family exhibiting heteroplasmy in the human mitochondrial DNA control region reveals both somatic mosaicism and pronounced segregation of mitotypes. *Human Genetics*, 1997; 100: 167–171.

844. Melton, T. Mitochondrial DNA heteroplasmy. *Forensic Science Reviews*, 2004; 16(1): 1–20.

845. Melton, T., C. Holland, and M. Holland. Forensic mitochondrial DNA analysis: Current practice and future potential. *Forensic Science Reviews*, 2012; 24(2): 101–122.

846. Brandstatter, A. and W. Parson. Mitochondrial DNA heteroplasmy or artefacts—A matter of the amplification strategy? *International Journal of Legal Medicine*, 2003; 117: 180–184.

847. Budowle, B., M.W. Allard, and M.R. Wilson. Critique of interpretation of high levels of heteroplasmy in the human mitochondrial region I from hair. *Forensic Science International*, 2002; 126: 30–33.

848. Budowle, B., M.W. Allard, and M. Wilson. Characterization of heteroplasmy and hypervariable sites in HV1: Critique of D'Eustachio's interpretations. *Forensic Science International*, 2002; 130: 68–70.

849. Stoneking, M. Hypervariable sites in the mtDNA control region are mutational hotspots. *American Journal of Human Genetics*, 2000; 67: 1029–1032.

850. Melton, T., et al. Forensic mitochondrial DNA analysis of 691 casework hairs. *Journal of Forensic Sciences*, 2005; 50(1): 1–8.

851. Calloway, C.D., et al. The frequency of heteroplasmy in the HVII region of mtDNA differs across tissue types and increases with age. *American Journal of Human Genetics*, 2000; 66: 1384–1397.

852. Bai, U., et al. Mitochondrial DNA deletions associated with aging and possibly presbycusis: A human archival temporal bone study. *The American Journal of Otology*, 1997; 18: 449–453.

853. Lagerstorm-Fermer, M., et al. Heteroplasmy of the human mtDNA control region remains constant during life. *American Journal of Human Genetics*, 2001; 68: 1299–1301.

854. Bandelt, H.-J. and W. Parson. Consistent treatment of length variants in the human mtDNA control region: A reappraisal. *International Journal of Legal Medicine*, 2008; 112: 11–21.

855. Anderson, S., et al. Sequence and organization of the human mitochondrial genome. *Nature*, 1981; 290: 457–463.

856. Behar, D.M. et al. A "Copernican" reassessment of the human mitochondrial DNA tree from its root. *The American Journal of Human Genetics*, 2012; 90(4): 675–684.

857. Behar, D.M. et al. A "Copernican" reassessment of the human mitochondrial DNA tree from its root. *The American Journal of Human Genetics*, 2012; 90(4): 675–684.

858. Malyarchuk, B.A. Improving the reconstructed sapiens reference sequence of mitochondrial DNA. *Forensic Science International: Genetics*, 2013; 7(3): e74–e75.

859. Salas, A., et al. A cautionary note on switching mitochondrial DNA reference sequences in forensic genetics. *Forensic Science International: Genetics*, 2012; 6(6): e182–e184.

860. Ohno, S. *Sex Chromosomes and the Sex Linked Genes*. Berlin: Springer; 1967.

861. Skaletsky, H., et al. The male specific region of the human Y chromosome is a mosaic of discrete sequence classes. *Nature*, 2003; 423: 825–837.

References

862. Rozen, S., et al. Abundant gene conversion between arms of palindromes in human and ape Y-chromosomes. *Nature*, 2003; 423: 873–876.
863. Quintana-Murci, L., C. Krausz, and K. McElreavey. The human Y chromosome: Function, evolution and disease. *Forensic Science International*, 2001; 118: 169–181.
864. Lange, J., et al. Intrachromosomal homologous recombination between inverted amplicons on opposing Y-chromosome arms. *Genomics*, 2013; 102(4): 257–264.
865. Tyler-Smith, C. and G. McVean. The comings and goings of a Y polymorphism. *Nature Genetics*, 2003; 35(3): 201–202.
866. Repping, S., et al. Polymorphism for a 1.6-Mb deletion of the human Y chromosome persists through balance between recurrent mutation and haploid selection. *Nature Genetics*, 2003; 35(3): 247–251.
867. Saxena, R., et al. Four DAZ genes in two clusters found in AZFc region of human Y chromosome. *Genomics*, 2000; 67: 256–267.
868. Tilford, C., et al. A physical map of the human Y chromosome. *Nature*, 2001; 409: 943–945.
869. Jobling, M.A. The Y chromosome as a forensic tool: Progress and prospects for the new millennium. In *First International Conference on Forensic Human Identification in the Millennium*, London, 1999.
870. Roewer, L., et al. Simple repeat sequences on the human Y chromosome are equally polymorphic as their autosomal counterparts. *Human Genetics*, 1992; 89: 389–394.
871. Butler, J.M., et al. A novel multiplex for simultaneous amplification of 20 Y chromosome STR markers. *Forensic Science International*, 2002; 129: 10–24.
872. Betz, A., et al. DYS STR analysis with epithelial cells in a rape case. *Forensic Science International*, 2001; 118: 126–130.
873. Henke, J., et al. Application of Y-chromosomal STR haplotypes to forensic genetics. *Croatian Medical Journal*, 2001; 42(3): 292–297.
874. Honda, K., L. Roewer, and P. De Kniff. Male DNA typing from 25-year-old vaginal swabs using Y-chromosome STR polymorphisms in a retrial request case. *Journal of Forensic Sciences*, 1999; 44(4): 868–872.
875. Jobling, M.A., A. Pandya, and C. Tyler-Smith. The Y chromosome in forensic analysis and paternity testing. *International Journal of Legal Medicine*, 1997; 110: 118–124.
876. Kayser, M. and A. Sajantila. Mutations at Y-STR loci: Implications for paternity testing and forensic analysis. *Forensic Science International*, 2001; 118: 116–121.
877. Sibille, I., et al. Y-STR DNA amplification as biological evidence in sexually assaulted female victims with no cytological detection of spermatozoa. *Forensic Science International*, 2002; 125: 212–216.
878. Klintschar, M., et al. Persisting fetal microchimerism does not interfere with forensic Y-chromosome typing. *Forensic Science International*, 2004; 139: 151–154.
879. Kayser, M., et al. Evaluation of Y chromosomal STRs: A multicentre study. *International Journal of Legal Medicine*, 1997; 110: 125–133.
880. Ge, J., et al. US forensic Y-chromosome short tandem repeats database. *Legal Medicine*, 2010; 12: 289–295.
881. Roewer, L., et al. Online reference database of European Y-chromosomal short tandem repeat (STR) haplotypes. *Forensic Science International*, 2001; 118: 106–113.
882. Willuweit, S. and L. Roewer. Y chromosome haplotype reference database (YHRD): Update. *Forensic Science International: Genetics*, 2007; 1(2): 83–87.
883. White, P.S., et al. New, male-specific microsatellite markers from the human Y-chromosome. *Genomics*, 1999; 57: 433–437.
884. Redd, A.J., et al. Forensic value of 14 novel STRs on the human Y chromosome. *Forensic Science International*, 2002; 130: 97–111.
885. Iida, R., et al. Characterization and haplotype analysis of the polymorphic Y-STRs, DYS443, DYS444 and DYS445 in a Japanese population. *International Journal of Legal Medicine*, 2002; 116: 191–194.
886. Bosch, E., et al. High resolution Y chromosome typing: 19 STRs amplified in three multiplex reactions. *Forensic Science International*, 2002; 125: 42–51.
887. Berger, B., et al. Molecular characterization and Austrian Caucasian population data of the multi copy Y-chromosome STR DYS464. *Forensic Science International*, 2003; 137: 221–230.
888. Sinha, S.K., et al. Development and validation of a multiplexed Y-chromosome STR genotyping system, Y-PLEX™ 6, for forensic casework. *Journal of Forensic Sciences*, 2003; 48(1): 93–103.
889. Shewale, J.G., et al. Y-chromosome STR System, Y-PLEX™ 12, for forensic casework: Development and validation. *Journal Forensic Sciences*, 2004; 49(6): 1–13.

890. Krenke, B.E., et al. Validation of a male-specific, 12-locus fluorescent short tandem repeat (STR) multiplex. *Forensic Science International*, 2005; 148(1): 1–14.

891. Mulero, J.J., et al. Development and validation of the AmpFlSTR Yfiler PCR amplification kit: A male specific, single amplification 17 Y-STR multiplex system. *Journal of Forensic Science*, 2006; 51(1): 64–75.

892. Roewer, L. Y Chromosome STR typing in crime casework. *Forensic Science, Medicine, and Pathology*, 2009; 5: 77–84.

893. Gusmao, L., et al. Alternative primers for DYS391 typing: Advantages of their application to forensic genetics. *Forensic Science International*, 2000; 112: 49–57.

894. Kuroki, H., et al. Spermatogenic ability is different among males in different Y chromosome lineage. *Journal of Human Genetics*, 1999; 44: 289–292.

895. Foster, E.A., et al. Jefferson fathered slave's last child. *Nature*, 1998; 396: 27–29.

896. Jobling, M. In the name of the father: Surnames and genetics. *Trends in Genetics*, 2001; 17: 353–357.

897. Paracchini, S., et al. Hierarchical high-throughput SNP genotyping of the human Y chromosome using MALDI-TOF mass spectrometry. *Nucleic Acids Research*, 2002; 30(6): e27.

898. Capelli, C., et al. A Y chromosome census of the British Isles. *Current Biology*, 2003; 13(11): 979–984.

899. Schneider, P.M., et al. Tandem repeat structure of the duplicated Y chromosomal STR locus DYS385 and frequency studies in the German and three Asian populations. *Forensic Science International*, 1998; 97: 61–70.

900. Caglia, A., et al. Increased forensic efficiency of a STR based Y specific haplotype by addition of the highly polymorphic DYS385 locus. *International Journal of Legal Medicine*, 1998; 111: 142–146.

901. Shepherd, C., J. Vintiner, and S. Harbison. Y STR haplotype data for New Zealand population groups using the Y-Plex™ 6 kit. *Forensic Science International*, 2004; 145(1): 69–72.

902. Ballantyne, K.N., et al. A new future of forensic Y-chromosome analysis: Rapidly mutating Y-STRs for differentiating male relatives and paternal lineages. *Forensic Science International: Genetics*, 2012; 6(2): 208–218.

903. Ballantyne, K.N., et al. Mutability of Y-chromosomal microsatellites: Rates, characteristics, molecular bases, and forensic implications. *The American Journal of Human Genetics*, 2010; 87(3): 341–353.

904. Pinto, N., L. Gusmão, and A. Amorim. Mutation and mutation rates at Y chromosome specific Short Tandem Repeat Polymorphisms (STRs): A reappraisal. *Forensic Science International: Genetics*, 2014; 9: 20–4.

905. Andersen, M.M., et al. Estimating stutter rates for Y-STR alleles. *Forensic Science International: Genetics Supplement Series*, 2011; 3(1): e192–e193.

906. Bright, J.-A., J. Curran, and J. Buckleton. Modelling PowerPlex® Y stutter and artefacts. *Forensic Science International: Genetics*, 2014; 11: 126–136.

907. Butler, J.M. Short Tandem Repeat (STR) loci and kits. In *Advanced Topics in Forensic DNA Typing*, J.M. Butler, Ed. San Diego, CA: Academic Press; 2012, pp. 99–139.

908. Butler, J.M., et al. Chromosomal duplications along the Y-chromosome and their potential impact on Y-STR interpretation. *Journal of Forensic Sciences*, 2005; 50(4): 853–859.

909. Kayser, M., et al. Melanesian and Asian origins of Polynesians: mtDNA and Y chromosome gradients across the Pacific. *Molecular Biology and Evolution*, 2006; 23(11): 2234–2244.

910. Promega. *Technical Manual: PowerPlex Y System*. Promega; 2012.

911. Sullivan, K.M.A.-G., et al. A single difference in mtDNA control region sequence observed between hair shaft and reference samples from a single donor. In *Proceedings from the Seventh International Symposium on Human Identification, Promega Corporation*, Scottsdale, AZ, 1996.

912. Hühne, J., H. Pfeiffer, and B. Brinkmann. Heteroplasmic substitutions in the mitochondrial DNA control region in mother and child samples. *International Journal of Legal Medicine*, 1999; 112: 27–30.

913. Siguroardottir, S., et al. The mutation rate in the human mtDNA control region. *American Journal of Human Genetics*, 2000; 66: 1599–1609.

914. Hühne, J., et al. Mitochondrial DNA in human hair shafts—Evidence of intra-individual differences? *International Journal of Legal Medicine*, 1999; 112: 172–175.

915. Tully, L.A., et al. A sensitive denaturing gradient-gel electrophoresis assay reveals a high frequency of heteroplasmy in hypervariable region 1 of the human mitochondrial DNA control region. *American Journal of Human Genetics*, 2000; 67: 432–443.

References

916. Scientific Working Group on DNA Analysis Methods (SWGDAM). *Guidelines for Mitochondrial DNA Analysis by Forensic DNA Testing Laboratories.* SWGDAM; 2013.

917. Scientific Working Group on DNA Analysis Methods (SWGDAM). Y-chromosome short tandem repeat (Y-STR) interpretation guidelines. *Forensic Science Communications,* 2009; 11(1).

918. Carracedo, A., et al. DNA commission of the international society for forensic genetics: Guidelines for mitochondrial DNA typing. *Forensic Science International,* 2000; 110(2): 79–85.

919. Scientific Working Group on DNA Analysis Methods (SWGDAM). *Interpretation Guidelines for Y-Chromosome STR Typing.* 2014. Available at: http://swgdam.org/SWGDAM_YSTR_Guidelines_APPROVED_01092014_v_02112014_FINAL.pdf

920. Parson, W., et al. DNA Commission of the International Society for Forensic Genetics: Revised and extended guidelines for mitochondrial DNA typing. *Forensic Science International: Genetics,* 2014; 13: 134–142.

921. Andersen, M.M., et al. Estimating trace-suspect match probabilities for singleton Y-STR haplotypes using coalescent theory. *Forensic Science International: Genetics,* 2013; 7(2): 264–271.

922. Andersen, M.M., et al. Identifying the most likely contributors to a Y-STR mixture using the discrete Laplace method. *Forensic Science International: Genetics,* 2015; 15: 76–83.

923. Andersen, M.M., P.S. Eriksen, and N. Morling. The discrete Laplace exponential family and estimation of Y-STR haplotype frequencies. *Journal of Theoretical Biology,* 2013; 329: 39–51.

924. Andersen, M.M., P.S. Eriksen, and N. Morling. Cluster analysis of European Y-chromosomal STR haplotypes using the discrete Laplace method. *Forensic Science International: Genetics,* 2014; 11: 182–194.

925. Andersen, M.M., P.S. Eriksen, and N. Morling. Corrigendum to "The discrete Laplace exponential family and estimation of Y-STR haplotype frequencies" [*J. Theor. Biol.* 329 (2013) 39–51]. *Journal of Theoretical Biology,* 2014; 350: 110.

926. Laplace, P.S. Mémoire sur la probabilité des causes par les évènmens. *Mémoires de l'Académie Royale des Sciences Presentés par Divers Savans,* 1774; 6: 621–656.

927. Todhunter, I. *A History of the Mathematical Theory of Probability from the Time of Pascal to that of Laplace—Reprinted 1949.* New York: Chelsea; 1865.

928. Andersen, M.M., P.S. Eriksen, and N. Morling. *A gentle introduction to the discrete Laplace method for estimating Y-STR haplotype frequencies.* arXiv:1304.2129 [stat.AP] 2013.

929. Andersen, M.M., et al. Identifying the most likely contributors to a Y-STR mixture using the discrete Laplace method. *Forensic Science International: Genetics,* 2015; 15: 76–83.

930. Andersen, M.M., et al. Identifying the most likely contributors to a Y-STR mixture using the discrete Laplace method. *Forensic Science International: Genetics,* 2015; 15: 76–83.

931. Kingman, J.F.C. The coalescent. *Stochastic Processes and their Applications,* 1982; 13(3): 235–248.

932. Wilson, I.J., M.E. Weale, and D.J. Balding. Inferences from DNA data: Population histories, evolutionary processes and forensic match probabilities. *Journal of the Royal Statistical Society: Series A,* 2003; 166(2): 155–188.

933. Roewer, L., et al. Signature of recent historical events in the European Y-chromosomal STR haplotype distribution. *Human Genetics,* 2005; 116(4): 279–291.

934. Clopper, C.J. and E.S. Pearson. The use of confidence or fiducial intervals illustrated in the case of the binomial. *Biometrika,* 1934; 26: 404–413.

935. Ivanov, P.L. Mitochondrial DNA sequence heteroplasmy in the Grand Duke of Russia Georgij Romanov establishes the authenticity of the remains of Tsar Nicholas II. *Nature Genetics,* 1996; 12(4): 417–420.

936. *Aytugrul v The Queen [2012] HCA 15.* S315/2011. 2012.

937. Taylor, D.A., et al. Knowing your DNA database: Issues with determining ancestral Y haplotypes in a Y-filer database. *Forensic Science International: Genetics Supplement Series,* 2009; 2(1): 411–412.

938. Bodner, M., et al. Inspecting close maternal relatedness: Towards better mtDNA population samples in forensic databases. *Forensic Science International: Genetics,* 2011; 5(2): 138–141.

939. Zimmermann, B., et al. Application of a west Eurasian-specific filter for quasi-median network analysis: Sharpening the blade for mtDNA error detection. *Forensic Science International: Genetics,* 2011; 5(2): 133–137.

940. Ge, J., B. Budowle, and R. Chakraborty. Interpreting Y chromosome STR haplotype mixture. *Legal Medicine,* 2010; 12(3): 137–143.

941. Ge, J., et al. Erratum. *Journal of Forensic Sciences,* 2012; 57(1).

942. Prinz, M., et al. Validation and casework application of a Y chromosome specific STR multiplex. *Forensic Science International,* 2001; 120: 177–188.

943. Sinha, S.K., et al. Development and Validation of the Y-PlexTM 5, a Y chromosome STR genotyping system for forensic casework. *Journal of Forensic Science*, 2003; 48: 985–1000.

944. Ge, J., B. Budowle, and R. Chakraborty. Comments on "Interpreting Y chromosome STR haplotype mixture." *Legal Medicine*, 2011; 13(1): 52–53.

945. Walsh, B., A.J. Redd, and M.F. Hammer. Joint match probabilities for Y chromosomal and autosomal markers. *Forensic Science International*, 2008; 174(2–3): 234–238.

946. Gjertson, D.W., et al. ISFG: Recommendations on biostatistics in paternity testing. *Forensic Science International: Genetics*, 2007; 1(3–4): 223–231.

947. Amorim, A. A cautionary note on the evaluation of genetic evidence from uniparentally transmitted markers. *Forensic Science International: Genetics*, 2008; 2(4): 376–8.

948. Buckleton, J. and S. Myers. Combining autosomal and Y chromosome match probabilities using coalescent theory. *Forensic Science International: Genetics*, 2014; 11: 52–55.

949. US Central Intelligence Agency, *The World Factbook*. New Zealand and United States estimates: 2.06 children born/woman. Available at: https://www.cia.gov/library/publicaqtions/the-world-factbook/fields/2127.html

950. Kreider, R.M. and J.M. Fields. Children's coresidence with half siblings, U.S. Census Bureau, Annual Meeting of the Population Association of America, Dallas, TX, April 15–17, 2010. Available at: http://www.census.gov/hhes/socdemo/children/data/sipp/children_coresidence-Halfsibsposter.pdf

951. Szibor, R., et al. Use of X-linked markers for forensic purposes. *International Journal of Legal Medicine*, 2003; 117: 67–74.

952. Lyon, M.F. Gene action in the X-chromosome of the mouse (*Mus musculus L.*). *Nature*, 1961; 190: 372–373.

953. Pinto N, Silva PV, Amorim A. A general method to assess the utility of the X-chromosomal markers in kinship testing. *Forensic Sci Int Genet*. 2012 Mar; 6(2): 198–207.

954. Morling, N. and A. Carracedo. International recommendations for paternity testing standards. *Forensic Science International*, 2002; 129: 147.

955. Thomson, J.A., et al. Analysis of disputed single-parent/child and sibling relationships using 16 STR loci. *International Journal of Legal Medicine*, 2001; 115: 128–134.

956. Whittle, M.R., E.C. Favaro, and D.R. Sumita. Paternity investigation experience with a 40 autosomal SNP panel. *Forensic Science International: Genetics Supplement Series*, 2009; 2: 149–150.

957. Johnson, D.J., et al. Isolation and individualization of conceptus and maternal tissues from abortions and placentas for parentage testing in cases of rape and abandoned newborns. *Journal of Forensic Sciences*, 2010; 55(6): 1430–1436.

958. Roberts, H.F.q.i.F., R.A. *Experiments in Plant Hybridisation*. London: Oliver & Boyd; 1965.

959. Walker, R.H., et al., Eds. *Inclusion Probabilities in Parentage Testing*. Arlington, VA: American Association of Blood Banks; 1983.

960. Robertson, B. and G.A. Vignaux. Unhelpful evidence in paternity cases. *New Zealand Law Journal*, 1992; 9: 315–317.

961. Fung, W.K., Y.K. Chung, and D.M. Wong. Power of exclusion revisited: Probability of excluding relatives of the true father from paternity. *International Journal of Legal Medicine*, 2002; 116: 64–67.

962. Morling, N., et al. Paternity testing commission of the International Society of Forensic Genetics: Recommendations on genetic investigations in paternity cases. *Forensic Science International*, 2002; 129: 148–157.

963. Poulsen, L., et al. A report of the 2009–2011 paternity and relationship testing workshops of the English Speaking Working Group of the International Society For Forensic Genetics. *Forensic Science International: Genetics*, 2014; 9: e1–e2.

964. Thomsen, A.R., et al. A report of the 2002–2008 paternity testing workshops of the English speaking working group of the International Society for Forensic Genetics. *Forensic Science International: Genetics*, 2009; 3(4): 214–221.

965. Hallenberg, C. and N. Morling. A report on the 2000 and 2001 paternity testing workshops of the English speaking working group of the international society for forensic genetics. *Forensic Science International*, 2002; 129: 43–50.

966. Lee, H.-S., et al. Motherless case in paternity testing. *Forensic Science International*, 2000; 114: 57–65.

967. Bacher, J.W., et al. Chromosome localization of CODIS loci and new pentanucleotide repeat loci. In *10th Promega International Symposium on Human ID*, 2000.

References

968. Rolf, B., et al. Paternity testing using Y-STR haplotypes: Assigning a probability for paternity in cases of mutations. *International Journal of Legal Medicine*, 2001; 115: 12–15.

969. Ayres, K.L. Relatedness testing in subdivided populations. *Forensic Science International*, 2000; 114: 107–115.

970. Drábek, J. Validation of software for calculating the likelihood ratio for parentage and kinship. *Forensic Science International: Genetics*, 2009; 3(2): 112–118.

971. Drábek, J. Use of animal/plant freeware for calculating likelihood ratio for paternity and kinship in complicated human pedigrees. *Forensic Science International: Genetics Supplement Series*, 2009; 2: 469–471.

972. Berry, D.A. and S. Geisser. Inference in cases if disputed paternity. In *Statistics and the Law*, M.H. DeGroot, S.E. Fienberg, and J.B. Kadane, Eds. New York: Wiley; 1986, pp. 353–382.

973. Crow, J.F. There's something curious about paternal-age effects. *Science*, 2003; 301: 606–607.

974. Walsh, P.S., N.J. Fildes, and R. Reynolds. Sequence analysis and characterization of stutter products at the tetranucleotide repeat locus vWA. *Nucleic Acids Research*, 1996; 24: 2807–2812.

975. Xu, X., et al. The direction of microsatellite mutations is dependent upon allele length. *Nature Genetics*, 2000; 24: 396–399.

976. Brinkmann, B., et al. Mutation rate in human microsatellites: Influence of the structure and length of the tandem repeat. *American Journal of Human Genetics*, 1998; 62: 1408–1415.

977. Jeffreys, A.J., et al. Complex gene conversion events in germline mutation at human minisatellites. *Nature Genetics*, 1994; 6: 136–145.

978. Rubinsztein, D.C., et al. Mutational bias provides a model for the evolution of Huntington's disease and predicts a general increase in disease prevalence. *Nature Genetics*, 1994; 7: 525–530.

979. Rubinsztein, D.C., et al. Microsatellite evolution-evidence for directionality and variation in rate between species. *Nature Genetics*, 1995; 10: 337–343.

980. Jeffreys, A.J., et al. Mutation processes at human minisatellites. *Electrophoresis*, 1995; 16: 1577–1585.

981. Kayser, M., et al. Characteristics and frequency of germline mutations at microsatellite loci from human Y chromosome, as revealed by direct observation in father/son pairs. *American Journal of Human Genetics*, 2000; 66: 1580–1588.

982. Primmer, C.R., et al. Unravelling the processes of microsatellite evolution through analysis of germline mutations in barn swallows *Hirundo rustica*. *Molecular Biology and Evolution*, 1998; 15: 1047–1054.

983. Cooper, G., et al. Markov chain Monte Carlo analysis of human Y chromosome microsatellite provides evidence of biased mutation. *Proceedings of the National Academy of Sciences of the United States of America*, 1999; 96: 11916–11921.

984. Ellegren, H. Heterogeneous mutation processes in human microsatellite DNA sequences. *Nature Genetics*, 2000; 24: 400–402.

985. Primmer, C., et al. Directional evolution in germline microsatellite mutations. *Nature Genetics*, 1996; 13: 391–393.

986. Huang, Q.-Y., et al. Mutation patterns at dinucleotide microsatellite loci in humans. *American Journal of Human Genetics*, 2002; 70: 625–634.

987. Sajantila, A., M. Lukka, and A. Syvanen. Experimentally observed germline mutations at human micro- and minisatellite loci. *European Journal of Human Genetics*, 1999; 7: 263–266.

988. Kimpton, C., et al. Evaluation of an automated DNA profiling system employing multiplex amplification of four tetrameric STR loci. *International Journal of Legal Medicine*, 1994; 106: 302–311.

989. Wierdl, M., M. Dominska, and T.D. Petes. Microsatellite instability in yeast: Dependence on the length of the microsatellite. *Genetics*, 1997; 146: 769–779.

990. Ellegren, H. Microsatellite mutations in the germline: Implications for evolutionary inference. *Trends in Genetics*, 2000; 16: 551–558.

991. Schlotterer, C., et al. High mutation rates of a long microsatellite allele in *Drosophila melanogaster* provides evidence for allele-specific mutation rates. *Molecular Biology and Evolution*, 1998; 15: 1269–1274.

992. Harr, B. and C. Schlotterer. Long microsatellite alleles in *Drosophila melanogaster* have a downward bias and short persistence times, which cause their genomewide underrepresentation. *Genetics*, 2000; 155: 1213–1220.

993. Crow, J.F. A new study challenges the current belief of a high human male: Female mutation ratio. *Trends in Genetics*, 2000; 16(12): 525–526.

994. National Association of Testing Authorities Australia. *ISO/IEC 17025 Application Document Supplementary Requirements for Accreditation in the Field of Forensic Science.* National Association of Testing Authorities Australia; 2000.

995. Pearman, C., Personal communication, 2002.

996. Dawid, A.P., J. Mortera, and V.L. Pascali. Non-fatherhood or mutation? A probabilistic approach to parental exclusion in paternity testing. *Forensic Science International*, 2001; 124(1): 55–61.

997. Ayres, K.L. Paternal exclusion in the presence of substructure. *Forensic Science International*, 2002; 129: 142–144.

998. Clayton, T., Personal communication. 2003.

999. Amorim, A. and J. Carneiro. The impact of silent alleles in kinship probability calculations. *Forensic Science International: Genetics Supplement Series*, 2008; 1(1): 638–639.

1000. Brenner, C.H. Multiple mutations, covert mutations and false exclusions in paternity casework. *International Congress Series*, 2004; 1261: 112–114.

1001. Weber, J.L. and C. Wong. Mutation of human short tandem repeats. *Human Molecular Genetics*, 1993; 2: 1123–1128.

1002. Rolf, B., P. Wiegand, and B. Brinkmann. Somatic mutations at STR loci—A reason for three allele patterns and mosaicism. *Forensic Science International*, 2002; 126: 200–202.

1003. Nutini, A.L., et al. Double incompatibility at human alpha fibrinogen and pents E loci in paternity testing. *Croatian Medical Journal*, 2003; 44(3): 342–346.

1004. Chakraborty, R. and D.N. Stivers. Paternity exclusion by DNA markers: Effects of paternal mutations. *Journal of Forensic Sciences*, 1996; 41(4): 671–677.

1005. Williams, E.D. and J.D. Crews. From dust to dust: Ethical and practical issues involved in the location, exhumation, and identification of bodies from mass graves. *Croatian Medical Journal*, 2003; 44(3): 251–258.

1006. Geneva Convention. 1949. p. Articles 130 and 136.

1007. Ferllini, R. The development of human rights investigations since 1945. *Science & Justice*, 2003; 43(4): 219–224.

1008. Ganswindt, M., et al. Bone finds: A challenge to forensic science. *Legal Medicine*, 2003; 5: 382–385.

1009. Skinner, M., D. Alempijevic, and M. Djuric-Srejic. Guidelines for international bio-archaelogy monitors of mass grave exhumations. *Forensic Science International*, 2003; 134(2–3): 81–92.

1010. Cox, M. A multidisciplinary approach to the investigation of crimes against humanity, war crimes and genocide: The Inforce Foundation. *Science & Justice*, 2003; 43(4): 225–227.

1011. Duhig, C. Non-forensic remains: The use of forensic archaeology, anthropology and burial taphonomy. *Science & Justice*, 2003; 43(4): 211–214.

1012. Gabriel, M.N., et al. Identification of human remains by immobilized sequence-specific oligonucleotide probe analysis of mtDNA hypervariable regions I and II. *Croatian Medical Journal*, 2003; 44(3): 293–298.

1013. Clayton, T.M., J.P. Whitaker, and C.N. Maguire. Identification of bodies from the scene of a mass disaster using DNA amplification of short tandem repeat (STR) loci. *Forensic Science International*, 1995; 76(1): 7–15.

1014. Minaguchi, K., et al. DNA analysis of neonatal human remains wrapped and kept in a vinyl bag for 15 years. *Legal Medicine*, 2003; 5: 183–186.

1015. Budimlija, Z.M., et al. World Trade Center human identification project: Experiences with individual body identification cases. *Croatian Medical Journal*, 2003; 44(3): 259–263.

1016. Takayama, T., et al. Quality and quantity of DNA in cadavers' serum. *Legal Medicine*, 2003; 5: 180–182.

1017. Barbaro, A., G. Falcone, and A. Barbaro. DNA typing from hair shaft. *Progress in Forensic Genetics*, 2000; 8: 523–525.

1018. Butler, J.M., Y. Shen, and B.R. McCord. The development of reduced size STR amplicons as tools for analysis of degraded DNA. *Journal of Forensic Sciences*, 2003; 48(5): 1054–1064.

1019. Smith, B.C., et al. A systematic approach to the sampling of dental DNA. *Journal of Forensic Sciences*, 1993; 38(5): 1194–1209.

1020. Malaver, P.C. and J.J. Yunis. Different dental tissues as a source of DNA for human identification in forensic cases. *Croatian Medical Journal*, 2003; 44(3): 306–309.

1021. Tahir, M.A. and N. Watson. Typing using DNA HLA-DQα alleles extracted from human nail material using polymerase chain reaction. *Journal of Forensic Sciences*, 1995; 40(4): 634–636.

References

1022. Uchida, S., et al. Utility of fingernail DNA for evaluation of chimerism after bone marrow transplantation and for diagnostic testing for transfusion-associated graft-versus-host disease. *Blood*, 1996; 87: 4015–4016.

1023. Fisher, D.L., et al. Extraction, evaluation, and amplification of DNA from decalcified and undecalcified United States Civil War bone. *Journal of Forensic Sciences*, 1993; 38(1): 60–68.

1024. Holland, M.M., et al. Development of a quality, high throughput DNA analysis procedure for skeletal samples to assist with the identification of victims from the World Trade Center attacks. *Croatian Medical Journal*, 2003; 44(3): 264–272.

1025. Evison, M.P., D.A. Smillie, and A.T. Chamberlain. Extraction of single-copy nuclear DNA from forensic specimens with a variety of postmortem histories. *Journal of Forensic Sciences*, 1997; 46(6): 1032–1038.

1026. Imaizumi, K., et al. The effects of decalcification and glass beads treatment on DNA typings from bone samples. *Reports-National Research Institute of Police Science: Research on Forensic Science*, 1998; 51: 19–28.

1027. Nakanishi, A., F. Moriya, and Y. Hashimoto. Effects of environmental conditions to which nails are exposed on DNA analysis of them. *Legal Medicine*, 2003; 5: 194–197.

1028. Meyer, H.J. The Kaprun cable car disaster—Aspects of forensic organisation following a mass fatality with 155 victims. *Forensic Science International*, 2003; 138: 1–7.

1029. Chakraborty, R. and L. Jin. Determination of relatedness between individuals using DNA fingerprinting. *Human Biology*, 1993; 65(6): 875–895.

1030. Ehm, M.G. and M. Wagner. A test statistic to detect errors in sib-pair relationships. *American Journal of Human Genetics*, 1998; 62: 181–188.

1031. Presciuttini, S., et al. Allele sharing in first-degree and unrelated pairs of individuals in the Ge.F.I. AmpFlSTR Profiler Plus™ database. *Forensic Science International*, 2003; 131: 85–89.

1032. Cockerham, C.C. Higher order probability functions of alleles by descent. *Genetics*, 1971; 69: 235–247.

1033. Hilden, J. GENEX – An algebraic approach to pedigree probability calculus. *Clinical Genetics*, 1970; 1: 319–348.

1034. Nadot, R. and G. Vayssex. Appartment et identite. Algorithme du calcul des coefficients d'identite. *Biometrics*, 1973; 29: 347–359.

1035. Fung, W.K., A. Carracedo, and Y.-Q. Hu. Testing for kinship in a subdivided population. *Forensic Science International*, 2003; 135: 105–109.

1036. Dawid, A.P., et al. Probabilistic expert systems for forensic inference from genetic markers. *Scandinavian Journal of Statistics*, 2002; 29: 577–595.

1037. Hugin. Available at: www.hugin.com

1038. GeNIe. Available at: www2.sis.pitt.edu/~genie

1039. XBAIES. Available at: www.staff.city.ac.uk/~rgc

1040. Brenner, C., Personal communication, 2003.

1041. Clayton, T. The WACO disaster, USA 1993. *Contact*, 1997; 25: 14–16.

1042. Ballantyne, J. Mass disaster genetics. *Nature Genetics*, 1997; 15: 329–331.

1043. Brenner, C. and B.S. Weir. Issues and strategies in the DNA identification of World Trade Center victims. *Theoretical Population Biology*, 2003; 63: 173–178.

1044. Vastag, B. Out of tragedy, identification innovation. *Journal of the American Medical Association*, 2002; 288: 1221–1223.

1045. Olaisen, B., M. Stenersen, and B. Mevag. Identification by DNA analysis of the victims of the August 1996 Spitsbergen civil aircraft disaster. *Nature Genetics*, 1997; 15: 402–405.

1046. Leclair, B., et al. Enhanced kinship analysis and STR-based DNA typing for human identification in mass disasters. In *Progress in Forensic Genetics 8*, G.F. Sensabaugh, P.J. Lincoln, and B. Olaisen, Eds. Elsevier Science B.V.; 2000, pp. 91–93.

1047. Egeland, T. and P.F. Mostad. Statistical genetics and genetical statistics: A forensic perspective. *Scandinavian Journal of Statistics*, 2002; 29: 297–308.

1048. Egeland, T., P.F. Mostad, and B. Olaisen. A computerized method for calculating the probability of pedigrees from genetic data. *Science & Justice*, 1997; 37(4): 269–274.

1049. Egeland, T., et al. Beyond traditional paternity and identification cases. Selecting the most probable pedigree. *Forensic Science International*, 2000; 110: 47–59.

1050. Cowell, R.G. and P.F. Mostad. A clustering algorithm using DNA marker information for sub-pedigree reconstruction. *Journal of Forensic Sciences*, 2003; 48(6): 1239–1248.

1051. Aulinskas, T.H., et al. No-suspect forensic casework: A one in five hit rate! In *Eleventh International Symposium on Human Identification*, Biloxi, MS, 2000.
1052. Coffman, D. Florida Department of Law Enforcement's convicted offender DNA database: Transition from RFLP to STR. In *Ninth International Symposium on Human Identification*, Promega Corporation, Madison, WI, 1998.
1053. Morrison, R. Databasing efforts in Alabama—Past and present. In *Tenth International Symposium on Human Identification*, Promega Corporation, Madison, WI, 1999.
1054. Hindmarsh, R. and B. Barbara Prainsack, Eds. *Genetic Suspects: Global Governance of Forensic DNA Profiling and Databasing.* Cambridge University Press; 2010.
1055. Werrett, D.J. and K. Sullivan. The national DNA database of England and Wales and the strategic use of DNA profiling. In *The First International Conference on Forensic Human Identification in the Millennium*, London, 1999.
1056. Werrett, D.J. and R.L. Sparkes. 300 matches per week—The effectiveness and future development of DNA intelligence databases—Parts 1 and 2. In *Ninth International Symposium on Human Identification*, Promega Corporation, Madison, WI, 1998.
1057. *Commonwealth of Virginia v Spencer*, 1989.
1058. Anonymous. DNA cold search execution. *Law & Order*, 2002; 50: 6.
1059. INTERPOL, *INTERPOL CHARTER—International DNA Gateway. Implementing Rules for the Interpol DNA Database.* 2005.
1060. Walsh, S.J., et al. The collation of forensic DNA case data into a multi-dimensional intelligence database. *Science & Justice*, 2002; 42(4): 205–214.
1061. Blakey, D. Under the microscope refocused. A revisit to the thematic inspection report on scientific and technical support. 2002. Available at: www.homeoffice.gov.uk/hmic/microscope
1062. Blakey, D. Under the microscope: Thematic inspection report on scientific and technical support. 2000. Available at: www.homeoffice.gov.uk
1063. Allman, D.S. and C.A. Pounds. Central Research and Support Establishment. *The Specificity of Diaminobenzidine for the Detection of Blood.* 1992.
1064. Asplen, C. and S.A. Lane. Considerations in the development of DNA databases. *Interfaces*, 2003; 36: 1–2.
1065. Hopwood, A., Personal communication: Masterclass lecture. 2003.
1066. Wasik, M. Legislating in the shadow of the human rights act: The criminal justice and police act 2001. *Criminal Law Journal*, 2001: 931–947.
1067. Attorney-general's reference (No. 3 of 1999) [2000] 2 Cr. App. R. 416 and [2001] 2 Cr. App. R. 475 (HL).
1068. Levitt, M. Forensic databases: Benefits and ethical and social costs. *British Medical Bulletin*, 2007; 83: 235–248.
1069. *S and Marper v United Kingdom.* 2008, ECHR 1581.
1070. *National DNA Database Strategy Board Annual Report 2013–14.* 2014. Available at: www.gov.uk/government/publications
1071. Jost, K. DNA databases. *CQ Researcher*, 1999; 9: 449–472.
1072. *Maryland v Kind*, in *Supreme Court of the U.S.* 2013.
1073. Meagher, D. The quiet revolution? A brief history and analysis of the growth of forensic police powers in Victoria. *Criminal Law Journal*, 2000; 24: 76–88.
1074. Walsh, S.J. and J.S. Buckleton. DNA intelligence databases. In *Forensic DNA Evidence Interpretation*, J.S. Buckleton, C.M. Triggs, and S.J. Walsh, Eds. Boca Raton, FL: CRC Press; 2005, pp. 439–469.
1075. Walsh, S.J., J.M. Curran, and J.S. Buckleton. Modeling forensic DNA database performance. *Journal of Forensic Sciences*, 2010; 55(5): 1174–1183.
1076. Bieber, F.R., C.H. Brenner, and D. Lazer. Finding criminals through DNA of their relatives. *Science*, 2006; 312: 1315–1316.
1077. Balding, D.J., et al. Decision-making in familial database searching: KI alone or not alone? *Forensic Science International: Genetics*, 2013; 7(1): 52–54.
1078. Curran, J.M. and J.S. Buckleton. Effectiveness of familial searches. *Science & Justice*, 2008; 48(4): 164–167.
1079. Murch, R.S. and B. Budowle. Are developments in forensic applications of DNA technology consistent with privacy protections? In *Genetic Secrets: Protecting Privacy and Confidentiality in the Genetic Era*, M.A. Rothstein, Ed. New Haven, CT: Yale University Press; 1997, pp. 212–230.

References

1080. Kaye, D.H. and M.E. Smith. DNA identification databases: Legality, legitimacy, and the case for population-wide coverage. *Wisconsin Law Review*, 2003; 3: 413–459.
1081. Goode, M. Some observations on evidence of DNA frequency. *Adelaide Law Review*, 2002; 23: 45–77.
1082. Weir, B.S. Matching and partially-matching DNA profiles. *Journal of the Forensic Sciences*, 2004; 49(5): 1009–1014.
1083. Budowle, B., et al. Source attribution of a forensic DNA profile. *Forensic Science Communications*, 2000; 2(3). Available at: www.fbi.gov/programs/lab/fsc/backissu/july2000/source.html
1084. Foreman, L.A. and I.W. Evett. Statistical analysis to support forensic interpretation of a new ten-locus STR profiling system. *International Journal of Legal Medicine*, 2001; 114: 147–155.
1085. *R v S*, in *Unreported*. 2006, NSWDC.
1086. Poetsch, M., et al. The problem of single parent/child paternity analysis—Practical results involving 336 children and 348 unrelated men. *Forensic Science International*, 2006; 159: 98–103.
1087. Gornik, I., et al. The identification of war victims by reverse paternity is associated with significant risks of false inclusion. *International Journal of Legal Medicine*, 2002; 116: 255–257.
1088. Birus, I., et al. How high should paternity index be for reliable identification of war victims by DNA typing? *Croatian Medical Journal*, 2003; 44(3): 322–326.
1089. Ungvarsky, E. What Does One in a Trillion Mean? *GeneWatch*, 2007; 20: 10–13.
1090. Curran, J.M., S.J. Walsh, and J.S. Buckleton. Empirical support for the reliability of DNA interpretation in Australia and New Zealand. *Australian Journal of Forensic Sciences*, 2008; 40(2): 145–154.
1091. Lauc, G., et al. Empirical support for the reliability of DNA interpretation in Croatia. *Forensic Science International: Genetics*, 2008; 3(1): 50–53.
1092. Balding, D.J. and P. Donnelly. Evaluating DNA profile evidence when the suspect is identified through a database search. *Journal of Forensic Sciences*, 1996; 41(4): 603–607.
1093. Dawid, A.P. and J. Mortera. Coherent analysis of forensic identification evidence. *Journal of the Royal Statistical Society. Series B*, 1996; 52(2): 425–443.
1094. Evett, I.W., L.A. Foreman, and B. Weir. Letter to the editor of biometrics. *Biometrics*, 2000; 56: 1274–1277.
1095. Dawid, A.P. Comment on Stockmarr's "Likelihood ratios for evaluating DNA evidence when the suspect is found through a database search." *Biometrics*, 2001; 57(3): 976–980.
1096. Donnelly, P. and R.D. Friedman. DNA database searches and the legal consumption of scientific evidence. *Michigan Law Review*, 1999; 97(4): 931–984.
1097. Evett, I.W. *A Discussion of Recommendation 5.1 of the Second NRC Report on DNA Profiling*. FSS report No. TN 821. 1996.
1098. Gittelson, S., et al. The database search problem: A question of rational decision making. *Forensic Science International*, 2012; 222(1–3): 186–199.
1099. Biedermann, A., S. Gittelson, and F. Taroni. Recent misconceptions about the 'database search problem': A probabilistic analysis using Bayesian networks. *Forensic Science International*, 2011; 212(1–3): 51–60.
1100. Stockmarr, A. Likelihood ratios for evaluating DNA evidence when the sis found through a database search. *Biometrics*, 1999; 55: 671–677.
1101. Stockmarr, A. The choice of hypotheses in the evaluation of DNA profile evidence. In *Statistical Science in the Courtroom*, J.L. Gastwirth, Ed. New York: Springer-Verlag; 2000, pp. 143–159.
1102. Devlin, B. The evidentiary value of a DNA database search. *Biometrics*, 2000; 56: 1276.
1103. Stockmarr, A. Author's reply. *Biometrics*, 2001; 57(3): 978–980.
1104. Morton, N.E. The forensic DNA endgame. *Jurimetrics Journal*, 1997; 37: 477–494.
1105. Research and Development Working Group. *The Future of Forensic DNA Testing: Predictions of the Research and Development Working Group*. 2000.
1106. Goldman, D. and J. Long. More on DNA typing dispute. Correspondence. *Nature*, 1995; 373: 99.
1107. Berger, C.E.H., P. Vergeer, and J.S. Buckleton. A more straightforward derivation of the LR for a database search. *Forensic Science International: Genetics*, 2015; 14: 156–160.
1108. Buckleton, J. and J. Curran, Personal communication, 2001.
1109. Champod, C. and O. Ribaux. Forensic identification databases in criminal investigations and trials. In *Harmonisation in Forensic Expertise*, W.J.J.M. Sprangers and J.F. Nijboer, Eds. Amsterdam: Thela Thesis; 2000, pp. 463–485.

Index

Note: Page numbers ending in "f" refer to figures. Page numbers ending in "t" refer to tables.

Index

Index

Index

For Product Safety Concerns and Information please contact our EU
representative GPSR@taylorandfrancis.com
Taylor & Francis Verlag GmbH, Kaufingerstraße 24, 80331 München, Germany

www.ingramcontent.com/pod-product-compliance
Lightning Source LLC
Chambersburg PA
CBHW080119220326
41598CB00032B/4888